FRAMES OF REFERENCE FOR
PEDIATRIC
OCCUPATIONAL
THERAPY
SECOND EDITION

FRAMES OF REFERENCE FOR
PEDIATRIC OCCUPATIONAL THERAPY
SECOND EDITION

PAULA KRAMER, PhD, OTR, FAOTA
Professor and Chair
Department of Occupational Therapy
Kean University
Union, NJ

JIM HINOJOSA, PhD, OT, FAOTA
Associate Professor
Department of Occupational Therapy
School of Education, Health, Nursing and Arts Professions
New York University
New York, NY

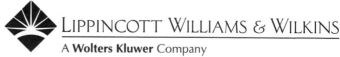

LIPPINCOTT WILLIAMS & WILKINS
A **Wolters Kluwer** Company
Philadelphia • Baltimore • New York • London
Buenos Aires • Hong Kong • Sydney • Tokyo

Editor: Eric P. Johnson
Managing Editor: Linda S. Napora
Marketing Manager: Debby Hartman
Production Editor: Ulita Lushnycky

Copyright © 1999 Lippincott, Williams & Wilkins

351 West Camden Street
Baltimore, Maryland 21201-2436 USA

227 East Washington Square
Philadelphia, PA 19106

Printed in the United States of America

First Edition, 1993

Library of Congress Cataloging-in-Publication Data

Frames of reference for pediatric occupational therapy / [edited by] Paula Kramer, Jim Hinojosa.
— 2nd ed.
     p.   cm.
Includes bibliographical references and index.
ISBN 0-683-30489-5
1. Occupational therapy for children.   I. Kramer, Paula.   II. Hinojosa, Jim.
   [DNLM: 1. Occupational Therapy—in infancy & childhood. 2. Occupational Therapy—
methods.   WS 368 F813 1999]
RJ53.025F73 1999
615.8'515—dc21
DNLM/DLC
for Library of Congress   98-44805
                                                               CIP

The publishers have made every effort to trace the copyright holders for borrowed material. If they have inadvertently overlooked any, they will be pleased to make the necessary arrangements at the first opportunity.

To purchase additional copies of this book, call our customer service department at **(800) 638-3030** or fax orders to **(301) 824-7390**. International customers should call **(301) 714-2324**.
                                               99 00 01 02 03
                                       1 2 3 4 5 6 7 8 9 10

We dedicate our collaborative efforts to the children and families with whom we have worked who have changed our lives and perspectives and to those children whose lives may be changed by this book.

Foreword

Until fairly recently, practice in occupational therapy was based on the use of imitated, stylized techniques and intuitive feelings about what was the best thing to do. Most therapists could not clearly articulate what exactly had been done to assist an individual in the process of problem assessment and problem remediation, nor were they able to identify what, if any, theoretical information supported and provided a foundation for the assessment/remediation process.

As the second edition of *Frames of Reference for Pediatric Occupational Therapy* demonstrates, this situation no longer exists. Occupational therapists now have frames of reference (theoretically based sets of guidelines for practice) to use as the basis for practice. Similar to the first edition, this text presents a variety of frames of reference that address the typical habilitation problems of infants, children, and adolescents.

Several changes have been made in this edition. Of particular note are changes that make the postulates regarding change (the principles used to guide problem remediation) of some frames of reference more succinct and thus easier to use in planning and implementing problem remediation. Another change has been the addition of several frames of reference that addresses many of the practical, daily life activities necessary for functioning in the home, school, playground, and community. Such additions highlight the need to maintain an optimal balance between assisting individuals to develop fundamental abilities and skills and assisting them to master daily life activities.

As Paula Kramer and Jim Hinojosa state in the text, frames of reference are a significant part of occupational therapy practice for a variety of reasons. Three of these reasons are worthy of special note. First, frames of reference give therapists a clear understanding of what they are doing, how they are doing it, and the theoretical rationale for their actions. Second, frames of reference are far more flexible than techniques. Thus, problem identification and remediation based on frames of reference can be tailored, within limits, to be compatible with the special characteristics of each individual such as his or her age, interests, likes and dislikes, and particular needs. Third, frames of reference allow us to determine whether, under what circumstances, and with whom our interventions are safe and lead to accurate problem identification and successful problem remediation. Such determinations could not be made in the past because the process of intervention was not sufficiently articulated to be examined. Only actions that can be described in words can be studied. The guidelines for problem identification and remediation contained in frames of reference are so stated that they can be subjected to the kind of applied scientific inquiry that is necessary for determining the efficacy of our interventions with individuals.

Frames of reference, of course, are only words on paper. It is how they are employed in practice that is of greatest importance. As the student reader is probably well aware of by this time, reading and understanding the material in a text is only the first step. Learning how to use frames of reference in a conscientious and consistent manner is the next step and one that is not particularly easy. It takes perseverance, self-discipline, proper supervision, and considerable practice. It is usual to feel inept at first. But in time, skilled use of the guidelines provided in frames of reference becomes a natural part of daily work with individuals.

And when that is accomplished, there is still more. Some of the frames of reference in this text, and those presented elsewhere, need to be further refined and better articulated. Most of the profession's frames of reference need to be assessed relative to their efficacy. Furthermore, additional frames of reference need to be formulated, refined, and assessed. Although learning how to do all of the above is far beyond the scope of this text, it is good to remember that such activities are necessary. It is only by continuing to develop adequate frames of reference that occupational therapy will be able to meet the ever-changing needs of the individuals we assist and the society to which we are responsible.

Finally, and on a more personal note, Paula, Jim, and several contributors to this text have studied with me at New York University. It is a great pleasure to see them continue to carry forward the work that we did together. But this is by no means an exclusive club . . . all are invited to join . . . there is plenty of work for everyone.

Anne Cronin Mosey, PhD, OT, FAOTA
Professor of Occupational Therapy
New York University
New York, NY

Preface

Pediatrics has been a major growth area for occupational therapy. Because of the increased need for skilled occupational therapists, curricula throughout the country have begun to place greater emphasis on teaching theory and developing practice materials relevant to pediatrics. The advent of laws that mandate occupational therapy services in early intervention programs and educationally-related services in the school system has added to the need for increased academic preparation. With the changing practice arena, it is essential that entry level curricula provide a foundation to address the shifting occupational therapy service delivery demands, emerging theories, and alternative practice settings.

Frames of Reference for Pediatric Occupational Therapy, Second Edition, provides comprehensive information regarding pediatric practice for the entry level occupational therapy student. Essential information is organized in a variety of frames of reference currently in use.

As set forth by Anne Cronin Mosey, PhD, OT, FAOTA, the frame of reference provides a methodical organization of theoretical and practical material in the sequence necessary for problem identification and solution in practice. The frame of reference provides an outline of essential theoretical information in particular areas of function, a guideline for assessing functional capacities in an individual, and a method of conceptualizing and initiating intervention—in essence, a blueprint for practice.

Frames of Reference for Pediatric Occupational Therapy, Second Edition, is unique in that it provides comprehensive pediatric information organized through the structure of frames of reference. The use of frames of reference as the structural scheme differs from the prevalent use of diagnostic categories or deficits in performance areas seen in most occupational therapy textbooks. Although a child's diagnosis provides some insight into that child's disabilities, occupational therapists are primarily concerned with the child's functional capacities. For this reason, a text organized around diagnostic categories does not address the essential focus of the occupational therapy process. In addition, a child may exhibit a variety of functional disorders that are not addressed through the specification of diagnostic category but are essential to intervention.

Insofar as a frame of reference is designed (1) to focus on the theoretical information critical to practice and (2) to relate that information for intervention strategies, it provides a blueprint for the occupational therapist seeking to improve the functional performance of the child.

This text is primarily intended for use in entry level occupational therapy education programs. It is appropriate for use in courses focusing on pediatric evaluation and intervention and developmental dysfunction, as well as in courses on occupational therapy theory and functional disorders of childhood. Postprofessional students who wish to specialize in pediatric practice may use this book as a basic text to provide an overview of commonly used frames of reference.

Pediatric occupational therapists will find the book helpful in understanding the theoretical concepts underlying intervention and the development of treatment planning according to a frame of reference approach. As such, therapists will be able to use this text to analyze their current practices. Those wishing to enter pediatric practice from other areas of practice will find it useful for updating their basic knowledge. Although the text is intended for occupational therapy education, anyone who works with children will find it to be an informative resource.

Frames of Reference for Pediatric Occupational Therapy, Second Edition, is designed to be a teaching tool devoted to instructional and lecture material and, to that end, presents frequently used frames of reference for pediatric practice. Each frame of reference clearly delineates the theoretical information that is critical to understanding and using that frame of reference. Essential terms are defined within the theoretical base in the context of the frame of reference. The reader who is interested in understanding a particular term should look for this term in the index. Through the index, the reader will be directed to the term as it is used and defined in that particular frame of reference. Flowing from the theoretical base, each frame of reference contains the information necessary for the student to move from theory to practice.

Those who have used the first edition of this text, and other expert reviewers, have provided feedback that was used to reorganize and update this new edition. Three frames of reference frequently used in pediatric practice have been added: the acquisition frame of reference, the motor skill acquisition frame of reference, and the occupational frame of reference. All of the frames of reference have been updated; some have been extensively revised.

In addition, Chapters 17 to 20 present four new case studies that illustrate the use of particular frames of reference. One of these case studies demonstrates the use of two frames of reference with one client. The case study chapters, with accompanying study questions, can be used as examples of the use of a frame of reference with a specific case. Instructors are encouraged to tailor the use of these examples to fit their courses.

We believe that the frames of reference presented here are representative of the best practice in pediatrics. We hope that you will agree.

Paula Kramer, PhD, OTR, FAOTA
Jim Hinojosa, PhD, OT, FAOTA

Acknowledgments

One would expect that writing a second edition would be significantly easier than writing a first edition. However, this was not the case, as we were committed to building on the first edition and having this second edition become an even stronger contribution to the occupational therapy literature in pediatrics. We hope that it is just that.

There are many people to thank who helped us, directly or indirectly, to make this possible. First and foremost, we thank our parents, Samuel and Rosalia Kramer and Ray and Rose Hinojosa. Although we have suffered some losses in the past few years, our parents contribution to our development remains critical to our success. Our families have always been there for us, providing love, support, and encouragement, most especially David L. Hunt and Steven A. Smith. And thanks to Andrew Litchfield Kramer Hunt, who reminded us of the wonder of normal development.

Dr. Anne Cronin Mosey has strongly influenced our thinking, organization skills, and professional development. We gratefully recognize her contribution to the body of knowledge of occupational therapy.

A special thanks to all the authors who contributed to this book and to their spouses, significant others, families, and friends who were supportive to them and thus assisted them in producing such fine work. We are fortunate that they consider us to be their friends as well as their colleagues.

The pictures are an essential part of this text. We are grateful to the Caring Center for Children in Chester, NJ, and Ken-Crest Developmental Center in Rosemont, PA, for helping us to create photographs that contribute to the text and provide interesting focal points for the reader. Further, we thank all the children and adults who allowed their pictures to be used, to name a few: Tamara Alfred, Jillian Alfred, Amy Antman, David Antman, Charles Antman, Victoria Buondonna, R. J. D'Agostino, Shane DeStefano, Courtney Dougherty, Paige Dougherty, Joseph E. Greenberg, Cheyenne Harrington, Andrew Litchfield Kramer Hunt, David L. Hunt, Al-Ameen Hussein, Eileen Hussein, Paul Johnson, Alex Kane, Suzanne Kane, Alexander LeGuillou, Jennifer Lubragge, Gaetano Mascara, Paula McCreedy, Samantha Miller, Samantha Myers, Alexandria Personeus, Devorah Leah Pruzansky, Taylor Jane Robinson, Dakota Swainson, and Zoe Swainson.

Our colleagues at Kean and New York Universities are thanked for their continuous encouragement and feedback throughout this project. The perspectives of our students and their questions and observations have always stimulated our growth. In particular, their comments about the first edition were invaluable in helping to shape this revision. Several people have kept us grounded in current practice issues, in particular Sol Ittah, Ruth Hansen, Flo Hannes, Arlene Kraat, Angela Peralta, and Angela Swainson. Many others have contributed to our professional growth and understanding of children; we wish we could individually thank all of you.

We are most appreciative of the efforts of the entire team at Lippincott Williams & Wilkins who have been tremendous supporters of this book, in particular Linda Napora who diligently reviewed every detail and provided us with ongoing guidance, John Butler who mentored us as authors during the first edition, and Eric Johnson who facilitated this edition.

Finally, we are indebted to the children and families with whom we have worked; they have enhanced our lives and taught us so much.

Contributors

JILL ANDERSON, MS, OTR
Occupational Therapy Supervisor
Step by Step Infant Development Center
Brooklyn, NY
The Herbert G. Birch Early Childhood Center
Springfield Gardens
Queens, NY

GARY BEDELL, PhD, OT
Coordinator, Post-Professional Program in Pediatrics/Developmental Disabilities
Department of Occupational Therapy
New York University
New York, NY

CHERYL ANN COLANGELO, MS, OTR
Occupational Therapist
North Salem Central School District
North Salem, NY

Adjunct Instructor
Department of Occupational Therapy
New York University
New York, NY

MAUREEN DUNCAN, OTD, OTR/L
Occupational Therapy Instructor
Creighton University
School of Pharmacy & Allied Health Professions
Omaha, NE
TheraPlayce Children's Developmental Center
Omaha, NE

BETH KORBY ELENKO, MA, OTR/L
Private Contractor, Early Intervention
Queens, NY

Doctoral Candidate and Teaching Fellow
Department of Occupational Therapy
New York University
New York, NY

KAY FARRINGTON, OTR/L
Occupational Therapist
Step by Step Infant Development Center
Brooklyn, NY
Women's League Jump Start Program
Brooklyn, NY

JANICE M. FERGUSON, MS, OT(C)
Halifax, Nova Scotia
Canada

JIM HINOJOSA, PhD, OT, FAOTA
Associate Professor and Director of Post-Professional Graduate Programs
Department of Occupational Therapy
New York University
New York, NY

MARGARET T. KAPLAN, MA, OTR/L
Acting Department Chair
Assistant Professor
State University of New York
Health Science Center at Brooklyn
Occupational Therapy Department
Brooklyn, NY

JUDITH GIENCKE KIMBALL, PhD, OTR/L, FAOTA
Professor and Chair
Occupational Therapy Department
University of New England
Biddeford, ME

PAULA KRAMER, PhD, OTR, FAOTA
Professor and Chair
Department of Occupational Therapy
Kean University
Union, NJ

AIMEE J. LUEBBEN, EDD, OTR/L, FAOTA
Director and Associate Professor
Occupational Therapy Program
University of Southern Indiana
Evansville, IN

MARY MUHLENHAUPT, OT/L, FAOTA
Occupational Therapist
Suburban Philadelphia Schools
Philadelphia, PA

LAURETTE J. OLSON, MA, OTR/L, BCP
Occupational Therapy Consultant
Mamaroneck Union Free School District
Mamaroneck, NY

Professional Associate
Graduate Program in Occupational Therapy
Mercy College
Dobbs Ferry, NY

LOREE A. PRIMEAU, PhD, OT(C), OTR
Assistant Professor and Chair
Department of Occupational Therapy
School of Allied Health Sciences
The University of Texas Medical Branch at Galveston
Galveston, TX

Formerly
Assistant Professor
School of Occupational Therapy
Dalhousie University
Halifax, Nova Scotia
Canada

CHANIE PRUZANSKY, OTR/L
Occupational Therapist
Step by Step Infant Development Center
Brooklyn, NY
Ocean County Health Department
Lakewood, NJ

CHARLOTTE BRASIC ROYEEN, PhD, OTR, FAOTA
Professor and Associate Dean for Research
School of Pharmacy and Allied Health
Creighton University
Omaha, NE

SARAH A. SCHOEN, MA, OTR/L
Supervisor, Occupational Therapy
Rose F. Kennedy Center
Children's Evaluation and Rehabilitation Center
Albert Einstein College of Medicine
Bronx, NY

Doctoral Candidate and Adjunct Instructor
Department of Occupational Therapy
New York University
New York, NY

MARGERY SZCZEPANSKI, MA, OTR
Pediatric Private Practitioner
Metropolitan New York

Instructor
Department of Occupational Therapy
New York University
New York, NY

VALORIE RICCIARDONE TODD, MA, OTR/L, BCP
Occupational Therapist, Kingston City Schools
New York, NY

Instructor
Infant/Early Childhood Specialist Interdisciplinary Studies
Rutgers University
Piscataway, NJ

G. GORDON WILLIAMSON, PhD, OTR/L, FAOTA
Director, Project Enhancing Resilience and Adaptation
Pediatric Rehabilitation Department
John F. Kennedy Medical Center
Edison, NJ

Associate Clinical Professor
Programs in Occupational Therapy
Columbia University
New York, NY

Contents

Foreword vii
Preface ix
Acknowledgments xi
Contributors xiii

SECTION I FOUNDATIONS OF PEDIATRIC PRACTICE

1 Developmental Perspective: Fundamentals of Developmental
Theory 3
JIM HINOJOSA / PAULA KRAMER

2 Domain of Concern of Occupational Therapy: Relevance to
Pediatric Practice 9
PAULA KRAMER / JIM HINOJOSA

3 Legitimate Tools of Pediatric Occupational Therapy 27
AIMEE J. LUEBBEN / JIM HINOJOSA / PAULA KRAMER

4 Perspective of Context as Related to Frame of Reference 41
MARY MUHLENHAUPT / JIM HINOJOSA / PAULA KRAMER

5 Structure of the Frame of Reference 67
PAULA KRAMER / JIM HINOJOSA

SECTION II FRAMES OF REFERENCE

6 NeuroDevelopmental Treatment Frame of Reference 83
SARAH A. SCHOEN / JILL ANDERSON

7 Sensory Integration Frame of Reference: Theoretical Base,
Function/Dysfunction Continua, and Guide to Evaluation 119
JUDITH GIENCKE KIMBALL

8   Sensory Integration Frame of Reference: Postulates Regarding
Change and Application to Practice 169
JUDITH GIENCKE KIMBALL

9   Visual Information Analysis: Frame of Reference for Visual
Perception 205
VALORIE RICCIARDONE TODD

10   Biomechanical Frame of Reference 257
CHERYL ANN COLANGELO

11   Psychosocial Frame of Reference 323
LAURETTE J. OLSON

12   Acquisition Frame of Reference 377
CHARLOTTE BRASIC ROYEEN / MAUREEN DUNCAN

13   Motor Skill Acquisition Frame of Reference 401
MARGARET T. KAPLAN / GARY BEDELL

14   Coping Frame of Reference 431
G. GORDON WILLIAMSON / MARGERY SZCZEPANSKI

15   Occupational Frame of Reference 469
LOREE A. PRIMEAU / JANICE M. FERGUSON

SECTION III   APPLICATIONS OF FRAMES OF REFERENCE

16   Frames of Reference in the Real World 519
JIM HINOJOSA / PAULA KRAMER

17   Case Study: NeuroDevelopmental Treatment Frame
of Reference 533
BETH KORBY ELENKO

18   Case Study: Motor Skill Acquisition Frame of Reference 551
GARY BEDELL / MARGARET T. KAPLAN

19   Case Study: Biomechanical Frame of Reference 573
CHERYL ANN COLANGELO

20 Case Study: Combined Sensory Integration and
NeuroDevelopmental Treatment Frames of Reference 589
CHANIE PRUZANSKY / KAY FARRINGTON
Index 609

FOUNDATIONS OF
PEDIATRIC PRACTICE

Developmental Perspective: Fundamentals of Developmental Theory

JIM HINOJOSA / PAULA KRAMER

As set forth by Anne Cronin Mosey, Ph.D., OT, FAOTA (1970), frames of reference provide an organization of theoretical material needed for problem identification and solution in practice. In the pediatric arena, the frame of reference offers an outline of fundamental theoretical concepts relative to particular areas of function. It likewise serves as a guideline for assessing functional capacities in the client and offers a method for conceptualizing and initiating intervention. The frame of reference has become an acceptable vehicle for organizing theoretical material in occupational therapy and for translating it into practice through a functional perspective. Frames of reference, therefore, enable the practitioner to shift from theory into practice.

This book is organized around major frames of reference used by occupational therapists. The frame of reference provides a structure for identifying relevant theories and then outlining the guidelines that occupational therapists use when assessing and intervening based on this information. Other occupational therapy texts are organized around diagnostic categories or intervention strategies. These textbooks link diagnostic categories with specific strategies for intervention, with the inherent premise being that one will choose an intervention based on the diagnosis of the client.

Although a diagnosis may provide insight into a child's disabilities, occupational therapists are concerned primarily with functional performance. Material organized around diagnostic categories does not always address the essential focus of the occupational therapy process. In addition, a child may exhibit several other needs not described in the diagnostic category but still essential to intervention. This textbook assumes that interventions are theory-based and thus is organized around articulated frames of reference that delineate the relationship between theory and practice. The frame of reference is designed first to highlight traditionally used theories, then to relate that information to function, and, finally, to organize that information for the purpose of intervention. The frame of reference essentially is a blueprint for evaluation and intervention.

DEVELOPMENTAL PERSPECTIVE

Occupational therapy intervention with a child is based upon an understanding and appreciation of normal development. Differences exist in the perceptions of development, yet everyone tends to describe patterns or sequences of development that are accepted as being characteristic for all children everywhere. In other words, there is a sequential nature to all theories of child development. Some theorists support the idea of linear progression—i.e., several components of a process must occur before the skill as a whole is acquired or learned (Freud, 1966; Gesell & Armatruda, 1947; Kohlberg, 1969). This is similar to the links in a chain, where each link provides an important piece toward the strengths of the whole chain. Other theorists view progression as being more pyramidal in nature (Ayres, 1972, 1979; Erikson, 1963; Llorens, 1976; Piaget, 1963; Reilly, 1974)—i.e., there must be a basic foundation from which skill development evolves. In this perspective, all blocks at the base of the pyramid must be strong and placed securely to provide support.

Those therapists who view development as linear are called reductionists. Their perspective on development is that it is made up of the components of a process and the resultant conditional responses. As the child develops, behavior represents a continual set of sequences. Other theories that support this perspective have been proposed by Pavlov (1927), Skinner (1974), and Kaluger and Kaluger (1984). Behaviorism and learning theory are included in this philosophy.

Those therapists who view development as pyramidal are called nonreductionists. Their concern is with the development of each level of function to provide the foundation for higher level skills. Processes that take place at lower levels only provide the foundation on which more sophisticated processes may develop. Inherent in this view is the idea that skills are stage specific—i.e., a skill that evolves in one stage forms a component part for the behaviors that take place at a later stage. These ideas have been proposed by Piaget (1963), Gagne (1970), and Maslow (1970). This perspective is summarized by Travers (1977):

> The development of complex behavior is analogous to the construction of a building. First the foundation has to be laid. The form of the foundation has much to do with the kind of building that can be constructed on it; a round building cannot be readily erected on a square foundation. The size and strength of the foundation has much to do with the structure that can be built. The walls determine the kind of roof that can be used to crown the structure (p. 25).

The reductionist viewpoint usually is not thought of as developmental in nature. Instead, the component parts of a process are considered first, followed by the conditional response. Some occupational therapists tend to think of this as creating a "splinter skill," which has a negative connotation; whereas others see it as creating learned or acquired behavior, which is a more positive connotation. Despite the negative or positive outlook, both groups believe that a certain set of conditions and skills exist before a new skill can be obtained. From our vantage point, this can be considered as developmental because there is a specified sequence that must take place, or that must be developed, before the actual skill can occur. When a child requires a specific piece of adaptive equipment, the therapeutic intervention usually involves choosing the appropriate device and teaching the child how to use it. The child's subsequent use of this device generally is thought of as learned behavior. In a pediatric setting, a therapist could not facilitate the successful use of a therapeutic device unless the child previously had obtained specific abilities that set the stage for using the particular piece of equipment. The sequential nature of the reductionist process, therefore, may be seen as one type of developmental process. On the other hand, the viewpoint that sees function as a pyramidal process (where each stage depends on the skills that have been preestablished) is traditionally considered to be developmental.

Within the pediatric context, the linear and pyramidal processes qualify as developmental, even though each differs greatly in its perspective of what development actually means. Development may occur through learning and skill acquisition, or it may occur through maturation, where subsequent skills are created based on preestablished foundations. Both viewpoints involve an attempt to understand the patterns of progression. Each of these theoretical perspectives describes a particular pattern of progression in a child's development differently, yet each shares the generally accepted principles of human development (Daub, 1988).

The developmental perspectives that we have discussed up until this point have drawn heavily on developmental psychology and human development. These perspectives point out the important stages of development and the sequences in which this development occurs. These developmental theories provide a foundational knowledge for pediatric occupational therapy, but our perspective is broader and more unique than basic development. As occupational therapists, we concentrate more on how development translates into functional performance rather than the pure sequential nature of development. The developmental theories previously discussed do not provide us with enough information about skill acquisition or the mastery of activities of daily living. Our perspective of development centers on how the child performs meaningful occupations within the context of the developmental foundation (Coster, 1995).

Although occupational therapists learn about all aspects of development, their major concern is with the child's ability to translate development into action. Pediatric occupational therapists share a unique viewpoint in their concern for development of performance skills. Occupational therapists are concerned with children being able to function within their own environments to the best of their abilities. This viewpoint requires consideration of the many different factors that can influence a child's overall development. Therapists, therefore, are inherently concerned with the child's abilities and how human and nonhuman influences affect the development of these abilities. The child's abilities may be seen as a composite of various specific skills. To address the development of these skills, therapists concentrate first on ascertaining the child's developmental level, which refers to a determination of each child's patterns and sequences of development and then on an evaluation of the level that has been attained.

A child does not develop in a vacuum. He or she is part of an ever changing dynamic process because changes occur continuously in internal and external environments. A child's body and mind represent the internal environment, and the child's body and mind are greatly influenced by growth and maturation. Human and nonhuman objects are part of the external environment. These two worlds influence the child's development separately and together. The importance of each environment varies with each child's capabilities, the specific demands of a situation, the objects involved, and the performance required. Although a child is considered to have many separate areas that develop independently, motor, psychological, and social development all are interrelated and interdependent. In reality, although a child's motor development may be discussed in isolation, it cannot be considered to be independent of the child's whole life. Some variables that affect motor development also involve the neurophysiological status, the orthopaedic status, early sensory and cognitive experiences, and the family situation. The child who is unable to walk may have limited access to interaction with his peers and, therefore, may have difficulty with age-appropriate social development.

Rates of development vary from child to child, with no two children being exactly alike. There is a range of normalcy within progression and rates of development. For example, it generally is accepted that a child creeps before walking. Usually, children spend several months mastering creeping, but some children progress very quickly through this stage and begin to attempt to walk soon after they have started to creep. When viewing normal development, however, it usually is orderly, predictable, and sequential. To be sure, there always is some degree of individuality with a child, with one aspect at times being more important than another. For instance, at an earlier stage in life, motor performance may be more imperative than cognitive performance. Finally, development does not always occur at a consistent rate but rather in spurts that alternate with rest periods, at which time consolidation of skills takes place. As a child begins to ambulate, he or she usually starts to ignore previous favored toys that required him or her to be sedentary. Instead, he or she now wants to explore his or her environment with his or her new found freedom.

Once a child's pattern, sequence, and level of development are determined, an occupational therapist can address needs in two ways. First, the therapist can establish the performance skills a child has or can develop at his or her current level of function. The child who cannot walk or talk still may be able to participate actively in self-feeding. Second, based on a pattern or sequence of development, a therapist can determine a child's deficits and the possible influencing factors. Based on some hypothesis, a therapist uses knowledge about normal growth and development, anatomy, neurophysiology, and life tasks to develop an intervention plan that is sensitive to any sequela of disease or to any known data about the development of the particular systems in which a child has deficits. In addition, occupational therapists are concerned with other areas that may influence development, such as family life, educational program, and other factors. Knowledge about the characteristic pattern of the development of a particular performance component must be balanced by the particular child's direction, rate, and sequence of development.

Perhaps the easiest area to understand is motor progression, which usually is presented in a format that identifies the sequence in which the child acquires the ability to move. This progression, like those of other systems, inherently includes the acceptance of two basic assumptions: (1) development has natural order and (2) development is sequential. Although affected by environment, stimulation, and the child's personal characteristics, motor development has a natural order that is consistent from child to child. Furthermore, the sequential order of each child seems to follow the same basic sequence to achieve similar basic skills. Some children develop faster in one area, some slower, but each child basically follows the same sequence. Mechanisms of the performance component cannot be observed directly, but evidence that change has occurred is obvious from developing skills.

IS THERE A DEVELOPMENTAL FRAME OF REFERENCE?

The developmental perspective forms a foundational knowledge that is important to all pediatric occupational therapists. The majority of the frames of reference presented in this text presume that the therapist has a firm knowledge of the developmental perspective and its impact on the skill acquisition of the child. However, there is no specific developmental frame of reference presented here. It is our viewpoint that there is no one specific developmental frame of reference for pediatric occupational therapy. We believe that what is commonly referred to as the developmental frame of reference is an acquisitional frame of reference that follows the sequence of normal development. In this situation, the therapist follows the normal developmental sequence, facilitating the development of those skills that are absent through a teaching learning process.

References

Ayres, A. J. (1972). *Sensory integration and learning disorders.* Los Angeles, CA: Western Psychological Services.

Ayres, A. J. (1979). *Sensory integration and the child.* Los Angeles, CA: Western Psychological Services.

Coster, W. (1995). What is the unique occupational therapy perspective on development? In Cermack, S., Henderson, A., and Ray, S. (Eds.) Proceedings of the Pediatric Occupational Therapy: Challenges for the future in education and research. U. S. Department of Health and Human Services, The Maternal and Child Health, Boston University, Boston, MA.

Daub, M. M. (1988). Occupational therapy—base in the human development process. In H. L. Hopkins and H. D. Smith (Eds.) *Willard and Spackman's occupational therapy* (7th ed.). Philadelphia, PA: J. B. Lippincott.

Erikson, E. H. (1963). *Childhood and society* (2nd ed.). New York: Norton & Co.

Freud, S. (1966). *Standard edition of the complete psychological works of Sigmund Freud.* London: Hogarth Press.

Gagne, R. M. (1970). *The conditions of learning* (2nd ed.). New York: Holt, Rinehart, & Winston.

Gesell, A., and Armatruda, C. S. (1954). *Developmental diagnosis* (2nd ed.). New York: Harper & Brothers.

Kaluger, G., and Kaluger, M. F. (1984). *Human development: the span of life* (3rd ed.). St Louis, MO: C. V. Mosby.

Kohlberg, L. (1969). *Stage and sequence: The cognitive developmental approach to socialization.* In D. Groslin (Ed.) Handbook of socialization theory and research. Chicago, IL: Rand McNally.

Llorens, L. A. (1976). *Application of developmental theory for health and rehabilitation.* Rockville, MD: American Occupational Therapy Association.

Maslow, A. H. (1970). *Motivation and personality* (2nd ed.). New York: Harper & Row.

Mosey, A. C. (1970). *Three frames of reference for mental health.* Thorofare, NJ: Charles B. Slack.

Mosey, A. C. (1968). Recapitulation of ontogenesis: A theory for practice of occupational therapy. *American Journal of Occupational Therapy,* 22, 426–432.

Pavlov, I. P. (1927). *Conditioned reflexes* (trans. by G. V. Andrep). London: Oxford.

Piaget, J. (1963). *Psychology of intelligence.* Paterson, NJ: Littlefield, Adams & Co.

Reilly, M. (1974). *Play as exploratory learning.* Beverly Hills, CA: Sage.

Skinner, B. F. (1974). *About behaviorism.* New York: Vintage Books.

Travers, R. M. W. (1977). *Essentials of learning.* New York: Macmillan.

Domain of Concern of Occupational Therapy: Relevance to Pediatric Practice

PAULA KRAMER / JIM HINOJOSA

In most professions, a continuous evolution of the concerns within the profession defines its focus and explains why it is important to society. Society rarely stays the same; as society changes, the professions need to respond accordingly. All helping professions evolve and change to meet a unique need of the society that they serve.

It is virtually impossible to define a profession in discrete terms because of this constant change. To remain viable, a profession must be dynamic, continuously developing and modifying to meet the changing needs of society. Those persons who study or enter a profession may struggle, however, with this concept because they usually strive for one constant definition of their profession.

One group of caretakers, the health professions, must adapt to changes in social priorities and in the ways that they deliver health care. Society tends to have different trends during different eras, when one age group or particular category of disability receives more attention than others. This leads to an increased professional focus on those particular groups and may lead to specialized practice. This has been the case in occupational therapy in the United States. For example, pediatric occupational therapists have been affected dramatically by societal changes. In the early 1970s, federal laws emphasized and supported the educational needs of special children and required that occupational therapy be a related service (Gilfoyle & Hayes, 1979; Hanft, 1990; Ottenbacher, 1982). This idea was expanded during the 1980s when the needs of infants and toddlers became an area of concern, and occupational therapy was identified as a primary service (Hanft, 1990). During the 1990s, there has been an increasing trend toward more community-based services and natural settings for intervention such as the home (Anderson & Schoelkopf, 1996) and school (Johnson, 1996). Early intervention services have increased with a family-centered orientation (Case-Smith, 1993). The use of assistive technology is a major innovation in practice

(Bain & Leger, 1997). In response, occupational therapy practice has evolved to address and focus on these priorities. Understandings of community-based and emerging models of practice have become essential. Today, occupational therapists can be found in a wide variety of settings, including well-baby clinics, neonatal intensive care units, early intervention centers, preschool and headstart programs, and school systems.

DOMAIN OF CONCERN

Occupational therapy's domain of concern defines the breadth of the profession and areas of expertise of the therapist. It is beyond the scope of this book to identify the entire domain of concern for the profession of occupational therapy. This chapter focuses, therefore, on the domain of pediatric practice.

The profession has identified the performance areas, performance components, and performance contexts that enable the individual to engage in meaningful occupation. It is recognized that these may change over time, depending on the needs of society and the focus of practice as it adapts to societal change. The profession has developed Uniform Terminology to meet this need. In 1979, a document called Uniform Terminology was approved by the American Occupational Therapy Association (AOTA) Representative Assembly to promote a uniformity of definition for practice within the profession. To respond to the evolution of practice, AOTA then recognized the need to update the document continually to reflect current practice and to reemphasize the need for uniformity of definitions. In 1989, the second edition of this document was adopted and revised to reflect current practice with a clarification of categories and refinement of definitions. In 1994, the third edition of this document was revised and expanded to include the context and environments that influence performance.

The domain of concern for pediatric occupational therapists incorporates a description of all areas of life that concern therapists when working with children and their families. The following discussion of the domain of concern of occupational therapy is primarily structured around AOTA's Uniform Terminology, 3rd edition. The discussion is focused only on how this relates to pediatric practice, and, in some cases, augmentations have been made to reflect the most current state of practice.

Performance Areas

Performance areas are broad categories of human activity that are typically part of daily life. They are activities of daily living, work and productive activities, and play or leisure activities (American Occupational Therapy Association, 1994, p.1047).

Performance areas are arbitrary divisions or classifications of occupations in which people engage. Performance areas include activities of daily living, work and productive activities, and play or leisure activities. The primary concern of occupational therapists is that a child can function in the performance areas.

Activities of Daily Living

Activities of daily living include the child's ability to perform the tasks needed for self-care. These include grooming, oral hygiene, bathing or showering, toilet hygiene, dressing, feeding and eating, medication routines, socialization, functional communication, functional mobility, and sexual expression (Figure 2.1). Depending on the individual situation of the children, the therapist may intervene with either the child, the care provider, or both to address these areas. The ability to perform activities of daily living independently is crucial to an individual's dignity. Therefore, this is a primary area of concern for pediatric occupational therapists and should not be overlooked in intervention.

Although it may be difficult for therapists to work with some areas of activities of daily living, it is critical that they do so because this may enable the child to become as independent as possible and to develop a positive sense of self. Although some frames of reference in this text do not address this area directly, it is understood that they are laying the foundation that allows the child to become independent in activities of daily living.

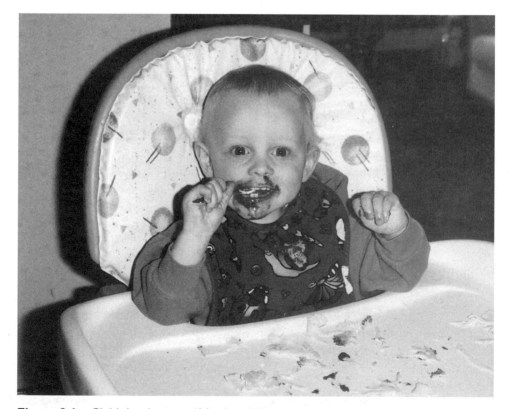

Figure 2.1 Child developing self-feeding skills.

Work and Productive Activities

Work activities include home management, care of others, educational activities, and vocational activities. Work and productive activities refer to involvement and accomplishment of activities in the home, school, and community. For children, home management may relate to household chores, maintaining one's room, and keeping clothes neat. Care of others may include looking after a younger sibling or care of a pet. Educational activities may include day care, nursery and preschool routines, or after school learning activities, such as religious education and traditional school involvements around classroom performance. The term "vocational activities" generally does not apply to young children. It may relate to older children who begin to be involved in work activities, such as paper routes, mowing lawns, or shoveling snow.

Within the document of Uniform Terminology, this area seems to be somewhat limited. However, school-based practice has become an important area of pediatric occupational therapy. In order for a child to function well within a school situation, the role of the occupational therapist can be broad, varying from something as obvious as developing handwriting skills to something more subtle as assisting the child in the transition from one setting to another (American Occupational Therapy Association, 1997).

Play or Leisure Activities

Play or leisure activities include exploration and performance. Although Uniform Terminology refers to this area as play or leisure activities, the term "leisure" does not generally apply to younger children. Professionally speaking, play is divided into two parts: play exploration and play performance. Play exploration relates to the identification of play interests that promote skills and opportunities. Play performance includes physical and social activities that are inherently gratifying. Play or leisure activities are those things in which a child chooses to engage. They are selected for a child's amusement, enjoyment, or self-expression (Figure 2.2). Intrinsically, play should be pleasurable, promoting the child's enjoyment or relaxation. Play should encourage skill development through involvement with objects and interaction with others.

Play is a natural part of a child's life, and the child without disabilities has many opportunities to engage in play. However, the child with disabilities may not have as many occasions to become involved in play activities. The primary exposure that the child has to play may be in the context of a therapeutic experience. The expertise of the occupational therapist can be used to assist the child in playing as a means of self expression and fun and as a means of assisting parents to strengthen their interaction with their child to provide a typical childhood experience (Hinojosa & Kramer, 1997).

Play or leisure activities are those things chosen by the child because they are amusing, enjoyable, relaxing, or self-expressive. Play often promotes skill develop-

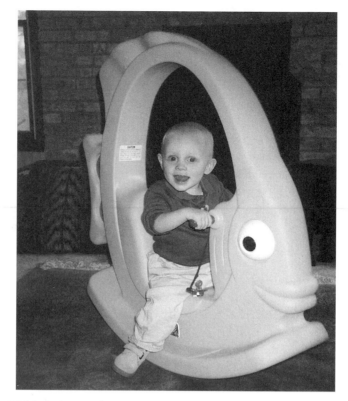

Figure 2.2   Child playing, exploring movement on a rocking fish.

ment and interaction with others. The occupational therapist uses play in two separate ways. First, the therapist tries to facilitate play exploration so that the child can try out various types of play and decide which ones he finds enjoyable. Second, the therapist uses play as a therapeutic modality to facilitate the performance and development of the child. This aspect of play is addressed later (as part of the legitimate tools of occupational therapy).

Performance Components

Performance components are fundamental human abilities that—to varying degrees and in differing combinations—are required for successful engagement in performance areas. These components are sensorimotor, cognitive, and psychological (American Occupational Therapy Association, 1994, p.1047).

Performance components are arbitrary divisions of human functioning with sensorimotor components; cognitive integration and cognitive components; and psychosocial skills and psychological components being the areas of major concern for occupational therapy (American Occupational Therapy Association, 1994). Separating human function into basic parts allows the occupational therapist to understand the individual sections that make up the whole. By looking at the small sections, a therapist gains a better understanding of how the child processes information in these discrete areas. Through this specific examination of each discrete area or performance component, a more comprehensive understanding of the child's skills and deficits can be gained. A therapist's knowledge and understanding of the complex human organism increases by examining and understanding the component parts.

Performance components are closely interrelated, and each performance component embodies an area of the child's development. Occupational therapists have expertise in all of the performance components. Understanding performance components and their interrelation provides basic information about the child. From this point, the occupational therapist can develop appropriate interventions after considering the child's biological potential and developmental status.

Pediatric occupational therapy tends to emphasize particular aspects of each performance component (i.e., a subset of each performance component). As growing human beings, children mature and develop skills in each of the performance areas, making them more sensitive to any condition that may interfere with their development. It is important then that a therapist also understand the various subparts of each performance component. For example, the sensorimotor performance component is divided into three units: sensory, neuromusculoskeletal, and motor. Based on the condition of the child who is being treated, the therapist may need to focus on one or two of these subcomponents. For example, with a child who has rheumatoid arthritis, the therapist may be more concerned with the neuromusculoskeletal and motor subcomponents than with the sensory subcomponents.

Sensorimotor Performance Component

A child's sensorimotor performance component includes those parts of human function that depend on the processing of sensory input. This performance component is comprised of sensory, neuromusculoskeletal, and motor subcomponents.

The *sensory* subcomponent encompasses sensory awareness, sensory processing, and perceptual processing. In this conceptualization, the critical concepts are the ability to take in sensory information, process this information, and produce an appropriate response or output. Motor skills are included because refined motor function is often the output based in the adequate processing of sensory information.

Sensory awareness involves receiving and differentiating sensory stimuli. Sensory awareness is based on the status of the central nervous system (CNS). It encompasses alerting to sensory information and arousal as a potential response to sensory input. Sensory processing involves interpreting sensory stimuli from tactile, proprioceptive, vestibular, visual, auditory, gustatory, and olfactory systems. Sensory processing is also based on the status of the CNS and the child's neurophysiological responses. Sensory processing responses are thought to develop from a generalized response to a more sophisticated discrete response to specific stimuli. The tactile system, for example, develops the ability to recognize internal as opposed to external sensation, such as interpreting light touch and pressure. The visual system likewise develops more sophisticated responses through recognition of pattern and color. Perceptual processing involves organizing sensory input into meaningful patterns. Subcomponents in this area involve various levels of processing ranging from the automatic subconscious level to the skill level. At the automatic unconscious level are stereognosis, kinesthesia, and pain response. At the cognitive understanding level are body scheme, depth perception, form constancy, and left-right discrimination. Finally, at the higher skill level are position in space, visual-closure, figure ground, spatial relations, and topographic orientation. This subcomponent is thought to be essential to the development of higher intellectual skills, such as academic abilities. It should be noted that others may classify these concepts differently, however, this classification is based on Uniform Terminology and the definitions included in that document.

The sensory subcomponent is critical to understanding the sensory integration, neurodevelopmental treatment frames of references, and, to a lesser extent, the visual perception frame of reference. The student should be aware when reading each of these frames of reference that theoretical bases of each may conceptualize these subcomponents somewhat differently.

The *neuromusculoskeletal* subcomponent involves areas of development that underlie the motor aspects of behavior. This depends on the maturity of the CNS and the neurophysiological system. Neuromusculoskeletal subsumes reflex, range of motion, muscle tone, strength, endurance, postural control, postural alignment, and soft-tissue integrity (American Occupational Therapy Association, 1994). When these subcomponents are considered by pediatric occupational therapists, each is considered relative to the typical development of the child. It is not simply a case of whether the child has reflexes, for example, but at what level are the reflexes relative to the child's chronological and developmental age, and how are they influencing performance. Most often these areas are looked at relative to motor behaviors and skills. This is particularly true in the neurodevelopmental, biomechanical, and motor skill acquisition frames of reference.

The *motor* subcomponent involves performance of the motor aspects of behavior. Generally, motor performance is viewed as sequential development with generalized rules: cephalo to caudal, proximal to distal, and gross control to fine control (Figure 2.3). Motor functioning subsumes gross coordination, crossing the midline, laterality, bilateral integration, motor control, praxis, fine coordination/dexterity, visual-motor integration, and oral-motor control. Subcomponents in this area involve various levels of processing ranging from foundational levels to the highly integrated skill levels. Those concepts that are at a foundational level are gross coordination, crossing the midline, laterality, and oral-motor control. Those concepts that are at the highly integrated skill level are bilateral integration, motor control, praxis, fine

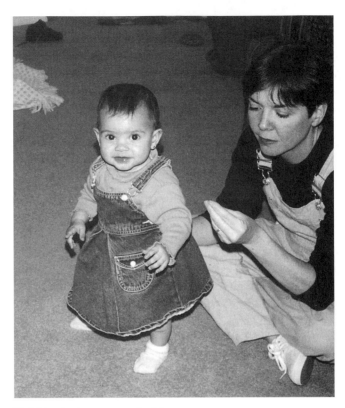

Figure 2.3   Child beginning to stand with support.

coordination/dexterity, and visual-motor integration. All of these subcomponents are critical to pediatric practice and are addressed in a multitude of frames of reference.

Cognitive Integration and Cognitive Performance Components

For children, cognitive integration and cognitive performance components involve the mental processes needed to comprehend or understand. At the basic level, this involves the child's conscious awareness and knowledge of objects through perception, memory, and reasoning. Included within this extensive performance component are level of arousal, orientation, recognition, attention span, initiation of activity, termination of activity, memory, sequencing, categorization, concept formation, spatial operations, problem solving, learning, and generalization of learning. Again, the subcomponents in this area involve various levels of cognition. At the foundational level, pediatric therapists are concerned with the child's level of arousal, orientation, recognition, and attention span, which underlie the ability to engage in activities. At the higher cognitive level, therapists are concerned with skills of concept formation, memory, sequencing, categorization, and spatial orientation. At an intellectual level, problem solving, learning, and the generalization of learning are the focus of the pediatric therapist. Finally, therapists at all levels of development are concerned with the child's ability to initiate and terminate activities.

These subcomponents are particularly important in the motor skill acquisitional, visual perception, and human occupation frames of reference.

Psychological Skills and Psychological Performance Components

Psychological skills and psychological performance components are the abilities to interact in society and process emotions. They are arbitrarily divided into the child's psychological, social, and self-management subcomponents.

The *psychological* subcomponent involves values, interests, and self-concept. This allows the child to develop a self-concept and the ability to handle life situations. The development of adequate psychological abilities allows a child to express and control himself or herself.

Social involves role performance, social conduct, interpersonal skills, and self-expression. This subcomponent allows the child to develop abilities and skills in relation to other people (Figure 2.4).

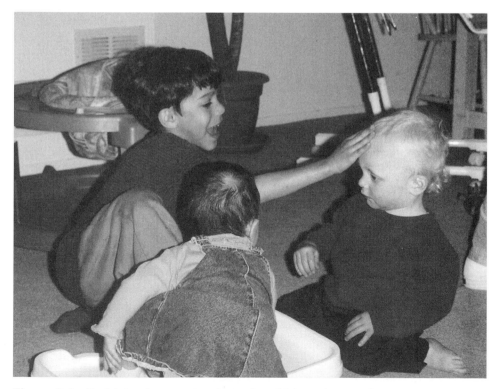

Figure 2.4   Social development is enhanced as children play together.

Self-management skills allow children to deal with their daily life routines in a way that supports their psychological and social development. Involved in this subcomponent are the child's coping, time management, and self-control skills.

These subcomponents appear to be directly related to the human occupation and coping frames of reference. However, its importance is much broader because it affects every area of the child's life. The natural milieu of the child is to be with other children and be able to interact and play in a way that enhances growth and development. Further, it is critical for the therapist to understand this component when working with families. The therapist often focuses on the child as an individual unit. However, this component allows the child to interact and be socialized as a family member, and so the therapist must broaden his or her focus to view the children within the structure of the family.

Performance Context

Performance contexts are situations or factors that influence an individual's engagement in desired and/or required performance areas. Performance contexts consist of *temporal* aspects (i.e., chronological age, developmental age, place in life cycle, and health status); and *environmental* aspects (i.e., physical, social, and cultural considerations) (American Occupational Therapy Association, 1994, p. 1047).

While performance areas and performance components are internal to the child, performance contexts are external to the child. These external factors have an impact on the child's ability to engage in performance areas. These factors may have a positive or negative effect. Performance contexts are divided into temporal and environmental aspects.

Temporal aspects of performance contexts include chronological and developmental age, place in the life cycle, and health status. The pediatric occupational therapist continually considers temporal aspects. The child is viewed relative to typical development and through an understanding of his or her mastery of developmental milestones. Another important consideration is the relationship between the child's skills and his or her chronological and developmental age. Within the context of pediatrics, place in the life cycle is a moot point; however, health status may be a real concern. This varies from child to child, depending on the diagnosis and sequela. For example, the therapist would not have the same approach or expectations for play for a child who is in a wheelchair because of muscular dystrophy, as for a child who has attention deficit disorder with hyperactivity.

Environmental aspects of performance context encompass physical, social, and cultural considerations. The physical environments include the surrounding materials, objects, and structures that are part of the child's life space. The structural environment ranges from the home in which the child lives, to the school he or she attends, to the playground where he or she plays, to the community settings that he or she frequents. The materials and objects range from toys to personal self care items to assistive devices. The social environment refers to all people and other living things with whom the child interacts. This includes family members, peers, significant others, and pets (Figure 2.5). The social environment shapes the child through opportunities for support, interaction, challenges, and encouragement.

Culture includes customs, beliefs, activity, patterns, behavior standards, and expectations. Culture has an impact on the child's expectations of self and the parents' expectations of the child. Subsequently, this may reflect on the child's performance. For example, in some cultures, it is acceptable for a child to use a bottle until he or she is ready to enter preschool, whereas in other cultures a child is weaned from the bottle once he or she becomes a toddler. This would impact on the child's exposure to a cup and his or her ability to drink from it. This is an example of a cultural expectation that affects performance. Throughout life, culture influences what a person considers to be typical and what constitutes expected patterns of behavior. Within the process of intervention, the therapist needs to be aware of and sensitive to the cultural background of each child encountered.

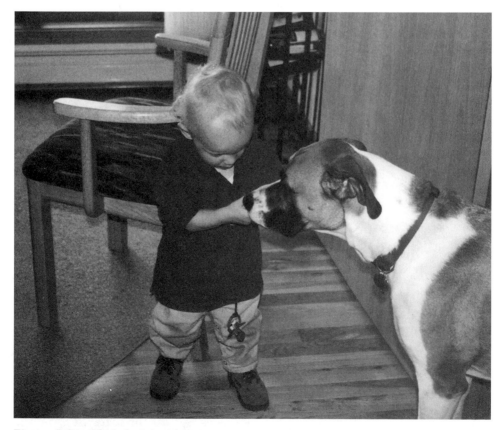

Figure 2.5   Child playing with a pet.

The interrelationship between culture and family is circuitous. Culture provides a backdrop for the family and influences the values and beliefs of family members. Family provides the background for the child. For the developing infant, family defines culture. As the major setting for family, culture is discussed first.

Culture

Culture refers to accepted patterns of behaviors shared by a group. These groups are defined by what they have in common—religion, ethnic background, nationality, or some other characteristic. Cultural groups also share common beliefs, customs, values, and attitudes. Aspects of culture that affect a child's development include family structure, marital status of the parents, parent/child rearing practices, and educational background (Krefting & Krefting, 1991). Cultural patterns influence the child's behaviors by defining what is acceptable, what rules prevail in physical interactions, and how to communicate. Culture influences the kinds of toys, games, foods, and objects that are part of daily life (Hopkins & Tiffany, 1988). The backgrounds of the authors serve as an example of this point. The child of Mexican heritage who lives in the West eats beans and tortillas as a regular part of his diet. He may listen to Spanish or country-western music as well as rock and roll. A common pastime may include tossing horseshoes, bicycle riding, and going to the playground. A little boy in this culture would not be expected to do kitchen chores or play with kitchen utensils. A child from a Jewish family in the Bronx may eat chicken soup with matzo balls as part of a traditional dinner. The music in the household could be classical or Broadway music as well as rock and roll. A young girl would be encouraged to pretend to "cook" and "bake" as well as play with Barbie dolls. She would also play in the playground and ride a bicycle. The shared experiences of these two children include rock and roll music, playing in the playground, and riding bicycles, all of which are part of the "American culture." The child's culture must be defined in terms of family background yet combined with the culture of community.

The effects of culture on intervention are multifaceted. Views on health and illness may be influenced by culture. The ways in which people feel and act toward persons who have disabilities reflect cultural views or biases. This may be true of family members and therapists alike. It is important for the therapist to respond to cultural identity. One way is to delineate how culture affects the selection of goals and the establishment of rapport (Levine, 1984). The perception of therapist and client may be "filtered through the screen of culture" (Hopkins & Tiffany, 1988, p. 108). For the pediatric occupational therapist, culture may outline the therapist-child-parent interaction. Consistent with the frame of reference, culture determines the choice of goals and the selection of legitimate tools and activities. "In every culture . . . some activities are regarded as proper, some inappropriate, and other unacceptable for specific ages, social status, economic class, men or women, times of day, days of week, or seasons of the year" (Cynkin & Robinson, 1990, p. 10). Culture also determines acceptable levels of performance so that the therapist can decide on expected outcomes.

Family

A family consists of two or more persons who provide the environment in which the child develops and learns to become a member of society. Families usually include parents and children and may include other significant people. Current American society has many different family configurations, including the nuclear, extended, expanded, and single-parent households. The nuclear family consists of a couple who shares the responsibility for raising a child. The extended family is a group related through family ties or mutual consent who share some part in child rearing. The expanded family is a complex combination of family configurations, involving a nuclear family, children, and significant others from previous relationships (Mosey, 1986). The configuration of this relationship among these different people is defined by the current and previous relationships. The single-parent household is one in which an adult assumes all the parental responsibilities.

The primary function of the family is to provide a supportive and nurturing environment for the child's development. The family shapes the child's ideological system and provides opportunities to develop interpersonal relationships (Turnbull, Summers, & Brotherson, 1986). All family member's needs are recognized and supported in a well-functioning, healthy family.

Temporal Adaptation

Another aspect of the temporal subcomponent is temporal adaptation (Mosey, 1986). Temporal adaptation encompasses three major areas: (1) the child's learned ability to structure himself or herself to accomplish tasks and to interact with others; (2) the ability to structure daily activities to fulfill social roles; and (3) the ability to assume responsibility for the organization of time, allowing the child to enjoy being a family member and taking on the culturally expected roles of work and play. Each of these three areas is determined by the child's cultural background and environment.

Temporal adaptation that involves the child's ability to structure himself or herself to accomplish tasks and to interact with others relates to the understanding of time as an external factor that regulates daily activities. As determined by his or her culture, the child learns that each day has its own cycle. This includes proscribed times to eat, to engage in activities, and to sleep. This structure gives the child a routine that allows him to predict what will happen each day and how to construct his or her interaction with others.

The ability to structure daily activities to fulfill social roles builds on the child's learned ability to structure himself or herself (i.e., his or her behavior). Through the child's understanding of time, he or she is now able to behave according to his or her needs and personal priorities. Often, however, the structure is controlled by external factors such as family or school. Again, building on the previously discussed areas, the child develops the ability to assume responsibility for the organization of time, allowing him or her to enjoy family, work, and play. As the child matures, he or she develops his or her own time plan based on the influences of his or her family, community, and school. As these routines develop, the child takes more responsibility for organizing his or her time and for developing and refining his or her roles as a family member, peer, student, and worker. The child now can take into account his or her internal needs as well as the demands of the culture, environment, and society. He or she also has to establish a balance between those needs and the demands of those around him or her (Pratt, 1989).

Within the intervention process, it is important for the therapist to take temporal adaptation into account; this way, the child will develop appropriate age and cultural routines as well as patterns of behaviors and will be able to satisfy his or her own needs while becoming a responsible member of his or her community.

The Relationship of the Occupational Therapy's Domain of Concern to Intervention

The domain of concern of a profession defines the scope and focus of practice. However, Uniform Terminology only provides an outline of our domain concern. It does not provide any in-depth information on the theoretical knowledge that underlies the practice of occupational therapy. Through looking at the broad categories of Uniform Terminology, therapists are able to identify areas that require further assessment and possible attention. Once these areas have been identified, the therapist can choose a frame of reference that will address these specific areas in more depth. Frames of reference address different areas of practice. No one frame of reference addresses all areas of practice fully. Some frames of reference focus more on performance areas, some on performance components, and some on performance context. Consequently, in order to adequately treat all areas of concern with a particular child and family, the therapist may have to use more than one frame of reference.

Regardless of the specific frame of reference chosen when working with a particular child, pediatric occupational therapists draw from their expertise to view the child from various theoretical perspectives. This involves looking at a child relative to typical development and relative to that individual child's mastery of developmental milestones, which involves considering the child's chronological and developmental age.

Often, pediatric occupational therapists begin by attending to the developmental aspects of the performance components that often are important in determining the frame of reference to be used to guide intervention. This attention to performance components is based on the therapist's understanding and appreciation for each performance component based on the appreciation for typical development. As defined by Uniform Terminology (3rd ed), the performance components are rather broad categories, and sometimes they are too broad for dealing with a specific child. Because of the specific types of intervention, therapists need to divide these performance components into even smaller entities. When a therapist deals with a child who has grasp problems for example, the categories of gross and fine coordination are not sufficient to understand and analyze these deficits. In this situation, the therapist needs to divide the child's motor performance into even more discrete and specific aspects of performance.

At other times, therapists begin by focusing on the performance areas. This requires looking at the overall performance and determining in what areas the child is functioning well and in what areas the child may need assistance. To some, this is considered a more holistic or global view of the child's performance. Additionally, some frames of reference concentrate on specific performance areas more than others or to the exclusion of others. Again, therapists are concerned with how the child functions within the performance area relative to his or her chronological and developmental levels. For example, the therapist may first determine how the child is performing activities of daily living and how that performance relates to the child's chronological and developmental level and then explore what performance components may be contributing to any deficits in functioning. In this situation, the therapist again understands that functioning within the performance areas is not independent of the performance components.

Finally, therapists may focus on the performance context. When looking at the context, the therapist may first determine what are the demands on the child based on this environment or how a particular disability status may impact on performance overall. Once the therapist has determined the relationship of context to the child's performance, then he or she can focus more specifically on performance areas or performance components. Pediatric occupational therapists are primarily concerned with the child's ability to function within his or her performance contexts. Therefore, it is acknowledged that performance components and performance contexts interact and may have an impact on performance areas.

When an occupational therapist uses a specific frame of reference, certain aspects of the domain of concern of the profession are the focus. Although individual therapists may divide human function in different ways, what remains important is that the whole of what is considered to be human function still remains the same. More discrete and specific performance components, performance areas, or performance contexts serve a specific need for the therapists' understanding of the children with whom they work. However, they are arbitrary divisions of human function that allow therapists to understand the parts of the whole to which children respond and then interact with their own environments. By understanding the component parts, a therapist has a better perspective for analyzing the child's overall function. On another level, this information gives the therapist a clear picture of how the child responds to situations and interacts with his or her environment.

OCCUPATION

Occupation is the core concept of the profession of occupational therapy. "Occupation, a collection of activities that people use to fill their time and give life meaning, is organized around roles or in terms of activities of daily living, work and productive activities or play/leisure" (Hinojosa & Kramer, 1997, p. 865). Occupations serve a multitude of purposes; people become involved in them for survival, necessity, pleasure, and for their personal meaning. Each individual's occupations are comprised of a unique combination of activities that are meaningful to that person.

Another way of looking at the domain of concern is using the concept "occupation" to organize and define the profession. This broad conception of occupation is the focus, and the subcategories of work, self care, and play/leisure have less importance. "Occupations are the ordinary and familiar things that people do every day" (Christiansen, et al., 1995, p. 1015). People engage in occupations throughout their daily lives to fulfill their time and give life meaning. An individual's unique occupations define that person. Depending on life situation and circumstances, the occupations that are important to the individual may change over time (Hinojosa & Kramer, 1997).

SUMMARY

All helping professions evolve and change to meet the needs of society. Within each of these professions, the profession's areas of expertise are considered their domain of concern. Occupational therapy's domain of concern encompasses human performance components that serve as the bases of performance areas. Performance components and performance areas are influenced strongly by the performance context.

Activities of daily living, work activities and education, and play or leisure activities constitute the performance areas. Occupational therapists are always concerned with the occupational performance of their clients. The focus in pediatric occupational therapy is the child's ability to function within a variety of environments. The child's culture provides that setting for intervention and must be taken into account by the therapist.

Performance components include sensorimotor components; cognitive integration and cognitive components; and psychosocial skills and psychological components. Performance components are significant in the way in which the occupational therapist views intervention. Although these component parts are essential to intervention, it is important for the therapist to maintain the perspective of the total child.

Occupational therapists are always concerned with the performance context. With children, the focus is to enable the child to function effectively within various environments (i.e., family, school, and community). To address the child's ability to function effectively within the occupational performance areas, the therapist should become sensitive to the child's life situation. Occupational therapists usually are aware of the child's developmental levels. It is also necessary, however, for the therapist to develop a sensitivity to the child's cultural and social background. The cultural and social background affects the child's everyday routines through parental and societal expectations. It is to the therapist's advantage to understand each case at these levels to ensure a good therapist-client association (with optimal outcome).

References

American Occupational Therapy Association. (1979). *Occupational therapy output reporting system and uniform terminology system for reporting occupational therapy services.* Rockville, MD: Author.

American Occupational Therapy Association. (1989). Uniform terminology for occupational therapy (2nd ed.). *American Journal of Occupational Therapy, 43,* 808–814.

American Occupational Therapy Association. (1994). Uniform terminology for occupational therapy—Third edition. *American Journal of Occupational Therapy, 48,* 1047–1054.

American Occupational Therapy Association. (1994). Application of uniform terminology to practice. *American Journal of Occupational Therapy, 48,* 1055–1059.

American Occupational Therapy Association. (1997). *Occupational therapy services for children and youth under the individuals with disabilities act.* Bethesda, MD: Author

Anderson, J., and Schoelkopf, J. (1996). Home-based intervention. In J. Case-Smith, A.S. Allen, and P. N. Pratt (Eds.) *Occupational therapy for children* (pp. 758–765). St. Louis, MO: Mosby.

Bain B., and Leger, D. (1997). *Assistive technology: An interdisciplinary approach.* New York: Churchill Livingstone.

Case-Smith, J. (1993). *Pediatric occupational therapy and early intervention.* Boston: Andover Medical.

Christiansen, C. (1991). Occupational therapy: Intervention for life performance. In C. Christiansen, and C. Baum (Eds.), *Occupational therapy: Overcoming human performance deficits* (pp.3–43). Thorofare, NJ: Slack.

Cynkin, S., and Robinson, A. M. (1990). *Occupational therapy and activities health: Towards health through activities.* Boston, MA: Little, Brown & Company.

Gilfoyle, E., and Hayes, C. (1979). Occupational therapy roles and functions in the education of the school-based handicapped student. *American Journal of Occupational Therapy, 33,* 565–576.

Hanft, B. E. (1991). Impact of Federal policy on pediatric health and education programs. In W. Dunn (ed.) *Pediatric occupational therapy: Facilitating effective service provision* (pp. 273–284). Thorofare, NJ: Slack.

Hinojosa, J., and Kramer, P. (1997). Statement: Fundamental concepts of occupational therapy: Occupation, purposeful activity, and function. *American Journal of Occupational Therapy, 51,* 864–866.

Hopkins, H. L., and Tiffany, E. G. (1988). Occupational therapy—a problem solving process. In H. L. Hopkins, and H. D. Smith (Eds.). Willard and Spackman's occupational therapy (7th ed.) (pp. 102–111). Philadelphia, PA: J. B. Lippincott.

Johnson, J. (1996). School-based occupational therapy. In J. Case-Smith, A.S. Allen, and P. N. Pratt (Eds.) *Occupational therapy for children* (pp. 693–716). St. Louis, MO: Mosby.

Krefting, L. H., and Krefting, D. V. (1991). Cultural influences on performance. In C. Christiansen, and C. Baum (Eds.). Occupational therapy: Overcoming human performance deficits (pp. 101–122). Thorofare, NJ: Slack.

Levine, R. E. (1984). The cultural aspects of home care delivery. *American Journal of Occupational Therapy, 38,* 734–738.

Mosey, A. C. (1986). *Psychosocial component of occupational therapy.* New York: Raven.

Ottenbacher, K. (1982). Occupational therapy and special education: Some issues and concerns related to PL 94–142. *American Journal of Occupational Therapy, 36,* 81–84.

Pratt, P. N. (1989). Occupational therapy in pediatrics. In P. N. Pratt, and A. S. Allen, (Eds.) *Occupational therapy for children* (2nd ed.) (pp. 121–131). St. Louis, MO: C. V. Mosby.

Turnbull, A. P., Summers, J. A., and Brotherson, M. J. (1986). Family life cycle: Theoretical and empirical implications and future directions for families with mentally retarded members. In J. J. Gallagher, and P. M. Vietze (Eds.). Families of handicapped persons (pp. 45–65). Baltimore, MD: Paul H. Brooks.

Legitimate Tools of Pediatric Occupational Therapy

AIMEE J. LUEBBEN / JIM HINOJOSA / PAULA KRAMER

As previously stated, the frame of reference provides organized theoretical and practical material in a methodical and sequential way for therapists' use in intervention. The frame of reference is an outline of essential theoretical concepts relative to particular areas of function, a guideline for assessing those areas of function, and a method for conceptualizing intervention. The frame of reference tends to be more global and general in a particular area of function to be applicable to larger groups and populations. Not specific, the frame of reference generally proposes how the therapist can create an environment to promote change. Although the frame of reference discusses the tools available to the therapist in a general sense, it is assumed that the therapist has a firm understanding of the various tools of the profession and is competent in their use. Tools are defined as those items, means, methods, or instruments used in the practice of a profession.

LEGITIMATE TOOLS

Every health profession has a specific set of tools or instruments to use in bringing about change. These are referred to as the profession's legitimate tools. Society accepts the professional as that person who is expert in the use of these specific legitimate tools. Legitimate tools change over time because these tools are based on the knowledge of the profession, technological advances in society, and the needs and values of the profession and society. To bring about change, occupational therapists use various legitimate tools.

Most professions hold their legitimate tools in high regard. For some practitioners, legitimate tools are symbolic of the profession. Used daily as a means of interacting with clients, legitimate tools may be considered more tangible than the body of knowledge or domain of concern (Mosey, 1986). Many practitioners feel that the tools of their professions are unique, and, in some cases, this may be true. Although various professions often share legitimate tools, the uniqueness to each profession exists in the way the tools are used in the application of the frame of reference.

Each frame of reference addresses the process of change or the way in which the therapist promotes change in the client. Occupational therapy has a variety of frames of reference that relate to many areas of practice. Legitimate tools are chosen by the therapist to match the particular frame of reference that he or she has determined to be appropriate for the particular client. Furthermore, specific legitimate tools are chosen based on their compatibility with the client's developmental level and the environment in which intervention is provided. Some legitimate tools are used by the profession as a whole but may be applied uniquely in pediatric occupational therapy. There have been extensive discussions about the tools of the profession as they relate to the profession and about specific areas of practice (Ayres, 1979; Christiansen & Baum, 1997; Mosey, 1986; Neistadt & Crepeau, 1998; Pedretti, 1996; Trombly, 1995). One should keep in mind that the ultimate goal in using legitimate tools is so the individual can engage in occupations that are important and meaningful to him or her. Although some people consider occupations to be a tool and an end product of intervention, occupation is a broad concept that encompasses many of the legitimate tools of our profession.

This chapter presents an overview of selected legitimate tools for pediatric practice, including the conscious use of self, nonhuman environment, purposeful activities, activity analysis and adaption, activity groups, and the teaching/learning process. In addition to those presented here, other tools exist that are specialized and often are specific to one frame of reference. These may be discussed in the theoretical base of the frame of reference. Often, however, such specialized tools require advanced education and training and, therefore, are beyond the scope of this chapter.

Conscious Use of Self

Conscious use of self involves the therapist's use of his or herself as an agent to effect change within the therapeutic process. The establishment of a positive therapeutic relationship between therapists and clients is a major part of the conscious use of self. An important characteristic of this relationship is the therapist's ability to develop comfortable rapport (i.e., to make the child aware that the therapist cares about him or her and to accept the child at his or her current level of performance). In addition, it requires that the therapist controls his or her own responses so that he or she acts in a way that promotes the child's ability to function or operate in his or her world. This is actively used in many frames of reference in this book, particularly the psychosocial and sensory integration frames of reference.

The conscious use of self can also be thought of in a physical context. Therapists can consciously use themselves physically in the intervention process (e.g., handling and some of the neuromuscular facilitation techniques, particularly used in the neurodevelopmental treatment frame of reference).

The pediatric occupational therapist continually uses him or herself as an agent for positive change in the child, which involves entering the child's world. The therapist needs to emotionally, physically, and developmentally relate to the child at his or her own level. If the child is at the developmental level at which he or she spends most of his or her time on the floor, then the therapist needs to work with the child on the floor. For the same child, objects and directions may have to be presented in a specific and concrete manner so that the child can understand them and respond. The conscious use of self in this example is the therapist's awareness of the child's level and the therapist's ability to adapt his or her posture and behavior to that level. Toys and therapeutic tools also need to be at the child's developmental level or slightly higher to stimulate the child's growth. The therapist has to have a clear understanding of the child's developmental level and skills so that he or she can intervene at that same level or above. Otherwise, the intervention may be less than successful.

The therapist's conscious use of self can be extended to interactions with the family and other care providers. The therapist needs to gauge the family's understanding of the child to be able to collaborate successfully. He or she cannot dictate to them, talk down to them, or be judgmental. The therapist needs to interact with the family in a positive manner. This entails language, posture, gestures, and tone of voice that engages family members (e.g., discuss things that they can understand and ensure that all family members can play an effective part in the therapeutic process). The conscious use of self in this sense therefore may mean that the therapist provides an appropriate role model for the family. The therapist's role with the family is flexible and needs to be open to change over time depending on need.

The skillful application of the conscious use of self develops with practice. To the master clinician, this becomes a natural part of his or her repertoire.

The Nonhuman Environment

The nonhuman environment includes everything that the child comes in contact with that is not human (Mosey, 1986; Searles, 1960). A child's nonhuman environment includes the community, school, and home as well as pets, objects, play things, and transitional objects (e.g., a blanket, preferred stuffed animal, favored doll, diary), which can be anything that is not human that has meaning for the person. The nonhuman environment of a child is influenced, to some extent, by his or her cultural background and developmental level (e.g., it may be considered unacceptable for some male children of Italian or Hispanic descent to play with kitchen utensils or pots and pans because that may not be considered appropriate to the role for male children in these cultures). In some cultures, gender roles are clearly delineated for children.

When working with children, particular aspects of the nonhuman environment are significant to the pediatric therapist. First, the physical, nonhuman environment changes as the child grows. The child starts out primarily in the crib, playpen, and, in some cultures, in an infant seat. As the child grows older, he or she may have a more varied nonhuman environment, moving onto the floor and into a playpen, walker, or activity stander. Second, the facets of the child's physical, nonhuman environment vary depending on culture. Some parents are eager to expose their children to a wide variety of environments, whereas others feel more secure in limiting their children's environment. The child's interaction and awareness of the nonhuman environment changes as the child's physical environments change and as he or she adapts to the different things around him or her.

As the child develops, he or she relates differently to toys and other objects that are part of his or her nonhuman environment. At first, the child may be unaware of a stuffed animal placed in his or her crib. As the child matures, however, he or she becomes aware that the same stuffed animal, a teddy bear perhaps, is always in his or her crib and that the animal has become important to him or her, separate from the environment of the crib. Regardless of the child's surroundings, that animal is important, and the child may be reluctant to engage in any new tasks without the presence of "Teddy" at his or her side. In this case, the stuffed animal may be a transitional object, helping the child move from one stage to another. Transitional objects often help to make a child feel secure, especially in a new environment. For example, a young child will often take a favorite toy with him or her when moving from a crib to a bed.

Toys

Toys are particularly important learning tools in the nonhuman environment. They provide children with basic stimulation, enjoyment, and an initial sense of mastery over their environments. Children learn a sense of competency from toys; they learn that they are able to do things. Children develop their initial understanding of task performance through interaction with toys. The occupational therapist is skilled at the use of toys in intervention and at matching toys with the child's developmental level (Blanche, 1997; Shepherd, Proctor, & Coley, 1996). Toys may "grow" with the child, having different meanings at various ages and stages. For example, the child may first throw blocks, then at a later stage stack the blocks, and still later build structures that are used in imaginary play (Figure 3.1).

Pets

Pets also are significant parts of the nonhuman environment, especially for children at the preschool level and older. Serving a function similar to transitional objects, pets also may help children to develop nurturing qualities and assist in the move away from the natural egocentrism of early childhood. Pets can teach the child how to relate to other living organisms and then to generalize that knowledge to interaction with another person. When the child is older, a pet can help the child to learn responsibility and the importance of providing care to another person or living thing. Throughout life, pets can be a source of pleasure and companionship (Figure 3.2).

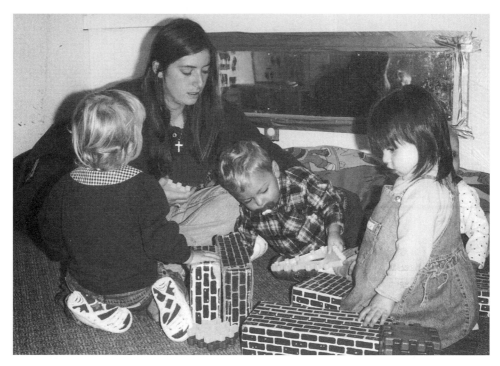

Figure 3.1   Blocks and constructional toys are here used by children in different ways.

Technology

Technology, in this age of information, has become readily available for everyone. In the occupational therapy profession, pediatric therapists often utilize assistive technology to maximize children's potential. Previously called *adaptive equipment*, before federal legislation provided new terminology and definitions, assistive technology can be used in a variety of frames of reference in occupational therapy practice. Additionally, assistive technology can play a role in other selected pediatric practice tools discussed in this chapter; however, this specialized type of technology is most often characterized as nonhuman environment.

The first legislation to provide terminology and definitions, Public Law 100–407: The Technology Related Assistance for Individuals with Disabilities Act of 1988 ("the Tech Act"), separated assistive technology into assistive technology services and assistive technology devices. Assistive technology services encompasses almost every aspect of occupational therapy practice, from the occupational therapy process (evaluation, intervention planning, intervention implementation, etc.) to caregiver training and peer education. Assistive technology device, according to the Tech Act, is any item, piece of equipment, or product system whether acquired commercially off the shelf, modified, or customized that is used to increase, maintain, or improve functional capabilities of individuals with disabilities.

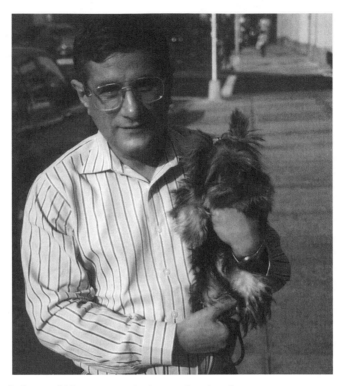

Figure 3.2   A dog and his owner enjoying each others' company.

Assistive technology devices are available across a spectrum of levels. For most people, the phrase "high tech" is synonymous with electronics-based devices such as computers. Because occupational therapists require specialized backgrounds to work with high tech equipment (which is beyond the scope of this chapter), additional assistive technology information can be found in Angelo (1997), Anson (1997), Bain and Leger (1997), Cook and Hussey (1995), or Galvin and Scherer (1996).

At the other end of the spectrum, less expensive nonelectronic (low) technology continues to provide functional solutions for many children. Low tech devices, under the guise of adaptive equipment, have been a primary staple in occupational therapists' practice repertoire for decades.

Adaptive equipment catalogs are packed with low tech equipment, primarily in the performance area, activities of daily living. Catalogs have numerous pages of spoons and forks with built-up handles, non-spill drinking cups, and one-way straws to assist in feeding and eating; button hooks, elastic shoe laces, and long-handled shoe horns for dressing as well as various devices for grooming, oral hygiene, bathing and showering, and toilet hygiene. Many work-related and play or leisure low tech devices are also available.

For children, high tech devices generally are used for work and productive activities and for play or leisure activities. Electronic augmentative communication systems can assist children in functional communication, and seating and wheeled mobility systems (commonly called wheelchairs) can help with functional mobility. Computers often provide assistance with educational activities and vocational exploration in addition to offering opportunities to explore or perform various play or leisure activities. Also, robotic devices can provide children with additional independence in activities of daily living such as eating or grooming in addition to educational and vocational activities and play or leisure activities.

Although high tech counterparts may be available, low tech solutions often work best. During crucial times such as taking tests in school, children have been known to ask that expensive augmentative communication devices be removed from wheelchair mounts in order to access homemade manual language boards on laptrays. For a quick trip to the mall, caregivers may substitute the ease and handling of a manual wheelchair for the child's independence in his power wheelchair.

Physical Agent Modalities

Physical agent modalities are nonhuman physical agents that "use the properties of light, water, temperature, sound, and electricity to produce a response in soft tissue" (McGuire, et al, 1991 p. 6). They include physical agents such as paraffin baths, hot packs, cold packs, fluidotherapy, contrast baths, ultrasound, whirlpool, and electrical stimulation. Some frames of reference delineate how and under what circumstances physical agent modalities are used with children. For example, the application of a heat modality is often used to reduce pain and stiffness and improve tissue healing or a cold modality is used to reduce acute or post exercise edema, reduce pain, or reduce inflammation (Hinojosa & Poole, 1995). Thus, pediatric occupational therapists sometime use physical agent modalities in conjunction with or in preparation for a child to engage in a purposeful activity. It is believed that use of a specific physical agent modality will support the child's ability to participate or engage in a task or activity. When used, physical agent modalities must be applied within the context of a frame of reference. It should be noted that none of the frames of reference in this text specifically use physical agent modalities. Therefore, pediatric therapists who choose to use physical agent modalities should obtain appropriate postprofessional training beyond their basic professional education (Hinojosa & Poole, 1995).

Nonhuman Environment Summary

The nonhuman environment often is used by pediatric occupational therapists in the intervention process. The therapist selects objects appropriate to the child's age, developmental level, and culture as part of the intervention. The therapist works to facilitate the child's mastery of the nonhuman environment. This mastery involves the child's ability to learn from his or her toys and to experiment with objects in his or her physical environment. The therapist also uses the nonhuman environment to facilitate the child's development of performance component skills. For example, a specific toy used in therapy may contribute to improvement in fine motor coordination.

Although the nonhuman environment is often thought of in an emotional context, it can also be considered in a physical sense. The therapist may adapt or manipulate the physical nonhuman environment to use it in the process of intervention. Examples of this include changing the child's equipment, using adaptive devices, and positioning. Low technology (such as assistive devices for feeding and writing, and adaptive and positioning equipment) would be used for such purposes. High technology devices for intervention include adapted computers, page-turning devices, environmental controls, and augmentative communication devices.

Whether the nonhuman environment is used from an emotional or physical perspective, it always should be taken into account when planning intervention so that the intervention is meaningful to the child within the context of his or her environment.

Purposeful Activities

Purposeful activities are those that have meaning to the child and that involve interaction with the human and nonhuman environments (King, 1978). Many purposeful activities for children revolve around play and schoolwork. Erikson (1963) proposed the idea that play is the work of the child. Play is one category available among the tools of purposeful activity. Children learn through play. The various types of play include sensorimotor play, constructional play, imaginary play, and group play. Sensorimotor play is characterized by the use of sensory stimulation with a motor component. Constructional play promotes pleasure through building and creating things. Imaginary play entails cognition combined with fantasy and creativity. Group play is an interactional process where children work together with a relatively common theme (Figure 3.3). Based on the developmental level, culture, and needs of the child, the pediatric occupational therapist uses and adapts the types of therapeutic experiences to the benefit of that child. Through the skilled therapeutic use of play as a tool, the therapist can enhance the child's enjoyment and success in therapy.

Purposeful activities need to be viewed within the context of the child and his or her environment. Some contextual aspects of a purposeful activity are culture, temporal adaptation, and socioeconomic climate. Each activity becomes modified because of how the child interacts with and performs that activity. Purposeful activities are an inherent part of occupational therapy. The pediatric occupational therapist must take care in selecting activities so that they are meaningful to the child. The activities should be developmentally appropriate and motivating to the child, meshing comfortably with the child's lifestyle and environment.

Activity Analysis and Adaptation

Activity analysis is the identification of the component parts of an activity. Occupational therapists are continually fascinated by the parts that make up an activity. Even activities that seem simple because of their familiarity may actually be com-

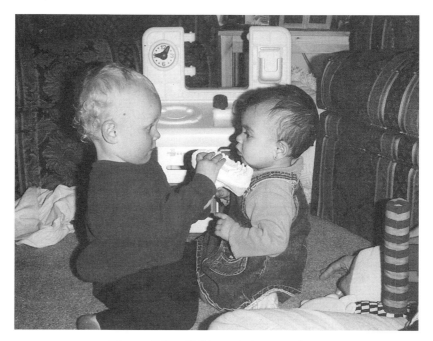

Figure 3.3   Children playing together.

plex. The occupational therapist analyzes activities so that they can be used to treat a client. Through the use of this tool, the therapist identifies whether the child has the necessary skills to perform or complete the activity. Activity analysis also enables the therapist to teach the activity more successfully through a clear understanding of its component parts.

When working with children, activity analysis is a constant focus of the intervention process. The pediatric occupational therapist continually divides activities into component parts to determine which skills are necessary to complete the task or activity. This is just the first step in the intervention process. The next step involves observation of how the child reacts and interacts with the activity or its component tasks. The therapist then analyzes the activity and the child's participation in and reaction to it. This process provides the therapist with the information he or she needs to adapt, grade, or combine activities to make them effective in intervention (Hinojosa, Sabari, & Pedretti, 1993).

The complexity of the activity analysis process is illustrated in the simple activity of stacking blocks. The preliminary analysis entails gaining an understanding of the skills required for the child to stack blocks. The child needs to have beginning fine motor skills, the ability to grasp the blocks, and controlled release for stacking the blocks (Figure 3.4). Then, as the child begins to stack the blocks, the therapist observes the child's behavior and response to the blocks. The next step involves analyzing the child and activity in combination. The questions that follow are examples of what the therapist may ask to start this analysis:

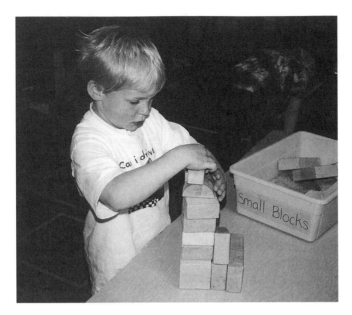

Figure 3.4 A child stacking blocks, grasping each block one at a time.

1. Can the child pick up the blocks?
2. Can the child place the blocks neatly on the stack?
3. Does the child have difficulty letting go of the blocks?
4. Does the child exhibit other compensatory body movements when engaged in the task?
5. Is the child more interested in building the tower or knocking it down?
6. What is the level of the child's fine motor skills in this task?

The therapist answers these questions based on his or her preliminary analysis combined with the knowledge gained from observing the child perform the activity. The therapist needs to look at the answers to all these questions before he or she proceeds to know how to modify this activity to make it therapeutic for the child. Furthermore, the same activity may be different with another child because the reactions of the child and the answers to the previously stated questions would be different. Any activity becomes modified by the way a particular child interacts with the environment and how he or she performs the activity.

The next step in the use of this tool involves adaptation. Activity adaptation means elements of the activity are modified to meet the needs of the client and to facilitate positive change. Activities are adapted by modifying the child's position, the presentation of the materials, or the characteristics of the materials (i.e., shape, size, weight, or texture). Adaptation may also involve modifying the procedure or sequence of events for the activity, nature, and degree of interpersonal contact (Hinojosa, Sabari, & Pedretti, 1993).

The therapist continually adapts activities for the child in pediatric practice. As discussed previously, an example of adaptation is the modification of stacking blocks. The therapist may use larger blocks, seat the child at a small table rather than on the floor, present one block at a time, or add Velcro to the blocks so that they may be attached more easily to each other. The possibilities of adaptation for this activity are endless, limited only by the therapist's creativity.

Activity Groups

Activity groups are those that have a common goal that involves purposeful activities. As a tool, activity groups are used more often in some frames of reference than in others. In this book, the psychosocial and coping frames of reference are more likely to use activity groups. Mosey (1986) has clearly described activity groups and their various levels.

In pediatric occupational therapy, activity groups are used as a tool to promote age-appropriate peer interaction in a therapeutic environment. Occupational therapists draw from their knowledge of child development, group dynamics, and a firm understanding of activities. Activity groups are used to develop play, task, social, and physical skills. The involvement of peers can be useful for facilitating motivation. The occupational therapist fosters group interaction in a safe and supportive environment.

Teaching/Learning Process

The teaching/learning process as a legitimate tool consists of two parts. Teaching gives instruction to a child or shows him or her how to do something, whereas learning promotes acquisition of knowledge or information from instruction, observation, or experience (Figure 3.5). Learning results in a relatively permanent change in behavior. As a tool, the teaching/learning process is more commonly used in some frames of reference than in others, such as acquisitional, motor acquisitional, and visual information analysis frames of reference. A therapist facilitates learning through the creation of an environment that encourages a positive change in the child.

A pediatric occupational therapist teaches through the careful selection of activities reflective of the child's developmental level, age, abilities, and interests. The learning process is enhanced through the use of positive reinforcement and feedback to the child based on his or her performance. The child is more likely to learn from therapeutic interventions that are enjoyable and interesting. Important aspects of learning include trial and error, shaping, modeling, repetition, and practice. The learning environment should be supportive and appropriate for the chosen activity.

OCCUPATION

Occupational therapy practitioners need to keep the individual's occupations in the forefront of their thoughts when using any legitimate tool. Interventions are always directed towards improving the child's ability to function within his or her oc-

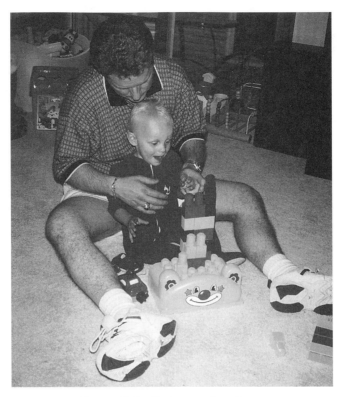

Figure 3.5 Father teaching his son.

cupations and in the roles as family member, sibling, player, or student. This is specifically dealt with in the human occupation frame of reference. However, within the context of using any frame of reference, it is important to address the overall occupations of the child and to focus on the occupations of the particular child (Hinojosa & Kramer, 1997).

SUMMARY

This chapter has outlined the current major legitimate tools for pediatric occupational therapy. Other legitimate tools exist that have not been presented here but that are specific to one frame of reference and may be highly specialized. These specialized tools often require advanced education and training. The tools of the profession can change over time, just as practice changes over time. Because these tools are used within a frame of reference to create an environment for change, each frame of reference has tools that are more relevant and acceptable to it than to others. Within each frame of reference, the change process is outlined, delimiting the tools that are viable.

References

American Occupational Therapy Association. (1994). Uniform terminology for occupational therapy (3rd ed.). *American Journal of Occupational Therapy, 48,* 1047–1054.

Angelo, J. (1997). *Assistive technology for rehabilitation therapists.* Philadelphia: F.A. Davis Company.

Anson, D. K. (1997). *Alternative computer access: A guide to selection.* Philadelphia: F.A. Davis Company.

Ayres, A. J. (1979). *Sensory integration and the child.* Los Angeles, CA: Western Psychological Services.

Bain B., & Leger, D. (1997). *Assistive technology: An interdisciplinary approach.* New York: Churchill Livingstone.

Blanche, E. I. (1997). Doing with—not doing to: Playing and the child with cerebral palsy. In D. L. Parham & Fazio, L. S. (Ed.) *Play in occupational therapy for children* (pp. 202–218). St. Louis, MO: Mosby-Year Book.

Christiansen, C., & Baum, C. (Eds.) (1997). *Occupational therapy: Enabling function and well-bearing.* Thorofare, NJ: Slack.

Cook, A.M., & Hussey, S.M. (1995). *Assistive technologies: Principles and practice.* St. Louis: Mosby.

Erikson, E. H. (1963). *Childhood and society* (2nd ed.). New York: Norton.

Galvin, J. C., & Scherer, M. J. (1996). Evaluating, selecting and using appropriate assistive technology. Gaithersburg, MD: Aspen Publishers.

Hinojosa, J. & Kramer, P. (1997). Statement: Fundamental concepts of occupational therapy: Occupation, purposeful activity, and function. *American Journal of Occupational Therapy, 51,* 864–866.

Hinojosa, J., & Poole, S. (1995). Modalities and domain of concern. In D. M. Baily & S. L. Schwartzberg (Eds.) *Ethical and legal dilemmas in occupational therapy* (pp. 95–111). Philadelphia, PA: F. A. Davis.

Hinojosa, J., Sabari, J., & Pedretti, L. (1993). Position paper: Purposeful activity. American Journal of Occupational Therapy, 47, 1081–1082.

King, L. J. (1978). Towards a science of adaptive responses. *American Journal of Occupational Therapy, 7,* 429–437.

McGuire, M. J., Fisher, T., Poole, S., Reitz, S., Schultz, K., Wilson, D., Hertfelder, S., & Ramsey, D. (1991). *Physical agent modality task group report.* Rockville, MD: American Occupational Therapy Association.

Mosey, A. C. (1986). *Psychosocial components of occupational therapy.* New York: Raven Press.

Neistadt, M. E., & Crepeau, E. B. (Eds.) (1998). *Willard and Spackman's Occupational Therapy* (9th ed.). Philadelphia: J. B. Lippincott-Raven.

Pedretti, L. W. (Ed.) (1996). *Occupational therapy practice skills for physical dysfunction* (4th ed.). St. Louis, MO: Mosby.

Searles, H. F. (1960). *The nonhuman environment.* New York: International Universities Press.

Shepherd, J., Proctor, S. A., & Coley, I. L. (1996). Self-care and adaptation for independent living. In J. Case-Smith, A. S. Allend, & P. N. Pratt (Eds.). *Occupational therapy for children* (3rd ed.) (pp. 461–503). St. Louis, MO: C. V. Mosby.

Trombly, C.A. (Ed.) (1995). *Occupational therapy for physical dysfunction* (4th ed.). Baltimore, MD: Williams & Wilkins.

Trombly, C.A. (1995). Occupation: Purposefulness and meaningfulness as therapeutic mechanisms. *American Journal of Occupational Therapy, 49*(10), 960–972.

20 U.S.C.1401 (a) (25) Public Law 100–407: The Technology Related Assistance for Individuals with Disabilities Act of 1988.

CHAPTER 4

Perspective of Context as Related to Frame of Reference

MARY MUHLENHAUPT / JIM HINOJOSA / PAULA KRAMER

Descriptions of pediatric occupational therapy can be traced back to the 1950's with programs located primarily in hospitals and other acute care medical facilities for children with biological impairments (Stephens & Tauber, 1989). In alternate environments, occupational therapy services evolved into specialized schools for children with neuromuscular and orthopedic impairments and outpatient clinics. Private practices in occupational therapy were also instituted. Current healthcare practice arenas include occupational therapy services in neonatal intensive care units, pediatric acute-care and rehabilitation units, intermediate and long-term care facilities, hospital- and community-based outpatient clinics, and children's homes.

A major shift in pediatric occupational therapy was facilitated in the mid-1970's when Public Law 94–142 (P.L. 94–142), the Education for All Handicapped Children Act (Federal Register, 1977), was enacted. For the first time in the United States, federal regulation mandated access to public schools, affording all children, regardless of their abilities, the right to equal educational opportunities. As school districts enrolled students with differing abilities, occupational therapy practitioners were among a variety of support personnel whose expertise assisted other educational team members to meet these children's specialized education needs. Occupational therapy practitioners affiliated with an educational system may provide interventions in children's homes, in public and private schools, in intermediate or long-term care facilities, in child care settings, or in other community-based environments, such as the library's weekly parent-child music group or a summer day camp program. Table 4.1 summarizes features that distinguish pediatric service settings.

LOCUS OF PEDIATRIC PRACTICE

Healthcare and education continue to represent two broad systems in which pediatric occupational therapy services are delivered today. Features of these two

Table 4.1 Distinguishing Features of Pediatric Service Settings

	Hospital	School System	Home-Based	Private Practice	Day-Care
Governance	Health-care, managed care organization, Board of Trustees	State Education Department, Local Board of Education, building administrator	Family culture and norms	Independent corporation, partnership, or individual owner	Corporation, partnership, individual owner or sponsoring agency
Funding	Public, private funds, endowment	State and federal government, local taxpayers	Third party payment, medical insurance, federal and state funding, out-of-pocket	Third party payment, private insurance, out-of pocket	Medical insurance, federal/state subsidies/ early intervention programs
Focus of Care	Treating acute or chronic disease/ conditions	Participation and progression within educational curriculum	Family system and child as part of the family	Specific to agency's mission	Nurturance, health and safety, develop-mental progression
Peer Relations/ Supervision	Occupational therapy is part of center-based rehabilitation department with other allied health professions	Principal is administrator of multi-disciplined staff. Occupational therapist may function solo within district or building	Traveling to homes on itinerant basis with periodic agency-based meetings with other service providers/ program administrators	Occupational therapist functions solo or with small group of related professionals	Occupational therapist functions solo, primarily interacting with child, day care providers, and supervisors
Treatment Setting	Simulated environment structured around dispensing care as a priority	Multiple school–based and community-based environment as determined by educational curriculum	Natural home and family setting and activities	Simulated settings in center-based practice	1:1 or small groups in settings that simulate home and preschool program environments

—continued

Table 4.1 Distinguishing Features of Pediatric Service Settings—(Continued)

	Hospital	School System	Home-Based	Private Practice	Day-Care
Provider/ Consumer Relations	Brief, intermittent contact, episodic in 1:1 relationship	Occupational therapist works with system, programs, education staff, students, and parents; short- to long-term contracts	Occupational therapist in 1:1 relationship with family/ child; short- to long-term contracts	Occupational therapist in 1:1 relationship with family/ child; short- to long-term contracts	Occupational therapist in relation to child and day care staff; short- to long- term contracts

systems and the practice environments associated with each, present a variety of contextual considerations that impact upon the effectiveness of the intervention process. Mosby's Dictionary (1994) defines systems theory related to health care as "a holistic medical concept in which the human patient is viewed as an integrated complex of open systems rather than as semi-independent parts. The health care approach in a systems view requires the incorporation of family, community and cultural factors as influences to be considered in the diagnosis and treatment of the patient."

As presented in this chapter, context has a critical relevance on the occupational therapy practitioner's roles and responsibilities and for the design and implementation of services. The holism views of systems theory (Bertalanffy, 1968; Capra, 1996) are presented to explain this relevance. Systems concepts help us to understand that an effective occupational therapy process requires considerations beyond viewing the child in relation to our profession-specific knowledge and expertise.

Understanding Health and Education Contexts Through Systems Theory

Bertalanffy (1968) described the open system as a complex of interacting elements that is characterized by relationships (1) within its internal environment and (2) between the system and external environments. An open system is defined not by its parts but by its relationships. One cannot understand the system by separating it from its environment or breaking it into component parts because, by doing this, the relationships that give the system its identity and attributes no longer exist. Interdependence between system components and between the system and external environments is an important concept in this approach. The open system receives and responds to information generated from exchanges (1) within itself and (2) with external environments. These responses provide feedback to which the system responds. The information flow from within and from outside of the system, along with the feedback mechanism, necessitate the view that a system's contextual features are not static but change and evolve over time.

As this view focuses on wholeness rather than segregated subsystems, it is important to be concerned with identity as it results from a constant exchange between subsystem-subsystem and system-environment interactions. It is as if the system is encased in a veil of relationships and one cannot see the system except through its relationships. A view that does not see the subject through these relationships is incomplete and may lead to an inappropriate or ineffective plan for intervention.

As an example, a school district is obligated by federal regulation that governs education for children with disabilities to provide occupational therapy when the service is needed to support a child's educational needs. By law, occupational therapy services that support education are available to every child with special needs who requires these services. At the same time, human factors in the district offer an influence concerning occupational therapy for enrolled students. When school staff members or someone familiar with a child are unaware of occupational therapy's potential relevance to that particular child's educational needs, the service will not be pursued.

To demonstrate how a systems view reveals a complete picture that aids in planning interventions, consider the following. The school district's annual quality control assessment process addresses the occupational therapy program. An analytical approach is taken to gather data concerning the number of occupational therapists providing services to district children, their credentials, relevant experiences, and recent continuing competency activity. Figures are gathered to reflect the total number of students with special needs in the district, the number of students receiving occupational therapy services during the year, the percentage of student objectives to which the service related, duration of students' occupational therapy programs, and so on. The data is collected, summarized, and reported to administrative personnel responsible for the curriculum and budgets.

However, from a systems perspective, in order to understand and improve the school district's occupational therapy program, the analysis must incorporate the contextual variables discussed (i.e., provisions in the federal regulation, knowledge by school staff concerning a particular student's needs, and lack of awareness of the potential contribution offered by occupational therapy services within the district's education programs). In the final systems analysis, one concludes a different answer to the question of how the district utilizes occupational therapy services. Further, a plan of action in response to this knowledge may now include a review of the district's assessment procedures and training efforts to increase parent and school personnel awareness of occupational therapy.

Similarly in healthcare systems, the provision of occupational therapy services is affected by the institution's mission and goals, the types of services provided, and the individual's reimbursement or payment system. In order to understand and improve services in healthcare systems, analysis must also consider federal and state regulations, classification of the institution for reimbursement purposes, and the types of clients most often served. The institution would have to decide what types of programs would be most beneficial to provide based on fiscal issues, the needs of the community or clientele being served, and the expertise of the staff. Studies would have to be done on the needs of the population and whether there is a demand for such a service. The focus is not on the context but more on the types of diagnostic groups being served. While the institution may have occupational therapy services, its administration may decide that it will focus on adult rehabilitation services rather than an outpatient pediatric clinic.

INFLUENCES THAT SHAPE HEALTH AND EDUCATION CONTEXTS

Culture, politics, economics, science, technology, and morality are some of the many factors that contribute to the makeup of large institutions (e.g., health and education systems, how they function, and how they influence individuals and society [Bellah et al, 1991]). The unique philosophical beliefs of medicine, health, and education blend with history and tradition to distinguish these two systems. Influences also come from system components or subsystems (e.g., the medical center's governance, the reimbursement or payment program, or the professional groups involved in service provision in the facility). A system's influential variables are human and nonhuman—as represented by people and their relationships, knowledge and information, ideals and beliefs, policies, norms and customs, events and activities, and objects and physical entities. These factors are all interrelated and woven together, contributing to each system's identity and creating a backdrop or context for individuals accessing that system.

Society's response to factors outside of health and education drive adaption and change within these systems. Califano (1994) and Ginzberg (1994) identify political and economic forces in our country that led to health care reform efforts designed to promote quality and cost-effective health care provision. Alston (1997) contends the resulting changes have occurred rapidly and have "completely reshaped the landscape of medicine and the allied professions" (1997, p. 5). Medical and health services are provided in a wide range of settings, varying from acute-care hospitals to the community. Occupational therapy practitioners are among many healthcare providers who have become affiliated as employees or contractors with independent provider groups under managed care initiatives. Shorter hospital stays, new treatment protocols, and changing patterns of therapist-client interaction can be traced through networks of events related to motivators outside of the intrinsic boundaries of healthcare.

Contemporary views of disability support the inclusion of all persons in society (Grady, 1994; Nagler, 1993). Disability rights movements have brought greater attention to consumer-focused care and the rights of all persons to define and choose lifestyles and the activities they pursue (Shapiro, 1993). These movements disband traditional views that held persons with disability to similar standards of process and performance attained by persons experiencing typical developmental accomplishments. The American Occupational Therapy Association (AOTA, 1996a; AOTA, 1996b) and other associations (Council on Exceptional Children, 1993; Association for Persons with Severe Handicaps, 1992) concerned with the rights of individuals with disabilities have adopted positions in support of inclusive practices for all persons.

Social problems, including homelessness, substance abuse, malnutrition, and poverty influence student performance and prompt education system change and adaptation. Crisis-oriented and prevention programs (Bucci & Reitzammer, 1992; Burnett, 1994) developed through school-community partnerships and the establishment of alternative teacher-roles to link health and social services to the classrooms are some examples of how the education system's context results from environmental influences.

In recent years, a look at short- and long-term educational outcomes for students has prompted educational reform initiatives to improve teaching and learning for all students (Fuchs & Fuchs, 1994; Lucas, 1997; O'Shea & O'Shea, 1997). These movements have suggested significant system change to affect the design and delivery of instruction in our nation's classrooms. Legislative amendments to P.L. 94–142 have changed its name to the Individuals With Disabilities Education Act (IDEA) (Federal Register, 1990), strengthened its requirements, and included family-focused early intervention services for children from birth through 2 years of age (Federal Register, 1991). Passage of early intervention components provided legal and financial support for major philosophical and practical shifts in the ways services for infants, toddlers, and their families are designed and delivered (Thompson, et al., 1997). Most recently, IDEA's federal reauthorization (Federal Register, 1997) incorporated a significant philosophical shift as an emphasis on outcomes related to life-long learning and employment was added to its original purpose to provide access to education. This change is designed to affect the results of education programs for children with special needs. Programmatic and curriculum modification from this change may be anticipated throughout school systems, offering potential new opportunities for occupational therapy's relevance in school programs across the country.

Considering Context When Planning Occupational Therapy Service

Systems theory continues to apply as one moves from a macro view and begins to look at subsystems relating to pediatric occupational therapy service delivery. Using systems theory, a child's behavior and performance are affected by influences from within the human system and those from the world in which the child exists. Bronfenbrenner's "ecology of human development" (1979) describes the relationship between the child and his or her environment. This approach can be used to examine the relevance of the child's environment to the provision of occupational therapy services. According to this view, the child is seen in the context of multiple layers of the environment that provide direct and indirect influence on the child's development and performance.

The macrosystem refers to culture, values, and beliefs and is an influence on all other ecological layers. At the core of his model, Bronfenbrenner (1979) identifies the microsystem, which he calls "a pattern of activities, roles and interpersonal relations experienced by the developing person in a given setting with particular physical and material characteristics" (p. 22). A young infant within the context of a family and home environment represents an early microsystem for many children. In one example, another microsystem evolves as the child grows and attends a community day-care setting for part of the day. The relationship between two or more microsystems is called the "mesosystem" and reflects additional contextual variables. The communication between a family and day-care staff and the compatibility or disharmony in discipline approaches between the two settings, influence that child's development. Both approaches must be considered when working with the child. The next level in Bronfenbrenner's ecology represents "settings that do not involve the developing person as an active participant, but in which events occur that affect, or are affected by, what happens in the setting containing the developing person" (p. 25). To illustrate, a parent's workplace, a sibling's elementary school classroom, or a grandparent's assisted living center are exosystem variables.

The importance of contextual features as key variables that influence human performance is emphasized when an ecological systems view is applied to occupational therapy practice (Dunn, Brown, & McGuigan, 1994). In this framework, context so influences behavior that it is impossible to interpret the child's performance abilities without understanding the unique physical, social, temporal, and cultural factors that serve as environmental cues to support or limit the child's task performance.

The world of a child is framed within the context of family and culture. Effective occupational therapy intervention requires that the therapist be sensitive to the child's environment, including family and culture (Figure 4.1). When a therapist conducts an evaluation or plans intervention without regard to the important people in the child's environment, the intervention may not be appropriate. Thus, the therapist may not be effective in treating the whole person. Occupational therapy intervention should be conducted in the human and nonhuman context of the child's life.

Some frames of reference include the family and the human environment as aspects of their theoretical bases. These frames of reference go so far as to involve family directly or indicate their influence in the application to practice. Examples of this are found in the human occupation frame of reference, the psychosocial frame of reference, and the coping frame of reference. Although the human environment may not be specifically mentioned in the theoretical bases of other frames of reference, it still is important for the therapist to consider this domain when designing and im-

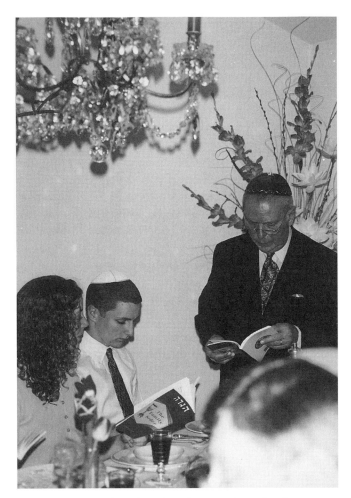

Figure 4.1   The observance of a cultural tradition within a family.

plementing a comprehensive intervention plan. It is vital that the child's culture and family be considered in the application of any frame of reference. For example, the neurodevelopmental treatment frame of reference does not address family issues in its theoretical base; however, practitioners who use this treatment frame of reference usually consider family support and education when implementing intervention. They recognize that their interventions will be less effective if they cannot be carried over into the child's home on a frequent basis.

For the purpose of this book, the primary function of the family is to provide a supportive and nurturing environment for the child's development (Figure 4.2). Consistent with its culture, the family shapes the child's ideological system and provides opportunities to develop interpersonal relationships (Turnbull, Summers, & Brotherson, 1986). In a well-functioning family, the needs of all family members are recog-

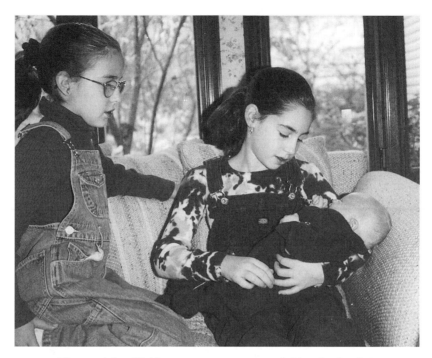

Figure 4.2   Children reacting to a new child in the family.

nized and supported. Each family is unique, and this must be considered by the therapist. When providing occupational therapy services to a child, the therapist usually is in contact with the parents, although the extent of this interaction generally is determined by the treatment setting and service delivery model. It also can be affected by the opportunities and willingness of the therapist and parent to collaborate.

Despite the setting or service delivery model, the therapist should make an effort to develop open communication with the family. Occupational therapists must strive to understand the way in which each family functions and the normal conflicts inherent in child rearing to work effectively with families of children who have disabilities. The entry-level therapist needs to gain some experience and sensitivity about the parenting process and must also understand that it is not always a positive experience. Conflict occurs naturally even in the most functional families.

Working with families requires specific knowledge and skills about effective communication. In addition, the therapist has to understand the dynamics of family function and what potential influence he or she may have on the family. Although the therapist should have a strong knowledge base related to occupational therapy, he or she may not have as much information about family operations and interactions. Such information can be gained primarily through experience and with the establishment of a relationship based on mutual trust. Each family has its own concerns and needs. To be responsive, the therapist must approach the family at their level, addressing their needs and concerns. To provide the most effective intervention, the therapist must work together with family members, being careful not to impose his or her values or concerns onto the family.

Therapists should approach families as partners in this endeavor. The communication between therapist and family should be nonjudgmental to meet the needs of all participants. The goal of communication is to establish a collaborative relationship in which the issues related to the child and family are discussed openly. This communication can provide the therapist with a clear perspective of the child's real-life world demands, how these things impact on the family, and what feedback occurs with regard to the therapist's own intervention and interactions.

It is beyond the scope of this text to discuss in-depth issues about working with families; however, the issues that follow have been identified as important whenever any frame of reference is applied in the context of the family. As the center of concern for the child, the family has the real power in the therapist/family relationship. Family members can facilitate or sabotage the intervention process. Therapists must be concerned with the expectations and responsibilities that they impose on families. Depending on the frame of reference chosen, therapists must be realistic about the role that the family plays in the intervention process. Furthermore, they need to recognize that family members are not experts in the use of the profession's legitimate tools. Therapists must be willing to accept that they do not have all the answers and adjust their interventions to meet the families' goals. The therapist needs to be open enough to discuss goals and types of interventions with family members. This may require an adjustment or change in the frame of reference. When interventions do not work, therapists must examine several areas. Reasons for failure may be the choice of the frame of reference; the cultural influence that impacts on the demands of the particular intervention; unrealistic expectations by either the therapist or the family; or the "fit" between the personalities of the therapist and family members. Therapists must be aware of how some families see the position of authority implied by the role of therapist, and they must be careful not to abuse that power.

Many professionals are sometimes apprehensive about working directly with parents and other family members. Often, family issues are overwhelming. The therapist may not feel adequately prepared to deal with family reactions or may feel uncomfortable with parent distress, anger, or frustration. Ironically, parental feelings of elation over achievements may also be overwhelming to the therapist. To understand this range of emotion, recognition of these feelings may contribute to the therapist's ability to develop a working relationship with families.

SOCIAL PARADIGMS IN PEDIATRIC HEALTH AND EDUCATION SYSTEMS

Capra (1996) defines a social paradigm as "a constellation of concepts, values, perceptions, and practices shared by a community, which forms a particular vision of reality that is the basis of the way the community organizes itself" (p. 6). The curative model, the palliative model, and the ecological model represent three social paradigms that incorporate a range of views that support occupational therapy services for children (Table 4.2).

Occupational therapy professional training is influenced by social paradigms as they exist within the sponsoring educational institution and clinical practice sites. Students adopt ways of thinking; later, as therapists, they bring these influences into the practice setting. In addition to influencing their expectations related to roles and relationships, social paradigms influence the way a particular frame of reference is implemented. As seen in the examples that follow, the types of interventions used by the therapist grounded in a curative model are different than those grounded in a palliative model.

No one of these paradigms as described is exclusive to practice in either system under consideration. In addition, there are many variations on these themes based on the unique experiences and inherent views of individual practitioners. As discussed earlier, a human service system creates a context, and certain contextual dimensions (human and nonhuman) may support or limit elements of these models for practice in that system. Scott, Aiken, Mechanic, and Moravcsik (1995) argue that cultural, organizational, and administrative contexts within the medical system impinge upon the characteristics of medical care that practitioners deliver, limiting what they refer to as "caring aspects" of medical care. Certain elements of the palliative care or ecological approaches discussed in this chapter may be difficult to implement within some hospital and medical care settings.

CURATIVE MODEL PARADIGM

Mosby's Medical, Nursing and Allied Health Dictionary (Mosby, 1994) defines the medical model as "the traditional approach to the diagnosis and treatment of illness . . . focuses on the defect, or dysfunction, within the patient, using a problem-solving approach. The medical history, physical examination, and diagnostic tests provide the basis for the identification and treatment of a specific illness. The medical model is thus focused on the physical and biologic aspects of specific diseases and conditions. . . ." The belief that the whole organism's function and operational behavior depend on the integrity of its underlying parts is a central concept in medical model thinking (Starr, 1982). In this approach, the presenting problem is examined by breaking the organism into its component parts and analyzing those underlying functions believed to contribute to the expression of observed behaviors. Testing is diagnostic to identify and defines symptomatology within components of the whole organism. Fox (1997) explains that the curative model of medical care is focused on curing symptomatology as its goal. As a result, symptomatology must be defined, and once determined, a patient's diagnosis must be treated. In this approach the body is separated from the mind. Psychosocial aspects are addressed separately

Table 4.2   Three Social Paradigms in Health and Education Systems

	Curative Model Paradigm	Palliative Model Paradigm	Ecological Model Paradigm
Goal	Cure	Improve function, reduce symptomatology	Achieve performance across relevant/desired environments
Method	Treat the diagnosis	Address person and environment; reduce undesired and enhance desired traits/ components	Create options for child's relationships between and within environments
Cause of the problem	Physical, biological phenomena	Multiple variables within human organism, environment, or both	Multiple variables in person-environment dimensions and dynamics
Model of thinking	Reductionistic; analysis	Incorporating mind-body connection; synthesis	Holistic; mind-body-environment interaction and interrelations
Assessment based upon	Pathophysiology, scientifically-based data, professional expertise	Pathophysiology, scientifically-based data, professional expertise, child/family's subjective views	Scientifically-based data, professional expertise, child/family/professional/ other relevant person's views of environment dimensions and dynamics
Relevance of human organism	A host for disease, compliance with treatment plan	Source for valuable information needed to supplement clinical findings and plan treatment	Child/family capable of making choices and influencing development
Intervention based upon	Professional discretion, individual's medical history, knowledge of clinical/hard science	Client-determined goals related to their life and diagnosis, in cooperation with professionals	Consensual decision making, family a peer on team
Service delivery	Subspecialties provided by multiple persons, each with focused perspective	Practitioners with diverse expertise, well-developed communication skills	Collaborative and consultative relationships with family and each other
Team process	Multidisciplinary	Interdisciplinary	Interdisciplinary/transdisciplinary
Intervention success measured by	Cure is achieved; symptomatology is eliminated/reversed	Patient/family perspectives combined with scientific data regarding symptom abatement	Sufficiency of environmental options to enable family/child to function in the community

from the condition. Similarly, environmental conditions that support or impede performance are not a central concern in the intervention plan. The medical cure model views selection of a treatment approach as a scientific question, best answered by the physician using objective, scientifically-based data (Fox, 1997).

Evolution in our medical system has included a shift from a "general practitioner approach" to the segregation of knowledge into specialties (Rosenberg, 1989), thus relying upon many professionals with varied educational and training backgrounds for service delivery. Different disciplines, each with a perspective toward a defined aspect of human function, contribute to care. As the model has ultimate respect for scientific and biomedical knowledge, the physician assumes a commanding position as the authority in the care process. Team operation in the medical model is based on principles of multidisciplinary function (Bailey, 1984; McGonigel et al., 1994). In practice, this approach is characterized by numerous disciplines, each assessing a component of the patient's function. To illustrate, a child's visit to the pediatric hospital clinic may include appointments with a neurologist, an orthopedist, an audiologist, a nutritionist, and an internist. Evaluation procedures often are completed in a specialized environment (e.g., the professional office or a "testing laboratory.") Each practitioner identifies pathology and outlines a plan of care to be managed by that discipline. Selection of the frame of reference that guides intervention is determined by the individual practitioner and his or her perspective relative to the diagnosis. Each professional carries out his or her intervention plan in isolation from other disciplines.

Applying a Curative Paradigm to Pediatric Occupational Therapy

Occupational therapy practitioners in a curative medical model practice arena function within discipline-specific departments in the agency. Along with their peers in medical, rehabilitative, and other allied health disciplines, they share similar values, beliefs, and interests in a specific domain of child function and behavior. The institution has a vested interest in generating scientific data so the agency encourages continued training by all staff members to update their knowledge about research into treatment approaches (Rosenberg, 1995). Conferences and continuing education events are frequently scheduled in-house for staff members' participation. As a result of these offerings, department members often acquire a similar knowledge base about interventions relevant to the population served by the agency.

In practice, the departmentalized arrangement provides the occupational therapist with direction and supervision concerning patient care. It gives ample opportunity for therapists to interact and collaborate with others who "speak the same language" and share similar interests. An occupational therapist working with a child who poses a treatment challenge may involve another department colleague to review the case and treatment regimen so additional or revised treatment strategies may be considered. This type of exchange may be facilitated by a department in-service structure reminiscent of "medical rounds" occurring in traditional hospital environments. This type of peer support is particularly valuable to an entry-level therapist. The collaborative opportunity is also rewarding for the therapist who enjoys a mentoring relationship with other colleagues.

Therapists using a medical curative model tend to select frames of reference based on neurophysiology and neuropsychology or on neuromotor and other theories explaining causal relationships between component parts within the human organism. These frames of reference stress the identification of pathology or dysfunction in any of the sensorimotor components that contribute to the child's task performance. The focus is on performance components. Although the therapist may not believe that he or she can "cure" the problem, the belief is that performance will be vastly improved by addressing underlying components. For example, when a child has a problem with shoe tying, the therapist operating within a curative model perspective may select a sensory integrative frame of reference concerned with performance components that enables the child to learn and master the tying process. The evaluation focus is on the analysis of the child's sensory and perceptual processing abilities and neuromuscular and motor functions. The therapist evaluates the way in which the child receives, processes, and organizes tactile, proprioceptive, vestibular, and visual stimuli; the therapist also addresses how that information is used as feedback to initiate, monitor, and adjust motor activity in the eyes, arms, hands, and fingers. Muscle strength, endurance, postural control, and the ability to automatically plan and carry out coordinated sequences of motor activity are also examined.

The underlying performance components that reflect dysfunction and are believed to contribute to the shoe tying difficulty are the subject of therapist's curative model interventions. Because the intervention plan is designed to remove the pathological processes identified through the diagnostic evaluation, once the dysfunction in performance components is resolved, intervention is deemed successful. As skill mastery is not the focus, the shoe tying task is not remediated in the therapy process. External factors in the environment, the method of shoe tying instruction chosen, frequency of training and practice opportunities, the physical and sensory properties of the shoes and laces used, or even the relative value of a child's independence in the task are not priorities from this perspective. The underlying performance components are the only concern rather than the ability to tie one's shoes.

When using a curative model perspective, the occupational therapist's focus is on underlying processes in the child that contribute to his or her observable behavior and not on environmental elements that influence performance abilities. To support programs that address this priority, usually space and equipment are needed for child-centered evaluation and intervention procedures. Locations for curative model interventions are chosen solely with the intervention in mind because treatment does not center on environmental components related to the child's performance. For example, a spacious environment with a supply of various sized positioning aids and an obstacle-free area for the therapist to use when handling the child in various movement planes is well-suited for therapy based on the neurodevelopmental frame of reference.

The following example demonstrates a situation in which the curative model approach is applied to occupational therapy practice in an outpatient clinic. In this case study, the therapist is using a frame of reference in a "pure" form without modification or using another frame of reference in a parallel or sequential manner.

> Kevin, an eight-year-old boy, was fidgety and had difficulty sitting still. His handwriting was also illegible. Kevin was referred to an outpatient clinic where the occupational therapist examined underlying sensory and motor processes believed to contribute to the handwriting task. Analyses of Kevin's body posture and control, ocular mobility, and tracking skills during various therapist-directed testing procedures were completed. Components of sensory integrative processing and visual perceptual function were measured through the administration and interpretation of the *Sensory Integration and Praxis Tests* (Ayres, 1989) and the *Test of Visual Perceptual Skills* (Gardner, 1996).
>
> Test results suggested a deficiency in tactile system functions that the therapist interpreted as being related to the referring problem (i.e., poor handwriting). A subsequent program of occupational therapy intervention included treatment sessions in the gymnasium that addressed gross motor areas. Interventions included play activities emphasizing deep pressure and touch sensory experiences, graded proprioceptive input, and calming movement stimuli. The therapist structured the sessions to encourage Kevin to initiate his own interaction gradually with various tactile stimuli, using and interpreting the sensory information as part of the session's adaptive tasks. During the course of his occupational therapy intervention, Kevin did not engage in any sedentary activities or writing or drawing activities other than finger painting or forming shapes with his finger in a wet sand tray.

In this example, the treatment program, based on sensory integration theory and practice (Fisher, Murray, & Bundy, 1991), does not appear to the casual observer to be related to a handwriting problem. Using this frame of reference, the occupational therapist plans intervention activities to develop mature central nervous system function. The focus is on changing the underlying neural functions that influence Kevin's ability to control and integrate sensory and motor systems. The structure and nature of the environment in which the handwriting performance is expressed are not the focus of treatment concerns for the occupational therapist using the frame of reference. The instructional materials, the teacher's directions or intervention approach, and the tools used are not addressed by the occupational therapist.

Frames of reference that have a curative perspective may be used more successfully within settings that are more medically-oriented or to address acute problems with the likelihood of resolution (e.g., a broken bone). The consistency between the model of the setting, the view of the therapist, and the perspective of the frame of reference is important and may contribute to the success of the intervention and the understanding by other professionals in the setting.

PALLIATIVE CARE PARADIGM

Palliative treatment is defined as "therapy designed to relieve or reduce intensity of uncomfortable symptoms but not to produce a cure" (Mosby, 1994). A recognized specialty in England, palliative care in medical systems has received attention in the United States in recent years (Billings & Block, 1997; Weissman, 1997). The hospice philosophy (Buckingham, 1996), which has been integrated into home, hospital, and community environments, incorporates palliative care components. This approach includes views that may be considered both opposing and complementary to the curative model just discussed. Palliative care does not espouse a cure as its primary goal, but rather it supports a variety of goals related to human function and quality of life.

Palliative care approaches incorporate broader goals of medicine and care in dealing with conditions or symptomatology that cannot be cured. This approach acknowledges a mind-body connection in relation to disease and illness. The focus is not on the disease but on the client and his or her family who become a part of the decision-making process. Value is placed on understanding the client's perceptions and knowing their goals and preferences related to their life and to intervention. Environmental factors, including psychosocial, cultural, and ethical concerns, are legitimate concerns within the evaluation and intervention processes.

Evaluation is based upon diagnostic tests and procedures, along with information from the client regarding a subjective assessment of his or her condition. Different possibilities are implied because this model acknowledges the importance of information from additional sources beyond those on which the curative care model depends. Practitioners using palliative care approaches adopt a more "generalist view" with more diverse expertise as they participate in a care process that deals with physical and social aspects of the human system along with influences from relevant environments. Team members share roles and responsibilities in the data-gathering process, which requires they address multiple sources for information. The analysis of information is accomplished through a team process with interdisciplinary components (McGonigel, et al., 1994). The provider's manner may be considered "more caring" or communicative as the person receiving service is asked to contribute information to the evaluation and treatment planning processes.

Applying a Palliative Model to Pediatric Occupational Therapy

Department structures in this model support interdisciplinary teamwork and collaboration. Frequently, separate, discipline-specific offices may be located in close proximity or designated work spaces may include accommodations for multiple disciplines. The need to learn important information from the client or family requires greater time allocation, different professional expertise, and, often, more coordination between service providers. The therapist's weekly schedule may include regular periods reserved for phone contact or face-to-face meetings with families. The occupational therapist may function in the role of case manager responsible for leading the team in working with the family to complete the evaluation and develop an intervention plan. Social workers and psychologists generally work closely with families, therapists, and other medical personnel throughout the care process.

Therapists in settings based on this approach choose a variety of frames of reference that emphasize operational theories, such as the biomechanical frame of reference. Evaluation procedures include clinical measures related to performance components, and these may be administered in isolated environments. The occupational therapist may evaluate the child's self-feeding skills on the hospital ward during breakfast or in the cafeteria during a lunch period. When this type of contextual opportunity is not available, permanently established simulated environments (e.g., a classroom renovated into a small apartment) may be available or else temporarily constructed by the therapist to evaluate performance areas.

The agency may have a predetermined assessment protocol that is the combined responsibility of occupational, physical, and speech therapists. Each therapist completes their own evaluation process in isolation of the other, and results are reviewed and discussed by all evaluators. Evaluation documentation may include perspectives from all three therapists combined into one report. Intervention priorities and recommendations are not determined until the team members meet together with family members to reach consensus.

Home and community visits may be a regular occurrence and serve as the primary venue for service delivery. Simulated environments that approximate the demands of "real-life" experiences may be used to support intervention. Practice environments may allocate intervention areas designed specifically for clinical procedures (e.g., the fabrication of daytime hand splints to support function in the child with juvenile rheumatoid arthritis and splints to promote comfort during sleeping).

The following example is based on palliative care approaches.

In the outpatient department in a community-based rehabilitation center, a young boy who has cerebral palsy and his parents meet with a physiatrist for an interview and examination procedures. Separate evaluation sessions are scheduled with the psychologist, the occupational therapist, the physical therapist, and the speech pathologist. Each professional completes assessment procedures during individual sessions with this child while his parents are present. On another date, after each evaluator has had the opportunity to collect and analyze assessment data, the professionals convene with the physiatrist to present and review their collective findings. A physiatrist often functions as team leader and summarizes the information presented. As a team including the family, the rehabilitation plan for the child and his family is developed. During the meeting, professionals and the boy's parents discuss the evaluation results and a final determination of services including occupational, physical, and speech therapy are made. Afterward, the family develops a schedule of visits with the therapists, and the therapy programs begin. The overall program and each professional's intervention plan address family, physical environment, and performance component strategies that address neuromusculoskeletal dysfunction and performance area limitations. Using a biomechanical frame of reference, the focus of occupational therapy in this example may be the types of equipment that will increase independence in performance areas.

ECOLOGICAL MODEL PARADIGM

Human ecology is defined as "the study of interrelations between individuals and their environments as well as among individuals within the environment" (Mosby, 1994). When an ecological perspective is applied to children's services (Peck et al., 1993; Rainforth et al. 1992), interactions with people and relationships within and across environments and settings are identified among the diverse influences that contribute to growth and maturation. This approach incorporates culture and society as important influences on the developing child. The child is viewed as an open system, evolving with the influence of intrinsic variables and from those within immediate and extended environments. Programs and services based on this model focus on child-environment interaction as a barometer of development and as a means to effect change. Many inclusive settings and programs that support services and interventions in "natural settings" espouse principles based upon ecological perspectives.

Reflecting assumptions in Bronfenbrenner's ecological framework (1979), a critical factor related to a child's development is the environment as it is experienced by the child. This points to the importance of individualized interventions that are tailored for each unique child rather than reliance on protocols of problem-solution strategies. Evaluations and intervention plans embrace strategies that facilitate knowing about the child's perceptions and interests and, when that's not possible, as in the case of a young infant, knowing the perceptions, interests, and priorities of persons relevant to the child's life.

Multiple methods are used to gather information about the child and environments, including formal tests and informal measurements. Quantitative and qualitative phenomena are considered. A fundamental difference in the evaluation process is evident in this model because it addresses any enabling and limiting influences in human and nonhuman environments to which the child relates. Early intervention programs that view family strengths and weaknesses as critical to the development of the Individualized Family Service Plan (Thompson et al, 1997) demonstrate this component.

In addition to identifying the current level of performance, the skills and environmental features the child needs to move forward to the next level of expected performance are a relevant concern. An ecological perspective values human development occurring in context. Understanding how changes in the environment can affect behavior is important in this model. The discrepancies between the child's performances and the demands and supports of the environment become the target of interventions. The creations of new options in the relationship between the child and his or her environments are valued intervention objectives. Teamwork is an important element in this approach, reflecting components of the interdisciplinary or transdisciplinary processes (McGonigel et al., 1994). Communication skills and interpersonal relations are important as individuals with varied backgrounds share their expertise related to the child. While each team member has an impression of the child based on one's own knowledge and data-gathering, a complete picture is possible when all come together and synthesize evaluation findings. Profession-specific language and concepts are translated to be understood by those without a similar professional background. Opportunities for team planning are an integral part of this perspective. The comprehensive picture that results, which reflects diverse expertise and attention to numerous variables, provides a meaningful and relevant approach that is designed within the context of the child's everyday activity.

Applying an Ecological Model to Pediatric Occupational Therapy

An occupational therapist in a setting based upon ecological perspectives works with family members and other persons relevant in the child's life. A service setting may be the community day care center where a child with cerebral palsy is integrated into the program's routine and activities. Team members cooperate to complete the evaluation that reflects all areas of expertise and may be combined into one summary report. Frequently, more than one discipline is present with family members to simultaneously observe the child's participation in a task or activity. Staff members may meet the child and parent in the day-care room over a period of parent-child play combined with other interactions between child and staff. They work together to identify the child's strengths and needs. A social worker may join in the classroom and informally meet with the parent to gain additional relevant information. An organized approach, such as the play-based assessment (Linder, 1993), may be used to facilitate the evaluation process. Afterwards, parents, professionals, and paraprofessionals meet to discuss and evaluate the performance from different perspectives. The child's performance is viewed in connection with the specific environmental supports and limitations that are present, with findings presented in behavioral statements that are relevant in the context of that child.

The occupational therapist works closely with families and members of other disciplines to reach consensus regarding program priorities and an appropriate intervention plan. This may mean that a particular area of concern identified by the occupational therapist is not accepted by the team for immediate attention. For example, the developing self-dressing needs of a 3-year-old boy may be weighed with less urgency as the team plans and implements a cohesive approach to facilitate oral communication in the preschool classroom.

Intervention is provided through functional activities that are environmentally-connected and applicable in a variety of situations. As the model emphasizes social contexts and relationships, activities may be structured for implementation in homogenous or heterogenous groupings within the classroom. Because adults in the child's life influence development, all persons working with the child in the preschool are given insight and information to positively influence the child's development. For example, the occupational therapist and other team members learn that one child needs to develop the "k" and "g" sounds at the start of words. With this information, all adults in the preschool environment are sensitive to the types of prompts and questions they can express to facilitate the child's developing articulation abilities as they are needed throughout the school routine. During a classroom activity when this child is playing "dress-up," the occupational therapist knows how to ask questions to facilitate articulation skill. Likewise, the occupational therapist looks to environmental cues that may be available throughout the child's day to support change and development. The specific presentation or placement of materials for the child in the classroom, use of modified tools, or altered sequences of activities may be recommended to the teacher and assistant in the classroom.

When a frame of reference is used that is consistent with an ecological perspective, information is presented in terms of end-product performance by using behavioral statements that reflect performance in context. Behaviors are defined as levels of achievement in positive terms, even though they relate to dysfunction in a child's performance components. Rather than define a problem by highlighting what the child cannot do, the therapist translates the child's dysfunction into statements of baseline performance abilities that are relevant in the environment. An example is demonstrated in the therapist's involvement with a student who needs physical support and assistance to accomplish positioning and movement throughout the day. The development of alternate systems to hold and activate classroom materials, the need for adapted equipment, recommendations regarding adult assistance required in the classroom for activity set-up, and the creation of modified activity sequences are all part of the occupational therapist's intervention plan. One IEP (Individualized Educational Program) objective related to the therapist's intervention may be written as follows: John will develop a repertoire of five different musical activities to enable his participation with classmates in the classroom group circle. The strategies to accomplish this objective may list the materials and interventions as described above.

Recent interest in including children with disabilities into all areas of community life has brought attention to the environmental discrepancies that exist for many children and families accessing new situations (Idol, 1997; Palmer, Borthwick-Duffy, & Widaman, 1998). An ecological perspective provides a framework that places relevance on those discrepancies and their relation to the child's development. Therapists may find this approach gaining momentum in a variety of children's services and programs.

Social Paradigms and Applying Frames of Reference in Context

Occupational therapists are responsible for carefully selecting and applying frames of reference in practice. In addition, throughout the occupational therapy process, they must consider the congruity between their own views of a setting's social paradigm along with reality in the setting. Therapists need to incorporate the setting's social paradigm into the chosen frame of reference in order to provide interventions within the system's context. When systems processes and influences are understood, an analysis can be made of the relationships between (1) a system's attributes, (2) a therapist's expertise and thinking approach, and, subsequently, (3) the ways in which an occupational therapy program may be designed and applied for a specific child. Using this information, the therapist may effectively integrate principles of occupational therapy evaluation, program planning, implementation, and outcome assessment for relevant and effective pediatric services.

PROFESSIONAL RELATIONSHIPS IN THE CONTEXT OF HEALTH AND EDUCATION SYSTEMS

A child does not operate in a vacuum, and occupational therapists should not operate in isolation. Almost all children who receive occupational therapy services are in contact with other professionals. Effective occupational therapy intervention requires that the therapist interact and communicate with any other professionals involved with the particular child.

Just as the therapist must establish rapport to work with families, lines of communication must be developed to collaborate effectively with other professionals involved with the child. Each professional who works with the child has a different educational background that lends a different viewpoint to the situation. The roles of each profession and their distinct perspectives, lead to unique concerns and goals for the child. Furthermore, these professionals often have different beliefs, values, and attitudes. Each person involved brings their own professional perspective to the work environment and a preconceived view of the other professionals involved. The one thing that all may have in common is a philosophy about the setting in which they are working.

Interaction among professionals requires mutual respect and support as well as a mutual understanding of different roles and goals. To achieve this rapport, professionals must communicate with each other and be willing to learn from one another. They must recognize and solve problems that arise when professionals from multiple disciplines interact and, ultimately, participate effectively in teams (Bailey, 1989).

Entry-level occupational therapists must become secure in their own roles to participate successfully with other professionals. They must understand their profession and the uniqueness that each contributes to the intervention process. This requires a firm understanding of the frames of reference and how they fit with the overall concerns for the child. The therapist must feel equal with the other professionals on the team. A reciprocal relationship enables the therapist to teach other team members about occupational therapy perspectives while learning about theirs.

It takes skills to collaborate effectively with other professionals. The following issues are important when using any frame of reference in the context of a professional team:

- All team members have equal status and should work toward facilitating positive change in the child and his or her family.
- Any one team member can sabotage team function and, therefore, negatively affect the intervention process.
- Therapists must be willing to accept the fact that they do not have all the answers and must be willing to modify their interventions to meet unified team goals for the child and his or her family.
- Therapists need to discuss and negotiate this openly with other team members. The result may require an adjustment or change in the frame of reference.
- Therapists cannot see themselves as being all things to all children. They must be aware of the strengths and limitations of their profession and understand the important contributions that can be made by other professionals.
- Therapists should be concerned about whether they are speaking the same language as other team members. They should avoid professional jargon for the sake of clarity. Each frame of reference has its own jargon, which should be translated for mutual understanding by all team members.

When interventions do not work, therapists must examine several areas. This requires communication with other team members and may require an exploration of overall goals for the child. All avenues need to be explored rather than looking for blame. Additional collaboration may be required to redefine the team's approach or another frame of reference may be used by the occupational therapist. Therapists should consider the possibility of "conflicting loyalties" (Purtilo, 1990). This occurs when a personal or professional view conflicts with the personal or professional views of other team members. Therapists should keep in mind that the overriding concern is how best to meet the needs of the child and his or her family.

Many entry-level occupational therapists initially feel insecure about working as a full-fledged team member. With experience, sensitivity, and self-examination of their own interactions, they rapidly acquire the skills needed to be an effective team member. Occupational therapists can draw from their educational background to facilitate the group process and psychosocial functioning to understand the workings of the team and become an important contributing member.

SUMMARY

A number of variables contribute to how a healthcare or education agency structures its programs and delivers services. Ultimately, the mix of influences and attributes that distinguish the system have implications for all phases of the occupational therapy process—from initial referral, throughout evaluation, to the selection of an appropriate frame of reference, treatment implementation, discharge planning, and termination of services. Intervention is also influenced by human interpretation of values, beliefs, and needs. To that extent, intervention becomes subjective because feelings color the definition of these systems. The occupational therapist must be aware, however, that although the therapist's feelings are important, the values and beliefs of the child and his or her family should take precedence.

Collaboration among occupational therapists, family members, and other professionals is essential to provide the most appropriate intervention services for children and families. A collaborative relationship is one in which issues are discussed openly, decisions are made mutually, and a foundation is built for effective working relationships.

References

Alston, R. J. (1997). Disability and health care reform: Principles, practices and politics. *The Journal of Rehabilitation*, (63)3, 5–9.

American Occupational Therapy Association. (1996a). Occupational Therapy: A profession in support of full inclusion. *American Journal of Occupational Therapy*, (50)10, 855.

American Occupational Therapy Association. (1996b). Occupational Therapy: White paper: The role of the occupational therapy practitioner in the implementation of full inclusion. *American Journal of Occupational Therapy*, (50)10, 856–857.

Association for Persons with Severe Handicaps (TASH). (1992). Endorsement of "full inclusion." Seattle, Washington.

Ayres, A. J. (1989). *Sensory integration and praxis tests*. Los Angeles: Western Psychological Services.

Bailey, D. B. (1989). Issues and directions in preparing professionals to work with young handicapped children and their families. In J. J. Gallagher, P. L. Trohanis, & R. M. Clifford (Eds.). *Policy implementation and PL 99–457* (pp. 97–132). Baltimore, MD: Paul H. Brooks.

Ballah, R. N., Madsen, R., Sullivan, W., Swidler, A., & Tipton, S. (1991) *The Good Society*. New York: Random House.

Bertalanffy, L. (1968). *General system theory: Foundations, development, applications*. New York: George Braziller.

Billings, J.A., & Block, S. (1997). Palliative care in undergraduate medical education. *Journal of the American Medical Association*, (278)9, 733–737.

Bronfenbrenner, U. (1979). *The ecology of human development*. Cambridge, MA: Harvard University Press.

Bucci, J.A., & Reitzammer, A. F. (1992). Collaboration with health and social service professionals: Preparing teachers for new roles. *Journal of Teacher Education*, 43(4), 290–295.

Buckingham, R. W. (1996). *The handbook of hospice care*. New York: Prometheus Books.

Burnett, G. (1994). *Urban teachers and collaborative school-linked services*. Washington, DC: Educational Resource Information Center (ED 371 108).

Capra, F. (1996). *The Web of Life: A new scientific understanding of living systems*. New York: Doubleday.

Califano, J. (1994). *Radical surgery: What's next for America's health care*. New York: Random House.

Council for Exceptional Children. (1993). *CEC Policy on inclusive schools and community settings*. Reston, VA: Author.

Dunn, W., Brown, C., & McGuigan, A. (1994). The ecology of human performance: A framework for considering the effect of context. *American Journal of Occupational Therapy*, (48)7, 595–607.

Federal Register. (1977). The Education for All Handicapped Children Act of 1975, P. L. 94–142, Vol. 42, No. 163, August 23, 1977.

Federal Register. (1990). The Education of the Handicapped Act Amendments of 1990, P. L. 101–476. #20, USC 1400. October 30, 1990.

Federal Register. (1991). The Individuals With Disabilities Education Act Amendments of 1991. P. L. 102–119. #20.

Federal Register. (1997). The Individuals With Disabilities Education Act Amendments of 1997. P. L. 105–117, Vol. 62, No. 204, October 22, 1997.

Fisher, A. G., Murray, E. A., & Bundy, A. C. (1991). *Sensory integration theory and practice.* Philadelphia, PA: F. A. Davis.

Fox, E. (1997). Predominance of the curative model of medical care. *Journal of the Amercian Medical Association,* (278)9, 761–763.

Fuchs, D., & Fuchs, L. (1994). Inclusive schools movement and the radicalization of special education reform. *Exceptional Children,* (60)4, 294–309.

Gardner, M. (1996). *Test of visual perceptual skills (non-motor),* Revised. Hydesville, CA: Psychological and Educational Publications.

Ginzberg, E. (1994). *The road to reform: The future of health care in America.* New York: The Free Press.

Grady, A. (1995). Building inclusive community: A challenge for occupational therapy, 1994 Eleanor Clarke Slagle Lecture. *American Journal of Occupational Therapy, 49,* 300–310.

Idol, L. (1997). Key questions related to building collaborative and inclusive schools. *Journal of Learning Disabilities.* (30)4, 384–394.

Linder, T. (1993). *Transdisciplinary play-based assessment: A functional approach to working with young children.* Baltimore, MD: Paul H. Brookes.

Lucas, C. (1997). *Teacher education in America: Reform agendas for the twenty-first century.* New York: St. Martin's Press.

McGonigel, M., Woodruff, G., & Rosmann-Millican, M. (1994). The transdisciplinary team: A model for family-centered early intervention. In L. Johnson, R. Gallagher, R. M. La Montagne, J. Jordan, J. Gallagher, P. Hutinger, & M. Karnes (Eds). *Meeting early intervention challenges.* Baltimore: Paul H. Brookes.

Mosby's Medical, Nursing and Allied Health Dictionary (4th ed.). (1994). Chicago, IL: Mosby.

Nagler, M. (Ed.). (1993). *Perspectives on disability.* Palo Alto, CA: Health Markets Research.

O'Shea, D., & O'Shea, L. (1997) Collaboration and School Reform: A twenty-first century perspective. *Journal of Learning Disabilities,* (30)4, 449–462.

Palmer, D., Borthwick-Duffy, S. & Widaman, K. (1998). Parent perceptions of inclusive practices for their children with significant cognitive disabilities. *Exceptional Children, 64*(2), 271–282.

Peck, C.A., Odom, S. L., & Bricker, D. D. (1993). *Integrating young children with disabilities into community programs.* Baltimore, MD: Paul H. Brookes.

Purtilo, R. (1990). *Health professional/patient interaction,* (4th Ed.). Philadelphia, PA: W.B. Saunders.

Rainforth, B., York, J., & Macdonald, C. (1992). *Collaborative teams for students with severe disabilities: Integrating therapy and educational services.* Baltimore, MD: Paul H. Brookes.

Rosenberg, C. E. (1995). *The care of strangers: The rise of America's hospital system.* Baltimore, MD: Johns Hopkins University Press.

Rosenberg, C. E. (1989). Community and communities: The evolution of the American Hospital. In: D. E. Long, & J. Golden (Eds.). (pp. 3–17). *The American general hospital communities and social contexts.* Ithaca, NY: Cornell University Press.

Scott, R., Aiken, L., Mechanic, D., & Moravcsik, J. (1995). Organizational aspects of caring. *The Millbank Quarterly*, (73)1, 77–95.

Shapiro, J. P. (1993). *No pity*. New York: Random House.

Starr, P. (1982). *The social transformation of American medicine*. New York: Basic Books.

Stephens, L. C., & Tauber, S. K. (1989). Early intervention and preschool programs. In P. N. Pratt, & S. S. Allen (Eds.) *Occupational therapy* (2nd ed.) (pp. 382–395). St. Louis: C. V. Mosby.

Thompson, L., Lobb, C., Elling, R., Herman, S., Jurkiewicz, T., & Hulleza, A. (1997). Pathways to family empowerment: Effects of family-centered delivery of early intervention services. *Exceptional Children*, (64)1, 99–113.

Weissman, D. E. (1997). Consultation in palliative medicine. *Archives of Internal Medicine*, (157)7, 733–737.

CHAPTER 5

Structure of the Frame of Reference

PAULA KRAMER / JIM HINOJOSA

There are various ways to intervene with any particular child. Each therapist uses clinical judgment to select an approach that will be beneficial and meaningful to that child. That approach needs to be significant to the child's life, relating clearly to the goals for that child and demands that will be placed on him or her. The approach chosen needs to relate to and be appropriate for the context of service delivery. In occupational therapy, one way to organize intervention approaches is the frame of reference.

Anne Cronin Mosey, Ph.D., OT, FAOTA (1968, 1972) proposed the frame of reference as a method of organizing knowledge so that it could be used for planning and implementing intervention. She presents the frame of reference as a linking structure between theory and application. Dr. Mosey's original components of a frame of reference are the theoretical base, function/dysfunction continua, behaviors indicative of function and dysfunction, and postulates regarding change. In 1996, Mosey revised the label of one of the sections of the reference, changing the label behaviors indicative of function and dysfunction to indicators of function and dysfunction.

Expanding on Mosey's work, we have highlighted the importance of evaluation guidelines and have added another component, application to practice. The purpose of the evaluation guidelines is to suggest to therapists methods and tools that may be used to evaluate a client's performance that would be compatible with the particular frame of reference. The application to practice component articulates for the therapist how the frame of reference is used for treatment. This component is meant to clarify how a therapist moves in practice clinically from a theoretical perspective through the process of evaluation and the identification of specific problem areas to intervention. It describes the legitimate tools that are used in each frame of reference and gives some specific examples as illustrations for the therapist. The physical environment in which this frame of reference may be used and the possible modifications to that environment are presented in this section. This allows the therapist to better understand the intervention process and give more attention to the context of intervention.

The challenge to any therapist is the application of theoretical knowledge to practice. Moving from theory to practice is a complex process; it entails taking ideas that are abstract and bringing them to a level at which they can be used. When choosing a frame of reference, the occupational therapist looks at the child's needs, strengths, limitations, and environment. With a comprehensive understanding of all these issues, the therapist chooses the most appropriate approach to the child and the context for service delivery. The frame of reference delineates the perspective of the occupational therapist when approaching the child.

These concepts are abstract and can be understood best through the use of examples. Examples are presented that are intended to clarify some of the ideas introduced while adding a note of levity to this complex topic. Our example of a frame of reference deals with adolescents making contact with persons of the opposite sex. It is not intended to be a completely developed frame of reference but, rather, a brief sample that exemplifies the various parts needed to understand the structure. This "frame of reference" can be found in marked sections throughout the chapter.

THEORETICAL BASE

Professional education provides occupational therapists with a broad knowledge base. One aspect of this educational process is the study of various theories. "A theory is concerned with how and under what circumstances those events happen and how they are related. The purpose of theory is to make predictions about the relationships between events or phenomena" (Mosey, 1981, p. 30). Theories provide therapists with ways of understanding the effects of their actions on the subsequent reactions of the child.

Generally, we talk about theory-based intervention in occupational therapy. If intervention is based on theory, a therapist is able to understand the relationship between the treatment and the subsequent reactions of the child. For example, if the theory states a relationship between tickling and laughter, when a child is tickled the therapist should then expect the child to laugh. If the child does not laugh, then the theory also should provide a means for the therapist to understand the lack of response. Most often, therapists do not use theories as a whole. Instead, they tend to select sections from a variety of theories and organize these pieces of information together in a way that it will be meaningful to assist an individual. During this process, therapists are creating a new conceptualization of theoretical information, not new theories themselves (Hinojosa, Kramer & Pratt, 1996). Intervention should be based on theoretical information because the therapist should be able to describe the postulated links between the intervention and the expected changes in the child.

Sometimes therapists have difficulty in moving from theory to practice. It is as if the theoretical knowledge is separated from practice. Sometimes therapists believe that practical knowledge constitutes a separate set of specific skills or techniques. Theoretical and practical levels of knowledge must be integrated. An organized, consistent treatment plan for the child flows from the clear understanding of the underlying theories. The underlying reasons for any intervention have to be clearly understood. The therapist's actions do not come from intuition but from a well thought out theoretical understanding. The frame of reference, therefore, provides the cohesion between theory and intervention in a practical manner, with the theoretical base providing the framework for the actual intervention.

The theoretical base provides the foundation of the entire frame of reference. The theoretical base may draw from one or more theories. If more than one theory is used, the theories must be consistent internally or operating from the same basic premises (Mosey, 1981). Most often, the theoretical base of a frame of reference includes constant and dynamic theories. Constant theories are those theories that are not concerned with change and only describe relationships between phenomena. For example, theories of anatomy describe the human body and the relationships of the various body parts to each other. Theories of anatomy do not concern themselves with explaining how the body develops or matures; therefore these theories are considered constant.

In order to be useful in a frame of reference, constant theories are used in combination with dynamic theories. Dynamic theories are those that are concerned with change and describe the theoretical information the therapist will use to promote change in the individual. The types of dynamic theories primarily used in pediatric practice are developmental, maturational, acquisitional, and operational. Change occurs in many ways. Developmental theorists believe that development is stage specific and one set of skills has to be mastered before the individual moves onto the next set of skills. Maturational theorists are concerned with the sequential changes that occur within the individual, with primary focus being on the progression in a specified pattern rather than stages. Acquisitional theories are based on learning and interaction with the environment, with change being dependent on the individual's ability to learn new skills or behaviors rather than on developmental stages or maturation. Operational theories are based on environmental changes that assist the individual to improve performance or function. These improvements in performance or function are dependent on environmental adaptions and are external to the individual (Hinojosa, Kramer, & Pratt, 1996). When an occupational therapist works with an individual, the ultimate goal is to improve the person's ability to function; therefore, the theoretical base needs to have a dynamic theory to explain how this change in function will occur. Included in the theoretical base are assumptions, concepts, definitions, postulates, and hypotheses. Furthermore, the theoretical base states the relationships between all these elements.

Making Contact with Persons of the Opposite Sex as An Adolescent: Theoretical Base

For those individuals who are heterosexually oriented, interest in developing relationships with the opposite sex generally begins around the preadolescent or early adolescent stage of development. It is normal and natural in early adolescence to begin to get interested in the opposite sex. It is somewhat difficult and uncomfortable, however, to make initial contact with an unknown person of the opposite sex. As one grows older, one usually finds it easier to initiate and maintain contacts with members of the opposite sex. Furthermore, as one gains more experience relating to the opposite sex, one becomes more interested in and comfortable with the idea of choosing a life mate. Persons become more focused about who they are and what they want, expect, and need from others.

The theoretical base of this frame of reference is drawn from several developmental theorists, including Blos (1962), Erikson (1968, 1982), Freud (1966), Rogers (1961), and Elkind (1967). Erikson (1968) describes development in terms of stages. The stages during preadolescence and early adolescence are industry versus inferiority and self identity versus role diffusion. Blos (1962) states that at the preadolescent stage, it is normal to begin to get interested in the opposite sex, although this interest may be expressed first in an inappropriate and somewhat hostile manner; however, this is still a means of making contact. Erikson (1968, 1982) further states that the beginning of interest in the opposite sex is a preparatory step toward young adulthood (intimacy and solidarity versus isolation), when one becomes involved in choosing a life partner. Elkind (1967) reinforces the concept that it is initially difficult to make contact with the opposite sex for the adolescent because he/she feels self-conscious. He states that adolescents presume that everyone around them is an "imaginary audience" and that they are the center of attention. Adolescents believe that everyone is looking at them. This presents some conflict to the preadolescent or early adolescent. They want to make contact with the opposite sex and yet it is difficult for them. Freud's (1966) contribution to this theoretical base is his theories about sexual development and the natural state of relationships between opposite sexes. Rogers' (1961) contribution is his theories of interpersonal communication and the ability to establish relationships. All these theories take the position that making contact with the opposite sex is normal and natural. Furthermore, they assume that a heterosexual orientation is natural at this stage of life.

There are various ways that people begin to make contact with the opposite sex during this stage of life. One way is generally referred to as flirting. Flirting is an attempt to get the attention of someone, usually a person that you do not know well, and generally has an underlying sexual connotation. It involves making eye contact, smiling, acting in a coquettish manner, and making actual contact in a socially appropriate way.

Flirting is frequently used to determine if the other party has any interest in the person doing the flirting. Making eye contact and smiling at the same time is an acceptable way of flirting. In many situations, flirting is a socially appropriate way of making contact with someone of the opposite sex. In some situations, however, it may be seen as forward or socially inappropriate behavior. Socially appropriate behavior refers to actions that are acceptable in a public situation based on age, sociocultural values, and norms.

Assumptions

Assumptions are ideas that are held to be true and are not questioned or tested in any way. In other words, they are basic beliefs. All theories have assumptions. If the theoretical base draws from several theories, then all the assumptions made must be accepted by all of those theories and the assumptions must not be in conflict with each other.

Assumption

It is normal and natural during early adolescence and preadolescence to want to make contact with the opposite sex.

Assumption

It is difficult initially to make contact with someone of the opposite sex.

Assumption

Preadolescents and early adolescents feel conflict because they want to make contact with the opposite sex and yet find it difficult.

Assumption

These theories assume that a heterosexual orientation is natural at this stage of life.

Concepts

Concepts describe phenomena that have been observed and have shared characteristics. The concept is a label that the theorist believes to be important. The following are concepts identified in this frame of reference.

Concept

flirting

Concept

behaving in a socially appropriate way

Definitions

Definitions explain the meaning of important concepts. Keep in mind that every concept in a theoretical base should be defined in terms of what it means to the particular frame of reference.

Definition

Flirting refers to getting the attention of someone, usually a person that you do not know well, in a coquettish manner that generally has an underlying sexual connotation. Flirting is frequently used to determine if the other party has any reciprocal interest. In some situations, it may be seen as forward or socially inappropriate behavior.

Definition

Socially appropriate behavior refers to actions that are acceptable in a public situation based on age, sociocultural values, and norms.

Postulates

Postulates state the relationship between concepts. Within the theoretical base, all concepts are related in some way. Within a theoretical base, the relationship between important concepts are made clear by postulates. The postulate serves as the linking mechanism between concepts.

Postulate

Flirting is usually a socially appropriate way of making contact with someone of the opposite sex.

Postulate

Making eye contact and smiling at the same time is an acceptable way of flirting.

Hypotheses

Hypotheses are a very specific type of postulate that are observable and should be measurable. Hypotheses are unique in that they predict expected behaviors. The hypothesis states the postulate in a way that it can be measured and tested. Usually the hypothesis will take a theoretical relationship and turn it into a real situation so that it can be seen and quantified. They are often not overtly written in the theoretical base but are implicit when the reader understands the meaning of the entire theoretical base. Hypotheses are based on concepts of the dynamic theory as they relate to the stated postulates. Hypotheses can be tested within a frame of reference.

Hypothesis

When adolescent boys and girls are together, they will look at each other and smile.

Hypothesis

When adolescent girls flirt with boys, the girls will make eye contact with the boys and then smile at them.

Organization of the Theoretical Base

When therapists begin to use a new frame of reference, they should be certain to understand the theoretical base and its component parts. The theoretical base sets the stage for the entire frame of reference. It usually is the most complex and abstract section in the frame of reference, but it is critical to understand it to move from theory to implementation of the frame of reference into practice.

The theoretical base broadly delineates the areas of concern of the frame of reference within the broader context of occupational therapy. The theoretical base also identifies the various theories on which the frame of reference is based. It identifies all assumptions being made, and it identifies the major concepts and defines them.

There usually is a design in the theoretical base that describes how each of the parts fit together to form a whole. When learning a frame of reference, it is important to understand its design or the way in which it is organized. The way that the theoretical base is organized should be reflected in all subsequent parts of the frame of reference. For example, if the theoretical base presents concepts in a particular order (as if one flows from the next), then that order should be reflected in all other parts of the frame of reference. This format enables the therapist to see the design of the frame of reference and follow this same order in the application of the theoretical base to intervention. This again highlights the importance of the theoretical base. In the sample frame of reference, a conceptual hierarchy related to flirting is making eye contact, smiling, acting in a coquettish manner, and, finally, making actual contact in a socially appropriate way.

When studying the theoretical base of a frame of reference, it may be helpful to keep the following questions in mind:

1. What are the assumptions?
2. What are the concepts?
3. What are the definitions of the concepts? Do you understand them?
4. What are the postulates? Do you understand these relationships?
5. How is the theoretical base organized? What is the design of the theoretical base? Do you understand the design?

FUNCTION/DYSFUNCTION CONTINUA

The next section in a frame of reference is referred to as the function/dysfunction continua. This section clearly identifies those areas of function with which the frame of reference is concerned. As you read through the theoretical base, you should be able to identify the specific areas of performance important to the child's development of skills and abilities. These are the areas that the therapist evaluates to determine whether the child is functional or dysfunctional. Concepts and their definitions from the theoretical base identify what therapists consider to be functional. Likewise, concepts and definitions identify what represents dysfunction. Each function/dysfunction continuum covers one area of performance important to the particular frame of reference. A frame of reference generally has several function/dysfunction continua, which are labeled as such because human performance rarely can be classified as good or bad, abled or disabled. The situation usually is not so clear cut. Function is at one end of the spectrum and dysfunction is at the other, and human performance may fall at any point along this scale:

Function————————————————————————————Dysfunction

The functional end of the continuum represents what the therapist expects the child to be able to do, whereas the dysfunctional end of the continuum represents disability:

Function————————————————————————————Dysfunction
Expected ability   Disability

Function/dysfunction continua come directly from the theoretical bases of the frames of reference and, thus, are specific to those frames of reference. They cannot be taken out of context.

Nonverbal contact and verbal contact are two function/dysfunction continua for the sample frame of reference (Charts 5.1 and 5.2).

Indicators of Function and Dysfunction

Underneath each function-dysfunction category are either lists of behaviors, physical signs, or some type of functional scale, such as a test score. These are called indicators of function. There is one list of expected abilities when the frame of reference uses lists of behaviors or physical signs. This is the functional end of the continuum. Another list identifies behaviors or physical signs that are considered areas of concern, which represent the dysfunctional end of the continuum. During the evaluation process, the therapist uses these lists of behavior and physical signs to identify strengths and areas of concern.

Sometimes a functional scale is used for evaluation. Some areas of human performance exhibit wide variations in acceptable performance. For example, grasping an

---

Chart 5.1   Function/Dysfunction Continua for Nonverbal Contact.

Communicating Nonverbally	Difficulty Communicating Nonverbally
FUNCTION: Nonverbal contact is the ability to communicate nonverbally with an unfamiliar person of the opposite sex	DYSFUNCTION: Inability to communicate nonverbally with an unfamiliar person of the opposite sex

---

Chart 5.2   Function/Dysfunction Continua for Verbal Contact.

Speaking Comfortably	Difficulty Speaking
FUNCTION: Ability to speak with an unknown person of the opposite sex	DYSFUNCTION: Inability to speak with an unknown person of the opposite sex

---

object involves many motoric steps. A child may have developed part of this and still be functional in relation to his or her age but may not have developed the whole sequence of grasping. This child, because he or she has not fully mastered grasping, still would not fall at the functional end of the continuum. In some frames of reference, a functional scale is used to identify acceptable ranges of behaviors or performance rather than specified abilities.

After the therapist performs an evaluation, he or she can then look at the results and check them against these descriptive lists or functional scales. The more behaviors or physical signs that the child exhibits indicative of dysfunction, the closer the child will be to the dysfunctional end of the continuum, showing that he or she needs intervention. Likewise, the fewer characteristics indicative of dysfunction that the child exhibits, the closer the child will be to the functional end of the scale.

The following are two function/dysfunction continuum and the indicators of function and dysfunction from the sample frame of reference:

Indicators of Function and Dysfunction: Nonverbal Contact

Nonverbal contact (i.e., the ability to communicate nonverbally with an unfamiliar person of the opposite sex) involves making eye contact with the opposite sex, smiling at the opposite sex, and appearing physically comfortable with people of the opposite sex. Problems in this area are evident when a person assumes childlike postures or has uncontrolled blushing in the presence of people of the opposite sex (Chart 5.3).

Indicators of Function and Dysfunction: Verbal Contact

Verbal contact, the ability to speak with an unknown person of the opposite sex, requires talking openly and smoothly with a person of the opposite sex and making

---

Chart 5.3 Indicators of Function and Dysfunction for Nonverbal Contact.

Communicating Nonverbally	**Difficulty Communicating Nonverbally**
FUNCTION: Nonverbal contact is the ability to communicate nonverbally with an unfamiliar person of the opposite sex	DYSFUNCTION: Inability to communicate nonverbally with an unfamiliar person of the opposite sex
INDICATORS OF FUNCTION	**INDICATORS OF DYSFUNCTION**
Able to make eye contact with someone of the opposite sex	Unable to make eye contact with someone of the opposite sex
Able to smile at someone of the opposite sex	Unable to smile at someone of the opposite sex
Appears physically comfortable with people of the opposite sex	Assumes childlike postures or has uncontrolled blushing in the presence of people of the opposite sex

---

Chart 5.4 Indicators of Function and Dysfunction for Verbal Contact.

Speaking Comfortably	**Difficulty Speaking**
FUNCTION: Ability to speak with an unknown person of the opposite sex	DYSFUNCTION: Inability to speak with an unknown person of the opposite sex
INDICATORS OF FUNCTION	**INDICATORS OF DYSFUNCTION**
Able to speak with an unknown person of the opposite sex	Unable to speak with an unknown person of the opposite sex or giggles when around members of the opposite sex
Able to talk openly and smoothly with a person of the opposite sex	Cannot talk openly and smoothly with a person of the opposite sex
Makes sense when talking to someone of the opposite sex.	Will call a person of the opposite sex and hang up before he or she answers
	Does not make sense when talking to someone of the opposite sex; may giggle or stutter

---

sense. A person who has difficulty in this area may giggle around members of the opposite sex, calls a person of the opposite sex and hangs up before he/she answers, or stutters when trying to talk with a person of the opposite sex (Chart 5.4).

GUIDE FOR EVALUATION

This section identifies how the therapist would approach the evaluation process within a particular frame of reference. It identifies potential assessment tools and methods and relates them to the indicators of function and dysfunction. This section may serve as an evaluation protocol in defining the areas of performance that the therapist should assess. It is not, however, a specific assessment tool or a specified evaluation protocol; it does not tell the therapist how to evaluate a child, but rather, it tells him or her the things he or she should be looking at to determine if the child needs intervention.

Through the evaluation process, the therapist determines where the child falls on the function/dysfunction continuum. Is the child closer to function, or does he or she have so much difficulty with this area of performance that he or she has to be considered in need of intervention?

Some frames of reference do not have specific assessment tools. In these situations, the therapist usually devises a set of tasks or observations that allow him or her to determine the child's performance in the various function/dysfunction continua. This is perfectly acceptable, as long as the tasks or observations chosen are directly related to the specified continua. Although it is often difficult to choose or devise evaluative tasks, the therapist should avoid falling back on "old favorites." A therapist needs to choose tasks that demonstrate the specific behaviors outlined. Tools should not be chosen based on the therapist's comfort level but on whether the tools follow the continua previously stated in the frame of reference.

Using the function/dysfunction continuum as the guideline for the evaluation, the therapist can determine whether the child can be considered functional or dysfunctional in terms of this specific frame of reference:

> In this sample frame of reference, observation of the early adolescent in a peer group situation could be used as an evaluation. This observation would provide the therapist with information about the adolescent's behavior and physical manifestations in a peer socialization experience.

POSTULATES REGARDING CHANGE

Postulates state the relationship between two concepts from the theoretical base of a frame of reference. Postulates regarding change also relate two concepts; however, these postulates are the guidelines for how the therapist should intervene with the child. Postulates regarding change, just like function/dysfunction continua, must relate back to the important concepts in the theoretical base. They use the dynamic theory stated in the theoretical base. The thread of continuity must be present from one section to another.

Postulates regarding change are critical because they move the frame of reference farther from the abstract level of theory to the more concrete level of practice. It may make it easier to think of the postulates as "if-then" statements. They state that if the therapist does something, then a resultant effect should occur. The statements are descriptive and guide the therapist's behavior and actions. As action-oriented statements, they convey to the therapist the type of environment that should be created to produce change or the type of technique needed to bring about change. The result can be a change in the child's behavior or an enhancement of normal growth and development that has been impeded by dysfunction.

The term "environment" within the context of a postulate regarding change encompasses more than the physical space of the intervention setting. It involves the emotional climate, the social interaction with the therapist and significant others, and the various activities to which the child is exposed. It is important to note that therapists do not actually create the change in the child, but they do create an environment that allows the change to take place (Mosey, 1981, 1986). The therapist may create an environment that should enhance normal growth and development by providing the child with specific activities that he or she has not engaged in previously.

When a postulate regarding change relates to the use of a specific therapeutic technique, it states the type of action the therapist should take to bring about an explicit response in the child. For example, if the therapist applies direct pressure to the insertion of a muscle, then the muscle should relax. Because an environment that allows for change is important, it is rare that a frame of reference will have only postulates that describe the use of specific techniques. Most frames of reference include postulates regarding change that discuss the environment and the therapist's direct actions.

Postulates regarding change are the turning points in the frame of reference. They apply the abstract material stated in the theoretical base to the practical actions that need to be taken by the therapists to facilitate change in the child. The postulates give the therapist a mechanism for using the frame of reference to plan the intervention.

Within the frame of reference for establishing a relationship with the opposite sex, postulates regarding change may be the following:

Postulate regarding change

The therapist creates an environment in which the adolescent will be in a social situation with members of the opposite sex.

Postulate regarding change

If the therapist creates a situation where the adolescent has more opportunity to talk with a member of the opposite sex, then he or she will begin to feel more comfortable.

Postulate regarding change

If the therapist puts male and female adolescents in a comfortable and natural social situation, then social interaction will be facilitated.

Postulate regarding change

If the therapist presents a group activity in which male and female adolescents have to work together, then they will learn to interact in a socially appropriate manner.

APPLICATION TO PRACTICE

The postulates regarding change have stated the important concepts that should be used by the therapist to facilitate that change in the child. Some frames of reference require a more in-depth explanation of the key concepts used to promote functional performance. Other frames of reference require additional descriptions of the actions to be taken by the therapist. Other frames of reference may require specific examples of the therapeutic process. Often it is difficult for even the most experienced therapist to make the move from the theoretical stage to practical application without additional explanation. This section eases that movement from theory to practice. In other words, this section is meant to provide added information for the therapist to put this frame of reference into practice effectively. In addition, this section may suggest guidelines for the selection of appropriate activities and describe how these activities may be graded so that the client can begin to interact and move from a state of dysfunction to one of function.

> For example, within the sample frame of reference presented in this chapter, Making Contact with Persons of the Opposite Sex as An Adolescent, intervention would have to be done in an environment that uses small groups because interaction could not be facilitated in individual treatment. An occupational therapist might develop an intervention plan that involved planning and carrying out a picnic. The group participants would have to work together to plan the food and the activities. The occupational therapist would guide the group to insure that activities selected would be appropriate for both sexes. For example, while the boys may suggest football, the therapist could guide the group to a more acceptable activity for all involved, such as volleyball. The therapist would use a client-centered approach focusing on interpersonal communication and the ability and importance of establishing relationships (Rogers, 1961). The therapist takes a non-directive approach encouraging the clients to define themselves. Following each group session, the therapist could lead a discussion where an open opportunity is provided for the participants to reflect on their own behaviors and provide feedback to each other.

This section is not meant to be a cookbook for application. Instead, it is meant to provide clarification, where necessary, by addressing the following questions:

1. Is there any additional information that the therapist needs to know to apply this frame of reference effectively?
2. Is there anything about the frame of reference that may not be immediately apparent?
3. Is there anything that has not been stated clearly, that the therapist should keep in mind when applying this frame of reference for intervention?

References

Blos, P. (1962). *On adolescence*. Glencoe, IL: Free Press.
Elkind, D. (1967). Egocentrism in adolescence. *Child Development, 38*, 1025–1034.
Erikson, E. H. (1968). *Identity: youth and crisis*. New York: Norton.
Erikson, E. H. (1982). *The life cycle completed: a review*. New York: W. W. Norton.

Freud, S. (1966). *Standard edition of the complete psychological works of Sigmund Freud*. London: Hogarth Press.

Hinojosa, J., Kramer, P., & Pratt, P. N. (1996). Theoretical foundations of practice: Developmental principles, theories, and frames of reference. In J. Case-Smith, A. S. Allen, & P. N. Pratt (Eds.) *Occupational therapy for children* (3rd ed.) (pp. 25–45). St. Louis, MO: C. V. Mosby.

Mosey A. C. (1968). Recapitulation of ontogenesis: A theory for practice of occupational therapy. *American Journal of Occupational Therapy, 22*, 426–432.

Mosey, A. C. (1970). *Three frames of reference for mental health*. Thorofare, NJ: Slack.

Mosey, A. C. (1981). *Occupational therapy: configurations of a profession*. New York: Raven Press.

Mosey, A. C. (1986). *Psychosocial components of occupational therapy*. New York: Raven Press.

Mosey, A. C. (1996). *Applied scientific inquiry in the health professions: An epistemological orientation* (2nd ed.). Bethesda, MD: American Occupational Therapy Association.

Rogers, C. R. (1961) *On becoming a person*. Boston: Houghton Mifflin Co.

FRAMES OF REFERENCE

NeuroDevelopmental Treatment Frame of Reference

SARAH A. SCHOEN / JILL ANDERSON

NeuroDevelopmental Treatment (NDT) is a sensorimotor approach widely used by occupational therapists in the treatment of neuromuscular disorders. Sensory motor techniques are applied to remediate the developmental sequelae of dysfunctions. These intervention techniques are designed to enhance the quality of the client's motor performance within the context of the functional environment. The use of this frame of reference requires a focus on active participation in goal-directed activities.

HISTORY

NDT has evolved and developed over 30 years, largely from the clinical experiences and personal views of Berta Bobath, a physiotherapist, and her husband, Karel Bobath, a physician, at the Western Cerebral Palsy Center in London now known as the Bobath Center. This approach originally was developed and used in the treatment of neurologically impaired children, primarily those diagnosed with cerebral palsy. It later was used with adults who had hemiplegia that resulted from cerebral vascular accidents. Application of NDT has expanded and currently is used for patients with various dysfunctions, including children who have neuromuscular disorders, immature central nervous system (CNS) disorders, such as found in some premature infants, and other developmental disabilities.

NDT has progressed through various phases from the early 1940s to today. Mrs. Bobath described the NDT approach as a "living concept" that is constantly changing, as a result of her observations of client reactions during treatment. An early focus was to decrease muscle tone through the use of reflex inhibiting postures (RIP). These postures were opposite to the primitive reflex patterns typically assumed by the child (Campbell, 1986). Later, the study of normal motor development led to the incorporation of hierarchical motor sequences into therapy, with one activity following another during facilitation (such as head control, rolling, sitting, quadruped, and kneeling). When this approach was used, the child was placed passively into these developmental positions. A major difficulty with this approach was that the child was unable to move actively from one position to another.

The primary focus in the next phase of NDT emphasized the facilitation of automatic movement sequences as opposed to isolated developmental skills. The development of righting and equilibrium reactions was considered essential for the ability to move against gravity. The therapeutic approach had two important components. The first was the reduction of the therapist's control over the child's movement while facilitating the child's active control. This was alternated with the second component, the use of inhibitory techniques to reduce the effects of increased tone. The primary criticism of facilitation of autonomic movement sequences was that the motor outcomes were not generalized by the child. The movements, therefore, did not lead to increased functional abilities or to greater independence in activities of daily living (ADL).

The most current phase of NDT incorporates the latest theories about the organization of the CNS and research related to the theories of motor control (Guiliani, 1991; Horak, 1991), motor development (Frank & Earl, 1990), and motor learning (Nashner & McCollum, 1997).

The organization of the CNS is described as a distributed model of control rather than a hierarchical model. Many systems impact on the production of human movement. NDT now emphasizes the active participation of the individual through participation in goal-oriented activities. Automatic and voluntary components of postural control and skill acquisition are learned through practice. Facilitation of functional skills must therefore be based on an appreciation of the interaction between the individual and the environment and the task and viewed from a biomechanical, kinesiological, musculoskeletal, and sensory-perceptual perspective.

THEORETICAL BASE OF NEURODEVELOPMENTAL TREATMENT

NDT is a developmental frame of reference and makes the same assumptions as other developmental frames of reference (i.e., the fundamental concepts of development constitute the building blocks of the theoretical base). It is expected that therapists who use this frame of reference have a comprehensive knowledge of normal development and the components of movement, a comprehensive understanding of atypical development, and a thorough understanding of the development of normal postural control. From this knowledge base, the occupational therapist can analyze functional skills in order to determine the motor components that are impeding function. This information also is critical to the development of an appropriate treatment plan.

Principles of Normal Motor Development

Formerly, general principles of normal motor development dictated that control precedes from cephalo-to-caudal, proximal-to-distal, and gross-to-fine. Rather, these principles are now interpreted as interactional rather than sequential. The interaction between cephalo and caudal is demonstrated by the achievement of head control. For example, head control is dependent on a certain degree of trunk control, and the head and trunk interact in achieving alignment and posture.

The hemiplegic child who attains control of the shoulder girdle before the elbow, wrist, and hand in the affected upper extremity illustrates the principle of proximal-distal control. In addition to this principle, it has been hypothesized that these two mechanisms of control interact. This is supported by research identifying a proximal system of control for the arms and a separate distal control system for the hand (Kuypers, 1963; Lawrence & Hopkins, 1972). Development reflects the child shifting between large movements and refined prehension based on the demands of the task. For example, the 7-month-old infant attempts to pick up a Cheerios with his or her palm and several fingers in a raking motion. Whereas the 2-year-old child can pick up Cheerios with a pincer grasp and translate them from finger tips to palm.

Feedback and Feedforward Mechanism

Feedback and feedforward are important concepts in this frame of reference. In earlier phases of NDT, feedforward was not recognized as having a role in movement and posture. Recent advances in motor sciences have endorsed the importance of feedforward, the anticipation of movement, and postural control as a foundation for functional activities. Sensory feedback is recognized as being important throughout the learning process. Once a movement is learned, an internal program precedes the interaction of a goal-directed activity in the form of postural preparation. This can be demonstrated by the muscle activation that occurs in the trunk and arm upon the intent to reach for a cup. Sensory feedback is only used to refine the skill as related to the success of the goal-directed movement. For example, the postural preparation for picking up a paper cup versus a heavy ceramic mug would involve a different degree of activation of these muscles. In addition, the proprioceptive feedback in the upper extremity would be different.

Postural Alignment, Postural Control, and the Base of Support

NDT defines postural control as the ability to assume and maintain postures during static and dynamic activity. Postural alignment precedes the development of postural control and is considered to be a prerequisite of postural control. Biomechanically, postural alignment is represented when the individual's center of gravity is over the base of support. The base of support is defined as that part of the body that makes contact with the support surface. For example, the pelvis and the lower extremities are the base of support in sitting. In quadruped, the hands, the knees, the calves, and the dorsum of the feet become the base of support.

Studies confirm that postural activity is initiated as the base of support (Hartbourne, Giuhani, & MacNeela 1987; Keshner, 1980; Cupps, 1997). Studies of postural responses in standing demonstrate activity at the ankles, followed by activity progressively more proximally. Cupps (1997) in a study of sitting of 4 to 5-month-old infants concluded that postural activity included muscle activation against the support surface. Fluid movement occurred with ongoing changes in the base of support (Cupps,1997).

Normal development is characterized by the ability to progressively narrow the base of support in conjunction with refinement of movement against gravity. Acquisition of postural control occurs developmentally through experience and practice. Changes in the base of support impact on the alignment of body segments. Children with abnormal postural tone and control may develop compensatory bases of support. For example, weightbearing on the dorsum of the hand will result in poor alignment of the shoulder girdle. In addition, sitting with a posterior pelvic tilt results in poor alignment of the head and trunk.

Components of Normal Development

The important components of normal movement are: 1) the interplay between stability and mobility; 2) postural tone and the development of postural alignment; and 3) the ability to dissociate movements. These basic components provide the foundation for specific treatment techniques.

Interplay between Stability and Mobility

The concepts of stability and mobility can be understood most effectively by defining dynamic movement. *Dynamic movement* refers to smooth, controlled, coordinated action based on a point of stability as its support. The part of the body in contact with the support surface can function as the point of stability. For example, the feet are the *point of stability* in a standing position. *Stability* is the ability to maintain a posture against opposing forces.

Mobility is then achieved through a weight shift in any direction. NDT assumes that normal movement requires the combination of stability and mobility. Each body part can perform a stabilizing and mobilizing function, depending on the activity. For example, when the infant rocks in quadruped, the arms and legs provide stability for the trunk. When this same infant reaches for a toy in quadruped, the baby gets stability from his or her legs, trunk, and one arm so that the other upper extremity can reach for the toy in space.

Postural Tone and the Development of Postural Alignment

For the purposes of this frame of reference, it is important to differentiate postural tone from muscle tone. Postural tone provides the background tone for normal movement and determines the muscle quality in overall patterns and distribution throughout the body rather than in specific muscles. Some clinicians use the term "stiffness" in place of postural tone. Muscle tone is more often used to refer specifically to the internal state of muscle fiber tension within individual muscles and muscle groups. Normal postural tone must be low enough to allow movement against gravity (mobility) yet high enough to maintain a stable position against gravity (stability).

The NDT frame of reference maintains that the acquisition of motor control occurs in the three body planes. Developmentally, motor control occurs first in the sagittal plane, with extension and flexion against gravity. The next phase of development occurs in the frontal plane, with lateral righting. The final phase of development occurs in the transverse plane, adding the component of rotation (Scherzer & Tscharnuter, 1990). For example, the child is able to shift weight anteriorly and posteriorly (the sagittal plane movement) in the prone position before shifting weight laterally (frontal plane movement). Control in the transverse plane, the last plane in which movement develops, is necessary for rotation (as in the transition from the prone position to sitting). This progression is then repeated in higher developmental positions such as sitting and standing.

Ability to Dissociate Movements

Dissociation, or the ability to differentiate movements between the various parts of the body, is indicative of maturation of the CNS. Dissociation of movement occurs in normal development within the first year of life and is characterized by separate movements between segments of the body and within a given segment. Following the principles of normal development, dissociation proceeds from cephalo-to-caudal and from proximal-to-distal. Dissociation of head movements from movements of the shoulder girdle and trunk precedes dissociation of the trunk movements from pelvic movements. The ability to creep reciprocally demonstrates dissociation of the lower extremities from pelvic movements and from each other, as well as the movements of the upper extremities from the shoulder girdle and from each other. The ability to perform bilateral hand activities that involve stabilization of a toy with one hand and manipulation of its parts with the other hand demonstrates a higher level of dissociation.

Variety of Movement

In normal development, infants show a variety of motor patterns when moving in and out of developmental positions and when interacting with objects. Infants rarely stay still. They move from one toy to another and are constantly changing their body positions. Transitions are performed in all directions. Infants never perform the same movement in the exact same way but rather utilize many different ways to approach an activity. For example, infants can transition into quadruped from a prone position in order to crawl across the room. When moving from a sitting position, they can accomplish this through a diagonal weight shift of the pelvis over the lower extremities into quadruped.

Relationship of Motor Development to the Performance of Functional Skills

NDT assumes that motor development interacts with the environmental context in the acquisition of functional skills. Originally, the Bobaths stated that normal development occurred sequentially and that the sequences overlapped. Currently, motor development is not considered to be a rigid sequence, rather it is considered to be dependent on multiple factors (e.g., genetic, environment, experience). During the acquisition of functional motor skills, the individual focuses on the goal rather than the specific motor components of the task. Normal movement allows for the use of the most efficient patterns to accomplish functional tasks, such as playing on the floor, sitting at a table, freely moving in and out of positions to explore the environment, feeding, and dressing oneself.

Atypical Motor Development

Previously, abnormal movements were characterized by the persistence of primitive reflexes or compensatory attempts to gain antigravity control. These views were described as stereotypical patterns of movement. Based on the specific type of tone of the child, varying clinical pictures of stereotypical patterns may be seen. Children with different types of neuromuscular disorders manifest different stereotypical patterns. An increased awareness of the impact of abnormal postural tone has influenced the analysis of abnormal movement.

Although there are many ways of looking at the basis for abnormal movement, the subsequent problems that result from the abnormal development are the same. Clinically, the problems may be seen in the child's postural tone, resulting in the lack of development of a variety of automatic movement patterns for functional skills. According to this frame of reference, there is a disruption in the feedback and feedforward mechanisms, which impairs the acquisition of postural control and alters the experience of learning movement skills.

Problems in postural tone are most often assumed to have a significant impact on the development of abnormal movement patterns. Postural tone, as previously discussed, refers to the state of muscle tension in the trunk or the extremities. Increased postural tone limits the movement around the joint. In kinesiological terms, this "fixing" or holding reduces the degrees of freedom at that joint. Prolonged use of fixing or freezing of joints, particularly when it occurs in the extremities, leads to shortening of muscle fibers, which can eventually cause decreased range of motion and contractures. Research has suggested that when phasic muscles are used for tonic stability, the intrinsic property of the fibers is altered (Keshner, 1990; Kuypers, 1963).

When an infant has problems with postural tone, patterns of extension tend to emerge first and appear to dominate the later motor patterns (Scherzer & Tscharnuter, 1990). As the infant matures, the pattern may become stronger because of habitual use. Differences may be observed in the trunk as compared to the extremities. The extensor patterns for most children are first seen as excessive cervical extension that then proceeds down the spine. This extension is not counterbalanced with flexion and abdominal control. Attempts to gain postural control through positional stability are also examples of fixing or reducing the degree of freedom. As the child continues to develop, differences in postural tone impact on the pelvis and hips, affecting sitting and the ability to pull to stand.

Habitual "fixing" precedes a lack of dissociation in movement. A lack of dissociation often is characterized by total patterns of movement, referred to as associated responses. For example, when movement of the head, shoulder girdle, trunk, and pelvis occurs in an associated pattern, there is a lack of independent movement of body parts and lack of rotation. This results in transitions from supine-to-prone or prone-to-supine positions being accomplished in a "log rolling" fashion, rather than rolling segmentally. Fixing also results in the lack of dissociation when hand motions cannot be performed independently but are completely controlled by movements made at the shoulder. When handwriting activities are controlled by movement of the shoulder, this prevents the use of the intrinsic muscles of the hand to control the writing tool. Another example can be seen in the lower extremities, where two primary patterns exist: complete extension of both legs or total flexion of both legs. Similar patterns also may be present in the upper extremities. These associated reactions limit the child's ability to perform independent functions, such as weight-shifting to the side in the prone position or reaching forward with the other arm.

The identification of patterns of atypical movements used by a child helps to guide the therapist in selecting appropriate intervention techniques. It is assumed that the resultant compensatory patterns will become habitual ways of moving, without intervention. For example, the infant with excessive head hyperextension who lacks the counteracting flexion control may also elevate his or her shoulders to stabilize his or her head in an effort to maintain midline head control. This pattern of head hyperextension and shoulder elevation soon may become the preferred method of achieving and maintaining head control (Bly, 1980).

Although infants and children who have abnormal patterns of movement certainly may attain some degree of independence in functional activities, their skill levels are compromised because of excessive reliance on compensatory patterns of movement. Compensatory patterns refer to those movements influenced by abnormal postural tone and habitual use. They are the abnormal movement patterns used repeatedly to achieve functional motor skills when normal movement patterns have not been established. For example, hyperextension of the head and neck is a compensatory movement pattern. The child who has poor trunk stability may attempt to improve visual orientation in space through hyperextension of the head and neck.

Sensory Input as a Means of Bringing About Change

Central to NDT is the assumption that abnormal patterns of movement may be changed by altering sensory input to the CNS, thereby altering motor output. Furthermore, this may be done through the therapist's use of various techniques referred to as "handling." Handling is when the therapist uses his or her hands on the child in a specified manner, using graded sensory input at key points of control. Key points of control are specific areas on the child's body selected for therapeutic handling. Key points may be proximal (such as the shoulder girdle, trunk, and pelvis) or distal (such as the hands and feet). Through handling, the therapist elicits and facilitates motor responses. Handling is used in preparation and facilitation. Preparatory activities are those techniques that involve mobilizing or elongating tight structures and promoting alignment of body segments to one another and in relation to gravity. For example, techniques may be used to promote mobility in structures that indicate limitations in passive movement. These techniques may also be used to promote stability through postural alignment of the body prior to the facilitation of active movement. These techniques or preparatory activities include:

- Deep pressure to the base of support can facilitate the initiation of movement at the base of support and mobility in tight structures.
- Elongation of tight pectoral muscles through the application of deep pressure before the scapula can be mobilized in a downwardly rotated position.
- The facilitation of proximal stability through weightbearing requires cocontraction around a joint.
- The facilitation of stability facilitated by applying intermittent compression directly to the muscles surrounding a joint.

Movement patterns facilitated by occupational therapists through handling must be goal-directed and incorporated into functional activities. For handling to be effective, the therapist must grade touch and other sensory input that are finely tuned to the child's individual needs (Scherzer & Tscharnuter, 1990).

Another central assumption is that the child must be actively involved in the change process. Change results from the therapist's handling of the child to facilitate postural control, initiation of movement, and a variety of movement patterns. The development of movement in a child is achieved without reliance on cognitive training methods or concern about skill development.

FUNCTION/DYSFUNCTION CONTINUA

Function/dysfunction continua provide therapists with descriptions of observable behaviors that are clinically relevant and identify the presence of function and dysfunction in children.

Indicators of Function and Dysfunction: Postural Tone

The term "postural tone" has been traditionally used in NDT literature to describe the background tone for movement. Increased and decreased stiffness are often used in place of increased or decreased postural tone. At the present time, the term "stiffness" is also being used to describe postural tone. The term "fixing" specifically addresses the muscle activity around a joint that is used to control movement. Therefore, "fixing" as a means of gaining control for movement will impact on the development of postural tone. Postural tone and degree of stiffness are terms that will be used synonymously in this chapter.

Normal postural tone allows the person to move against gravity with mobility and ease. This amount of muscle activation must be high enough to support the body against gravity and low enough to allow free movement. A predominance of trunk or extremity stiffness resulting in excessive stability and difficulty moving against gravity is seen in a child who has cerebral palsy with spastic quadriplegia. A lack of trunk or extremity stiffness resulting in excessive mobility and lack of control of movement is seen in the child who has cerebral palsy with hypotonia (Figure 6.1). The presence of varying degrees of stiffness at different joints is also possible. Postural tone can range from low to high, normal to high, or low to normal depending on the context and the nature of the task. Normal postural tone can be reflected in the pattern of distribution, adaptability in relation to the task and/or environmental stimuli, and degree of stiffness. In normal development, as the infant develops refined movement and stability, the degree and location of fixing patterns of the joints varies. For example, as the infant develops sitting balance, fixing patterns in the upper and lower extremities are initially used to maintain the position. As the infant develops sufficient postural tone in the trunk, these patterns are no longer necessary.

Normal postural tone may not be the same throughout the body. It is generally lower distally. In dysfunction, as seen in the child who has cerebral palsy resulting in spastic quadriparesis, tone may be higher distally than proximally. In addition, differences in the distribution of tone can be evident in the upper extremities, as seen in the child who has cerebral palsy that results in spastic diplegia. In these children, tone in the lower extremities is higher than in the upper extremities. Differences in tone also can be seen between the right and left sides of the body (e.g., the child who has hemiplegia) (Chart 6.1).

Indicators of Function and Dysfunction: Stability/Mobility

The normal child combines stability and mobility on a foundation of normal postural tone when weightshifting and moving from one position to another. The functional end of the stability/mobility continuum is reflected in a dynamic base of support and the ability to use any body segment as a base of support during transitional movement. The normal child who is able to maintain sitting and then weightshift to

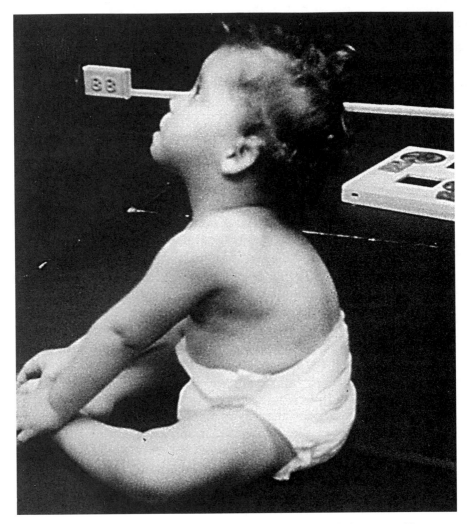

Figure 6.1 Hypotonic child in sitting position. Note the rounded spine and hyperextension of the neck.

the side to reach for a toy has enough stability in the pelvis and trunk to allow mobility and free movement of the upper trunk, shoulder girdle, upper extremity, and head to obtain a toy out of reach. A child who lacks dynamic stability uses other mechanisms or compensations to achieve function. One such mechanism is the use of positional stability (i.e., the use of the skeletal system rather than the neuromuscular system to achieve stability). The use of a posture with a broad base of support, such as the hips in marked external rotation and abduction or "W" sitting position (Figure 6.2), are examples of a child's attempt to provide positional stability. Another example is the compensatory pattern of high guard posturing of the arms during sit-

Chart 6.1 Indicators of Function and Dysfunction for Postural Tone.

Normal Postural Tone	Atypical Postural Tone
FUNCTION: Postural tone **INDICATORS OF FUNCTION**	DYSFUNCTION: Atypical postural tone **INDICATORS OF DYSFUNCTION**

Antigravity movement in and out of developmental positions
Developmentally appropriate use of limbs for support and
    finer adjustments during skilled activity
	Trunk or Extremities
	A predominance of trunk or extremity stiffness interfering with
	    antigravity movement
	Hypermobility and hyperextendability of joints
	Decreased degree of tension in muscles
	Limbs feel heavy on passive range of motion
	Limbs and body sink into any support surface
	Presence of varying degrees of stiffness in various joints
	    interfering with antigravity movement
	Presence of involuntary movements
	Increased degree of tension in muscles
	Resistance to passive range of motion
	Areas of the body with increased stiffness withdraw from contact
	    with the support surface
	Presence of stretch reflex, clonus, or tremors

ting or ambulation, used in an attempt to achieve stability (Figure 6.3). When high guard posturing is used to maintain balance, then the arms are not free to reach or grasp objects. Using an asymmetrical posture may also reflect the child's attempt to gain stability (Chart 6.2) (Figure 6.4).

Indicators of Function and Dysfunction: Postural Control

Postural control is expressed by an ability to assume and maintain positions during static and dynamic movement. Posture and control result from cooperative interaction of the sensorimotor system with other systems used such as musculoskeletal, cardiopulmonary, and the environment. Postural control develops through repeated movement patterns and experiences learned in relation to performing specific tasks under a variety of environmental conditions. Feedforward and feedback contribute to this process through preparation before the onset of functional movement (e.g., widening the stance in anticipation of [feedforward] picking up a large object and the resultant sensory feedback as the item is picked up). Postural control is initiated at the base of support and progresses to allow the individual to move to higher antigravity positions with a narrow base of support for the acquisition of skilled movement.

Problems in this area are evident at either end of the continuum. When children have mid-range control only (spasticity) with an inadequate base of support, they may have stereotypical movement patterns, lack accommodation of body segments to the base of support, and use an excessively narrow base of support. They often at-

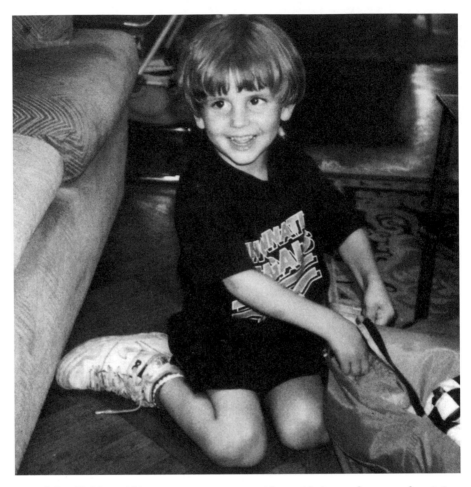

Figure 6.2 Child in a W-sitting posture to provide a wide base of support for sitting.

tempt to gain postural control by moving away from their base of support. Children at the other end of the continuum have difficulty with end-range control (athetosis and low tone). They have difficulty grading movement transitions, use excessive accommodation of body movements, and have difficulty maintaining their base of support. These children often use an extremely wide base of support and statically control their posture (Chart 6.3).

Indicators of Function and Dysfunction: Postural Alignment as Related to Three Planes of Space

A lack of postural alignment in any or all of the body planes is considered dysfunctional. For example, in the sagittal plane, a predominance of extensor patterns

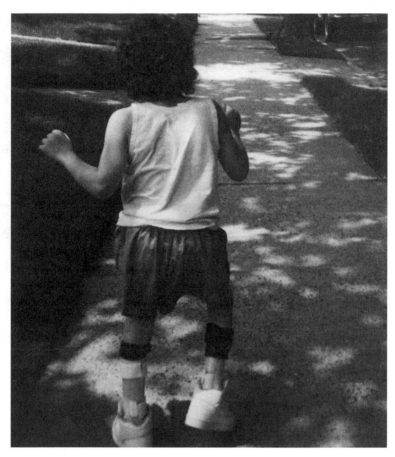

Figure 6.3   Child walking in high guard position.

Chart 6.2 Indicators of Function and Dysfunction for Stability/Mobility.	
Dynamic Stability	**Compensatory Stability**
FUNCTION: Dynamic stability	DYSFUNCTION: Compensatory stability
INDICATORS OF FUNCTION	**INDICATORS OF DYSFUNCTION**
Maintains and moves in and out of developmental positions	Use of a wide base of support
	Use of upper extremities for stability beyond developmentally appropriate age
	Use of compensatory patterns such as persistence of the upper extremities in high guard position for maintaining or regaining balance during a weight shift; excessive reliance on protective reactions during weightshifting; persistence of asymmetrical patterns; variety of fixation patterns present (i.e., toe clawing, hand fisting) (Figure 6.6)
	Exclusive use of "W" sitting position for sitting

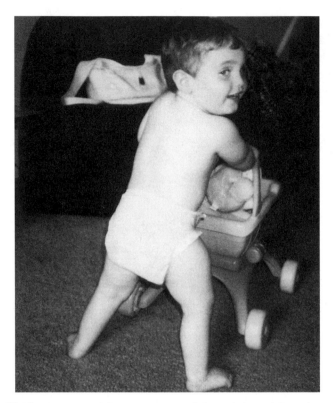

Figure 6.4 Child assumes standing position with legs abducted for a broad base of support. Note that toes are clawed for stability.

Chart 6.3 Indicators of Function and Dysfunction for Postural Control.

Atypical Postural Control	Postural Control	Atypical Postural Control
DYSFUNCTION: End-range control (athetosis and low tone)	FUNCTION: Postural control with a dynamic base of support	DYSFUNCTION: Mid-range control only (spasticity) with an ineffective base of support
INDICATORS OF DYSFUNCTION	**INDICATORS OF FUNCTION**	**INDICATORS OF DYSFUNCTION**
Inability to grade movement transitions Excessive accommodation of body Segments of the base of support Excessively wide base of support Postural control predominantly static	Refined movement for skilled activities that reflect a dynamic base of support in a variety of movement patterns	Presence of stereotypical movement patterns Lack of accommodation of body segments to the base of support. Excessively narrow base of support Attempts to gain postural control by moving away from the base of support

or an abnormal pull into flexion are considered dysfunctional. In the frontal plane, a lack of active elongation on the weightbearing side and shortening on the non-weightbearing side is also dysfunctional. A third example demonstrates that postural alignment may be present in the sagittal and frontal planes but still can be deficient in the transverse plane, evidenced by a lack of rotation within the body axis. Children who demonstrate this type of dysfunction are not able to rotate their trunks freely to reach for a toy. These children instead would use lateral flexion (i.e., sidebending of the head and trunk) as a substitution. In addition, these children may need to rely on a broad base of support to maintain balance in various positions, or they may use their arms in compensatory fashion to protect against falling (Chart 6.4).

Dissociation

Dissociation is the ability to differentiate movements among various parts of the body. Movement patterns performed in an associated or synergistic way are indicative of dysfunction. These patterns frequently involve muscle contractions at various joints that tend to occur in a predictable pattern of movement, such as the upper extremity flexor synergy. Persistence of these associated patterns also is dysfunctional. These associated reactions limit the child's ability to perform independent functions, such as weightshifting to the side in a prone position when reaching forward with one arm (Chart 6.5) (Figures 6.5, 6.6, and 6.7).

Indicators of Function and Dysfunction: Variety of Movement

In normal development, infants show a variety of motor patterns when moving in and out of developmental positions and when interacting with objects. The presence of stereotypical movement patterns, such as persistence of primitive reflexes, is one indicator of dysfunction. Another stereotypical pattern may include posturing of the

---

Chart 6.4   Indicators of Function and Dysfunction for Postural Alignment as Related to Three Planes of Space

Postural Alignment	Lack of Postural Alignment
FUNCTION: Postural alignment **INDICATORS OF FUNCTION**	DYSFUNCTION: Lack of postural alignment **INDICATORS OF DYSFUNCTION**
Alignment of body parts to one another and position in space	Excessive pull into flexion in upright positions Predominance of head and trunk hyperextension Inability to elongate muscles on weightbearing side of the body Asymmetry

---

Chart 6.5   Indicators of Function and Dysfunction for Dissociation.

Dissociated Movement Patterns Within and Between Body Parts Associated Movement Patterns

---

FUNCTION: Dissociated/differentiated movement patterns within and between body parts

INDICATORS OF FUNCTION

Rolls with rotation between shoulders and pelvis (Figure 6.5)
Use of reciprocal leg movements in creeping and crawling (Figure 6.7)
Orients head in all planes of space

When developmentally appropriate, holds a toy with one hand and manipulates its parts with the other

DYSFUNCTION: Associated or synergist movement patterns

INDICATORS OF DYSFUNCTION

Log rolling (Figure 6.6)
Bunny hopping
Pull to stand with lower extremities in extension, adduction, and internal rotation
Hand closing associated with flexion of the arm and hand opening with extension of the arm

---

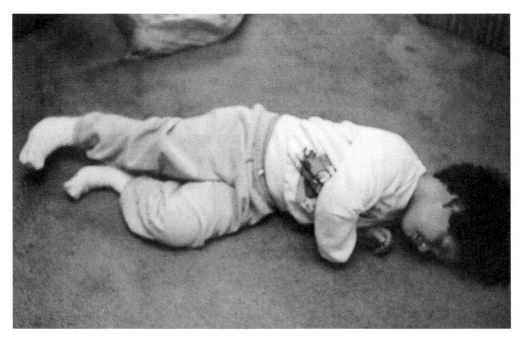

Figure 6.5   Normal segmental rolling.

lower extremities with internal rotation and adduction. This would make it difficult to perform the external rotation and abduction necessary for sitting or standing activities. A stereotypical pattern of the upper extremities is shoulder elevation with scapular retraction. This pattern would impede functional skill development. A limitation of the variety of movement can interfere with the acquisition of independence and hamper the child's ability to interact with the environment (Chart 6.6).

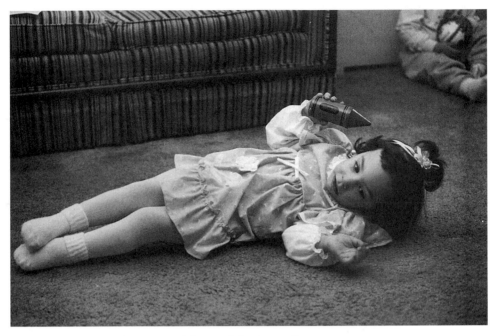

Figure 6.6   Log rolling.

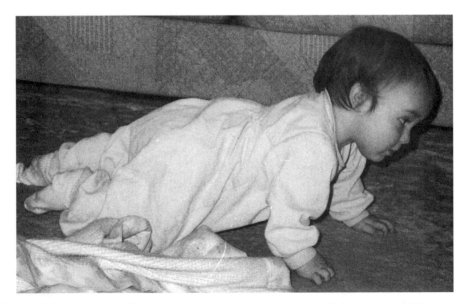

Figure 6.7   Normal child is able to dissociate movements of the upper and lower extremities in a reciprocal pattern.

Chart 6.6   Indicators of Function and Dysfunction for Variety of Movement.

Variety of Movement Patterns	Stereotypical Movement Patterns Reflexive Movement Patterns
FUNCTION: Variety of movement patterns **INDICATORS OF FUNCTION**	DYSFUNCTION: Stereotypical movement patterns **INDICATORS OF DYSFUNCTION**
Use of varied repertoire of movement patterns based on the demands of the activity	Stereotypically, one or both lower extremities persist with extension, adduction, and internal rotation in all positions Stereotypically, one or both upper extremities persist with shoulder elevation and retraction in all positions
Use of varied repertoire of movement patterns based on the demands of the activity	Stereotypical movement

---

Indicators of Function and Dysfunction: Full Passive Range of Motion

In this continuum, the child who has full range of passive movement and no contractures or deformities is at the functional end of the continuum. Children restricted by abnormal tone and stereotypical movement patterns may develop contractures and deformities. Compensatory patterns of movement that are used repeatedly and become automatic also may contribute to the development of contractures and, ultimately, to deformities. The child who shows contractures or deformities with limitations in passive range of motion (PROM) is evidencing dysfunction. Intervention may prevent or correct deformities; however, the more consistently that these limited movements are used by the child, the more likely that dysfunction will occur (Chart 6.7).

GUIDE TO EVALUATION

NeuroDevelopmental assessment is designed to identify and analyze characteristics of movement that may be associated with CNS dysfunction. It relies heavily on the therapist's ability to observe movement, categorize movement problems, elicit responses, and determine how possible deficits interfere with the child's ability to acquire functional skills. When evaluating, the therapist needs to be able to adapt to the functional level of the child, including the child's age, specific needs, and severity of dysfunction. A complete occupational therapy evaluation might include evaluation of oral-motor and feeding skills, gross and fine motor skills, sensory deficits, social-emotional factors, and cognitive skills. Not all of these areas, however, are addressed in this chapter. Other frames of reference in this book may be applicable to these areas.

Currently, no universally accepted format is available that uses the NDT frame of reference to evaluate a child who has CNS dysfunction. Numerous formats have

Chart 6.7   Indicators of Function and Dysfunction for Full Passive Range of Motion.

Full Passive Range of Motion	Contractures/Deformities
FUNCTION: Full passive range of motion	DYSFUNCTION: Contractures, deformities
INDICATORS OF FUNCTION	**INDICATORS OF DYSFUNCTION**
Full passive range of motion	Contractures
	Deformities

been suggested for evaluation in this frame of reference (Bly, 1980; Bobath, 1975; Campbell, 1981). The evaluation delineated here is adapted from evaluations proposed by Scherzer and Tscharnuter (1990) and Boehme (1984). Although similarities exist in the observations and activities performed within a widely accepted format, when assessing a child who has CNS dysfunction, the therapist looks specifically at atypical patterns of postural control and movement.

In the past, traditional developmental assessments used to assess children from birth to 5 years of age had several limitations. These standardized assessments have specific items or tasks to evaluate gross and fine motor skills and other areas of development. The motor items, however, tend to measure only the acquisition of motor milestones, such as the ability to sit, stand, or grasp. Most of these assessments do not analyze the specific factors that contribute to a child's inability to achieve a motor skill, nor do they address quality of movement issues.

For the most part, assessments using an NDT frame of reference rely on observation and the therapist's judgement when handling the child, as originally proposed by the Bobaths. Assessments are based almost exclusively on the observation of the child's spontaneous movements and on selectively elicited movements brought about through handling by the therapist or care giver. The NDT evaluation attempts to determine which motor components are interfering or missing in the performance of functional skills.

The entry-level therapist develops skills in this type of assessment by following a more structured evaluation approach under the supervision of an experienced therapist. The outline presented in Figure 6.8 provides some structured guidelines for NDT assessment.

Overall Assessment of Functional Skills

Functional skills explore what the child can do, without regard for the quality of movement. The therapist is concerned with the overall developmental picture of the child's functional skill performance with respect to the child's chronological age and his or her cognitive and sensory/perceptual levels. Another factor that should be considered, although it is not specific to this frame of reference, is the child's motivation.

I. Overall assessment of functional skills (What can the child do? At this point, the therapist is not concerned with the quality of movement but, rather, with the child's basic skills.)

   A. Gross motor abilities
   B. Upper extremity function
   C. Activities of daily living

II. Quality of movement

   A. Postural tone
   B. Describe functional postures and transitions from one position to another in terms of :
      1. Stability and mobility,
      2. Postural control and base of support,
      3. Dissociation of movement,
      4. Postural control in three planes of space, and
      5. Variety of movement patterns
   C. Structural limitations and deformities

Figure 6.8 Evaluation outline.

The therapist observes the child's desire and ability (on a gross motor level) to initiate and achieve balance in all developmental positions, the ability to initiate transitions from one position to another, and the desire to locomote.

The occupational therapist also is concerned with assessing upper extremity functional skills. These skills are described as they relate to the child's ability to use the arms for weightbearing, support, reaching and grasping, manipulating, and releasing objects in various positions.

Gross motor and upper extremity functional performance skills contribute to the ability to perform ADL. In this frame of reference, ADL is a discrete area of functional skills, an end result of gross motor and upper extremity function. ADL include participation in feeding, dressing, and self-care, as well as the ability to explore, play, and then learn from the environment. Again, this should be viewed in the context of the child's chronological age, cognitive level, and motivation as it relates to movement and interaction with the environment.

Often, when doing an assessment, it is best to start with the child's spontaneous movement in response to toys or equipment in the environment. Interview techniques are also extremely helpful to obtain a more thorough clinical picture of what the child can do at home or school relative to self-care, work, and play.

Quality of Movement

Following a detailed description of the child's functional skills, therapists analyze the quality of movement used to accomplish these skills. As described in the theoretical base, quality of motor behavior also may depend on the child's age and developmental level and may impact on the performance of functional skills. Certain behaviors considered age-appropriate for one child, may be immature or primitive for an older child. For example, the high guard posture in the sitting position at 5 or 6 months of age is normal, although it is abnormal for the 12-month-old child. Simultaneously, other behaviors may be observed in both these children, irrespective of age, that are abnormal, pathological, or not generally seen at any time in normal development.

Postural tone, as previously stated, is important in this frame of reference. It is examined with regard to three characteristics: the degree of stiffness, the distribution of tone, and the adaptability of tone in response to movement and handling. The child is evaluated in all functional positions and activities with respect to these characteristics. A detailed description is made of the child's posture at rest and the patterns used to achieve transitional movements (e.g., the progression of movement through space or when changing of positions). Consistent observations are then grouped together to develop summary statements about the child's functional limitations.

Postural alignment is assessed in the three body planes (sagittal, frontal, and transverse) in which movement occurs and also in every developmental position. For example, a child with spasticity while sitting with his or her head hyperextended is out of alignment in the sagittal plane. A child with hemiplegia while standing asymmetrically with weight primarily on one lower extremity is out of alignment in the frontal plane. A child with spastic quadriplegia and who cannot roll with dissociation or rotation exhibits lack of alignment in the transverse plane.

Dissociation is the ability of the child to perform a movement of one body part independent of another body part. An example is shoulder movement independent of pelvic movement or movement of one leg in isolation to the rest of the body. Frequently the child with spastic diplegia is unable to pull into a standing position through the use of the half-kneel position. This child may achieve standing through use of symmetrical extension of both lower extremities and by pulling to stand with both upper extremities. Again, a knowledge of typical development relative to age is critical in the analysis of appropriate dissociative movement patterns.

Stability and mobility are described in the various positions in which the child functions. Specifically, the therapist is concerned with the postures or patterns used to maintain a position or provide support for movement. For example, a child with decreased trunk control will often need to use the upper extremities as a compensatory form of stability. If the upper extremities are habitually used for stability either through elevation of the shoulders and/or hyperextending the arms, there will be reduced opportunities for use of the arms and hands for play. In addition, a child who does not have the stability to maintain balance in a sitting or standing position may use a broad base of support by abducting and/or externally rotating the lower extremities in order to maintain balance.

Postural control affects the child's ability to coordinate movement smoothly and accurately throughout range with a varying base of support. This ability to assume and maintain positions against gravity incorporates initiation of movement at the base of support and accommodation of those body parts to the support surface.

Variation of movement patterns constitute the repertoire that a child uses to perform functional tasks. Lack of variety may result in stereotypical patterns. This should be observed in the way a child moves and reaches for objects during functional tasks.

Of critical importance to occupational therapists is the impact of abnormal movement and posture on the child's use of his or her upper extremities for function and independence in self-care activities. Assessment of the upper extremities includes the child's habitual postures and the influence of tone in weightbearing and non-weightbearing positions. This may be reflected in the child's ability to orient his or her limbs in space and to use a full range of motion when reaching in varied planes of movement. Specific observations of grasp, release, prehension, and in-hand and bilateral manipulation should be included.

Standardized Evaluations

Recently, attempts have been made to standardize observations that address the quality of movement in young children. Standardized evaluations such as the *Movement Assessment of Infants* (MAI) (Chandler, Andrews, & Swanson, 1980), the *Posture and Fine Motor Assessment of Infants* (PFMAI) (Case-Smith, 1991), *Toddler Infant Motor Evaluation* (TIME) (Miller & Roid, 1994), and the *Tufts Assessment of Motor Performance* (Gans, Haley, Hallenberg, Main, Inacio & Fass, in press) attempt to assess the quality of movement. For example, the MAI addresses muscle tone, primitive reflexes, automatic reactions, and volitional movement. This is accomplished through observation. For these assessments, quality of movement is viewed separately from the developmental and functional behaviors of the child. These tests assess many of the concepts outlined in the previously identified function/dysfunction continua. It should be noted, however, that the criteria for provision of services in occupational therapy is less concerned with quality of movement and more concerned with magnitude of delay in functional skill development. When using standardized assessments in this frame of reference, it is important to use an observational guide as an accompaniment.

NDT as a frame of reference is primarily concerned with motor behaviors. A thorough occupational therapy evaluation can supplement an NDT oriented evaluation and should include sensory, oral-motor, perceptual, cognitive, and fine motor skills. Specialized assessments beyond the format discussed in this chapter, such as the *Developmental hand dysfunction: Theory, assessment, treatment* (Erhardt, 1982) and *The development of oral-motor skills in children receiving non-oral feedings* (Morris, 1990), may provide more in-depth information on the development of fine motor and oral-motor skills. As-sessment of sensory, perceptual, and cognitive functions also do not relate specifi-cally to the NDT frame of reference and therefore were omitted here.

POSTULATES REGARDING CHANGE

Postulates regarding change delineate the therapeutic environment that needs to be created and suggest the methods used by the therapist to facilitate change. For the NDT frame of reference, 14 postulates have been identified. When the results of evaluation indicate dysfunction, intervention focuses on the qualitative aspects of movement that interfere with the child's ability to develop skills or functional abili-ties. Different postural problems require different handling approaches. As previ-ously described, the primary mode of intervention in NDT is handling by the ther-apist. Handling, which refers to techniques and methods to promote active movement in a child, assists the child in moving as independently as possible in functional in-teractions with the environment. Beyond hands-on interaction in individual treat-ment, handling also refers to lifting and positioning during other activities that oc-cur throughout the child's day. Effective handling relies on the therapist's ability to understand and interpret the child's reactions and then to respond appropriately.

Four postulates are related to postural tone:

1. If the therapist is able to feel the child's muscle activation and the therapist can grade his or her touch accordingly, then the child will receive the optimum level of input to promote active participation in movement.
2. If the therapist is able to monitor the child's reactions to handling on input, then handling techniques may be modified easily.
3. If the child has atypical postural tone, then the therapist needs to provide graded therapeutic input. This may consist of various combinations of tactile and proprio-ceptive stimulation provided at different rates and speeds. Distal and proximal key points of control can be used with varying range and speed and a variety of move-ments. The goal of this handling is to reduce excessive fixation patterns through specific techniques.
4. If therapeutic handling is used by all professionals and family members who have contact with the child, then the child has the most opportunities to move with dynamic postural tone and a variety of patterns of movement.

Postural control as it relates to the base of support is the next general area within the sequence of intervention, with postulates:

5. To promote postural control in relationship to the base of support, the therapist must provide a sequence of intervention beginning with preparatory activities. These activities may include techniques that promote mobility in structures that indicate limitations in passive movement or techniques that promote stability through postural alignment of the body before active movement.

- Deep pressure to the base of support will facilitate the initiation of movement at the base of support and mobility in tight structures.
- Proximal stability may be facilitated through weightbearing, which requires cocontraction around a joint.
- Stability may be facilitated by applying intermittent compression directly to the muscles surrounding a joint.

6. If the therapist facilitates postural control during functional movement and the child has ample opportunity to repeat these movement patterns, then these patterns will become integrated into his or her repertoire of motor behaviors. If the therapist uses handling techniques, then the child will develop greater stability and control over more complex movement sequences.

Two postulates relate to postural alignment. They are as follows:

7. If the therapist facilitates postural alignment in preparation for the initiation of movement, then the child will have the potential to use appropriate muscle activation to maintain postural control during activities.
8. If the therapist facilitates a smooth interplay between the agonist and antagonist muscles, then the child will be able to achieve postural control.

There is one postulate that relates to dissociation:

9. If the therapist provides handling on either static or dynamic surfaces to facilitate differentiated motor responses, then dissociated movements will occur. The therapist uses handling techniques to provide a dynamic and varying base of support so that the child will develop greater stability and control over more complex movement sequences.

The development of a wide variety of movements is influenced by the child's human and nonhuman environment. The occupational therapist's use of objects and activities maximizes the child's motivation to engage in therapy and, ultimately, improve motor abilities. The following five postulates relate to this area:

10. If movement achieved through handling is used in functional interaction within the environment, then the child has the greatest opportunity to develop functional skills.
11. If the therapist adapts the environment to take into account the child's developmental level, needs, and interests, then the maximum amount of stimulation will be provided to encourage motor skills.
12. If the therapist uses handling techniques when a child's attention is focused on a play activity, then it often is easier for the child to respond with an automatic movement pattern.

13. If the occupational therapist is responsive to the child's needs (i.e., sensitivity to movement, familiarity with situation or environment) and encourages the child to initiate movement during treatment, then therapeutic handling will be an interactive and meaningful process and the child will be more likely to initiate active movement to engage in purposeful activities.

14. If preventative measures such as adaptive equipment and orthotic devices are provided, then the child will receive consistent input to prevent or reduce the occurrence of deformities and limitations.

APPLICATION TO PRACTICE

The theoretical base and concepts of NDT as presented in this chapter constitute essential knowledge for entry-level occupational therapists who work with children who have neurological impairment. The application of these concepts requires skill and practice. Translating these concepts into treatment also may be learned effectively through supervision from an experienced therapist. Specialized training, through continuing education workshops—ranging from 2-day introductory courses to 8-week basic courses that lead to NDT certification—provide a comprehensive understanding and application of this frame of reference (Further information can be obtained from the NeuroDevelopmental Treatment Association, Inc. P.O. Box 70, Oak Park, IL 60303).

Occupational therapists have a unique perspective on the quality of life of each child within the context of his or her family. This includes placing a high priority on functional ability. Within each intervention then, it is critical for the therapist to analyze the motor components of activities needed to accomplish the practical skills. This activity analysis assists the therapist in the development of functional and realistic goals for the child.

The ideal application of NDT uses a team approach that includes occupational therapy, physical therapy, speech therapy, special education, and the family. In each setting, such as school, home, clinic, or private practice, the occupational therapist must establish treatment priorities. The role and responsibilities of the occupational therapist may vary, depending on the setting and the other disciplines involved and the therapist's individual skills.

PRINCIPLES OF INTERVENTION

Previously, NDT intervention systematically followed the normal developmental sequences. At present, a child's movement requirements are assessed relative to a specific task. Therefore the performance of specific tasks is more important than following the normal development sequence. Carry over to other areas of development occurs as the child successfully masters each task. Motor control is believed to develop sequentially in the three body planes (i.e., sagittal, frontal, transverse). This sequential view of motor control in the three planes is no longer rigidly followed.

Preparation techniques may address range of motion or mobility issues occurring in the sagittal plane. Frontal and transverse plane movement helps develop a balance between flexors and extensors. In other clinical situations, sagittal plane movements may be introduced after frontal and transverse plane movements have achieved a balance between flexors and extensors.

Sequence of Intervention

Within this frame of reference, handling, preparation, and facilitation are ongoing segments of the intervention process. All three are going on simultaneously and are interactive, although at any given time, one of these three may take precedence over the other two segments. Handling is the broadest type of intervention; it is innately part of preparation and facilitation, although it may occur on its own.

Handling

Handling is graded sensory input provided by the therapist's hands at key points of control on the child's body. Handling includes any contact that the therapist's hands have with the child's body resulting in active control or movement. Handling is used in preparation and to facilitate active postural control and movement patterns.

Handling is used to facilitate active postural control and movement patterns. The therapist's decision to facilitate at proximal or distal key points of control often depends on the child's tone. For example, low-tone children frequently benefit from input at distal points of control. This encourages active movement by the child while simultaneously preventing the child from depending on support from the therapist's hands and body. Some degree of proximal control is necessary for use of distal hand placement. Handling at proximal key points often is used with the child with high tone (Figure 6.9). Alignment is central to the objective of providing the child with greater stability and control over more complex movement sequences. It is important to note that the therapist must maintain a constant awareness of his or her touch or degree of pressure to be responsive to the child's needs.

When applying deep pressure, the therapist's hands are shaped to the child's body contour. During light or intermittent touch pressure, the therapist's hands follow the movement of the child and gently intervene to prevent abnormal responses.

The child with high tone benefits from therapeutic handling that uses full range of movement and a variety of movement patterns. Generally, handling of the child with spasticity involves an interplay of techniques to reduce tightness and facilitate active movement. The child with low tone benefits from slow, controlled movements in limited ranges. This child frequently is treated in higher level antigravity positions, such as sitting and standing, to promote increased activation of proximal musculature. One of the specific concerns of the occupational therapist is upper extremity movement and function. Specific handling techniques need to be used with children who have stiffness and stereotypical movement patterns in the upper extremities and

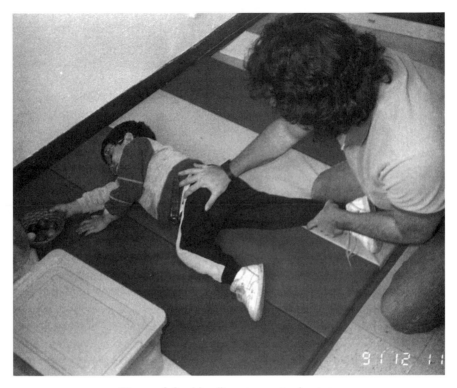

Figure 6.9 Handling at proximal points.

trunk. These problems often manifest in difficulty with bilateral movements, reaching, grasping, releasing of objects, and in-hand manipulation skills (Exner, 1989). Another priority for the occupational therapist is to use handling techniques during self-care activities, including feeding, dressing, toileting, and personal hygiene.

Therapeutic handling also may require additional equipment, such as various sized balls, rolls, or benches. This equipment provides a static or dynamic surface, allowing the therapist to use his or her hands and body effectively (Figure 6.10).

Preparation and Facilitation

A recommended sequence of intervention begins with preparatory activities. These activities may include techniques to promote mobility in structures that indicate limitations in passive movements or techniques that facilitate alignment of the body before active movement. Then the therapist selects specific areas of the child's body for therapeutic handling. These key points may be proximal (e.g., the shoulder girdle, trunk, and pelvis) or distal (e.g., the hands and feet). The specific key points used depend on the child's therapeutic needs. The end result of preparation is the establishment of improved body alignment, which allows for more efficient movement and postural control. Alignment allows for the most efficient form of

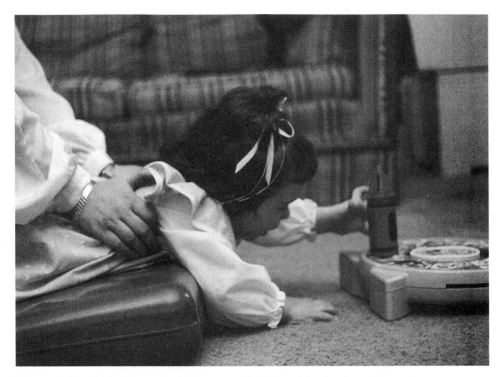

Figure 6.10 Use of a wedge facilitates positioning while the therapist applies pressure to the child's torso in an inward and downward motion to facilitate reaching.

muscle cocontraction around a joint for stability and mobility. The purpose is to produce a desired motor response. Preparation and facilitation utilize selective tactile and proprioceptive input to produce alignment, gain elongation of muscles, or facilitate normal muscle contraction and movement (Boehme, 1988; Neurodevelopmental Association, 1990) (Figure 6.11).

Compression and traction are employed throughout this process. Compression can be utilized to promote body alignment and activate muscles for functional use. Traction can be used to elongate tight muscles or in the process of facilitating the initiation of movement. These facilitation techniques are used repeatedly throughout the process of handling. They serve to maintain the child's alignment and active participation in movement. Following preparatory activities, active or automatic movement patterns should be facilitated, using continued therapeutic input at necessary key points of control. Facilitation techniques involve direct input to stimulate muscle activity.

Most often, preparation and facilitation techniques are used in combination. For example, heavy compression can be applied to the scapula in a downward rotated position to promote alignment of the scapula on the rib cage. At the same time, facilitatory techniques are evident when the occupational therapist uses gentle trac-

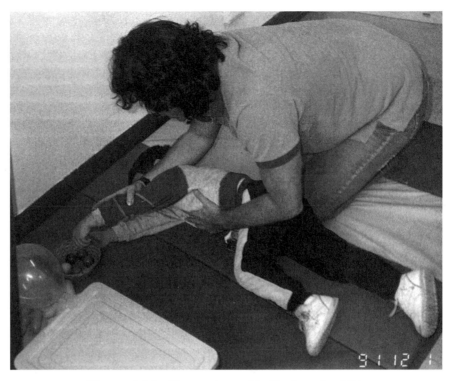

Figure 6.11 Preparation and facilitation of a child.

tion on the humerus in the direction of external rotation in order to obtain increased range of reaching.

Graded compression to the large muscles of the trunk can increase stability and postural control. In working with a low-tone child to maintain an upright posture in sitting, the therapist's hands are placed on either side of the trunk. The hands apply a compressive force and remain in contact with the child's body with input toward the weightbearing surface. In this example, the therapist applies pressure to the child's torso in an inward and downward motion (Figure 6.12). On observation, the child then begins to hold his or her trunk more independently or move his or her limbs actively.

In a sitting position, preparation may involve deep pressure to the base of support and activation of trunk muscles in order to free the upper extremities for self-feeding. The child who sits with a posterior pelvic tilt lacks sufficient contact of the lower extremities with the support surface. Preparation may include mobilizing the pelvis in an anterior direction to achieve trunk alignment. The therapist can follow-up with facilitation of an anterior weightshift as the child reaches to the table for eating utensils.

Weightbearing and weightshifting may be used throughout the process of preparation and facilitation. The goal of weightbearing and weightshifting is to promote

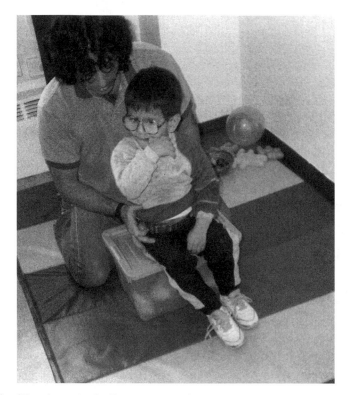

Figure 6.12   The therapist facilitates a neutral sitting posture.

postural alignment and facilitate the child's ability to move in and out of positions and move through space.

All postural movements, whether gross or subtle, occur with a shift in weight. Shifts in weight, therefore, may occur in degrees of amplitude and in various planes (e.g., anterior-posterior, laterally, and diagonally). Children who have problems in postural tone often have difficulty initiating, controlling, or grading a shift in weight. For example, the hypertonic child has difficulty initiating a weight shift, whereas the hypotonic child has difficulty grading a weight shift.

Weightbearing is when a child's body part or extremity maintains contact and exerts pressure against a surface such as the ground, therapy equipment, or, possibly, the therapist's body. Through weightbearing, cocontraction around a joint can be achieved, allowing for the development of greater proximal stability. This can be seen when children weight bear in quadruped and weight shift over extended arms as they move in and out of sitting. Weightshifting also occurs when children creep forward through space (Figures 6.13 and 6.14).

Weightbearing and weightshifting are important in the development of proximal and distal control; therefore, weightbearing may be alternated in a treatment se-

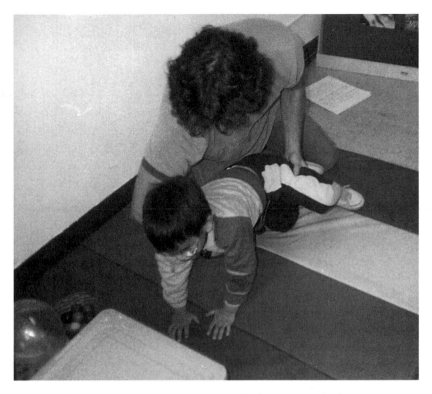

Figure 6.13   Weightbearing with postural alignment to facilitate creeping.

quence with graded reaching or hand activities. If movement is not initiated by the child, the environment is altered to encourage motivation or the therapeutic input is changed. For example, a more visually stimulating toy can be used to facilitate the child to reach. In addition, graded therapeutic stimulation can be provided at different rates and speeds in order to stimulate more active participation.

When the therapist incorporates specific preparatory activities and facilitation techniques while engaging the child in a functional activity, this requires the child to initiate or attempt to initiate the movement with the therapist's assistance. Practice of the task ensures that the movement will be learned. Gradually the therapist releases the hands-on contact so that the child can perform the functional movement more independently.

Integration of Activities

Activities that facilitate functional skills are essential for occupational therapists. Play activities are especially important for children. Children who have motor impairments frequently have limited participation in play activities. The therapist who

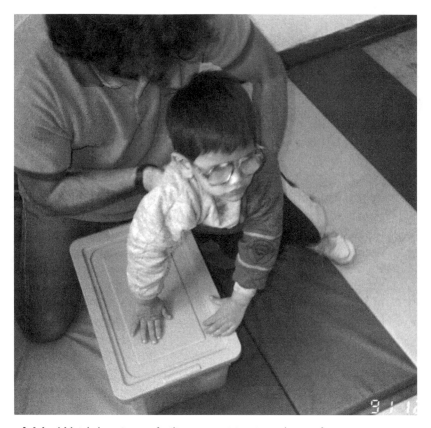

Figure 6.14 Weightbearing to facilitate transition in and out of various positions.

applies NDT therefore needs to be sensitive to the use of play activities during treatment (Anderson, Hinojosa & Stauch, 1988). Incorporating play fulfills a variety of therapeutic goals. Play motivates or engages the child during therapy and develops specific cognitive and perceptual skills.

It is essential to promote movement patterns when a child's attention is focused on a play activity. Handling techniques on the rib cage can be used to activate the abdominal as the child weightshifts in sitting or prone to reach a toy. The therapist carefully selects the play activity to avoid the influence of excessive effort by the child, which may result in associated reactions. The therapist can use increased contact to the base of support to prevent or minimize these reactions.

Movements used during play often are similar to movements used in other aspects of life. The use of play activities during treatment, therefore, may encourage the use of the same movements in other activities such as ADL. For example, facilitating a bilateral hand pattern in play with lotion or powder may involve future movements necessary for personal hygiene, feeding, and dressing. Such activities could include hand-to-hand contact for hand washing, hand-to-feet for donning socks, or hand-to-face for eating. Reaching with external rotation can only be achieved with alignment of the scapula in a downwardly rotated position. Preparation for the child with excessive scapular abduction, shoulder internal rotation, and forearm pronation may involve mobilizing the scapula into a position of adduction depression and downward rotation. Facilitation at the humerus and forearm in the direction of external rotation and supination positions the arm for grasp. An important element in this frame of reference is the facilitation of movement patterns during the performance of ADL.

The next challenge is for the therapist to change the demands of the environment so that the child learns to perform the movement in a variety of contexts. Activities refined in the therapy situation can then be practiced in the home or school environment.

Positioning and Adaptive Equipment

Positioning and equipment may be used as adjuncts to handling. They facilitate postural alignment and stability without hands-on contact by the therapist. The assumption is that this external stabilization allows more independent movement elsewhere. In addition, equipment reduces the likelihood of deformities and contractures that develop with habitual abnormal posturing and movement. Through the use of positioning, adaptive equipment, and orthotic devices designed specifically for the child's needs, the goals of therapy can be reinforced by parents and other professionals (Whiteside, 1997). This is discussed further in Chapter 11.

SUMMARY

The NDT frame of reference is based on the work of Berta and Karel Bobath in the 1940s. Other professionals in the field of pediatric rehabilitation have contributed extensively to this body of knowledge. This approach uses a "hands-on" method to facilitate movement patterns necessary for the acquisition of functional skills. Clinically, the approach is adapted and modified for use with children of varying ages and diagnoses.

The theoretical basis of NDT has continued to evolve with the emergence of new information, models, and theories in the movement sciences. Functional movement involves the interaction between the individual, the environment, and the task. Practice and experience are essential to the learning and adaptation of motor skills. An in-depth analysis of individuals' motor dysfunction is necessary to determine their functional limitations. Treatment focuses on increasing function, and therapeutic handling is one method utilized to help the individual achieve functional goals.

There are seven key function/dysfunction continua that provide therapists with descriptions of observable behaviors essential for the clinical assessment of most children. These continua provide the foundation for an NDT assessment, which is designed to identify and analyze dysfunction characteristics of movement associated with CNS dysfunction. The entry-level therapist is encouraged to follow a structured approach under the supervision of an experienced therapist to elicit the child's movement repertoire, categorize the movement problems, and determine how these deficits interfere with the child's ability to acquire functional skills (Figure 6.15).

Postulates regarding change delineate the environment that needs to be created and the techniques used by the therapist to facilitate change. These postulates emphasize the importance of consistent handling, active participation on the part of the child, responsibility of the therapist to the child's needs, creation of a motivating environment, use of ongoing assessment, incorporation of movement into functional activities, maximization of the therapist's sensory feedback through handling, and use of preventative strategies such as adaptive equipment and orthotic devices.

Application of the frame of reference requires practice, which is learned most effectively through the supervision of an experienced therapist. Specialized training also is available through continuing education. Specific techniques used in this frame of reference include handling for preparation and facilitation of muscle activity during functional interaction with the environment.

These techniques involve graded sensory input and incorporation of weightbearing and weightshifting to elicit automatic, active control. Play activities provide an

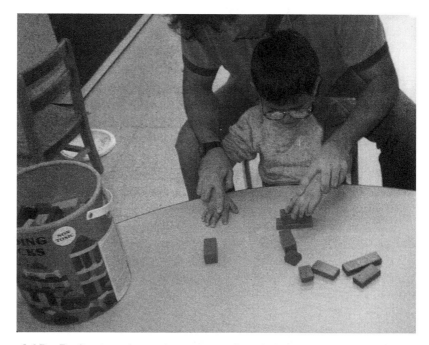

Figure 6.15 Facilitation of wrist extension and graded digital release of blocks.

essential component of motivation and cognitive and perceptual stimulation. Adaptive equipment and positioning provide an adjunct to achieving the goals of therapy. The result is that the child acquires the movement components needed to achieve the greatest independence in developmentally appropriate areas of play, self-care, and school performance.

The NDT frame of reference provides the occupational therapist with a repertoire of handling techniques designed to improve a child's postural control. It requires an ongoing process of problem solving to determine the movement components necessary for the performance of these functional skills and to analyze the child's responses to determine any interfering factors and missing components. It is a dynamic process in which the therapist may perform a range of activities, including elongating tight muscles, promoting mobility, and inhibiting spasticity and abnormal posturing within the context of goal-directed activity. The aim is for the child to achieve mastery in selected developmentally appropriate areas of play, self-care, and, ultimately, beginning school skills. Optimum achievement is possible when individual treatment is combined with activities at home and in school.

Acknowledgments

Figures 6.5, 6.6, and 6.8 were taken by Steven A. Smith of New York.

References

Anderson, J., Hinojosa, J., & Strauch, C. (1987). Integrating play in neurodevelopmental therapy (NDT). *American Journal of Occupational Therapy, 41,* 421–426.

Birkmeier, K. (July–August 1997). Curriculum and theoretical base committee update. *NDTA Network,* 1–6.

Bly, L. (1980). Abnormal motor development. In D. Slaton, (Ed.). *Development of movement in infancy.* University of North Carolina at Chapel Hill, Division of Physical Therapy, May 19–22, 1980.

Bly, L. (1991) A historical and current view of the basis of NDT Pediatric. *Physical Therapy, 3,* 131–135.

Bly, L. (September/October 1996). What is the role of sensation in motor learning? What is the role of feedback and feedforward? *NDTA Network,* 1–7.

Bobath, B. (1971a). *Abnormal postural reflex activity caused by brain lesions* (2nd ed.). London: William Heineman Medical Books, Ltd.

Bobath, B. (1971b). Motor development, its effect on general development and application to the treatment of cerebral palsy. *Physiotherapy, 57,* 526–532.

Bobath, B. (1975, February). Sensorimotor development. *NDT Newsletters.* 7(1).

Boehme, R. (1984, May). Advanced NDT course in occupational therapy. New York: Long Island. Unpublished notes.

Boehme, R. (1988). *Improving upper body control.* Tucson, AZ: Therapy Skill Builders.

Campbell, P. (1981). Movement assessment of infants: An evaluation. *Physical and Occupational Therapy in Pediatrics, 1*(4), 53–57.

Campbell, P. (1986). Introduction to neurodevelopmental treatment. Pamphlet. Cuyahoga Falls, OH: Children's Hospital Medical Center of Akron.

Case-Smith, J. (1991). *Posture and fine motor assessment of infants* (research edition). Ohio State University.

Chandler, L. S., Andrews, M. S., & Swanson, M. W. (1980). *Movement Assessment of Infants: A manual.* Rolling Bay, WA.

Cupps, B. (January–February 1997). Postural control: a current view. *NDTA Network,* 1–7.

Erhardt, R. P. (1982). *Developmental hand dysfunction: Theory, assessment, treatment.* Laurel, MD: Ramsco.

Exner, C. E. (1996). Development of hand skills. In J. Case-Smith, A. S. Allen, & P. N. Pratt (Eds.) *Occupational therapy for children* (3rd ed.) (pp. 268–306). St. Louis, MO: C. V. Mosby.

Frank, J. S., & Earl, M. (1990). Coordination of posture and movement. *Physical Therapy, 70,* 855–863.

Gans, B. M., Haley, S. M., Hallenberg, S. C., Mann, N., Inacio, C. A., & Faas, R. M. (in press). Description and inter-observer reliability of the Tufts Assessment of Motor Performance. *American Journal of Physical Medicine and Rehabilitation.*

Guiliani, C. (1991). Theories of motor control: New concepts for physical therapy. In *Contemporary management of motor control problems: Proceedings of the II Step Conference.* (pp. 29–35). Alexandria, VA: American Physical Therapy Association.

Hartbourne, R., Giuhani, C. A., & NacNeela, J. (1987). Kinematic and electromyographic analysis of the development of sitting posture in infants. *Developmental Medicine and Child Neurology, 29,* 31–32.

Horak, F. (1991). Assumptions underlying motor control for neurological rehabilitation. In *Contemporary management of motor control problems: Proceeding of the II Step Conference* (pp. 11–27). Alexandria, VA: American Physical Therapy Association.

Keshner, E. (1990). Coordinating stability of a complex movement system. *Physical Therapy, 70,* 844–854.

Kuypers, H. G. J. M. (1963). Organization of the motor systems. *International Journal of Neurology, 4,* 78–91.

Lawrence, & Hopkins. (1972). Developmental aspects of pyramidal motor control in Rhesus monkey. *Brain Research, 40,* 117–118.

Loria, C. (1980). Relationship of proximal and distal function in motor development. *Physical Therapy, 60,* 167–172.

Miller, L. J., & Roid, G. H. (1994). *Toddler Infant Motor Evaluation.* Tucson, AZ: Therapy Skill Builders.

Morris, S. E. (May, 1990). *The development of oral-motor skills in children receiving non-oral feedings* (rev. ed.). Faber, VA: New Visions.

Nashner, L. M., & McCollum, G. (1985). The organization of human postural movements: A formal basis and experimental system. *Behavioral Brain Science, 8,* 135–172.

Neurodevelopmental treatment 8-week certification course manual. Oak Park, IL: Neurodevelopmental Association.

Scherzer, A. L., & Tscharnuter, I. (1990). *Early diagnosis and treatment in cerebral palsy* (2nd ed.). New York: Marcel Dekker.

Short-DeGraff, M. A. (1988). *Human development for occupational and physical therapists.* Baltimore, MD: Williams & Wilkins.

Whiteside, A. (September–October 1997). Clerical goals and application of NDT facilitation. *NDTA Network,* 1–14.

CHAPTER 7

Sensory Integration Frame of Reference: Theoretical Base, Function/Dysfunction Continua, and Guide to Evaluation

JUDITH GIENCKE KIMBALL

Sensory integration is the process of organizing sensory information in the brain to make an adaptive response (Ayres, 1972a). An adaptive response occurs when a person successfully meets an environmental challenge. The sensory integrative frame of reference is applied when sensory system processing deficits make it difficult for a child to produce an appropriate adaptive response. In this chapter, the child's physical adaptive response and his or her reactions and behaviors, which include emotional and ideational adaptive responses, are addressed. The primary consideration in sensory integration is that processing problems are related to subtle yet definable differences in neurologic functioning, often called soft signs by physicians. The sensory integration frame of reference is complex, requiring an in-depth understanding of the functions of the central nervous system (CNS). This chapter will introduce the theoretical base, function/dysfunction continua, and guide for evaluation for the frame of reference. The following chapter will address intervention by presenting the postulates regarding change and application to practice.

A. Jean Ayres, Ph.D., OTR, FAOTA, the originator of the theory of sensory integration, began work on the theory in the late 1950s. Dr. Ayres was an occupational therapist with a doctorate in educational psychology; she did a postdoctoral fellowship at the Brain Research Institute of the University of California at Los Angeles. Her research is most commonly identified with children with learning disabilities; however, it has been extended to include many other forms of neurobehavioral development, including mental retardation, autism and pervasive developmental disorders, sensory defensiveness, numerous behavioral disorders, and other neurosensory-based problems.

Dr. Ayres made major contributions to the field of occupational therapy with the publication of the Southern California Sensory Integration Tests (SCSIT) in 1972 (1972b, 1980). The SCSIT was based on factor analytic studies that focused on the components of sensory integration and other tests commonly used at the time with learning disabled children (Ayres, 1965, 1966a, 1966b, 1969, 1972a, 1972b, 1972c, 1972d, 1975a, 1975b). Her 1977 study, which used the Southern California Postrotary Nystagmus Test (SCPNT) (Ayres, 1975a), supported the role of the vestibular system in sensory integrative dysfunction (Ayres, 1978). Earlier studies had already identified several deficit areas seen in children who had sensory integrative dysfunction, notably, tactile discrimination problems, tactile defensiveness, perceptual difficulties, bilateral integration dysfunction, and dyspraxia (poor motor planning abilities). Later, factor analytic studies pinpointed left-hemisphere dysfunction, including auditory language disabilities, and right-hemisphere dysfunctions, such as deficits in perception and a lack of awareness of the left side of the body (Ayres, 1976). Cumulatively, all the factor analytic studies resulted in a topology for identifying and treating sensory integrative problems. The topology included vestibular and bilateral integration problems, dyspraxia, left-hemisphere disorders, right-hemisphere disorders, and generalized sensory integrative dysfunction. These categories were used by occupational therapists until the late 1980's. (For a summary of Ayres' factor analytic studies and their contributions to the theory of sensory integration, the reader is advised to see Clark, Mallioux, and Parham [1989]).

During the 1980's, Ayres developed and standardized the Sensory Integration and Praxis Tests (SIPT). These tests, published in 1989, were more specific to praxis and more in-depth than the SCSIT. Research using the SIPT indicates that the areas of dysfunction are similar to those already identified by the SCSIT. Because the SIPT tests are more complex and specific to praxis, test research findings expand the knowledge of the complexity and interrelationships in the CNS (Kimball, 1990). According to Fisher, Murray, and Bundy (1991, p. 10), "the patterns that were delineated by both cluster and factor analysis in the SIPT data include:

1. Somatosensory processing deficits
2. Poor bilateral integration and sequencing
3. Impaired somatopraxis
4. Poor praxis on verbal command
5. Visual praxis factor, more appropriately considered poor visual perception and visuomotor coordination
   a. Poor form and space perception
   b. Visual construction deficits
   c. Visuomotor coordination deficits
6. Generalized sensory integrative dysfunction."

The SIPT is scored by computer and generates a profile of the child's abilities compared against six patterns that emerged from SIPT standardization. These patterns include the following:

1. Low average bilateral integration and sequencing
2. Low average sensory integration and praxis
3. General sensory integrative dysfunction
4. Dyspraxia on verbal command
5. Visuo- and somatodyspraxia
6. High average sensory integration and praxis

Figure 7.1 is a chromagraph report that shows a child's scores on each of the SIPT tests and the relationship to the six diagnostic clusters (SIPT, 1989).

Work on the theories of sensory integration continued to develop after Dr. Ayres' death in 1988. A major contribution to the theory is the work by Wilbarger and Wilbarger. They expanded Dr. Ayres' work on tactile defensiveness into an evolving theory about how sensory system modulation difficulties can lead to a cluster of behavioral symptoms they call "sensory defensiveness." Their work includes neurophysiologic correlates that explain the possible causes and presentations of these CNS differences in functioning and suggest treatment strategies (Wilbarger & Wilbarger, 1991; Wilbarger, 1991).

Other occupational therapists have applied these modulation theories and traditional sensory integration theories to populations other than children with learning disabilities. Those populations include children and adults with autism spectrum disorder (i.e., autism, pervasive development disorder, Asperger syndrome), mental retardation, behavioral disorders, anxiety disorders among others. Anecdotally, treatment results have been promising, but research is still limited. Much of the theory and practice that deals with the therapeutic use of sensory systems modulation and sensory-motor input comes under the sensory integration umbrella. This new work expands and clarifies Ayres' original work and is presented within this frame of reference.

THEORETICAL BASE OF SENSORY INTEGRATION FRAME OF REFERENCE

A knowledge of human development provides a starting point for understanding sensory integration. Sensory integration is far more complex, however, than the outward signs of function and skill development often associated with human development. The sensory integration frame of reference focuses on the influences of the integration of the sensory systems that underlie the development of function and skills—i.e., those sensory systems that organize the nervous system for actual acquisition of function (Figure 7.2). This classic chart devised by Ayres is the starting point for understanding that function and skill are based on sensory system integration.

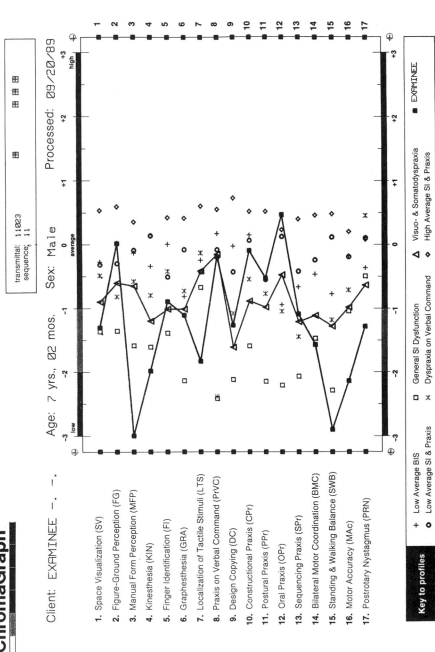

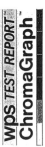

Figure 7.1   Chromagraph report that shows a child's scores on each of the SIPT tests and the relationship to the six diagnostic clusters (SIPT, 1989). SIPT = Sensory Integration and Praxis Tests.

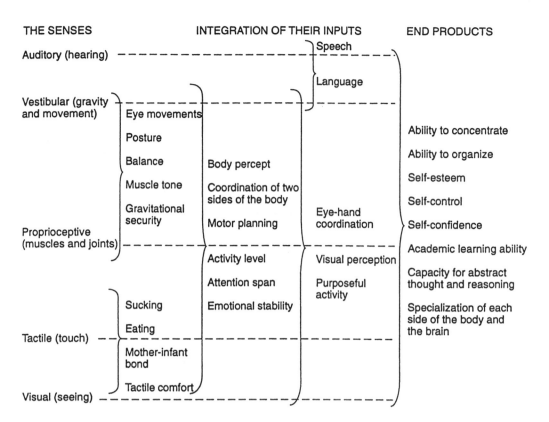

Figure 7.2   The senses, integration of their inputs, and their end products. Reprinted by permission of the publisher, Western Psychological Services, 12031 Wilshire Boulevard, Los Angeles, CA.

The sensory systems—"senses" as they are labeled on Figure 7.2—that are important in the theoretical base of the sensory integrative frame of reference are the auditory, visual, vestibular, proprioceptive, and tactile systems. The vestibular, proprioceptive, and tactile systems are highlighted as the precursors to development of the auditory and visual systems. They are thought to be the precursors to the development of most end-product abilities. This perspective is different from the theoretical bases of other frames of reference, particularly those involved with cognitive development, which focus on the auditory and visual systems.

As Figure 7.2 is followed from left to right and the sensory systems integrate (i.e., "integration of their input"), the results are "end-products" that reflect function and skills. The goal of occupational therapists who use a sensory integration frame of reference is to facilitate the development of these end-products. The therapist is primarily concerned, however, with the integrity and integration of underlying sensory systems and the functional support capabilities that contribute to these end-products. The occupational therapist directs the intervention at the sensory system and functional support capability levels (middle level of figure—"integration of their input") in combination with facilitating an adaptive response, all of which result in the development of end-product abilities.

Basic Concepts

The theoretical base of the sensory integration frame of reference is unique in that it deals specifically with the contributions of the subcortical areas of the brain to human behavior. Dr. Ayres specifically stated that the brain stem was the primary area of integration and therefore played the greatest role in sensory integration. Structures of particular interest in the brain stem include the thalamus (viewed as the master integrator of the brain), the vestibular nuclei and their interconnectors, and the reticular formation (particularly important in alerting and arousal). Dr. Ayres also postulated that the cerebellum plays a major role in sensory integration because of its processing of input related to gravity and movement. As this theoretical base evolved, the importance of other structures of the CNS was recognized. The limbic system has been identified because of its association with sympathetic arousal, which results in the survival (fight-or-flight) response often seen in people who exhibit sensory defensiveness (Ayres, 1979; Wilbarger & Wilbarger, 1991).

The cerebral cortex also is important to the theoretical base of sensory integration because of its contribution to praxis, particularly in the areas of ideation or a person's understanding of the need for movement. The entire CNS and the interplay or integration of all its systems are considered in sensory integration.

There are six basic assumptions that underlie CNS organization in sensory integration:

1. The CNS is hierarchically organized. Cortical processing relies and depends on adequate organization of inputs supplied by the lower brain centers.
2. Meaningful registration of stimuli must occur before the CNS can make a response to it and, therefore, allow for higher functioning to occur.
3. The brain is innately organized to program a person to seek out stimulation that is organizing or beneficial in itself.
4. Input from one sensory system can facilitate or inhibit the state of the entire organism. Input from each system influences every other system and the whole organism.
5. There is plasticity within the CNS.
6. Normal human development occurs sequentially.

The CNS is hierarchically organized. Cortical processing relies and depends on adequate organization of sensation supplied by the lower brain centers. Phylogenetically, as the brain developed, newer and higher level structures, like the cerebral cortex, remained interconnected and depended on the adequate functioning of the older and lower level brain structures. The integration of sensory input provided by the lower brain centers allows the cortical or higher centers to process more complex and specialized information.

Meaningful registration of the stimuli must occur before the brain can make a response to it and, therefore, allow higher functioning to occur, including adaptive responses. The registration of sensory input must occur to signal a change in the environment, and this must be meaningful enough to alert the person. For example, if a child is not alerted to the possibility of falling when he or she starts to tip over, a balance response that is adaptive to the environmental situation cannot occur. In this example, the lack of registration may be caused by one of three things: (1) an inefficiency in the detecting mechanism—in this case, the vestibular system; (2) underarousal of the whole system; or (3) a masking of the response by overarousal of many other systems.

The brain is innately organized to program the person to seek out stimulation that is organizing or beneficial in itself. Accomplishing an adaptive response reinforces integration in sensory systems, but it also is based on input from those sensory systems. Children naturally seek out and engage in activities that optimally promote neural integration. This is referred to as the inner drive for sensory integration. For example, the jumping, climbing, and falling activities seen in most 2-year-old children are related to the incipient understanding of gravity. At this age, the child needs to experience his or her ability to move against gravity and needs to challenge gravity at all levels. Even adults seek out activities to give themselves a balanced "sensory diet." For example, when an adult works at a desk, he or she may ski, jog, or participate in aerobics to make him or herself feel better.

Input from one sensory system can facilitate or inhibit the state of the entire organism. Input from each system influences every other system and the whole organism. In other words, facilitation and inhibition of a specific system do not have to occur within that system alone but also can be achieved through the influence of inhibition and facilitation of other sensory systems. This powerful assumption provides the basis for the occupational therapist to treat dysfunction of one sensory system through intervention with another sensory system. It also demonstrates the vast interconnection between the function and structure of the CNS.

There is plasticity within the CNS. Brain processing and structure can be modified to bring about more optimal functioning. Using the sensory integration frame of reference, intervention is directed at sensory systems and functional support levels to facilitate changes in the child's ability to produce an adaptive response. In many cases, this change is permanent and reflects a processing difference that cannot be attributed to learning alone. Although younger children are thought to have the most neural plasticity, experience has shown that change can occur throughout adulthood.

Normal human development occurs sequentially. The sensory integration frame of reference is based on an understanding of the sequence of human development and on an understanding of the adaptive responses that children should be able to accomplish at each age level. If sensory system modulation and functional support capabilities are not integrated, then adaptive responses will not reach optimum levels. Splinter skills develop out of a need in specific situations, but their transferability to other situations is limited. The sensory integration frame of reference focuses on developing integration, not on teaching splinter skills.

These assumptions, basic to CNS organization, are the foundation for the theoretical base of sensory integration.

Sensory Systems

Important to the theoretical base of sensory integration is an understanding of the sensory systems, particularly the vestibular, proprioceptive, tactile, auditory, and visual systems. Although the neuroanatomy and neurophysiology of the systems are beyond the scope of this chapter, the chapter assumes a basic understanding of neuroscience. Functional connections will be emphasized, with reference made only to the neuroscience that underlies these connections. (For a synopsis of neuroscience, the reader is referred to Moore in Gilfoyle, Grady, & Moore, 1990).

Tactile System. This system has several different functions. Of particular interest is the ongoing interaction between the two major divisions of the body's tactile system: the dorsal column medial lemniscal and the anterolateral systems. (The head is served by the cranial nerves, particularly the trigeminal nerve).

The dorsal column medial lemniscal system carries discriminative touch (specifically two-point discrimination), conscious proprioception, touch pressure, and vibration for the body. Of the two tactile systems, the dorsal column medial lemniscal system is the newer phylogenetically. It plays a major role in the development of praxis. Wall (1970) identified an expanded role for the dorsal medial lemniscal system that is particularly pertinent to the development of praxis. He identified deficits in motor performance, especially voluntary exploratory movements, and deficits in attention, orientation, and anticipation with dorsal column lesion. (For a detailed discussion of this and related research the reader is referred to Cermak in Fisher, Murray & Bundy [1991, p. 151–154].)

The anterolateral system—composed of spinothalamic, spinoreticular, and spinotectal pathways—is a nonspecific, protective system that can produce sympathetic arousal. It also is a diffuse system that directs input into the reticular formation. It is responsible for the body sensations of pain, temperature, and crude touch (tickle and itch) and plays a major role in tactile defensive responses, such as an aversive response to light touch that results from overarousal. Phylogenetically, this system is older than the dorsal column medial lemniscal system.

Adequate functioning of both major divisions of the tactile system is necessary for appropriate sensory integration. Problems in interpreting tactile input may result in difficulties in the end-products, such as touch discrimination or praxis. Praxis is the ability to motor plan a new, nonhabitual motor act. In addition, the child may have difficulty in modulating tactile input. This can result in over- or underregistration of the tactile system. Overregistration is called tactile defensiveness.

Proprioception. Proprioception is the understanding of where joints and muscles are in space. Proprioceptors include the muscle spindles, the Golgi tendon organs, and mechanoreceptors of the skin. Proprioceptors work in conjunction with the vestibular system to give a sense of balance and position in space. All the muscles and joints are involved in this process; however, the neck joints and proximal limb joints, such as shoulders and hips, are of primary importance and give the most feedback to the CNS. Proprioception is a powerful system therapeutically.

Vestibular System. The vestibular receptors, located in the inner ear, are composed of three semicircular canals at right angles to each other and the utricle and saccule. These structures are filled with endolymph and contain hair cells called cilia that send the signals concerning direction of movement when they are displaced within the endolymph because of head movement. The semicircular canals are responsible for detection of angular, fast, short bursts of motion, and results in phasic limb movements and momentary head righting. The utricle and saccule, which contain the otoliths (calcium carbonate crystals or the "rocks in your head") as well as endolymph and hair cells, are responsible for the detection of gravity (the "rocks" fall "down") and linear acceleration. Utricle stimulation results in tonic input to the limbs and maintained head righting.

According to Ayres (1979), the child's relationship to gravity is "more primal than the (child's) relationship to mother" (p. 40); or, Mother Earth's gravity is more important for security than a child's biological mother. Furthermore, Ayres described gravity as ". . . the most constant universal force in our lives" (Ayres, 1979, p. 40). She pointed out that all living things must relate to the earth's gravitational pull. Humans appear to be endowed with a strong drive to master gravity and to attain an upright position. This ability to move against gravity is one of the key movements a therapist looks for in a child because it indicates a well-organized nervous system. Movement against gravity develops over time, as in (1) an infant's ability to raise its head off the mat at 1 month of age; (2) an infant's ability to raise his head, shoulders, and legs off the mat at 4 months of age; (3) a 1-year-old child's ability to stand upright and walk; (4) a 4-year-old child's ability to remain on a swing; and, (5) a school-aged child's love of movement activities that involve the challenge of gravity, such as jumping horses, skiing, or skateboarding.

The vestibular system makes connections through the vestibular nuclei in the brain stem and then sends information to higher levels in the brain. Dysfunction of the vestibular system, as seen in developmental problems, usually is caused by deficits in the integration of the vestibular input rather than by deficits in the vestibular receptors. Developmental vestibular problems can be functional, such as balance and coordination, or modulational (under- or overarousal), such as gravitational insecurity or intolerance to movement.

The *auditory and visual* systems have received less emphasis in sensory integration than the other sensory systems. Although Ayres did incorporate them into her work, the emphasis on subcortical, automatic processing led her successors away from these two systems. Ayres made theoretical and research connections between ear preference, laterality and crossing the midline, and midline stability and vestibular processing. She used dichotic listening and the Illinois Test of Psycholinguistic Abilities (ITPA) in her research. Today there is a renewed interest in the auditory and visual systems, and their levels of integration should also be understood. On the sensory system modulation level, the association between the auditory system and the vagus nerve is important as is the importance of the visual system in modulating vestibular processing, especially the stability of the visual field (Kandel & Schwartz, 1985). The visual and vestibular systems work together to produce visual perception and perceptual motor integration skills.

sensory integrationFunctions. The five systems previously discussed (auditory, visual, vestibular, proprioceptive, and tactile) provide the basis for development of the functional support capabilities that lead to the end-product abilities noted in Figure 7.2.

Table 7.1 shows the sensory integrationfunctions addressed in the sensory integration frame of reference. To produce the desired adaptive response in an end-product ability, the person must have sensory system modulation within normal levels and reasonable functional support capabilities. Optimal functioning means that all systems and capabilities work integratively.

Sensory System Modulation

The manner in which the sensory systems process input affects the quality of a child's ability to respond adaptively. Figure 7.3 shows the classic arousal curve commonly associated with the autonomic nervous system. Note that moderate arousal results in an optimal adaptive response, whereas high arousal results in behavioral disorganization and even anxiety or a negative emotional response. The key point often overlooked by health professionals is that arousal initiates a sympathetic, fight, flight, or freeze response. This reaction is the primary survival response of the organism. When arousal gets too high, the body responds as if to a serious survival threat. If it is not possible to fight or flee, then arousal does not dissipate easily, causing stress, anxiety, and difficulty in completing other adaptive responses. Persons who have sensory system modulation problems have more changeable arousal or reaction levels than normal. This results in problems with adaptive responses because their systems lack stability.

The sensory systems do not function independently. Arousal in several systems can combine, therefore, to increase arousal, and inhibition in several systems can combine to decrease arousal. The 12 sensory system responses that are considered to be contributors to modulation of arousal are listed under Sensory System Modulation in Table 7.1.

Table 7.1   Sensory Integrative Functions

Sensory System Modulation

Tactile
Auditory
Relationship to gravity
Movement level
Oral arousal
Olfactory arousal
Visual arousal
Attention level
Postrotary nystagmus
Sensitivity to movement
Proprioceptive sensitivity
Emotional level

Functional Support Capabilities

Suck-swallow-breathe
Tactile discrimination
Other discriminative abilities
Cocontraction
Muscle tone
Proprioception
Balance and equilibrium
Developmental reflexes
Lateralization
Bilateral integration

End-Product Abilities

Praxis
Form and space perception
Behavior
Academics
Language and articulation
Emotional tone
Activity level
Environment mastery

Sensory system modulation is influenced by the child's "sensory diet." Sensory diet is "related to the essential but changing need of all humans to have an optimum amount of organizing and integrating sensation being registered by one's central nervous system at all times" (Wilbarger, 1984, p. 7). Sensory diet is the accumulation of the child's total sensory input and its effect. In normal children, the sensory diet acts as the only external modulating force that the nervous system needs under usual circumstances. Normally, a child seeks out varied sensory inputs to maintain normal modulation levels (Figure 7.4).

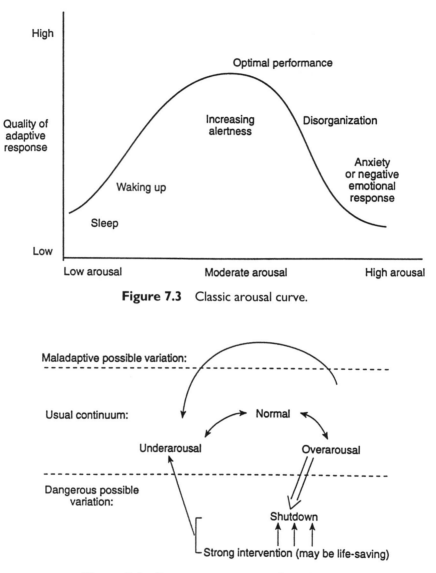

Figure 7.3   Classic arousal curve.

Figure 7.4   Sensory systems arousal continuum.

Usually, sensory system modulation fluctuates within a range of normal. Children who have sensory system modulation problems are much more variable than normal. A few children even react in a dangerous way and go from overarousal to physiological shutdown (Figure 7.4). "Shutdown" appears to be an autonomic nervous system response that can result in respiratory and cardiac irregularities and alterations in blood pressure that may produce decreased consciousness or shock. Shutdown results from severe overarousal that the nervous system cannot respond to in normal ways (Kimball, 1976; Kimball, 1977a). Other children may experience a dangerous possible variation in the pattern, which is also maladaptive, and go quickly from overarousal to underarousal but not to shutdown. This is thought to be a protective mechanism against severe sensory overload. This occurs before shutdown, but does not necessarily progress to shutdown except in rare cases.

The severe physiological responses seen in shutdown are infrequent but have been documented medically in at least two cases (Kimball, 1991). The more usual pattern is for a severely sensory overloaded person to shut off input and appear to be under-aroused. When intervention that looks inhibitory is initiated with such a child, he or she may quickly go to overarousal rather than stay in underarousal. Because treatment strategies are different for under- and overaroused children, this variation must be anticipated. A child who looks underaroused does not necessarily need excitatory input. Such input may be detrimental.

New research on neurotransmitters, particularly glutamate, and the finding that excess glutamate leads to cell death under extremely stressful conditions certainly will contribute to a new understanding of the development of sensory defensiveness in cases of abuse. This research indicates that sensory defensiveness can be "acquired" later in life and that the mechanism is not psychological but physiological. Cell death leads to lessening the ability of the cortex to inhibit. Research has shown that rats lose cortical sensing cells in their hippocampus under abusive conditions and that abused women who experience increased anxiety, depression, and trouble with stress also show hippocampal differences (Dubner, 1991; Fitzgerald, 1991; Gold, Goodwin, & Chrousus, 1988a, 1988b; Wilcox, 1991; Woolf, 1991).

Each of the sensory systems also has an information processing component that discriminates appropriate aspects of the environment. Modulation problems mask the information components of the systems, often resulting in the less than optimal ability to use the information processing systems. When sensory systems are well modulated, normal information processing is possible.

Normal tactile arousal/reactivity and integration allow children to differentiate among the types of tactile input that they experience. Ayres (1972a, 1975b) felt that the interplay between the two divisions of the body's tactile system gave the child a signal about being alert to a dangerous situation (anterolateral system) or differentiating what touch might imply (dorsal column medial lemniscal system). If this interplay is inaccurate, the anterolateral system may overarouse and cause the child to react as if in a survival situation when the stimulus warranted orientation only. When survival situations alert the nervous system, a fight-flight-freeze reaction might occur. Because most children react normally to touch, this overreaction could be interpreted as a behavior problem when it actually is a variation in tactile system functioning called *tactile defensiveness*. It is apparent that much more than an interplay between the anterolateral and dorsal medial lemniscal systems is involved. Numerous ascending and descending controls exist on the two systems from many areas of the brain including the raphe spinal system, the reticular system, the limbic system, the hypothalamus, and the cortex (Caseate, 1979; Daube, Reagan, Sandok & West-moreland, 1986; DeGroot and Chusid, 1988; Fisher et al., 1991; Kandel & Schwartz, 1985; Melzak & Wall, 1965; Nieuwenhuys, Voogd, & Van Huijzen, 1988; Pribram, 1975; Royeen, 1985). Important for treatment is the fact that all these functions in the head are served by cranial nerves, especially the trigeminal nerve, so that body input does not influence the head directly (Wilson-Panwels, Akesson, & Stewart, 1988).

Children who are *oral defensive* can have difficulty in eating as they cannot tolerate the textures of foods. These difficulties can range from mild to so severe that they compromise the child's nutrition.

Sounds, which are interpreted by the auditory system, alert children to changes in their environment that may need attention and action. Usually, the only sounds that alert the child are those that need to be attended to. These differences may be caused by sound level, type, or novelty. Once the child has registered a sound and has been aroused to the sound, he or she decides if action is necessary. If not, the sound can be ignored. When a child with normal hearing is not alerted by sounds that may signify important changes in the environment, a state of underreactivity may exist. Because the child has not been alerted, changes in the environment are not registered, and, therefore, the child does not react adaptively.

In a state of overreactivity or defense, the child may be alerted to any environmental sounds, including those that do not require a response. Often the child is not able to habituate to a sound; therefore he or she continues to be alerted long after the sound is no longer novel. This state of overreactivity is called *auditory defensiveness*.

The gravity receptors in the vestibular mechanism, the otoliths in the utricle and saccule, normally alert children to changes in the relationship of their head position to gravity (Figure 7.5). A change in head position that results in loss of equilibrium produces a compensatory response in the trunk and limbs to maintain balance. Children who are underreactive to gravity appear to be unaware of these changes in head position. They frequently seek out strong movement input that can even be dangerous to them. Conversely, the child who is overreactive to changes in head position in relationship to gravity has a real fear or strong emotional response to situations that normally require only a balance reaction. This overreactivity is thought to be an otolithic response that is not being integrated appropriately. It is referred to as *gravitational insecurity*.

Movement level refers to a child's need for nonpurposeful movement or much higher than normal levels of movement. Colloquially, this is described as the child "fidgeting" or being "motor driven." Normal children use movement to accomplish an end-product, such as relocating from one place to another. The child who constantly needs to move to maintain a normal arousal level is referred to as being "motor restless." The child's need for movement probably is related to an overinhibition in the integration of vestibular input. This leads to a need to seek out more movement input to maintain a normal arousal/ reactivity level (Kimball, 1988). Sometimes

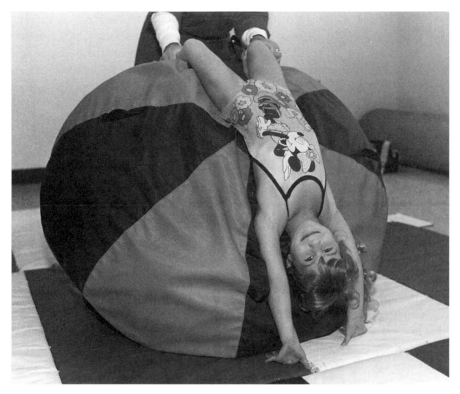

Figure 7.5 A gravitationally secure child; no fear responses noted.

it is difficult to differentiate between movement level and attention level. The child who has a movement level modulation problem is motor restless and not necessarily distracted. He or she needs to move his or her body constantly and continually seeks out motor input. Conversely, the underreactive child may be slow moving and appear to conserve movement.

Infants put objects in their mouths to learn about such things as texture, size, and shape and to fulfill the psychological need to mouth. This is referred to as oral arousal. Some children are adverse to putting certain textures in their mouths. They refuse foods based on texture, not on taste. In severe cases, this can eliminate important foods from the child's diet, affecting nutrition. This overreactivity to textures is called *oral defensiveness*.

Odors can register powerfully because they go directly to the limbic system, referred to as the "smell brain," or the seat of emotions in the brain. Olfaction is the only sensory modality that does not have a synaptic connection in the thalamus before reaching higher centers. This primitive brain connection makes it a powerful system for sympathetic arousal. Many strong danger signals are delivered by the environment through the olfactory system (e.g., the smell of smoke, the memory of smells associated with dangerous situations that persons have experienced, the smell of fear given off by animals and humans). *Olfactory defensiveness* is the negative response to certain odors. An example is the inability to tolerate scented soaps. An example of olfaction used as a positive sensory input is the development of "aroma therapy" and its attempts to influence mood through olfaction. Other examples include the practice of baking something with cinnamon or burning a cinnamon scented candle prior to showing a house in order to positively influence the purchaser.

Children respond to visual stimuli by orienting to novel situations, checking them out, and then acting as required. The child who underregisters visual stimuli may not react appropriately in a situation that requires arousal and response. The child who is overreactive to visual stimuli might not be able to habituate; hence, he or she reacts to the visual stimulus as if it were constantly novel. An example of this is the fascination an autistic child may have with a revolving record. Children who dislike certain visual inputs such as sunny days or who overreact to increase visual input such as too many people or too many colorful objects are said to be *visually defensive.*

If the child's attention level to all environmental input is too high or too low, education will be difficult because his or her focus probably is not on academics. *Attention level* is modulated by the reticular system, and this system is influenced by all the other sensory systems. Moderate attention is required to interact effectively with the environment. Overreactivity to environmental input leaves the child deficient in his ability to screen out enough to attend to the "important" things, and underreactivity leaves the child with inadequate arousal for input to which he or she should respond. A child who has an overreactive attention level may be labeled as having "attention deficit disorder with or without hyperactivity." It is important to note that the label "attention deficit disorder" refers to the ability to attend cognitively, whereas the term "hyperactivity" often refers to motor restless behavior. These two terms sometimes are used interchangeably, but they really are distinctly different and should be defined separately (Kimball, 1986).

Postrotary nystagmus is an ocular response attributed to the semicircular canals of the vestibular mechanism. It consists of rhythmic back and forth eye movement (nystagmus) following body rotation. This response is related to arousal/reactivity of the vestibular system (Ayres, 1976; Kimball, 1981; Kimball, 1986; Kimball, 1988). Underreactivity is thought to be related to excess inhibition in the lower brain centers. Conversely, overreactivity is thought to be caused by inadequate inhibition from the cerebral cortex. Underreactivity and overreactivity are considered to be problematic.

Sensitivity to movement is thought to be mediated by the vestibular system. In sensitive persons, movement often triggers an autonomic reaction of nausea or vomiting. Sensitivity to movement may be caused by an intravestibular conflict in which the semicircular canals and the otoliths send conflicting messages. Another possibility is a vestibular-ocular conflict in which the vestibular mechanism and the eyes send conflicting messages. This may be the mechanism involved in carsickness and seasickness. For example, in carsickness, sitting in the front seat appears to lessen the sensitivity to movement because the person does not have to refocus the eyes constantly in relation to the moving environment. This is thought to reduce vestibular-ocular conflict.

Proprioceptive sensitivity refers to the child's response to joint or muscle movement, especially movement that is initiated by someone else. When movements are not self-initiated, no feed-forward mechanisms are involved; only the less efficient feed-back systems are used (see Praxis Section discussed later). Therefore no neurophysiological warning is given that the body is going to move. Movement by someone else could cause a negative response.

Emotional tone often is thought of as a purely psychological response; however, the sensory system antecedents of these behavioral responses need to be addressed. Children may have more or less than normal emotional variability because their sensory systems are not interpreting input in a normal fashion. All the systems we have discussed contribute to emotional tone. Overreactivity may lead to hyperactivity, anxiety, or chronic stress. Underreactivity may mimic depression (Table 7.2).

Functional Support Capabilities

These physical capabilities underlie and provide support for the end-product abilities. Functional support capabilities help integrate and modulate the input from the

Table 7.2   Sensory System Arousal Continues

Sensory System Arousal Levels	Functional Support Capabilities		
	Low	Normal	High
High	Hyperactive Sensory defensive Poor end-product ability levels	Hyperactive Sensory defensive Behavior problems No motor problems	Hyperactive Sensory defensive Cortical signs
Normal	Normal sensory modulation Normal attention Few behavior problems Motor problems	Normal sensory modulation Normal attention Good end-product ability levels Good motor skills	Normal sensory modulation Cortically based attention problems
Low	Underaroused to pain, etc. Poor end-product ability levels Poor motor skills May be hyperactive	Normal motor skills Slow adaptation	Slow adaptation Cortical problems

arousal/reactivity components of the sensory systems. They also integrate the information/discriminative components of these systems. The ten functional support capabilities are listed in Table 7.1.

Suck-swallow-breathe synchrony is a vital but often overlooked part of motor development. Appropriate muscle tone and stability need to develop in the tongue and jaw to allow nursing to occur with proper force as well as synchronization of swallowing and breathing. This process proceeds to development of intercostal and diaphragm stability for good breath support for articulation. Neck and eye stability also are involved. The initial coordination of eye muscles with regard to focusing and coordinating bilateral movements occurs during feeding, stimulated by the heavy work of sucking. Besides the muscles of the mouth, sucking also involves neck muscles as well as the diaphragm and intercostals. All these things provide support for biting, chewing, phonation, vocal abilities, and postural control.

A child who does not develop these abilities may show a pattern of shallow, rapid breathing because of poor development of or low tone in breathing musculature. This breathing pattern results in a sympathetic response resulting in increased arousal. Other problems include drooling, poor eating (bite, chew, and swallow), poor stability in the neck and trunk, poor articulation, and misuse of the large proximal muscles that fixate (to help with breathing) rather than move freely to develop skilled motion. Remember that the head is controlled by the cranial nerves—different sensory pathways than the rest of the body—so, each of these problems must be evaluated and treated separately (Oetter, Richter, & Frick, 1992).

Tactile discrimination is the ability to perceive through touch and to define the spatial and temporal qualities of the environment by touch. As previously discussed, tactile discrimination is thought to be mediated largely by the dorsal medial lemniscal system (body) and trigeminal system (head). It helps to provide a basis for the normal development of praxis.

Other discriminative abilities are involved. All the sensory systems have an information processing component that provides discriminative information to the CNS. Constant discriminative input from all sensory systems orients the person to the environment and defines the way to modify or change behavior.

Cocontraction (i.e., the simultaneous contraction of agonist and antagonistic muscles) stabilizes joints for action and use. Cocontraction contributes to balance and also is believed to help form the basis for the development of movement patterns for praxis (Figures 7.6A and 7.6B).

Muscle tone is the background level of muscle tension that is normal in everyone. Normal muscle tone also provides a basis for equilibrium, movement, and praxis.

Proprioception is the understanding of the body's position in space (consciously and unconsciously) based on feedback from joint, muscle, and skin receptors. Proprioception contributes to balance and equilibrium, muscle tone, and cocontraction.

Balance and equilibrium, as modulated by the vestibular system, is responsible for the ability to maintain posture and to move through the environment. Balance and equi-

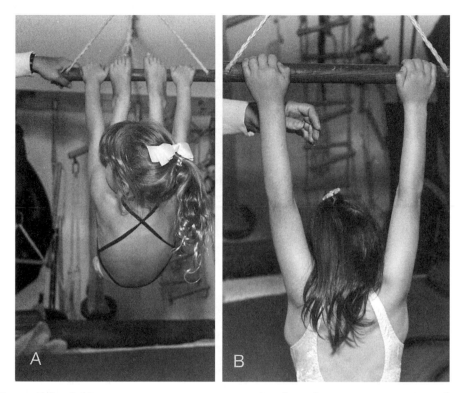

Figure 7.6 A, Mature response: note cocontraction throughout upper extremity and stable scapula; B, immature response: note holding on only with fingers and winging of scapular, indicating poor stability.

librium contribute significantly to all end-product abilities (Figures 7.7, 7.8A, and 7.8B).

Developmental reflexes are species-dependent movement patterns evoked by sensory input. Some human examples are protective extension of the arms when falling and the asymmetrical tonic neck reflex (Figures 7.9A and 7.9B). Developmental reflexes can contribute to integration of movement by being present or absent, appropriately. They depend on the age and developmental stage of the child and are influenced by arousal/registration level.

Lateralization involves the development of dominance in a hand, foot, and eye. The emergence of a dominant hand by the age of 5 or 6 years can signal that the brain has lateralized other functional abilities (e.g., language to the left hemisphere, perceptual abilities to the right hemisphere). The lack of a dominant hand may signal lack of lateralization.

Bilateral integration is the ability to use both hands together in activities. One indicator of bilateral integration is the ability to cross midline efficiently.

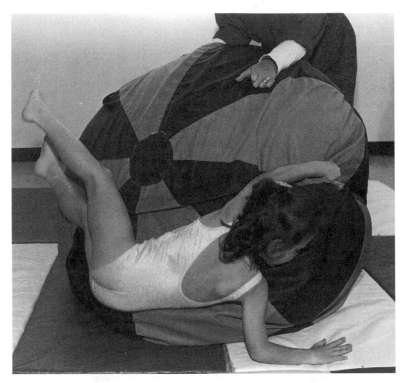

Figure 7.7 Less than optimal equilibrium response in prone position.

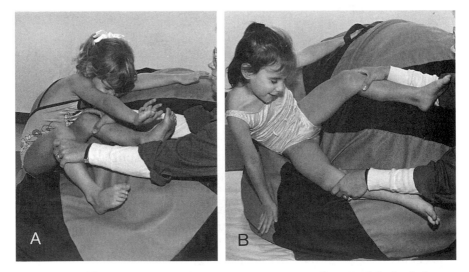

Figure 7.8 A, Mature response: balance reaction occurs in all parts of the body (even toes and trunk rotation) in response to balance challenge; B, immature response: only head responds to balance challenge (note low tone in legs, winging of scapula, and holding on with upper hand).

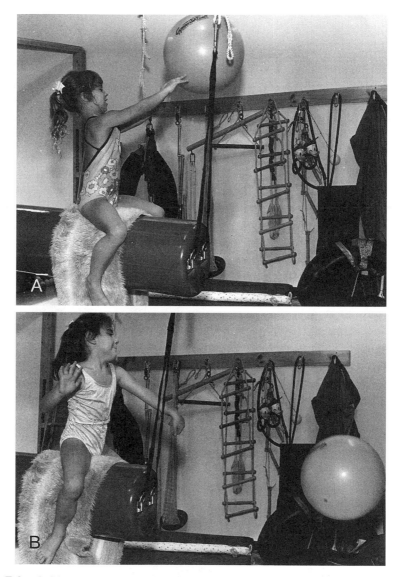

Figure 7.9 A, Mature response: child swinging on bolster swing can rotate trunk and use hands bilaterally and symmetrically to push large ball away; B, immature response: child swinging on a bolster swing uses straight plane movement (less mature than rotation), and asymmetrical tonic neck is apparent in arms on attempting to push ball away.

All functional support levels are rated on a scale, from poor to good to excellent, with the exception of muscle tone and developmental reflexes. Muscle tone is rated low, normal, or high, with low and high being abnormal. Developmental reflexes are rated hyporeflexive, normal, or hyperreflexive, with both extremes being abnormal.

End-Product Abilities

End-product abilities reflect integration of the sensory system modulation levels and functional support capabilities. The eight end-product abilities are listed on Table 7.1.

Praxis is often defined as motor planning, but it is much more. It is the ability to accomplish a nonhabitual motor act or the ability to coordinate the body through a complex movement that requires an adaptive response. According to Ayres (1985), "Praxis is a uniquely human skill that enables us to interact effectively with the physical world. It is one of the most critical links between brain and behavior. Praxis is to the physical world what speech is to the social world. Both enable interactions and transactions" (p. 1).

Praxis is complex and has been equated to motor intelligence. All aspects are detailed on the praxis figure (Figure 7.10) and include ideation or conceptualization; planning the course of action, including sequencing the actions; and, execution of adaptive responses.

This frame of reference assumes that praxis provides one basis for the development of academic abilities, behavior, articulation, emotional tone, and environmental mastery. Praxis probably is the most important organizational aspect of function

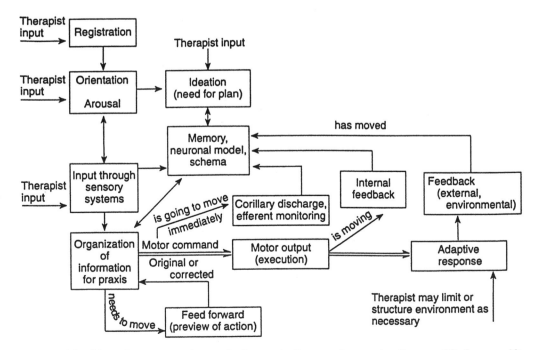

Figure 7.10 Neural processes that underlie praxis: Sensory Integration Frame of Reference. Kimball, 1988.

that a person is able to accomplish. Children who have praxis problems are said to show "developmental dyspraxia." Developmental dyspraxia is an impairment of ability during development and not a loss of praxic ability like a stroke patient might experience (apraxia).

Dyspraxic children are "clumsy," and the problem is based on a complex interaction of less than optimal sensory processing, less than optimal functional support capabilities, and less than optimal ideation. Praxis is not a question of whether the child can accomplish the movement but whether he or she can accomplish it with integration and quality.

In this frame of reference, dyspraxia is the major area of concern and is considered the most encompassing of all the problem areas. Specific knowledge of praxis, therefore, is important for understanding the client who has sensory integration problems. Children who have dyspraxia have difficulty with the initial planning of a nonhabitual movement. They then have trouble internalizing the plan for the movement and, finally, have difficulty transferring the motor learning to a new situation and extracting the common components from previous learning so that they need only learn the differences or additions. A common example for adult readers would be learning to drive. Initially, attention must be given to all movements, then the process becomes internalized, and, finally, it transfers to the ability to drive any car (with modifications made only for differences among cars). Compare this to the dyspraxic child who learns to roller skate. The child works much harder than a normal child to learn the skill. Long after the other children have learned, the dyspraxic child is still not as fluent in his or her movements and has difficulty with unexpected situations that require a "new wrinkle" in the movement pattern (e.g., a quick change in direction to avoid a child who has fallen in front of him while skating). The transferability of this skill to a new, similar situation, like ice skating, is more limited than with the normal child.

The praxis process (Figure 7.10) starts with the child's registration of, or his or her attention to, some change in the environment. Once the child has registered a change in the environment, orientation and arousal must take place. Orientation occurs after registration—a change in the environment—alerts the system to gather more information. This orientation is accompanied by a change in the arousal state and increased perceptual sensitivity. The child's system automatically makes a judgment about the significance of the stimuli being registered. This includes reallocation of attention and preparation for action.

Once the registration, orientation, and arousal have occurred, the situation is compared with established neuronal models by the CNS, allowing the child to move to ideation or to the realization of a need for a plan. At this point, the child begins organizing the information for movement—praxis—and may take in more input through the sensory systems to facilitate a better plan for action.

The first neuromechanism of the praxis sequence, that of feed-forward or a preview for action, comes at the point of organizing for praxis. Feed-forward is a neuromechanism that alerts the CNS to the need to move and compares the planned action with previous models to ascertain the possibility of success. Feed-forward is an important piece in the building of motor patterns. It contributes speed and efficiency to movement because "old" motor learning is utilized in a non-conscious way, which allows changes or additions to an established pattern. This makes movement more efficient, rather than moving as if each time were the first time the movement was made. After feed-forward, the CNS organizes a motor command and sends it forward. As the motor command is sent, afferent monitoring and corollary discharge occur. These signals alert the system that the child is going to move immediately. It is a preview monitoring of the command to move or an alerting of higher cortical centers that a command has been sent. Again there is a comparison with previous experience, and a decision is made whether to continue with the motor command as sent or to correct it before the execution has begun, which is again an efficient way for the nervous system to monitor itself to increase motor abilities quickly. Feed-forward and corollary discharge allow a child to use previous motor learning efficiently and only add or change what is needed for the new situation, rather than having to "relearn" movement each time he or she moves or only benefit from feedback after the fact. An example would be a child trying to learn to ski by falling. Feed-forward and corollary discharge are the systems a child uses when skiing along in a nice rhythm and suddenly seeing a rock right in his or her path where his or her movement patterns planned to take him or her. Without pausing to think about it, a child's body can change course so that his or her next movement pattern is a new one to avoid the rock. Feed-forward and corollary discharge have alerted the child's nervous system to the fact that changing the movement pattern would be a positive thing and enabled him or her to do this automatically, rather than taking time to think about it. If this neurologic mechanism did not occur, the child would hit the rock, and then receive "feedback" too late.

Once the motor execution has begun, internal feedback occurs. The CNS realizes that the body is moving, and, again, a comparison is made with previous experience. Neural models of organization for praxis are rechecked, and, if necessary, the motor command can be corrected midstream. For example, a child may speed up his or her steps because he or she notices that a door is closing fast; the child is aware that if he or she didn't speed up, the door may hit him or her. After the motor command is completed by accomplishing an adaptive response, feedback of an external or environmental nature occurs. The CNS realizes it has moved in a particular way and understands that it has or has not achieved the desired or adequate response (oops, I fell, what did I do wrong here?). The whole process is then stored in the neural model or memory for future use. The above process is mostly nonconscious and may take only milliseconds.

The building up of neuronal models through this sequence is an active process. If the child does not organize himself or herself for movement and does not originate and carry out the motor command and movement himself or herself, then the only mechanisms that will be called into action are external and environmental feedback. Feedback is an inefficient system and could be equated to learning how to rollerblade with the learning occurring only from falling down or "doing it wrong." Neuronal models are formed slowly and inefficiently with feedback only. This frame of reference assumes that if a child does not build neural models efficiently, then practicing a motor skill sometimes improves that motor skill but not the child's overall ability to coordinate or to extrapolate to other situations. In this frame of reference, the therapist's goal is to facilitate an active response from the child to build neuronal models. To achieve this, the therapist may add input at the following levels: registration, orientation, arousal, sensory systems, or ideation to facilitate a more appropriate adaptive response. The therapist also structures the environment to limit the complexity of the adaptive response to one within the child's developmental level.

The therapist must keep in mind at what level the problem occurs in the dyspraxic child. For example, if the problem is one of registration or arousal, the child may (1) not pay attention to the need to act on the environment, or (2) continually pay attention to the same stimulation so that no level of importance is assigned to it. This often is seen in autistic children who continually register an environmental stimulus (such as a moving object) without assigning significance.

Dyspraxia also may involve a problem in the ideation or understanding of the need for a plan. This may be seen in a child who attempts to accomplish an environmental action and accomplishes only a small piece of it. For example, a child swinging on a bolster swing has a ball thrown at him or her and allows the ball to hit him or her. The arousal may have occurred but the child did not understand that something needed to be done with the ball. Often, input through sensory systems, such as the vestibular, proprioceptive, and tactile systems, heightens the child's CNS ability to respond by summation over sensory systems. This assumption leads to one of the key treatment principles in sensory integration: Input from several sensory systems may be needed to achieve a registration or integration level sufficient for an adaptive response. For example, a child who has low muscle tone may not be able to balance himself or herself on a moving surface, but after linear swinging on a bolster swing, jumping on a trampoline, and receiving heavy proprioceptive activity to proximal limb joints and neck, the child may be able to balance and also catch a ball while balancing.

Although praxis is viewed as the most encompassing of the end-products in the sensory integration frame of reference, this does not mean that others are not important. When using the sensory integration frame of reference, therapists view all other end-product issues first through the sensory integration lens. For example, sensory defensiveness definitely influences behavioral issues such as compliance, socialization, and activity level. Activity level influences ability to attend; therefore sensory defensiveness affects academic mastery.

Praxis issues influence acquisition of ability to start, stop, and sequence, which influences all parts of academia. Praxis based on vestibular inefficiencies as reflected in low tone and poor cocontraction especially influences fine motor skills such as writing and skilled tool use. Poor praxis based on a combination of vestibular and tactile discrimination difficulties influences the development of form and space perception. All of these can lead to difficulty with environmental mastery and emotional tone.

Form and space perception skills are end-product skills that are thought to provide some basis for academic skills. Visual form and space perception can be broken down into various types, most of which are based on sensory motor processing deficits. Some children, however, show discrete visual spatial perception problems that are thought to be mediated by the right hemisphere.

Behavior as an end-product cannot be analyzed completely without the inclusion of the antecedent effects of sensory system modulation and functional support capabilities. Contrary to this perspective, psychologists view behavior mainly as an end-product of cognitive, social, and environmental interactions. In sensory integration, the sensory system antecedents must be evaluated for their own contributions before the psychosocial aspects are addressed. For example, a child who "loses it" and has a tantrum in the school cafeteria might be labeled as having a behavioral problem and be recommended for counseling with the school psychologist. An occupational therapist using a sensory integration approach might interpret at least some of the behavior to be indicative of sensory defensiveness, a response to being overloaded by the environment of the cafeteria. Another example is a child who "explodes for no apparent reason." A psychologist may recommend finding the issue that caused the explosion (the antecedent) and eliminate it, if possible. An occupational therapist using the sensory integration frame of reference may say that it does not matter what the antecedent was because any excitatory sensory input may set the child off because his or her nervous system is just below the threshold for overload. Intervention would involve decreasing the child's sensory defensiveness, thus keeping the nervous system modulated.

Academics—scholastic abilities—usually are viewed in relation to difficulties in other end-product abilities, such as language, form and space perception, behavior, activity level, and emotional tone. Recently, academics have begun to be studied in terms of the antecedent effects of sensory system modulation, functional support system capabilities, and praxis.

Language and articulation abilities usually are evaluated by speech therapists. Occupational therapists also can contribute understanding of the underlying antecedents for difficulties in language and articulation, which sometimes can be traced to problems in sensory system modulation, functional support capabilities, and end-product abilities. Muscle tone and cocontraction are areas of functional support capability that are related to language and articulation. If there are deficits in these two areas, the resultant effect can be a jutting forward of the chin, which makes articulation and swallowing difficult. The end-product component that is considered most important in this area is praxis. If the problem is one of articulation, the difficulty often lies in a praxis problem that can affect the speech musculature. This type of praxis problem includes difficulty in producing an appropriate adaptive response for sequencing. In addition, Ayres (1972a) has suggested that a pattern of language problems, particularly auditory language dysfunction, is related to left-hemisphere disorders.

Emotional tone, including stress level and self-esteem, is thought to be linked closely to sensory system modulation. If a number of components of sensory system modulation show overreactivity, then the person may be considered to be sensory defensive (Wilbarger & Royeen, 1987; Wilbarger & Wilbarger, 1991). Sensory defensiveness may result in behavioral and emotional problems, including anxiety. Some examples of this have been presented previously. Often seen is the need to remain extremely organized, bordering on compulsion, to keep the environment under control, and to add no more arousal to the already overaroused sensory systems.

Activity level, including self-control, relates to the person's ability to stay cognitively and motorically focused. Although activity level often is thought to be related only to cognitive attention behaviors by other frames of reference, in this frame of reference it is assumed to be related to modulation in all sensory systems. A high activity level can be functional and productive if the individual can remain focused. A dysfunctional activity level includes motor restlessness and lack of focus, which may be mistaken for impaired attention span or cognitive deficits.

Environmental mastery involves the ability to produce a suitable adaptive response with appropriate praxis, emotional tone, activity level, behavior, and academic level. Environmental mastery involves a total repertoire of adaptive responses that reflect the integration of all sensory systems, the functional support capabilities, and, to some extent, all components of the end-product abilities. The child who has environmental mastery also has sensory integration at all levels.

Most components of the end-product abilities are rated from poor to good to excellent. The exceptions are behavior and activity level. Behavior usually is rated as poor to good. Activity level is rated as underactive to normal to overactive. Over- and underactive activity levels are considered to be problematic.

POSTULATES OF THE SENSORY INTEGRATION THEORETICAL BASE

The evolving theoretical base of sensory integration presently includes 11 basic postulates. These postulates outline the elements that the occupational therapist must understand to apply this frame of reference. The postulates include the following:

1. Integration of sensory input is holistic (i.e., all systems influence each other and the whole).
2. The child's behaviors are influenced by the state of the CNS. There is a relationship between certain behaviors and underlying CNS dysfunctions or inefficiencies. Some behaviors can be related to a specific sensory system but

may be exhibited in a variety of ways. Unless the basic problems are addressed or treated, the resultant behaviors will continue. For example, in the tactile system, shirt tags may bother a child, but they may bother the child more when other sensory systems are overloaded (e.g., in a noisy cafeteria) because of a heightened sense of arousal.

3. The functioning of the underlying sensory systems determines the quality of adaptive responses.

4. For integration to occur, meaningful registration of sensory input is required. Integration is reflected in an adaptive response.

5. When the child makes an appropriate adaptive response, this contributes further to the development of general sensory integrative abilities.

6. The child needs to be self-directed to act on the environment for the greatest potential change to occur in the underlying neurologic organization and to result in an adaptive response.

7. Adaptive responses that are within the child's abilities should be used; therefore the child's developmental level must be assessed. These adaptive responses should be at the upper limits of the child's abilities to facilitate growth.

8. Sensory integration difficulties may arise from problems in two distinct areas: sensory system modulation levels and functional support capabilities. Either one or a combination of the two results in end-product ability problems.

9. Intervention is specific to the underlying deficits; it is not specific to behaviors. As adaptive responses become more organized, the child's behavior becomes more organized.

10. The child's behaviors can be modified through appropriate controlled sensory inputs that elicit or facilitate adaptive responses. Responses should be motor, emotional, and ideational ones.

11. Input from several sensory systems may be needed to achieve the registration level (arousal or inhibition) or integration level appropriate for an adaptive response.

FUNCTION/DYSFUNCTION CONTINUA

The theoretical base of sensory integration provides the basis for decision making in evaluation and intervention. In sensory integration, understanding function/dysfunction of sensory systems helps the therapist to determine the severity of the problem and to indicate the multiple systems that need to be addressed. Three function/dysfunction continua are (1) sensory modulation; (2) functional support capabilities; and (3) end-product abilities (see Table 7.1). This chapter will discuss function/dysfunction continua, guide to evaluation, and application to practice.

Indicators of Function and Dysfunction: Sensory System Modulation

The way in which the sensory systems process input affects the quality of a child's ability to respond adaptively. Moderate reactivity results in an optimal adaptive response. Overreactivity/high arousal results in disorganization and even in anxiety or a negative emotional response. Underreactivity/low arousal results in partial or ineffective responses. When arousal gets too high, the child responds as if to a serious survival threat. If it is not possible to fight or flee, then the arousal does not dissipate easily, causing stress, anxiety, and difficulty in completing other adaptive responses. Persons who have sensory system modulation problems have more changeable reactivity/arousal levels than normal persons. The result can be problems with adaptive response because their systems lack stability. The sensory systems do not function independently. Arousal in each of several systems can combine, therefore, to produce high arousal, just as inhibition in several systems can combine to produce low arousal. The arousal or reactivity levels as well as the information processing components of each system need to be assessed. Remember that in sensory systems either under- or overarousal is dysfunctional. It should be noted that the theoretical base as previously presented, the function/dysfunction continuum of modulation, guide to evaluation, postulates regarding change, and application to practice related to this continuum can stand alone as a frame of reference for treating children with sensory defensiveness and sensory modulation problems (Chart 7.1).

Indicators of Function and Dysfunction: Functional Support Capabilities

These physical capabilities underlie and provide support for the end-product abilities. Functional support capabilities help integrate the input from the sensory systems. Furthermore, they can be used to help modulate and provide balance to the sensory systems (Chart 7.2).

Indicators of Function and Dysfunction: End-Product Abilities

End-product abilities reflect integration of sensory system modulation and functional support levels. All these end-product ability levels can be scored on a poor to excellent continuum of function/dysfunction (Chart 7.3).

GUIDE TO EVALUATION

A therapist who uses the sensory integration frame of reference first filters the client's difficulties through that lens, then goes on to use other forms of remediation to compliment this frame of reference if a sensory integration problem is found. Few

Chart 7.1   Indicators of Function and Dysfunction for Sensory System Modulation.

Underregistration	Normal Response	Overregistration
INDICATORS OF DYSFUNCTION	**INDICATORS OF FUNCTION**	**INDICATORS OF DYSFUNCTION**
Tactile System May not feel pain May not be aware of injury May not differentiate among types of touch	*Tactile System* Likes light touch Differentiates types of touch Discriminates and integrates touch from people, objects, animals, and clothing	*Tactile System* Reacts negatively to light touch Perceives light touch as painful or irritating May not tolerate touch from certain types of clothing, objects, animals or people
Auditory System May not orient to noises; no startle to loud sounds	*Auditory System* Orients to noises, then reacts appropriately	*Auditory System* Overly distracted by noises Startles easily to sounds Upset at or appears annoyed by normal level sounds
Relationship to Gravity No respect for heights, falling or moving fast or moving in dangerous ways, even if caution is warranted	*Relationship to Gravity* Normal, respectful caution in dangerous-movement–related situations	*Relationship to Gravity* Real fear, anxiety or intense emotional reaction in response to movement situations that should only require alerting or changes in body/head position
Movement Level Slow moving or appears to conserve movement	*Movement Level* Normal amount of movement	*Movement Level* Appears to be moving constantly
Oral Arousal Will put anything into mouth Does not seem to be bothered by inappropriate items after the age at which he should be aware of inappropriateness	*Oral Arousal* Dislikes a few items because of texture but normally will allow food products to enter the mouth; reacts because of taste Discriminating with objects not appropriate for mouth	*Oral Arousal* Overly sensitive to texture of items placed in mouth Refuses many foods because of texture, not taste Dislikes objects in mouth (i.e., toothbrush, dentist's fingers or drill) Uses heavy chewing to calm self Chews on inappropriate things such as blankets
Olfactory Arousal Appears not to notice odors, even dangerous ones such as smoke	*Olfactory Arousal* Normal response to odors	*Olfactory Arousal* Very responsive to odors Odors may make child upset or nauseous Odor may give negative "flashbacks"
Visual System Underresponsive to changes in the visual field Underresponsive to objects that enter the visual field Underresponsive to changes in movement and color even though visual acuity is normal	*Visual System* Normally orients to changes in the visual field	*Visual System* Orients persistently to objects that are common (not unusual) in the visual field Difficulty habituating visually
Attention Level Appears to pay little or no attention to environmental changes that require an active intervention or response	*Attention Level* Normal level of attention	*Attention Level* Appears to be reacting constantly to stimuli Some reaction to stimuli may be movement-related but also includes all other sensory systems

—*continued*

Chart 7.1 Indicators of Function and Dysfunction for Sensory System Modulation—(Continued)		
Underregistration	**Normal Response**	**Overregistration**
INDICATORS OF DYSFUNCTION	**INDICATORS OF FUNCTION**	**INDICATORS OF DYSFUNCTION**
Postrotary Nystagmus Does not show dizziness or shows decreased dizziness after rotary movement (referred to as depressed postrotary nystagmus)	*Postrotary Nystagmus* Becomes dizzy normally after rotary movement	*Postrotary Nystagmus* Becomes overly dizzy after rotary movement (referred to as prolonged postrotary nystagmus)
Sensitivity to Movement Tolerates excessive amounts of rotary or angular acceleration without autonomic nervous system response	*Sensitivity to Movement* Tolerates some rotary or angular acceleration, and then needs to stop because of autonomic response	*Sensitivity to Movement* Tolerates little or no rotary or angular acceleration without having autonomic nervous system response (usually of nausea or "feeling funny")
Proprioceptive Sensitivity Does not appear to "feel" some limb and muscle positions or movements	*Proprioceptive Sensitivity* Normal registration and responses to proprioceptive input provided externally	*Proprioceptive Sensitivity* Overly sensitive to joint and muscle movement provided externally Very aware of movements of limbs
Emotional Arousal Shows decreased levels of emotions or the expression of them	*Emotional Arousal* Normal expression of emotions	*Emotional Arousal* Becomes upset by items that might be considered trivial by most other people

therapists use sensory integration exclusively but most would want to ascertain if sensory integration problems are present before using another frame of reference. An underlying sensory integration deficit frequently will not respond to other types of interventions. Sensory integration is a way of understanding the nervous system functionally, and its use helps make other treatment modalities more effective.

Children referred to occupational therapy for suspected sensory integrative problems may present particular behaviors that often are interpreted as aberrant or as cortically-based dysfunction. Such children are sometimes referred to physicians or psychologists before they are referred to an occupational therapist. These behaviors are presented in Appendix 7A. This is particularly true of sensory defensiveness where symptoms are often mistakenly diagnosed as psychologically-based behavioral disorders. The occupational therapist may be the first to identify sensory defensiveness. Only in the orderly association of apparently nonconnected symptoms can sensory defensiveness be clearly identified. It should be kept in mind that several symptoms together are indicative of sensory integrative dysfunction; one isolated symptom is not.

The evaluation of children for sensory integrative dysfunction is an intricate process. It requires that therapists be knowledgeable in this specific area and be well grounded in their understanding of development. Often children who are referred to an occupational therapist for evaluation already have been seen by several other professionals. The possible causes of the child's behaviors or motor deficits should be evaluated at all levels.

Chart 7.2 Indicators of Function and Dysfunction for Functional Support Capabilities.

Specific Functional Capabilities: Normal Response	Poorly Developed Capabilities
INDICATORS OF FUNCTION	**INDICATORS OF DYSFUNCTION**

Suck-Swallow-Breathe
Can synchronize suck-swallow-breathe patterns
Has good muscle tone stability and coordination in all
   suck-swallow-breathe mechanisms
	Suck-Swallow-Breathe
	Experiences difficulty with suck-swallow-breathe synchrony
	Muscle tone and stability are not developed enough to allow
	   good coordination of suck-swallow-breathe mechanisms

Tactile Discrimination Ability to identify various shapes, textures, sizes by touch alone Good two-point discrimination Good conscious proprioception (kinesthesia) Uses touch for information gathering	*Tactile Discrimination* Not able to differentiate objects haptically or cannot identify accurately by touch alone Poor two-point discrimination Poor conscious proprioception (kinesthesia) Poor differentiation of touch for information gathering

Other Discriminating Abilities
Auditory Discrimination
Ability to use auditory system for information gathering
Relationship to Gravity
Normal balance response to change in head/body position in
   relation to gravity
Postrotary Nystagmus
Discriminates amount of dizziness
	Other Discriminating Abilities
	Auditory Discrimination
	Poor ability to use auditory system for information gathering in
	   spite of normal hearing
	Relationship to Gravity
	Inefficient registration of change in head/body signaling;
	   equilibrium/balance response needed
	Postrotary Nystagmus
	Difficulty in discriminating amount of dizziness

Movement Level Movement goal-directed, focused	*Movement Level* Much non-goal-directed movement, unfocused
Oral Discrimination Can discriminate taste and texture	*Oral Discrimination* Poor oral discrimination of taste and texture
Olfactory Discrimination Can discriminate odors	*Olfactory Discrimination* Poor differentiation of odors
Visual Discriminate Good visual discrimination Good visual acuity	*Visual Discriminate* Poor acuity: uses glasses Poor discrimination

Proprioceptive Discrimination
Use proprioceptive abilities to discriminate force, velocity, and
   direction of movement
	Proprioceptive Discrimination
	Is unable to judge force, velocity, or direction of movements
	   accurately

Attention Level Can attend well to take in more/new information	*Attention Level* Unable to attend well to take in new information
Emotional Discrimination Discriminates meaning and expression of emotion in self and others	*Emotional Discrimination* Difficulty in using emotional expression as a guide for action

Cocontraction
Ability to cocontract muscles around the joint so that the joint
   may be stabilized for action
	Cocontraction
	Inability to cocontract muscles around the joints so that there is
	   less than normal stabilization

Muscle Tone Normal tone for stability of normal movement patterns	*Muscle Tone* Low muscle tone; floppy tone Tone does not provide enough stability for some normal movement patterns
Balance and Equilibrium Good balance abilities Usually exhibited in good overall coordination	*Balance and Equilibrium* Difficulties in catching balance

—continued

Chart 7.2 Indicators of Function and Dysfunction for Functional Support Capabilities—(Continued)

Specific Functional Capabilities: **Normal Response**	**Poorly Developed Capabilities**
INDICATORS OF FUNCTION	**INDICATORS OF DYSFUNCTION**
Developmental Reflexes	*Developmental Reflexes*
Reflexes are "integrated" into movement, and are not obligatory	Difficulty moving against gravity volitionally
	May be obligatory movements in postures (e.g., asymmetrical tonic neck reflex with head turning)
	Certain positions or movements may cause child to assume a particular posture (e.g., back arching in supine position)
Lateralization	*Lateralization*
Eye, hand, and foot dominance all the same	No or mixed dominance
Bilateral Integration	*Bilateral Integration*
Smooth crossing of midline with eyes and hands	Hands do not cross midline well
	Eyes blink, gaze shifts, or eyes jerk when eyes cross midline

---

The clinical observations suggested in this chapter should be conducted in a standardized procedure (Dunn, 1981; Harris, 1981; Wilson, Pollack, Kaplan, & Law, 1994). Clinical observations, histories, and checklists and some standardized tests can be done by entry-level therapists. It is suggested that therapists should have some educational background in test administration and measurement before using standardized evaluations. The administration and interpretation of the SCSIT (Ayres, 1972b), SCPNT (Ayres, 1975a), and SIPT (Ayres, 1980) require additional education. These are not considered entry-level occupational therapy skills and have been designed for therapists who have post professional degrees and clinical experience. There are extensive training programs, including certifications, that teach the administration and interpretation of these tests. Evaluation reports from other professionals may require interpretation by those specialized professionals. The occupational therapist is responsible, however, for interpreting the findings relative to this frame of reference.

When evaluating a child, the therapist may notice that problems in the sensory system modulation level often result in sensory defensiveness. Problems in functional support capabilities often result in decreased functional abilities. Both problems—those in the sensory modulation level and functional support capabilities—influence the end-product ability levels. Although all end-product ability levels are important to the occupational therapist, one of primary concern is praxis, with the second concern being behavioral problems.

Evaluation of sensory integrative problems involves a systematic appraisal of the child's functioning. Appendix 7B and Appendix 7C will help organize thinking during evaluation. The outline in Appendix B helps to organize results.

Chart 7.3   Indicators of Function and Dysfunction for End-Product Abilities.

Normal Response End-Product Abilities	Poorly Developed End-Product Abilities
INDICATORS OF FUNCTION	**INDICATORS OF DYSFUNCTION**
Praxis	*Praxis*
Ability to organize for nonhabitual movement to accomplish an appropriate adaptive response	Difficulty in organizing for movement or accomplishing an appropriate adaptive response
	Difficulty at any of the levels of integration may be seen in organization, sequencing, internalizing, or accomplishing the appropriate adaptive response
Form and Space Perception	*Form and Space Perception*
Able to use form and space perception effectively to produce adaptive responses	Difficulty in understanding and interpreting spatial relationships and figure-ground
	Contribution to difficulty with reading or math
Behavior	*Behavior*
Behaves appropriately in relationship to age, situation, and environment	Inappropriate behavior in relationship to age, situation, or environment
Academics	*Academics*
Functioning at or above ability level	Functioning below ability level
Language and Articulation	*Language and Articulation*
Language use is at age level	Language use is below age level
Articulation is at age-appropriate level	Articulation is worse than peers with no apparent structural cause
Emotional Tone	*Emotional Tone*
Emotional tone is balanced	Difficulty with emotional tone
Self-esteem is good and appropriate for age	Inadequate self-esteem
May be compulsively organized	May be sensory defensive
Activity Level	*Activity Level*
Normal activity level for age level	Low activity level that may look like depression
Demonstrates appropriate self-control for age level	High activity level without focus; poor self-control
Environmental Mastery	*Environmental Mastery*
Produces a suitable adaptive response with appropriate praxis, emotional tone, activity level, behavior, and academic performance	Demonstrates inappropriate adaptive responses or poor response with inappropriate praxis, emotional tone, activity level, behavior, or academic performance
Understands and functions within the environment at an age-appropriate level	Difficulty in understanding and functioning within the environment at an age-appropriate level

Evaluation of Sensory System Modulation Levels

Sensory modulation and defensiveness are the first areas that must be addressed during the evaluation. Once such problems are identified and intervention for these deficit areas has begun, other sensory integration problems identified in the evaluation process may appear to be as severe. Helping children to achieve an appropriate modulation level allows them to use all of their resources at an optimum level to achieve better results in functional support capabilities and end-products.

The following assessments are suggested for the sensory system modulation continuum.

General (all systems)
- Touch inventory for elementary school aged children (TIE) (Royeen, 1987; Royeen & Fortune, 1990)
- Sensory motor history (Ayres Clinic, 1971)
- Sensory history (Wilbarger & Oetter, 1989; Wilbarger & Wilbarger, 1991)
- Clinical Observation of Motor and Postural Skills (Wilson, Pollack, Kaplan, & Law, 1994)
- Clinical observations
- Tactile defensiveness checklist (Royeen, 1986)
- Overall sensory motor history
- Evaluation of sensory defensiveness (Wilbarger & Wilbarger, 1991)
- Sensory Profile (Dunn & Westman, 1997)

Specific

Relationship to Gravity
- Clinical observations, including equilibrium reactions in supine, sitting, and prone positions and reaction to moving equipment

Attention Level
- Observation
- Teacher report
- Parent report
- Physician report
- Postrotary Nystagmus
- SCPNT (Ayres, 1976; Kimball, 1981)

Sensitivity to Movement
- Clinical observations on the SCPNT
- Observations during other clinical observations
- Parent report

Emotional Arousal Level
- Psychological assessment

Evaluation of Functional Support Capabilities

The child with poor functional support capabilities will have difficulty with accomplishing end-products successfully. Identification of functional support problems results in helpful explanations as to why a particular child cannot accomplish something or achieve success in particular tasks. For example, a child with low muscle tone and poor cocontraction may appear weak in some situations and not in others. This can be baffling to parents until it is explained that the child looks weak in mid-range movements requiring the coordination of two muscle groups (cocontraction) but strong in activities where only one muscle group is used (as in full elbow extension or flexion).

The following assessments are suggested for the functional support capabilities.

Suck-Swallow-Breathe

- Evaluation of oral mechanisms (Oetter, Richter, & Frick, 1992)

Tactile Discrimination

- SIPT (Ayres, 1989)
- Teacher and parent reports

Cocontraction

- Clinical observations (Dunn, 1981; Fisher & Bundy, 1989)
- Muscle tone

Proprioception

- Clinical observations (Dunn, 1981)

Balance and Equilibrium

- Clinical observations (Dunn, 1981; Fisher & Bundy, 1989)
- Standing balance eyes open and closed, SIPT (Ayres, 1989)
- Bruininks Oseretsky Test of Motor Proficiency (Bruininks, 1978)

Developmental Reflexes

- Clinical observations
- Parent report

Lateralization

- Clinical observations
- Parent report

Bilateral Integration

- SIPT (Ayres, 1989)

Evaluation of End-Product Ability Levels

Dyspraxia is the key area of concern for the occupational therapist in the sensory integration frame of reference. It also is the most encompassing of the end-product problem areas and often influences other end-product abilities. Therefore, specific understanding of praxis is important in evaluating the child who demonstrates sensory integrative problems. The use of the praxis chart (Figure 7.10) and the clinical reasoning process (see Appendix 7D) helps the therapist to organize his or her thinking about the child's response. Furthermore, it helps the therapist to pinpoint where the problem occurs for the child. For example, using Figure 7.10, is the problem in registration, arousal, ideation, handling more or different sensory input, or responding to the limitation or structure of the environment?

The following assessments are suggested for end-product ability

Praxis

- SIPT (Ayres, 1989)
- Parent report
- Teacher report

Form and Space Perception

- SIPT (Ayres, 1989)
- Developmental Test of Visual-Motor Integration (DTVI) (Beery, 1989)
- Motor Free Visual Perception Test (MVPT) (Colarusso & Hammill, 1972)
- Parent report
- Teacher report
- Test of Visual-Perceptual Skills (nonmotor) (Gardner, 1988)
- Behavior
- Clinical observations
- Parent report
- Teacher report
- Psychological evaluation

Academics

- School reports, including report cards
- Teacher report
- Educational assessment done by teacher and/or school psychologist (i.e., Wechsler Intelligence Scale for Children Revised, 1974; Kaufman Assessment Battery for Children [Kaufman & Kaufman, 1983])

Language and Articulation

- Evaluation is done by the speech pathologist
- Observations

Emotional Tone

- Observations
- Psychological report
- Social worker report
- Parent report
- Teacher report

Activity Level

- Observation
- Psychologist report
- Physician report
- Parent report
- Teacher report

Environmental Mastery

- Observation
- Child self-report
- Parent report
- Teacher report

References

Ayres, A. J. (1965). Patterns of perceptual-motor dysfunction in children: a factor analytic study. *Perceptual and Motor Skills, 20,* 335–368.

Ayres, A. J. (1966a). Interrelations among perceptual-motor abilities in a group of normal children. *American Journal of Occupational Therapy, 20,* 288–292.

Ayres, A. J. (1966b). Interrelations among perceptual-motor functions in children. *American Journal of Occupational Therapy, 20,* 68–71.

Ayres, A. J. (1969). Deficits in sensory integration in educationally handicapped children. *Journal of Learning Disabilities, 2,* 160–168.

Ayres, A. J. (1971). *Sensory motor history.* Torrance, CA: Ayres Clinic.

Ayres, A. J. (1972a). *Sensory integration and learning disorders.* Los Angeles: Western Psychological Services.

Ayres, A. J. (1972b). *Southern California sensory integration tests manual.* Los Angeles: Western Psychological Services.

Ayres, A. J. (1972c). Improving academic scores through sensory integration. *Journal of Learning Disabilities, 5,* 338–343.

Ayres, A. J. (1972d). Types of sensory integrative dysfunction among disabled learners. *American Journal of Occupational Therapy, 26,* 13–18.

Ayres, A. J. (1975a). *Southern California postrotary nystagmus test manual.* Los Angeles: Western Psychological Services.

Ayres, A. J. (1975b). Sensorimotor foundations of academic ability. In W. M. Cruickshank & D. P. Hallahan (Eds.) *Perceptual and learning disabilities in children* Vol. 2 (pp. 301–338). Syracuse, NY: Syracuse University Press.

Ayres, A. J. (1976). The effect of sensory integrative therapy on learning disabled children: The final report of a research project. Los Angeles: University of Southern California.

Ayres, A. J. (1978). Learning disabilities and the vestibular system. *Journal of Learning Disabilities, 11,* 18–29.

Ayres, A. J. (1979). *Sensory integration and the child.* Los Angeles: Western Psychological Services.

Ayres, A. J. (1980). *Southern California tests of sensory integration tests manual: (Rev. ed.).* Los Angeles: Western Psychological Services.

Ayres, A. J. (1985). *Developmental dyspraxia and adult-onset apraxia.* Torrance, CA: Sensory Integration International.

Ayres, A. J. (1989). *Sensory integration and praxis tests.* Los Angeles: Western Psychological Services.

Beery, E. (1989). *The developmental test of visual-motor integration* (3rd rev. ed.). Cleveland, OH: Modern Curriculum.

Bender, L. (1938). *A visual-motor gestalt test and its clinical use* (Res. Mon. No.3). New York: American Orthopsychiatric Association.

Bruininks, R. H. (1978). *Bruininks-Oseretsky test of motor proficiency examiner's manual.* Circle Pines, MN: American Guidance Service.

Chusid, J.G. (1979). *Correlative neuroanatomy and functional neurology* (17th ed.). Los Altos, CA: Lange Medical Publishers.

Clark, F. A., Mailloux, Z., and Parham, D. (1989). Sensory integration and children with learning disabilities. In P. N. Pratt and A. S. Allen (Eds.). *Occupational therapy for children* (2nd ed.) (pp. 457–507). St. Louis: C.V. Mosby.

Colarusso, R. P., and Hammill, D. D. (1972). *Motor free visual perception test.* Novato, CA: Academic Therapy.

Daube, J. R., Reagan, T. J., Sandok, B. A., and Westmoreland, B. F. (1986). *Medical neuroscience.* Boston: Little, Brown.

DeGangi, G., and Greenspan, S.I. (1989). *Test of sensory functions in infants.* Los Angeles, CA: Western Psychological Services.

DeGroot, J. and Chusid, J.G. (1988). Correlative neuroanatomy (12th ed.). Connecticut: Appleton and Lange.

DeQuiros, J.B., and Schrager, O. L. (1979). *Neuropsychological fundamentals in learning disabilities* (rev. ed.). Novato, CA: Academic Therapy.

Dubner, R. (1991). Neuronal plasticity and pain following peripheral tissue inflammation or nerve injury. Proceedings of the VIth World Congress on Pain. New York, NY: Elsevier Science Publishers BV.

Dunn, W. (1981). *A guide to clinical observation in kindergartners.* Rockville, MD: American Occupational Therapy Association.

Dunn, W., and Westman, K. (1997). The sensory profile: The performance of a national sample of children with disabilities. *American Journal of Occupational Therapy, 51,* 25–34.

Farber, S. D. (1982). *Neurorehabilitation: A multisensory approach.* Philadelphia: W. B. Saunders.

Farber, S. D. (1989, May). Neuroscience and occupational therapy: Vital connections. Eleanor Clark Slagle Lectureship at the American Occupational Therapy Association Annual Conference, Baltimore, MD.

Fisher, A. G., and Dunn, W. (1983). Tactile defensiveness: Historical perspectives, new research: A theory grow. *Sensory Integration Special Interest Section Newsletter, 6*(2), 1–2.

Fisher, A. G., and Bundy, A.C. (1989). Vestibular stimulation in the treatment of postural and related disorders. In O. D. Payton, R. P. Fabio, S. V. Paris, E. J. Protas, and A. F. Van Sant (Eds.), *Manual of physical therapy techniques* (pp. 239–258). New York: Churchill-Livingstone.

Fisher, A. G., Murray, E. A., and Bundy, A. C. (1991). *Sensory integration theory and practice.* Philadelphia, PA: F. A. Davis.

Fitzgerald, M. (1991). The developmental neurobiology of pain. Proceedings of the VIth World Congress on Pain. New York, NY: Elsevier Science Publishers BV.

Gardner, M. F. (1988). *Test of visual-perceptual skills (non-motor).* San Francisco, CA: Health Publishing Co., Children's Hospital.

Gold, P. W., Goodwin, F. K., Chrousos, G. P. (August 11, 1988). Clinical and biochemical manifestations of depression: relations to the neurobiology of stress, (Part I). *New England Journal of Medicine.*

Gold, P. W., Goodwin, F. K., Chrousos, G. P. (August 18, 1988). Clinical and biochemical manifestations of depression: relations to the neurobiology of stress, (Part II). *New England Journal of Medicine.*

Harris, N. P. (1981). The duration and quality of the prone extension position in 4, 6, and 8 year old normal children. *American Journal of Occupational Therapy, 35,* 27–29.

Kandel, E. R. and Schwartz, J. H. (1985). *Principles of neural science.* New York: Elsevier.

Kaufman A. S., and Kaufman, N. L. (1983). *Kaufman assessment battery for children.* Circle Pines: American Guidance Service.

Kimball, J. G. (1976). Vestibular stimulation and seizure activity. Center for the Study of Sensory Integrative Dysfunction Newsletter (now Sensory Integration International), July, Torrance, CA.

Kimball, J. G. (1977). Case History Follow Up Report, Center for The Study of Sensory Integrative Dysfunction Newsletter (now Sensory Integrative International), Torrance, CA.

Kimball, J. G. (1981). Normative comparison of the Southern California Postrotary Nystagmus Test: Los Angeles vs. Syracuse data. *American Journal of Occupational Therapy, 34,* 21–25.

Kimball, J. G. (1986). Prediction of methylphenidate (ritalin) responsiveness through sensory integrative testing. *American Journal of Occupational Therapy, 40,* 241–248.

Kimball J. G. (1988). Hypothesis for production of stimulant drug effectiveness utilizing sensory integrative diagnostic methods. *Journal of the American Osteopathic Association, 88,* 757–762.

Kimball, J. G. (1990). Using the sensory integration and praxis tests to measure change: a pilot study. *American Journal of Occupational Therapy, 44,* 603–608.

Kimball, J. G. (1991). Personal case records, Scarborough, ME. Larson, K. A. (1982). The sensory history of developmentally delayed children with and without tactile defensiveness. *American Journal of Occupational Therapy, 36,* 590–596.

Melzack, R., and Wall P. D. (1965). Pain mechanisms: A new theory. *Science, 150,* 971–979.

Montagu, A. (1978). *Touching: The human significance of the skin.* New York: Harper & Row.

Moore, J. C. (1990). Highlights of neurological development and functioning. In. E. M. Gilfoyle, A. Grady, and J. C. Moore (Eds.) *Children adapt.* (pp.33–85) Thorofare, NJ: Slack.

Nieuwenhuys, R., Voogd, J., and Van Huijzen, C. (1988). *The human central nervous system.* New York: Springer-Verlag.

Oetter, P., Richter, E., and Frick, S. (1992). *MORE integrating the mouth with sensory and postural function.* Hugo, MN: PDP Products.

Pribam, K. (1975). Arousal, activation and effort in the control of attention. *Psychological Review, 82,* 116–149.

Routtenberg, A. (1968). The two arousal hypothesis: reticular formation and limbic system. *Psychological Review, 75,* 1, 51–80.

Royeen, C. B. (1985). Domain specifications of the construct tactile defensiveness. *American Journal of Occupational Therapy, 39*(9), 596–599.

Royeen, C. B. (1986). Development of a scale measuring tactile defensiveness. *American Journal of Occupational Therapy, 46,* 414–419.

Royeen, C. B. (1987). Test-retest reliability of a touch scale for tactile defensiveness in children. *Physical and Occupational Therapy in Pediatrics, 7*(3), 45–52.

Royeen, C. B., and Fortune, J. C. (1990). TIE: Touch inventory for school aged children. *American Journal of Occupational Therapy, 44,* 155–160.

Sagan, C. (1977). *Dragons of Eden.* New York: Random House.

Wall, P. D. (1970). *Sensory of impulses traveling in the dorsal columns.* Brain, 93, 505–524.

Wechsler, D. (1974). *Intelligence scale for children revised.* New York: Psychological Corporation.

Wilbarger, P. (1984). Planning an adequate "sensory diet"—application of sensory processing theory during the first year of life. *Zero to three,* Sept, 1991, 7–12.

Wilbarger, P. (1991). Occupational therapy: sensory defensiveness, 60-minute video, PDP Products, Hugo, MN.

Wilbarger, P., and Oetter, P. (October, 1989). Sensory processing disorders. Paper presented at the American Occupational Therapy Association Practice Symposium, St. Louis, MO.

Wilbarger, P., and Royeen, C. B. (May, 1987). Tactile defensiveness: Theory, applications and treatment. Annual Interdisciplinary Doctoral Conference, Sargent College, Boston University.

Wilbarger, P., & Wilbarger, J. (1991). Sensory defensiveness in children 2–12. Santa Barbara, CA: Avanti Education Programs.

Wilcox, G. L. (1991). Excitatory neurotransmitters and pain. In M. R. Bond, J. E. Charlton, & C. J. Woolf, (Eds). *Proceedings of the VIth World Congress on Pain.* New York, NY: Elsevier Science Publishers BV.

Wilson, B. N., Pollack, N., Kaplan, B., & Law, M. (1994). *Clinical observations of motor and postural skills.* Tucson, AZ: Therapy Skill Builders.

Wilson-Pauwels, L., Akesson, E., & Stewart, P. (1988). *Cranial nerves.* Philadelphia, PA: B.C. Becker, Inc.

Woolf, C. J. (1991). Central mechanisms of acute pain. In M. R. Bond, J. E. Charlton, & C. J. Woolf (Eds). *Proceedings of the VIth World Congress on Pain.* New York, NY: Elsevier Science Publishers BV.

Presenting Problems: Children with Suspected Sensory Integration Dysfunction

For the identification of sensory systems dysfunction, several symptoms must occur together.

INFANCY

Irritable baby
Low muscle tone
Poor sleep cycles
May dislike being held
May dislike being on back
May startle easily
Slow development or less than normal quality of movement

TODDLER

Above may continue with the addition of the following:
Short attention span
Clumsiness
Poor articulation
Overly upset by slight injury
Fear of walking on some surfaces
Fear of slides and other movements
Very messy eater
Slow language development
Rejects many foods because of texture

CHILDHOOD PRE KINDERGARTEN TO 3RD GRADE

Above may continue with the addition of the following:
Fine motor problems (i.e., hand writing, cutting, coloring)
Hyperactivity
Poor social skills
Impulsiveness
Cries easily
Dislikes textures (i.e., fingerpaint, food)
Difficulties in gross motor activities
Falls easily

Often accidentally breaks toys during play
Strong dislike for certain types of clothing

MIDDLE CHILDHOOD 4TH TO 6TH GRADE

Above continues with the additions of the following:
Increased academic problems and attention
Behavioral problems
Poorly or compulsively organized
Reversals in writing and reading
Trouble keeping up with peers in activities

PRE-ADOLESCENCE

Above may continue with the additions of the following:
Organization problems
Trouble finishing homework or maintaining attention to task
Immature in physical skills and social relationships
More pronounced behavioral problems (i.e., acts out, picks fights)
Loses or forgets things
Often socially isolated
Chooses individual sports (i.e., running, swimming)
Chooses heavy contact sports (i.e., football, soccer)
Avoids team sports (i.e., basketball, baseball)
May be overly emotional

A P P E N D I X   7 B

Occupational Therapy Evaluation of Sensory Integrative Abilities

Name_____   Referred by _____

Test Date _____

Date of Birth _____

Chronological Age _____

Presenting Problem _____

_____

_____

_____

_____

_____

_____

I. Sensory Systems Modulation/Sensory Defensiveness

System	Indicators	Summary	Sensory Defensiveness Present
Tactile			
Auditory			
Vestibular			
Relation to gravity			
Movement level			
PRNT			
Sensitivity to movement			
Oral			
Olfactory			
Visual			
Attention			
Proprioception			
Emotion			

II. Information/Discriminative System

System	Indicators	Summary	Contribution to what end-product Problem
Tactile			
Auditory			
Vestibular			
Relation to gravity			
Movement level			
PRNT			
Sensitivity to movement			
Oral			
Olfactory			
Visual			
Attention			
Proprioception			
Emotion			

III. Functional Support Capabilities

Area	Indicators	Summary	Contribution to what end-product Problem
Suck-swallow-breathe			
Cocontraction			
Muscle tone			
Proprioception			
Balance/equilibrium			
Integrated reflex development			
Laterality			
Bilateral integration			

IV. End-Product Abilities

Area	Indicators	Tests Used	Summary
Praxis			
Behavior			
Academics			
Language/articulation			
Emotional tone			
Activity level			
Environmental mastery			

PRNT = Postrotary Nystagmus Test

A P P E N D I X   7 C

Synthesis of Occupational Therapy Sensory Integration Evaluation

1. Presenting problems:
   a. What are the presenting problems?
   b. Can they be grouped into clusters such as:
      — Sensory system modulation problems,
      — Information/discrimination problems,
      — Functional support capability problems, or
      — End-product problems?
   c. What are the child's particular strengths?
2. Sensory systems modulation/sensory defensiveness
   a. What evidence of modulation problems do you have?
      — Sensory history,
      — Presenting problems,
      — Parent/teacher report, or
      — Your evaluation?
   b. Is the child sensory defensive?
      — What sensory systems are involved?
      — How severe are the problems?
      — Would you rate them as mild, moderate, or severe?
   c. What end-product abilities might be affected by these problems?
3. Information/discriminative systems
   a. What evidence of information/discriminative system problems do you have?
      — Presenting problems
      — Parent/teacher report
      — Reports from other professionals
      — Your evaluations
   b. What systems are involved?
      — Do modulation problems interfere with processing?
   c. What end-product abilities might be affected by these problems?
   d. What are the child's particular strengths?
4. Functional support capabilities
   a. What evidence of problems with functional support capabilities do you have?
      — Presenting problems
      — Parent/teacher report
      — Reports from other professionals
      — Your evaluations

    b. What capabilities are involved?

    c. Do modulation or information system problems contribute to the problems?

    d. What end-product abilities may be affected by the functional support capability problems?

    e. What are the child's particular strengths?

5. End-product abilities

    a. What evidence of end-product ability problems do you have?
      — Presenting problems
      — Parent/teacher reports
      — Reports from other professionals
        — IQ assessments
        — Educational assessments
        — Psychological assessments
        — SIPT results (see explanation below)[a]
        — Your evaluations

    b. What end-product abilities are involved?

    c. Do modulation, information system, or functional support problems contribute to the end-product problems?
      — How do they contribute?

    d. What are the child's particular strengths?

6. Summary

    a. What are the major end-product ability problems?

    b. Are they contributed to by modulation, information, or functional support problems?

    c. How does your evaluation relate to the presenting problems?

    d. Are the child's problems based in sensory integrative processing deficits of inefficiencies?

    e. What are the child's particular strengths?

    f. What treatment do you recommend?
      — Occupational therapy using a sensory integrationframe of reference
      — Occupational therapy using another frame of reference
      — Educational intervention (for cortically-based problems)
      — Psychological referral (for nonsensory defensive behavior problems)
      — Others

---

[a] The SIPT may be given only by therapists who have advanced training and certification in its administration. Most therapists who give the SIPT hold Master's degrees. The beginning therapist may use the SIPT evaluations done by other therapists in their evaluation process. Therapists may refer children to SIPT-certified therapists for SIPT evaluation and then consult with them concerning treatment planning. See Fisher et al (1991) for an in-depth analysis of the interpretation of the SIPT.

Clinical Reasoning: Causal Explanation and Prediction of Patient Treatment Outcomes

CRITICAL THINKING PROCESS:	*QUESTIONS TO BE CONSIDERED BY THE THERAPIST:*
1. Brainstorm causes for the unexpected	What are the possible causal explanations for the child's inability to produce an adaptive response?
2. Focus	Based on brainstorming, identify general categories or multiple factors to focus on.
3. Find evidence for and against each possible cause	What additional information is needed to identify which factors are more likely responsible to explain the child's inability to produce an adaptive response?
	At this point, what is inadequate in your knowledge base? Where can you get adequate information?
4. Theoretical perspective	Based on the theoretical base of the frame of reference, consider which neural processes are most likely to produce deficits in the system. Consider the complexity of the CNS and limitation on knowledge.
5a. Evaluate evidence	Assess the child's and therapist's performance (on videotape if possible).
	What relevant evidence shows up?
	Which possible explanation does it support?
	"What is the best thing about my evaluation/treatment?" "What did I do well?" "What can I do differently to facilitate a better adaptive response in my client?" Develop treatment objectives. Return to number 1 and use process to evaluate treatment.
	Continue process during treatment.

5b. Evaluate evidence continued

How do we know treatment is/is not working?

What evidence has been overlooked or not fully understood?

6. Look at possible default patterns

Can normal "blind spots" or default patterns be identified? How can they be guarded against? Who can help me in this area?

7. Gather more evidence

Try other hypotheses.

8. Make decision

Make judgment on most likely factor or set of factors responsible for client's behavior.

9. Prediction

Predict change that would occur if therapist changes input to client.

What should effect be on client if therapist is right; exactly what should happen?

10. Evaluation

How would you evaluate your treatment/evaluation session?

Sensory Integration Frame of Reference: Postulates Regarding Change and Application to Practice

JUDITH GIENCKE KIMBALL

The focus of this chapter is the intervention process within the sensory integration frame of reference. Building on the theoretical base, function/dysfunction continua, and guide for evaluation presented in Chapter 7, this chapter will identify and describe the postulates regarding change and application to practice of this frame of reference.

POSTULATES REGARDING CHANGE

Postulates regarding change focus on the therapeutic environment needed to facilitate change. The occupational therapist does not create change in the child but facilitates optimum conditions in the environment so that change is most likely to occur. The interplay among the occupational therapist, the child, and the environment is complex and requires constant clinical reasoning. The clinical reasoning process is based on the therapist's observational abilities and on the organization of theoretical knowledge in the frame of reference.

In the sensory integration frame of reference, 20 postulates have been identified. When the evaluation indicates dysfunction, intervention should be directed at the sensory system modulation level first and then at the functional support capabilities and end-products.

There are eight general postulates related to the use of the sensory integration frame of reference:

1. If intervention involves several sensory systems and requires intersensory integration, then it will be more powerful and more likely to bring about an adaptive response.

2. If the therapist provides a situation in which the child can act on his or her environment, then the child will be more likely to produce adaptive responses. The child's self-initiated actions also use the *more efficient feed-forward neurological mechanisms that build motor patterns rather than only the neurologically less efficient feedback.*

3. If the child moves his or her own body volitionally during therapy rather than being moved by someone else, then effective motor patterns are more likely to develop.

4. If the therapist provides a situation that requires an adaptive response that is developmentally appropriate, then the adaptive response is more likely to occur and more likely to promote growth.

5. If the activity presented to the child is challenging yet achievable, then it will facilitate an improved adaptive response.

6. If the therapist provides the child with a sense of emotional safety, then the child will be more likely to engage actively in the therapy process.

7. If the therapist provides the child with constant feedback during the therapy session, then the child will gain a greater understanding of what he or she is doing and what he or she has done.

8. If the therapist provides activities that involve controlled change and variety, then the child is more likely to make an adaptive response rather than develop a learned behavior.

If there are deficits in the sensory system modulation level, it is important to bring modulation within normal levels. There are six postulates regarding change related to sensory system modulation:

9. If sensory system modulation is within normal levels, then an adequate adaptive response is more likely to occur.

10. If the child's sensory diet is modified, then sensory system modulation is more likely to occur.

11. If a child is underreactive, then sensory system input may have to be of greater intensity or duration or more intentional for the child to be able to produce an adequate adaptive response. (Exception: those children who look underaroused but are really shut off because of severe over-registration.)

12. If a child is overreactive, then the usual adaptive response will reflect survival needs and not integration; therefore, the sensory system input will have to be modified for the child to produce an adequate adaptive response.

13. If modulating input is given to one system, then influence is seen in all systems because they are interdependent.

14. If the sensory system modulation level is brought closer to normal levels, then functional support capabilities and end-product abilities will be facilitated.

Functional support capabilities must be activated sufficiently to provide a base for organizing and supporting the adaptive responses. If perceptions, abilities, or feedback are faulty in these areas, they lead to partially accurate adaptive responses. The partially accurate response is not even stable (always partially accurate in the same way) because of the inconsistent nature of the input from sensory systems and functional support capabilities; therefore, the client has inconsistent or inadequate information on which to base an adaptive response, leading to faulty motor patterns and learning.

There are three postulates regarding change related to functional support capabilities:

15. If the therapist provides opportunity for input to the functional support areas at a level intentionally more intense or prolonged than that found in the environment, then functional support abilities are more likely to improve. (Remember that the body and head must be treated separately because of separate innervations.)
16. If the therapist provides opportunity for active, spontaneous, child-initiated movement incorporating functional support capabilities, then these capabilities are more likely to improve than if these skills were specifically practiced.
17. If the therapist provides opportunity for several functional support capabilities to be reinforced (integrated) simultaneously, then the capabilities are likely to improve.

There are three postulates regarding change related to end-product abilities:

18. If the therapist encourages the child to verbalize what he or she is doing during the therapy session, then he or she is more likely to build ideation.
19. If the child is to build motor plans, then he or she must self-initiate the adaptive response process.
20. If the child develops increased practic abilities and increased organization, then there will be a positive effect on other end-product abilities.

APPLICATION TO PRACTICE

The specific techniques of the sensory integration frame of reference differ from the techniques identified in other frames of reference used by occupational therapists. Intervention in this frame of reference is mainly child-directed. That is, the child needs to act on his or her environment to produce the adaptive responses. This action by the child also produces the more efficient feed-forward mechanisms necessary for optimum adaptive response, rather than relying on the less-efficient feedback. In this frame of reference, the therapist is often nurturing and playful and is involved as an active participant in the treatment activities.

One goal of sensory integration is to achieve an effective adaptation to the environment through an improvement of central nervous system (CNS) processing. The therapist encourages a large variety of activities and exploration, rarely repeating an activity. Activities should not be geared toward specific skill development through practice but should elicit an adaptive response.

General Considerations

In this frame of reference, therapy is often individually-based because the child's responses are watched continually and modifications must be made in treatment. Sometimes, small group activities may be used with several children. This limits the activities, however, to only those beneficial to all children and may limit the intensity of the therapy session. If therapy is school-based, group activity and classroom consultation may necessitate activities of lesser intensity but will provide opportunity to use the natural environment for a longer period of time (duration) and increased frequency, which can have the same effect as increased intensity. The therapist must constantly observe the child's autonomic nervous system responses during therapy so that overarousal- and underarousal/registration do not occur. As discussed previously, severe overarousal/registration can lead to shutdown or even shock. Some specific sensory integrative techniques have the potential to affect the nervous system positively. Conversely, some specific sensory integrative techniques also have the possibility of having strong negative effects if used incorrectly or carelessly.

During the therapy session, the therapist needs to give constant feedback to the child. Verbal feedback helps the child understand what he or she is doing and what has been done. Eliciting verbalization from the child about what he or she is doing is also helpful in building ideation. Any praise given to a child should be a real compliment because children are attuned to fake praise. Consider positive comments on the process rather than on the end-product. For example, use phrases such as "you really tried," "you must be proud of yourself for working so hard," and "that was the biggest jump you ever made."

The child needs to be self-directed or no feed-forward or corollary discharge will occur. The role of the therapist is to entice the child to want to act on the environment. This can be done with organization of the environment to help the child choose the most beneficial activities. When the therapist cannot set up the environment to eliminate some distracting activities, the therapist should then guide the child's choices while still allowing him or her to have some control. One method is to ask questions such as "Would you like to go ride on the bolster swing or on the scooter board?" This offers the child an opportunity to be involved in making choices and to build self-esteem.

Therapists often fall into the pattern of using particular pieces of equipment to get particular responses from the child and thereby insisting the child use those pieces of equipment. If the child comes into the room and immediately gravitates toward another activity or equipment, fast thinking on the part of the therapist can modify the activity to get the type of feedback and adaptive response the child needs. The occupational therapist needs to be always vigilant for creative possibilities to facilitate the adaptive responses while still using the child's desires and choices. Observing typically developing children on equipment can broaden the therapist's ideas about how equipment may be used. Intervention that involves several sensory systems and requires intersensory integration is more powerful than intervention that uses just one system. For example, an activity that involves only swinging on a bolster swing is not nearly as integrative as an activity that involves swinging on a bolster swing and getting heavy proprioception by catching and throwing a three-foot ball. Tactile input can be added by putting a piece of fleece over the bolster and having the child sit on the bolster swing in shorts (see Figure 7.9 A, B).

In the sensory integration frame of reference, the aim is not to teach skills but to facilitate appropriate physical and emotional adaptive responses. The goal is to facilitate an adaptive response that can be used at any time in the child's life and can be adapted when the child needs it in other situations. The therapist should help build the child a motor and emotional repertoire.

In this frame of reference, intervention uses an environment organized to help guide the therapy. Any activity in which the child wishes to engage can be used therapeutically if structured appropriately by the therapist. The child's spontaneous ability to produce an adaptive response and transfer it to other environments is one of the expected outcomes of a well-planned occupational therapy program.

Intervention is based on the therapist's knowledge of the child's developmental level. Furthermore, activities are selected that require the adaptive responses within the upper levels of the child's capacity. To require only adaptive responses that are easy will not help the child to integrate new abilities. Conversely, to require a response that is too hard can cause disintegration, which could result in the child's loss of what he or she had gained previously in that particular therapy session.

Methods Used to Facilitate Adaptive Responses in Sensory Integration

Based on the identified needs of a child, the therapist selects appropriate activities and develops an actual plan for the sequence of the therapy session. The specific activities are not always planned; rather, the desired response is planned, such as flexion activities or two-step sequences. For example, a basic treatment sequence over time could include activities to (1) develop overall extension and flexion to achieve a balance in the use of the two patterns; (2) develop the ability to cross the midline of the body with the upper and lower extremities; (3) develop the ability to rotate the trunk during activities; and, (4) develop the ability to follow three-step directions. Before the activities are initiated, the therapist must prepare a child appropriately for success at each adaptive response. Listed below are some guidelines for facilitating an adaptive response:

- Avoid complex motor planning activities early in a session because functional support capabilities should be facilitated first. Build up to complex motor planning activities through appropriate input and intermediary adaptive responses to ensure success.

- Get the child involved actively in the activities and help him or her to succeed. Do not impose yourself as a therapist on the child (other than possibly in treating sensory defensiveness with brushing). Rather, it is helpful to elicit the desired response through interaction.

- Intervention should be specific to the underlying sensory system deficits; it is not specific to behaviors. Practice may improve particular skills but does not improve the generalization of abilities.

- Balance the treatment session with structure and freedom. Neither free play nor total structure is therapeutic in the sensory integration frame of reference. Some children come to therapy very self-directed (e.g., children with learning disabilities). Other children come to therapy not self-directed at all (e.g., some children with autism and mental retardation). For those who are not self-directed, the therapist may need to impose structure first and then work into more freedom.

- As a therapist, hypothesize about what the child understands and what is happening in his or her CNS. Answer the following questions: Does he or she know what he or she is going to be doing in the activity? Is he or she able to articulate it? Does he or she have the idea of what is required in the activity?

The therapist must capture the child's attention and motivation through his or her personality and through the activity. In this frame of reference, the occupational therapist is expected to have fun, act a little silly, and actually engage in play with the child. The best "problem" to have is that the child does not want to go home at the end of a therapy session and that the parent or care provider wonders why occupational therapy is so much fun for the child. Often, the therapist needs to explain to parents or care providers the importance of the child's having fun during therapy. Some parents or care providers may think that therapy should be hard work and that they are not getting their money's worth if it appears to be otherwise.

When selecting activities, the therapist must be sure that the activities are within the child's reach, but that they also extend that reach just a little to the "achievable challenge." An activity that is too easy is not organizing; one that is too hard is disorganizing.

For children who are very dyspraxic or distractable, the therapist should avoid changing the whole activity. Instead, the therapist should change only part of the activity so that the required adaptive response is modified and neuronal models can be built. The therapy session should always end with the child's successful completion of an activity. (Go back to an activity that you know the child can execute successfully. If possible, give him or her a choice.)

The therapist must be infinitely flexible. In addition to changing adaptive responses quickly, the therapist often must change his or her treatment plan because the child's sensory system modulation may be different from session to session. Activities that work at one time may not work at another. At all times, the therapist must keep in mind the child's treatment goals. In addition, the therapist must realize that a specific activity is not essential to meet these goals and that many activities will work. Flexibility will get the most positive results in a particular session.

It is critical that a therapist provides emotional safety for the child. The child must trust the therapist so that he or she can push him or her a little for better results. Part of the emotional adaptive response is laughter. Often music and singing can help integration. Some controlled fear also is appropriate. Young children, when learning about gravity and movement, often will challenge themselves by jumping off things (such as stairs) that are just a little higher than the ones they have tried before. This small element of fear can be arousing and exciting in therapy. The therapist must be careful, however, not to go overboard so that the fear becomes disintegrating.

Finally, it is important that a therapist recognize that improvement may not be linear but may be stepwise with plateaus. Sometimes, especially in older children who have praxis problems, only small motor improvement occurs, but the children become much more organized. The child may retreat at times or refuse to do things previously done. He or she may be bored with the activity, have had a bad day, just not feel like doing the activity, or may hold back just before a large improvement. After significant change, children often need a chance to adjust or integrate to the new level of learning. Demands from school or home or a change in schedule also may intrude and could distract the child from a therapy session.

Intervention Considerations

Occupational therapists who use a clinic-based sensory integrative approach need to be cognizant of three particular areas of treatment: the intervention environment, the child's responses, and the sequence of intervention.

Intervention Environment

The intervention environment is important in this frame of reference because it is organized to help guide the therapy. Any activity in which the child wishes to engage can be used therapeutically if structured appropriately by the therapist. The child's spontaneous ability to produce an adaptive response and transfer it to other environments is an expected outcome of a well-planned occupational therapy program.

Occupational therapists who use this frame of reference need to be "environmental engineers." The safety of the child must be of primary importance. Some elements of physical safety in a treatment setting include the following:

1. Sufficient space is needed to allow swinging movements as well as running and jumping activities, and space for a scooter board ramp.
2. Mats must provide sufficient padding for a fall from a height of up to 4 feet. Mats should be made of dense foam for the bottom 2 to 4 inches, topped by thick crash mats. Checking with the gymnastic association in the area will help determine the

legal liability for numbers of inches of matting required for falls from particular heights.

3. The floor of the clinic is also extremely important. If the clinic is built on a concrete floor, additional mats will be required. If possible, the clinic should have a wooden floor with a tile covering. Or, if wooden floors are not part of the structure, a wooden suspension floor can be built over the concrete floor to allow some give during falls. The tile on the clinic floor should be of a nondistracting color and pattern. This will reduce optokinetic nystagmus when the child is moving on the equipment.

4. An overhead suspension system is necessary to allow safe suspension of swings such as net hammocks suspended by one point, trapezes, and bolsters and inner tubes suspended as swings. The overhead suspension must be capable of holding at least 500 pounds (to hold an adult therapist and a large client at the same time on equipment). This 500-pound suspension needs to be safe during a swinging movement. There are many varieties of suspensions. Consult a professional engineer or an occupational therapy equipment supplier who also sells suspension equipment.

Clinical equipment includes materials with which children readily engage yet perceive as fun and challenging. Essential equipment includes scooter boards, a ramp, a trapeze, a net (pocket or sportsman's) hammock, assorted large therapy balls, a bolster swing, inner tube swings, a mini trampoline, an assortment of foam rubber pillows, cardboard stacking blocks, boxes, balls, bean bags, hula hoops, Theraband mouth toys, and sucking and chewing (oral motor) items, to name a few. Additional equipment may include a waterbed mattress or air mattress on the floor of the clinic, a bubble ball bath or a large box filled with Styrofoam packing material, a "Play all roll," and a Whizwheel. Almost any active toy can be used in treatment. It is not the toy itself that is important but the way in which the toy is used to obtain an optimal adaptive response (Figures 8.1 and 8.2).

Although treatment is often done in a clinical setting, the child's activities in any environment may be orchestrated to contribute to a positive outcome through the "sensory diet." All the child's environments (including community, family, and school) should be involved in the intervention process. The community can offer modulating "sensory diet" activities such as gymnastics, dance, karate, or roller skating. The family can carry out a home program to decrease sensory defensiveness and provide emotional support and monitoring of the sensory diet (Figure 8.3). Also, once school personnel understand the contribution of sensory system's functioning to the end-products, they can assist in the intervention process and reinforce improvement in academic skills.

Sensory integration intervention carries over into the child's natural environment. Of greatest importance have always been the play and school environments. Sensory integration techniques, especially those involving sensory defensiveness, are becoming regular components of school-based intervention. Of particular interest are

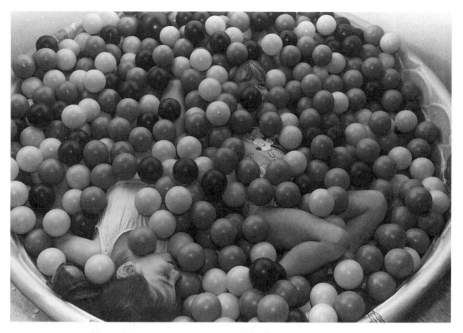

Figure 8.1   Inhibitory activity—bubbleballs. Photograph courtesy of J. Kimball.

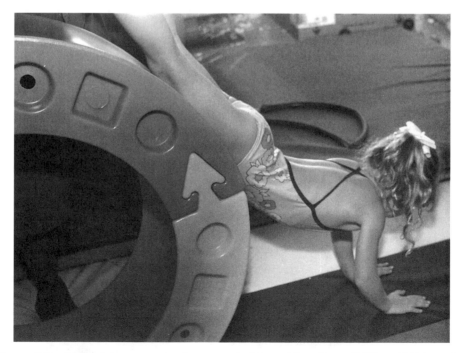

Figure 8.2   Maintaining extension in prone position while rolling off "Play-all." Note that therapist is holding feet for safety. Photograph courtesy of C.C. Church.

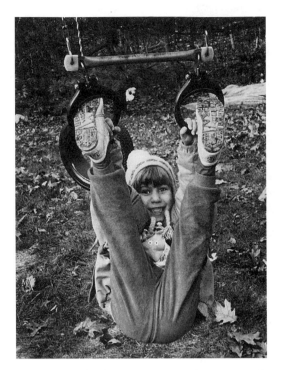

Figure 8.3 Sensory diet activity for home: trapeze and rings; provides proprioceptive and vestibular input. Photograph courtesy of C.C. Church.

those principles and resultant techniques that fit with teachers' frames of reference around classroom management.

The Child's Responses

The goal of intervention is to obtain a complex adaptive response that is integrated and results from multisensory input. What follows are some characteristics of an adaptive response in the sensory integration frame of reference:

- An adaptive response is meaningful to the child; appropriate developmentally, socially, and psychologically; and specific to the situation. An adaptive response is not a taught skill or a rigid pattern of behavior but is elicited when needed.
- An adaptive response is reinforced by elicitation; therefore, adaptive responses are self-reinforcing, especially if they are integrated and work. An adaptive response requires active involvement of a child's CNS.
- An optimal adaptive response is achieved when the therapist interacts with the child, rather than instructing the child.
- An adaptive response should be within the child's developmental level. These adaptive responses should be at the upper limits of the child's abilities to promote growth. Care

should be taken by the therapist not to push the limits of the child's abilities because this may result in disorganization.

Raw sensory stimulation (such as spinning a child for 10 minutes) is not sensory integration and will not elicit an integrated adaptive response.

Beyond the adaptive motor response, a therapist must address the adaptive emotional responses and the ideational responses. It is important that a child know what he or she is trying to do. Sometimes a therapist needs to initiate an activity by asking the child to verbalize what he or she is about to do. The therapist may need to provide the child with the first part of the sequence and then ask him or her to verbalize the next part. At other times, the therapist may need to demonstrate or actually help the child move through the activity before the child can take over for himself or herself.

It is important to keep in mind that oral motor abilities must be facilitated separately from other motor abilities because of their separate neural systems (cranial nerves) (Figure 8.4).

Sequence of Treatment

In sensory integration, the sequence of treatment is (1) to modulate the sensory systems, (2) to work on the functional support capabilities within the adaptive responses, and (3) to require adaptive responses necessary to build the end-product

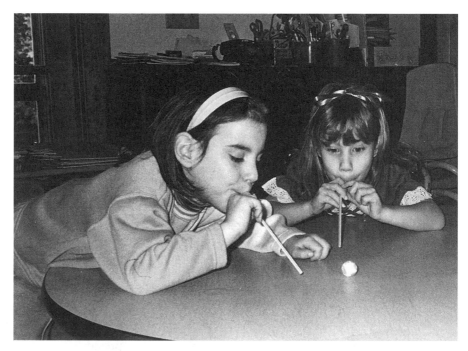

Figure 8.4   Oral-motor game: blowing ball with straws. Photograph courtesy of J. Kimball.

abilities. In the sensory integration frame of reference, intervention follows the sequence of development. First, sensory modulation levels should be normalized to facilitate functional capabilities, bringing about adaptive responses.

SENSORY SYSTEM MODULATION

Sensory system modulation may be influenced in several ways. It is critical to keep in mind that arousal in one system can raise the set point (baseline) for the entire CNS. According to Wilbarger and Wilbarger (1991), a child who has sensory system modulation problems is called "sensory defensive" (SD). Sensory defensiveness can be rated as mild, moderate, or severe. Children with *mild sensory defensiveness* are described as "picky," "overly sensitive," or "slightly controlling." They can be irritated by some sensations but not by others. They achieve at school and socially but need enormous control and effort to do so. When this control becomes too hard to maintain, they "fall apart."

The child with *moderate sensory defensiveness* is affected in several areas of life (i.e., difficulty with social relations, self-care skills, or attention and behavior in school). The child with *severe sensory defensiveness* is affected in every aspect of life. According to Wilbarger and Wilbarger (1991), these children usually have other diagnostic labels like "severe developmental delay" or "emotionally disturbed." All children with sensory defensiveness need intervention to deal with this primary problem and to enable other forms of treatment to be more effective.

Treatment of sensory defensiveness can take several avenues:

1. Just identifying the problem can increase understanding of the child,
2. Sensory systems can be influenced through a planned "sensory diet," and
3. Treatment with a touch pressure brush may be needed.

Sensory diet inputs can raise or lower the modulation level. What follows are some examples of excitatory and inhibitory activities that may be used with a child who is experiencing sensory defensiveness:

Excitatory Activities	Inhibitory Activities
Amusement park rides	Staying alone in a quiet room
Fast driving	Dimming lights
Fast skiing	Soft music
Loud music	Heavy joint and muscle work (such as
Noisy parties	jogging, bike riding, slow weight lifting,
Fast dancing	karate, tap dancing, tackle football)
Rock concerts	Heavy touch pressure (such as massage)

Excitatory Activities	Inhibitory Activities

Fast-moving sports (i.e., basketball
   and soccer)
Worrying and anxiety
Scary movies
Riding on motorcycles

Children who have sensory system modulation problems also may need to have their sensory activities modified to help control modulation. More opportunity for activities that contribute to modulation may need to be provided. It seems apparent that some activities are calming and others are excitatory. Sometimes excitatory-appearing activities have an inhibitory effect because of the type of dysfunction in some sensory systems.

Children who have one type of hyperactivity and who respond to stimulant medications (e.g., Ritalin, Cylert) to calm them are considered to be experiencing underarousal to parts of the CNS (Kimball, 1986, 1988). Excitatory input, especially fast vestibular input, can override the underarousal and lead to modulation. In these children, the hyperactive behavior is believed to be caused by low arousal, and this activity level serves to increase arousal. Fast vestibular activities, particularly combined with proprioception, can normalize the sensory system functions in some children at least for short periods of time and can reduce the "hyperactivity." There is mounting evidence that these changes may be more permanent. Another group of children, those who do not respond to Ritalin and Cylert by calming (and become more stimulated by these medications), can become more stimulated by fast activity. These children appear to have less than optimal cortical inhibitory mechanisms (Kimball, 1986, 1988).

Children who are not hyperactive but who have preferences for fast, intense movements (e.g., carnival rides, fast skiing, motorcycles, fast swinging, spinning) also have apparent underarousal or overinhibition in the lower brain centers, as discussed with depressed nystagmus. These fast movements actually modulate arousal to a more normal level.

Another way in which sensory systems are influenced for sensory defensive children is through a treatment approach called the Wilbarger Protocol (Wilbarger & Wilbarger, 1991). The method of treatment involves direct sensory input to decrease sensory defensiveness through the use of a specific type of nonscratching pressure brush followed by proprioceptive input to all joints (Wilbarger & Wilbarger, 1991). Only one particular surgical scrub brush, available through PDP products, has been found to provide the right input to effect the modulating response quickly (Wilbarger & Wilbarger, 1991). The fast, very firm, long-stroke brushing should be applied quickly on each extremity (hands, feet) and on the back but never on the stomach or face. This is then followed by 10 quick compressions of each joint. The joints can be compressed in groups by pushing the hands together, by jumping up and down, or by having another person push firmly (but not with too much pressure) on each set of joints 10 times. This treatment should take a total of approximately 1 minute and should be repeated 8 to 12 times per day for 1 to 2 weeks. The treatment should be monitored at all times by a specifically trained occupational therapist. If appropriate, maintenance treatment may need to be continued. Because the mouth is controlled by a different part of the nervous system (the cranial nerves), oral defensiveness must be treated separately with short, quick applications of firm pressure to the hard palate (with the finger covered by a face cloth or by a plastic nipple) (Wilbarger & Wilbarger, 1991).

This pressure-proprioceptive treatment represents a departure from other treatments in this frame of reference in that it is "imposed lovingly" on the child (and most children love it). Some problems with sensory defensiveness are so resistant to change and have such a pervasive effect on a child's life that the imposition of input is the only way to "break through" and to begin normalizing the system. The person with true sensory defensiveness rejects all therapeutic contact (Wilbarger & Wilbarger, 1991). In 1972, Ayres stated: "Occasionally a therapist may be justified in applying stimuli in spite of discomfort for a few days in an effort to bring a sufficient shift in balance between the protective and discriminative response systems to enable development of tolerance to some stimuli" (p. 219). The pressure brushing proprioceptive program that is part of the Wilbarger Protocol can result in a decreased sensory defensiveness and more appropriate responses to sensory input. The parent or care provider may provide the program. This treatment must be closely monitored, however, by a therapist who has experience in sensory system dysfunction. For more information, the reader is directed to the videotape "Occupational Therapy: Sensory Defensiveness" (Wilbarger, 1991).

Another method of sensory input, a "sensory diet," can be self-selected by the child or constructed with family consultation (Figure 8.5). Proprioception is important in sensory modulation and may consist of joint compression or traction; thus, any heavy work, along with motor activity, that a child engages in will have a normalizing effect on the child's nervous system. Slow movement activities combined with proprioception are helpful for almost every child. Fast movement activities may have varying effects, depending on the child's nervous system. The neck joints and proximal limb joints, the shoulders and hips, are most responsive to proprioceptive input. A quick proprioceptive activity that can be used in a school classroom is 10 slow pushups. Other easy proprioceptive activities that can be done at home are chin-ups with a chin-up bar, bouncing on a mini-trampoline, doing pushups against the wall, slow wrestling with others, jogging, bike riding, and roller-skating. One method of providing heavy proprioception to a child's neck joints is to lean couch cushions against the front of the couch and have the child kneel on all fours and push his or her head firmly, slowly, back and forth into the couch cushions. The therapist needs to be careful not to injure the neck.

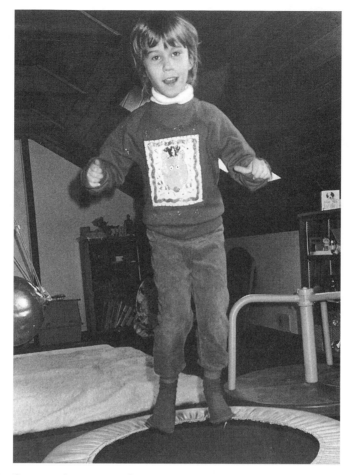

Figure 8.5 Sensory diet activity for home: mini-trampoline. Photograph courtesy of J. Kimball.

If the child is oral defensive, intervention can involve deep pressure to the roof of the mouth; changing the foods the child eats to choices that have increased resistance so the child has to work his or her oral muscles more to eat; sucking activities that increase oral muscle work such as using a crazy straw; increasing the resistance of the liquids sucked through the straw by thickening them with yogurt, apple sauce or a pureed banana; and increasing the tartness of the thick liquids (tart and sour have the effect of increasing modulation) by adding or starting with grapefruit, cranberry, or orange juice or lemonade or strawberries (Oetter, Richter, & Frick, 1992).

Functional support capabilities and end-product abilities can be worked on once sensory system modulation is "normalized," or the arousal level is reduced at the beginning of the treatment session. It is important to remember that different types of input can influence the nervous system for varying lengths of time as a modulator.

The therapist should be aware that tactile input can last up to 2 hours, propriocep-tive input up to 2 hours, and vestibular input up to 4 hours or more.

Though the auditory system is generally considered the domain of the speech pathologist, a better understanding of this system can be helpful to the occupational therapist. New information on the auditory system indicates that sounds in the en-vironment are not regulated enough to get a modulating effect, but specifically en-gineered sounds and types of music delivered through high impedance earphones can be an effective addition to a sensory diet (Workshop, Frick, Quechee, VT, 1997). There are numerous anecdotal reports of auditory training and "listening programs" having improved auditory processing, attention, and even coordination in many types of children, particularly children with autism. Though little research exists on auditory training, and it is controversial, the emphasis auditory training places on the auditory system's contribution to language, sensory processing, and coordination is intriguing. Shiela Frick, an occupational therapist who has studied auditory training extensively, has modified and refined this work and placed it under the umbrella of "methods to influence sensory system modulation." Her "therapeutic listening" pro-grams hold great promise. The important difference in what Frick is doing lies in its functional integration with sensory integration activities. While auditory training uses special equipment and special sounds, Frick uses real music and integrates it as part of the "sensory diet." The music she uses is specially configured to heighten the high frequency sounds, to eliminate static, and to add overtones. It is delivered with high intensity but very low volume through high impedance earphones while the child is involved in functional activity, especially sensory integration movement-based work (Frick, Queechee, VT, 1997).

Therapists working in school systems are noticing that their referral base is chang-ing. Typically, children with learning disabilities and gross and fine motor problems leading to academic difficulties were frequently referred; recently there have been in-creases in referrals of children with severe behavioral disorders who need a constantly reinforcing environment. The reason for this change in the referred population is not apparent. Also, there appears to be an increase in cases with autism spectrum disor-der. Many of these children have primary difficulties with sensory defensiveness, and many respond well to interventions for their sensory defensiveness.

Of particular benefit is explaining sensory defensiveness to teachers and parents who are then able to make a shift in thinking away from behavioral or psychologi-cal reasons for the aberrant behaviors and toward investigating whether there is a neurophysiologic basis (sensory defensiveness). Once the sensory defensiveness is ruled in or out, appropriate behavior management programs can be constructed that honor and utilize sensory processing theory. It should be noted that behavior man-agement programs constructed without regard to sensory systems issues will not be as successful as those that treat the sensory systems problems first.

There are many excellent ways to treat sensory defensiveness in schools. All of these programs are aimed at increasing the student's awareness of his or her problems so he or she can become responsible for his or her own nervous system and its responses. This can be done by utilizing the Wilbarger Protocol when appropriate and by providing ongoing sensory diet through the school day. It should be noted that some schools do not wish to use such treatment in the classrooms. The sensory diet can either be on a timed schedule or at the request of the student. Another program that has been used successfully to teach students about their nervous systems is the Alert program or "How Does Your Engine Run" (Williams & Shellenberger, 1994). It can be easily used in schools by teachers under the supervision of an occupational therapist and helps the children be responsible for their own behavior and the teacher to understand the antecedents of that behavior.

Sensory diet activities for the classroom can be constructed with the teacher to take into account what is acceptable to him or her. The major components of sensory diet are heavy touch pressure, heavy work (including heavy work with the mouth and breathing work), and rhythmic vestibular or movement input. Included may be a sensory corner in the classroom containing:

- a large box (washer or refrigerator box) filled with pillows; have the children paint it
- bean bags for sitting on or under
- a rocking chair
- a physioball for sitting on and bouncing or lying on
- many hand fidget toys such as squish (stress) balls, silly putty, kooshes, flour- or pea-filled balloons, vibrating toys, and squiggle pens

Other activities for a sensory diet that may work in a classroom situation are use of the Alert program (Williams & Shellenberger, 1994), have periodic (half hourly or hourly) "sensory breaks" including activities such as standing up and stretching or bounce on heels, or timing recess just before the most important academic work of the day. For children who get "overdone" by unstructured play time, end recess with structure requiring heavy work such as stomping like elephants from playground to class. In order to have children begin to take responsibility for their own nervous systems and sensory needs, it may be helpful to encourage them to ask for sensory diet activities as needed. Heavy work that can be done in the classroom includes starting the day with an exercise program and marching with stomping (such as pretending to be animals). It is also helpful to use the environment by letting the students move the desks out of the way and put them back.

Mouth input tends to help children to concentrate. It should be noted that the teacher's approval should be obtained before using mouth input activities in the classroom. Activities for mouth input would include the following:

- chewing sugar-based gum, which is more resistant than sugarless gum
- chewing on sour candies such as Sweetarts

- chew necklace (made from theratubing, either one color with plastic beads attached or short lengths of many colors—each color is a different resistance—strung on string)
- blowers or noisemakers (be sure to use ones with plastic mouth pieces and ones that can make sounds to be able to grade the activity)

Families can be helpful in carrying on sensory diet activities when the child is not in school. The following activities can be done in any environment and can be used to modulate behavior at any time. To increase work done by the mouth:

- switch to bagels from white bread
- add carrots, apples, and beef jerky
- change candy from mushy chocolate to resistant candy like Twizzlers, regular gum, or carmels
- add tartness with Sweetarts, sourballs, or hot balls
- increase sucking with crazy straws or thickened, tart beverages
- chew bubble gum
- blow whistles, party blowers, or balloons (be careful of popping noises)
- make chewy necklaces

Other suggestions include:

- having a pet
- sleeping in a sleeping bag or under heavy blankets or in blanket sleepers (two pairs work best)
- using playground equipment: hang up an inner tube swing and a trapeze bar outside or in the basement (be sure to have lots of old mattresses under the equipment for safety)

FUNCTIONAL SUPPORT CAPABILITIES

Once the sensory systems modulation is under control, the functional support capabilities and end-product issues may be worked on. There is anecdotal evidence that when the sensory systems become modulated, the functional support capabilities and end-product deficits appear less severe without direct intervention to these deficit areas (Wilbarger, 1991). The sensory systems modulation problems appear to have overridden the children's ability to access their other capabilities. Please be reminded that the sequence of treatment is (1) sensory systems modulation, (2) functional support, and (3) end-products. It should be noted that (2) and (3) may be treated simultaneously.

Activities to develop functional support capabilities are numerous and most activities incorporate more than one area. Cocontraction and muscle tone are best worked on with proprioception and balance equilibrium activities. The therapist needs to be reminded that in all interventions in which activity uses several sensory modalities, it is more likely that change will occur than when an activity is based on a single modality. Doing a proprioceptive activity while challenging equilibrium, therefore, can affect those two systems as well as cocontraction, muscle tone, and even the developmental reflexes and bilateral integration.

The more muscles and joints involved in the activity, the more input the child will receive from the activity. The lower to the ground the activity (e.g., not standing), the more joints and muscles involved and the more elemental balance is required. Rather than the skill development approach of walking on a balance beam to enhance balance and equilibrium, a sensory integrative approach looks at the underlying integration inefficiency and treats it. Another example involves the use of a waterbed. If a therapist has a child kneel in the quadruped position on a waterbed so that his or her hands and knees are touching the surface and are weight bearing, then the adaptive response may be to keep from falling over. If the therapist pushes on the waterbed and says "don't fall over," the adaptive response of the activity may be elemental and be more of a learned rather than a developmental skill. Whereas, if the therapist states "you are a boat in the ocean, and I am the hurricane. I am trying to sink you," and the therapist gets involved with making hurricane-type noises, blowing air at the child's face, and bouncing the waterbed around, then the child has an emotional and physical adaptive response. Because the child concentrates on the fun of the game, the equilibrium reactions become more automatic and integrated (Figure 8.6 A). The environment and activity have been set up for success, and the most mature adaptive response possible. Involved in the activity, in addition to

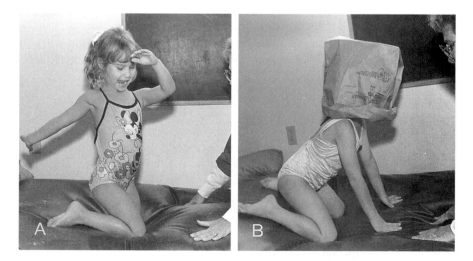

Figure 8.6   A, Mature response during equilibrium challenge (hurricane game) on waterbed; note rotation of trunk; B, Challenge to equilibrium with vision occluded by bag (less upsetting than a blindfold). Photograph courtesy of C.C. Church.

the equilibrium, are proprioception, cocontraction, and muscle tone. The activity can be changed if the therapist changes places with the child so that he or she becomes the hurricane and tries to sink the therapist. Another adaptation is to pretend that it is night—the child then has to "close his or her eyes" so that darkness ensues or a paper bag can be placed over the child's head so that his or her vision is occluded (Figure 8.6 B). This makes the balance and equilibrium responses even more spontaneous because optical righting has been eliminated.

A common activity in an occupational therapy clinic—swinging on a bolster swing—can be used for balance, equilibrium, cocontraction, muscle tone, and proprioception at the same time. An adaptation of this activity consists of using a large three-foot ball thrown at the child (see Figures 7.9 A, B). This requires additional joint/muscle work to catch and throw. The ball can be thrown from various angles as the bolster swing is moved. To change the activity, balls of different sizes and shapes or balloons can be thrown so that the child must make constant modifications and adaptations because of the different weights of the objects being caught or thrown. The constant change in this activity ensures an adaptive response and not a learned behavior. The swinging of the bolster swing also contributes greatly to making this an adaptive response that builds praxis rather than a learned behavior (as would be the case with practicing catching on a stationary surface).

The development of the ability to assume and maintain the prone extension posture is an indication of vestibular proprioceptive functioning. This position can be facilitated by placing a child prone on a scooter board and by doing many activities that require heavy proprioception and movement at the same time. Any activity down a scooter board ramp facilitates prone extension if a child is prone on the scooter board (Figure 8.7). Another activity, scooter board basketball, which requires the prone child to throw the ball with two hands into a target approximately 1.5 feet off the floor, also facilitates prone extension, whereas throwing with one hand does not. Activities done from a prone position in a net hammock are also appropriate (Figures 8.8 A, B).

For the inexperienced therapist, judging the quality of another antigravity response—the flexion response—is a difficult concept. It often appears that the child can do the response, but, if observed closely, the quality is not the same as that of a child without deficits. Supine flexion is tested in the supine position on a mat where the child flexes his or her neck and knees off the floor at the same time. This often results in the knees being drawn up toward the stomach appropriately, but the neck is being lifted with a chin jut. In other words, extension occurs in place of flexion. This needs to be watched for and, if seen, indicates that the child is not producing a mature antigravity flexion response (Figures 8.9 A, B). The flexion response is extremely important in survival and in articulation and swallowing. If the chin is jutted forward slightly in extension, this makes it difficult for the child to articulate clearly, chew, and swallow effectively. Neck proprioception activities help greatly to reinforce the flexion response (Figure 8.10).

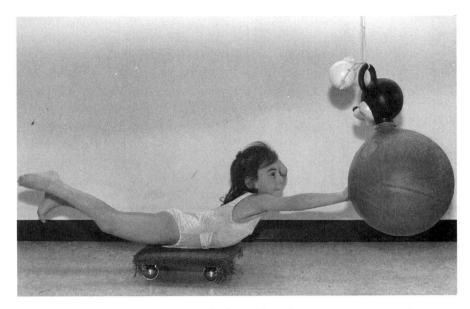

Figure 8.7   Prone extension position facilitated by ride down scooter ramp in prone position and reaching for suspended ball; note asymmetrical tonic neck reflex. Photograph courtesy of C.C. Church.

Supine flexion is often a deficient response in children who are dyspraxic. The flexion pattern is extremely important to the child's development and is seen by Carl Sagan (1977) as being a primary survival pattern for mankind. Flexion follows a specific sequence of development that needs to be facilitated in a child who does not have a good flexion response. The first point is to maintain flexion, which can be facilitated in occupational therapy by placing a child on a flexion swing and having him or her maintain position as he or she swings. Holding flexion against gravity (e.g., holding onto the bottom side of a bolster swing) is the most difficult way to maintain flexion (Figures 8.11 A, B). Sitting in an inner tube and hugging it is also a way to facilitate flexion. The second level in developing flexion is to have a child assume the flexion position. In this case, a child can leave the flexion response momentarily by reaching for something while on the flexion swing and then can reassume the position (Figures 8.12 A, B, and 8.13 A, B). The third point in the development of flexion is being able to release flexion at the appropriate time. This can be seen in a child who can swing on a trapeze, lift his or her knees up over a barrier, and then jump into an inner tube or land on a desired space or swing on a trapeze and kick only the top box off from a pile (Figure 8.14). This activity assumes that the child can initiate flexion, maintain it, and release it at appropriate times.

In a sensory integrative approach, the therapist needs to work through a typical motor developmental sequence of stability on which to build mobility. The particular sequence that can be followed is: (1) ability to assume the basic starting position;

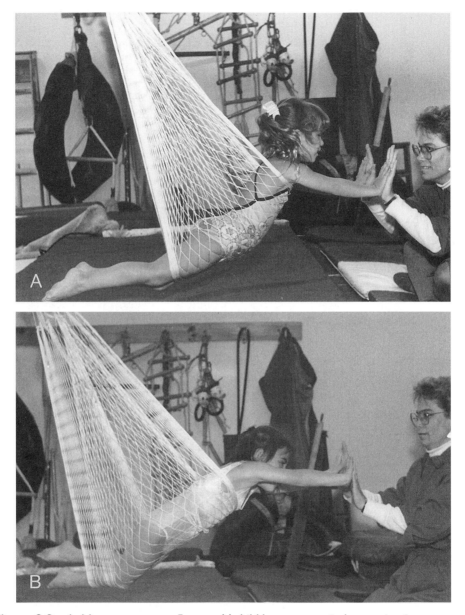

Figure 8.8   A, Mature response: 5-year-old child has symmetrical extension in prone position against gravity; B, Immature response: 6-year-old child has some asymmetry and flexion of hips in prone position, indicating difficulty moving against gravity. Pushing the therapist's hand with resistance adds proprioceptive reinforcement to this vestibular activity.
Photograph courtesy of C.C. Church.

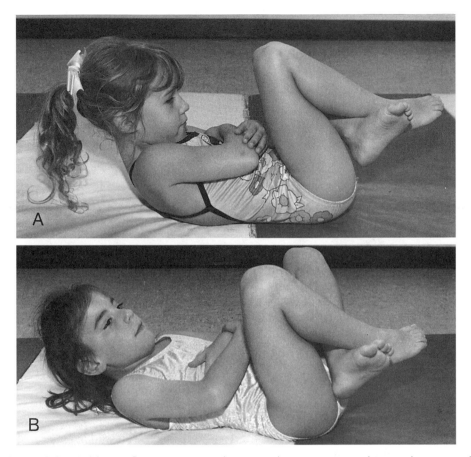

Figure 8.9 A, Mature flexion in supine (antigravity) position; note chin on chest, scapula off mat; B, Subtle immaturity in flexion in supine (antigravity) position; note chin not quite on chest and scapula on mat. Photograph courtesy of C.C. Church.

(2) develop stability in that position; (3) ability to move from the position in a straight plane movement; and (4) integration of the movements and the addition of rotation.

An example of a typical motor developmental sequence is creeping in an infant. The child first gets up on all fours and generally falls down; then the child gets up on all fours and rocks back and forth, giving stability to the joints and strength to the muscles needed for the movement; after the rocking phase, the child begins a creeping movement in a straight plane; and then, eventually, the child is able to add rotation, in that he or she can move around corners, pick up one hand, and turn to grab something all in the quadruped position. The same thing occurs in learning how to walk, where the child pulls up and sits down, then pulls up and cruises along the furniture in a straight plane motion, and then stands and walks in a somewhat controlled

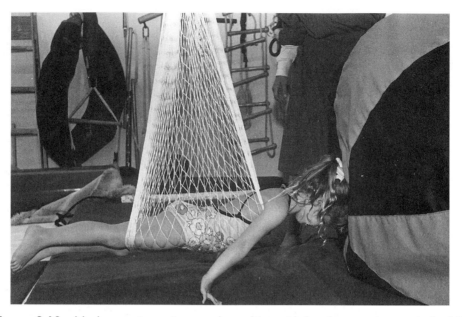

Figure 8.10 Neck proprioception; gentle pushing with head on mushroom ball while prone in net hammock. Photograph courtesy of C.C. Church.

fall method with hands held up. Finally, as a more mature walker, the child adds some rotation in the upper body to the movement. (The same process can be seen in learning to ski.)

Lateralization and bilateral integration also are addressed in functional support capabilities. Integrated movement in two planes is necessary for bilateral integration and in three planes for rotation (Oetter, Richter, & Frick 1992). One method used to address this is the inclusion of rotation in an activity. Many children who have been identified as having sensory integrative dysfunction can be seen to be "straight plane" movers, that is, children who do not rotate their bodies but tend to move in straight, linear styles. Linear motion is indicative of earlier developmental organization. Beginning therapists need to be aware of the sequence, particularly rotation, because some children are able to accomplish a basic motor activity but the quality is worse than normal because of the lack of integration of rotation. *Remember that when using sensory integration intervention, it is not about whether the child can do an activity but about the quality of the movement (see Figures 7.9 A, B, and 8.6 A, B).*

Getting children who have sensory integrative dysfunction to rotate can be a difficult task. The therapist must be creative in incorporating rotational movements into the adaptive responses. For instance, have a child catch a bean bag with his or her hands on one side of the bolster swing, and then rotate around to throw the bag into a target placed far back on the child's other side. Often, the therapist observes that the child will switch hands to avoid crossing midline or rotating.

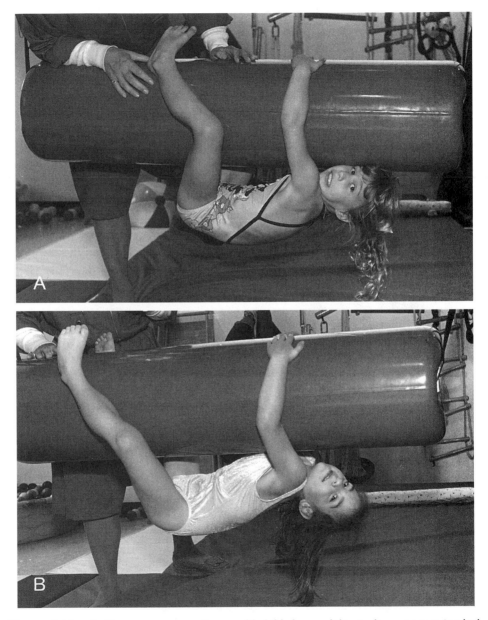

Figure 8.11   A, Mature response: 5-year-old child shows ability to hang on moving bolster swing in total flexion with good cocontraction (although expressing some fear—she was flipped over suddenly without warning); B, Immature response: extension in neck and back showing influence of gravity. Photograph courtesy of C.C. Church.

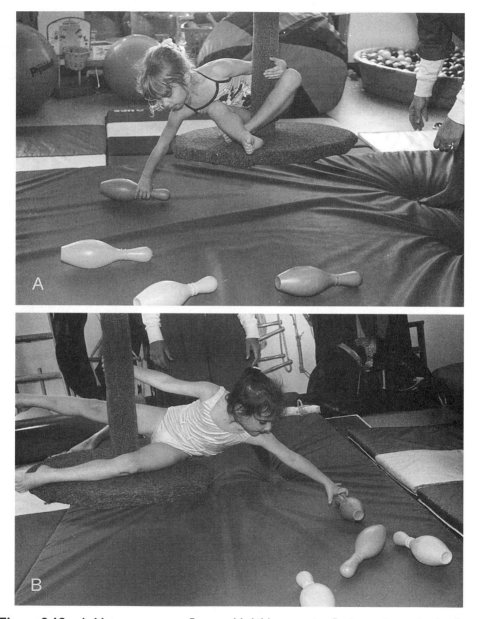

Figure 8.12   A, Mature response: 5-year-old child on moving flexion swing maintains flexion in lower body while extending arm to pick up bowling pin; B, Immature response: 6-year-old child on moving flexion swing extends whole body while arm extends to pick up pin. Photograph courtesy of C.C. Church.

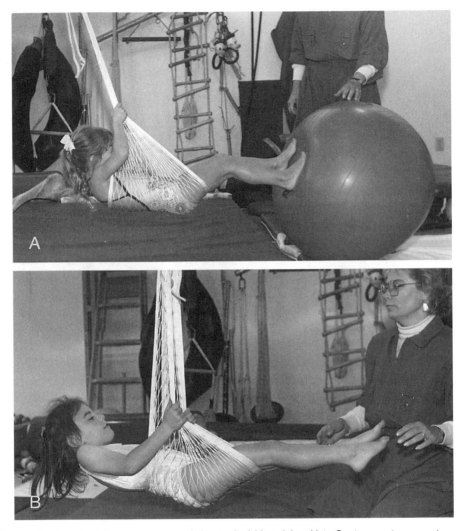

Figure 8.13   A, Mature response: ability to hold head (neck) in flexion against gravity and move legs into extension and flexion as needed to kick ball; B, Immature response: difficulty holding head (neck) and knees in flexion against gravity. Photograph courtesy of C.C. Church.

The development of the suck-swallow-breathe sequence is vital for the integration of good breathing and phonation, the development of muscle tone in the tongue and jaw, and stability and integrated movement of the head, neck, and trunk. The first place that midline stability and bilateral integration occur is in the eyes when a newborn sucks. Activities follow a sequence of suck-blow to bite-crunch to chew-lick (Oetter, Richter, & Frick, 1992). Examples of suck-blow would be to encourage

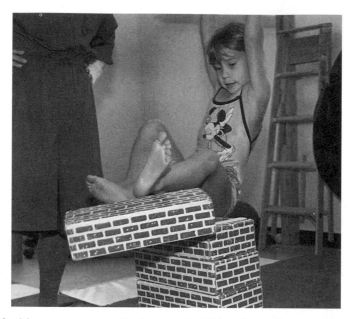

Figure 8.14   Mature response: this 5-year-old child is able to flex selectively to kick the number of blocks desired off the pile, showing mature use of flexion abilities.

the child to use a narrow straw for normal drinking but also to provide heavy things to suck through the straw such as pudding, sherbet, or fruit shakes. Strong flavors that stimulate the bitter and sour receptors at the back portion of the tongue help develop muscle tone in the back of tongue and jaw stability. Mouth toys such as fancy, unusual whistles and blowing games are encouraged (Figure 8.15), and musical instruments are good for older children. Treatment of oral defensiveness also may need to be incorporated.

Biting and crunching activities include eating crunchy foods like carrots or popsicles (ice). Chew-lick activities include chewing bagels, gum, resistant candy (like caramel and licorice), and ice cream in a cone. Providing something for children to chew on between meals is indicated. Aquarium tubing can be tied in a knot and worn around the neck so that the child can reach it easily and put it into his or her mouth to chew on. Theratubing has better resistance to chewing but has a bad chemical taste; therefore, it needs to be soaked a long time before use (Oetter, Richter, & Frick 1992).

End-Product Abilities

The end-product abilities are the combination of the child's sensory system modulation and functional support capabilities and his or her cognitive capabilities. Without the lower systems, the end-product abilities are difficult to develop at the

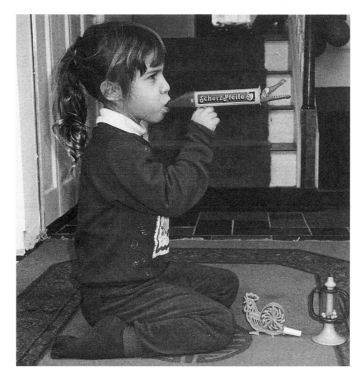

Figure 8.15   Mouth toys/whistles. Photograph courtesy of J. Kimball.

highest level possible. It is often said of children who have sensory integration problems that they work so much harder than other children for inferior results.

Praxis

The occupational therapist who uses the sensory integration frame of reference is concerned primarily with praxis. The other end-product abilities may also be worked on directly in a treatment session but may be influenced indirectly in five major ways.

1. The heightened organization gained by increasing practice abilities may affect other end-product abilities.
2. The increased feelings of mastery and self-esteem gained by producing and reinforcing appropriate adaptive motor responses may transfer to other end-product abilities.
3. The increased awareness of space and spatial perception gained by getting consistent internal feedback about the body in space impacts on the development of other end-product abilities.
4. Articulation may be improved by incorporating head and neck movements in coordination activities.

5. Increased motor sequencing abilities improve general sequencing abilities that then improve academics (because all academic activity involves a sequence).

The end-product abilities often are addressed in other frames of references, like those that focus on skill development and can be used as adjuncts to sensory integration, where the purpose is to change the child's nervous system responses. There are nine major guidelines for increasing a child's practicabilities:

1. Therapists need to be sure that a child's sensory systems are modulated. A nervous system on overarousal/reactivity will produce any adaptive response focused mainly on survival (Figure 8.16).
2. Whenever possible, therapists should use functional support capabilities in activities (Figures 8.17 A, B).
3. Therapists should organize the treatment session so that sensory system modulation occurs first, followed by functional support capabilities. Next, the therapist focuses on using functional support capabilities in conjunction with basic adaptive responses to achieve more integrated adaptive responses. For example, if the end-product practice response is to hit a ball with a bat while swinging on a bol-

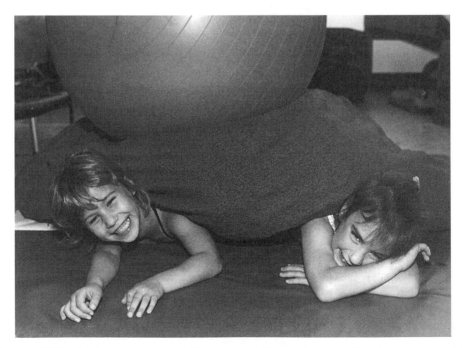

Figure 8.16 Inhibitory activity: children pretending to be pizza dough are covered in sauce (mat pillow), and the cheese (ball) is rolled on with pressure. Photograph courtesy of C.C. Church.

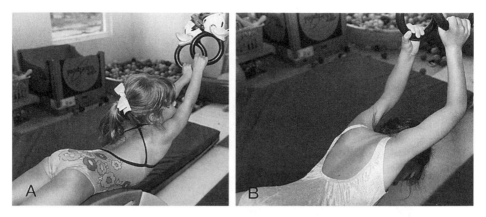

Figure 8.17 A, Mature response: head up against gravity, good cocontraction in arms, strong proprioceptive input is used; B, Immature response: head down, influenced by gravity. Photograph courtesy of C.C. Church.

ster swing, then the preliminary activity may involve vestibular and proprioceptive input. These systems may be activated by having the child swing himself or herself in the bolster by pushing and pulling on the bolster suspension rope (Figure 8.18 A, B, C). Or, a therapist may select an activity that would require a more integrated adaptive response, such as having the child go down the ramp prone on a scooter board and pick up certain bowling pins whose colors are called out once the scooter has started, calling out "right-hand blue, or left-hand red." The preliminary activity may be to propel along prone on a scooter board by placing hands on the floor and pulling back hard or by using both hands on a plunger to pull along. These preliminary activities activate the proprioceptive and vestibular systems so that they are more available to support the praxis activity. The probability of success is improved, and the nervous system has a better chance of using correct pathways to accomplish the activity, thereby building more accurate neuronal models for future use.

4. Therapists need to have the equipment and space to provide appropriate sensory input, particularly vestibular input. Suspended equipment is necessary to give the child the opportunity to experience strong vestibular/proprioceptive input.

5. Therapists should provide proprioceptive input whenever appropriate. Proprioception has been underused in treating sensory integrative dysfunction. Joint compression or traction (especially on the neck and proximal limb joints, the shoulders and hips) provides important input to help the child improve practice abilities. If a child is having difficulty with a praxis activity, the therapist may stop the activity and give 10 quick compressions to the child's joints involved in the activity (e.g., the arms, hands, and shoulders in a catching activity). Then the child should be asked to try the activity again. Often the therapist will observe significant changes in the child's ability to succeed at the activity.

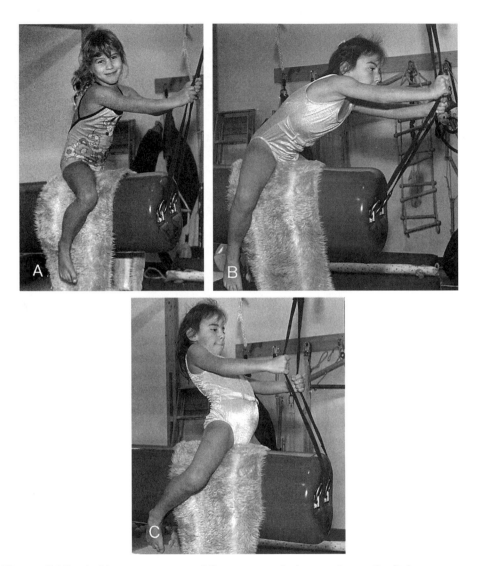

Figure 8.18 A, Mature response: ability to move bolster swing easily; B, Immature response: use of total body pattern to move bolster swing, note low tone in leg; C, immature response: use of total body pattern to move bolster swing; note lack of elbow flexion. Photograph courtesy of C.C. Church.

6. Therapists need to set up the treatment environment so the child can succeed. As stated previously, therapists should provide children with achievable challenges.
7. When a child is inner directed and wants to do activities that a therapist had not anticipated, the therapist should use quick clinical reasoning to use the child's ac-

tivity to get an integrated adaptive response. For example, if a therapist has a bolster swing set up and the child arrives and wants to play on the large mushroom ball by throwing himself or herself over it, rather than tell the child to get off the mushroom and get on the bolster, a therapist may make an adapted game out of being prone on the mushroom. The therapist could be King Kong, complete with roars, and try to knock the child off the mushroom. Or, bean bags or bowling pins could be scattered on the floor, and the child could be asked to pick them up and throw them into a target while still prone over the mushroom.

8. Neuronal models may be built by changing a small portion of the required adaptive response. The whole activity does not have to change. This allows the adaptive response to remain adaptive and not become a learned activity. Furthermore, a small change gives a child a good chance to succeed because the activity is similar to a previous one and, therefore, does not require total reorganization. For example, if the activity is for a child to swing on a trapeze holding on with his or her hands, flexing his or her knees and hips so as not to knock down a pile of large blocks or boxes while he or she swings over, the activity could be graded by increasing the height of the boxes each time or by having the child kick boxes off the pile (Figure 8.13). The activity of swinging on a trapeze to increase flexion abilities is being repeated, but it is not the same as practicing a skill because the adaptive response is changed each time, requiring the flexion pattern to be incorporated into a slightly different practice response.

9. Finally, therapists must be constantly inventive to change adaptive responses asked of the child. This poses a challenge for the therapist and also keeps things interesting for the therapist and the child.

Other End-Product Abilities

This frame of reference assumes that most other end-products, including academics (Ayres, 1976), are improved by addressing the child's sensory integrative problems. Other than praxis and incorporation of some form and space perception, the occupational therapist may not address other end-product abilities individually in his or her intervention. At times, when there are language and articulation problems, occupational therapists work with speech therapists during the same session because many articulation problems may be related to low muscle tone and poor co-contraction, sometimes causing the chin to jut. Additionally, poor praxis can affect the coordination of the mouth. Most of the end-product abilities, though, are gained through sensory integration by combining sensory modulation, the development of functional support capabilities, and praxis. Some therapists feel that other end-products are best worked on toward the end of an occupational therapy session using the sensory integration frame of reference because the child has been "prepared" for success by the earlier portions of the session. Other therapists incorporate other end-products as they naturally occur and can be facilitated during the session. All methods are appropriate and based on the therapist's own skills and judgments. It is important for environmental mastery to become apparent for the child during occupational therapy using the sensory integration frame of reference.

Clinical Reasoning Process

Occupational therapy has long been considered an art as well as a science. Part of the art of occupational therapy is the clinical reasoning process that assists the therapist in developing and implementing the sequence of intervention. Appendix 7D explains this process. This table acts as a guide for the therapist to interpret the child's responses to evaluation or intervention, and it is grounded in the therapist's knowledge base, careful evaluation of the child, and ongoing evaluation of the intervention. What is best for the child today may be different tomorrow, based on new information about the child and his or her family or on additional theoretical information. One strength of the occupational therapist is his or her ability to change treatment as the situation shifts. Rarely does only one way exist to interact with a child.

The clinical reasoning chart (see Appendix 7D) can be used individually but is used best with another therapist. The critical thinking process (on the left side) is guided by the client-centered questions on the right. This involves the process of looking for causal explanations for behavior so that predictions can be made about clinical outcomes.

The clinical reasoning process may be used for evaluation and assessment of treatment outcomes. Steps 1 through 5 are used for evaluation and then are repeated, with the addition of steps 5A through 10 for assessment of treatment. Step 6—a critical one—often is overlooked by therapists. Therapists all have "default patterns" in their thinking or areas that they ignore or do not pay as much attention to. If they can identify the type of default patterns that they have, then default patterns can be guarded against through consultation, peer review, case conferences, or just plain awareness. For example, the author discovered her default pattern to be an overconcern with safety that limited client activity choices. In one instance, the author's students produced a major improvement in one client by allowing an activity that the author had thought would be too dangerous but that was not. Becoming cognizant of her default pattern allowed the author to let clients experience the more intense activities they needed while still addressing safety issues.

SUMMARY

The occupational therapist who uses a sensory integrative approach may be called on to explain that approach in terms of its effect on the end-product abilities, especially in school systems. Many children who are referred to occupational therapy within a school setting have been identified as having handwriting problems, praxis problems, or behavior problems. When the therapist determines that the child has or may have a problem with sensory integration, the therapist can best serve the child by explaining sensory system modulation to his or her parents and teachers.

Some major behavior problems that become apparent in the school are related to sensory system modulation. For example, a child who has been identified as having sensory defensiveness may (1) hit out at another child who bumps him or her in the playground or in the lunch line, (2) refuse to use any sticky materials such as paste or finger paint, (3) become outraged if pushed off balance, (4) be fearful of walking down stairs, (5) cover his or her ears during public system announcements, (6) act out, mainly in the cafeteria, or (7) become upset if the class schedule is changed for a special event. If the teacher understands these things as sensory defensiveness and not solely as behaviors, he or she could respond in a more effective way.

When the occupational therapist provides consultation about a child who has problems with sensory integration, the therapist helps the teacher solve problems that affect his or her classroom. Poor handwriting could be related to poor praxis, poor muscle tone, or poor cocontraction. Poor attention span could be the result of sensory defensiveness. Poor perceptual skills contribute to problems in reading and mathematics. The most important contribution that the occupational therapist can make in the school environment is to explain to school personnel what these problems mean in terms of behavior, how changes in input to the child's nervous system can change behavior, and how the therapist and school personnel can work together to help the child succeed.

As with school personnel, the occupational therapist can assist the families of children who have sensory integrative problems to understand the child and his or her behavior. At times, increased understanding may allow parents or other care providers to shed their blame for "causing" the child's problems. The understanding of sensory system modulation alone should produce a major difference in dealing with a child's behavior. The change in environment that a parent can influence can also result in beneficial changes well beyond the reach of a therapy session. It can also give parents the opportunity to interact optimally with their children, thereby increasing self-esteem for children and parents alike. This can also produce successful coping strategies. To explain sensory integration to parents or care providers can be one of the most empowering roles for a therapist.

Acknowledgments

The author is grateful to Glen Ellen Roth for her patient preparation of numerous drafts of this chapter; to Pat Wilbarger for her review of portions of the manuscript and her helpful suggestions for content revisions; to Patty Oetter, Sheila Frick, Eileen Richter, and Pat Wilbarger for their insight into the newest sensory integrative theory; and to Emily Sarah Kimball (then age 5), my daughter, who posed for the mature responses and to her special friend who graciously posed for the contrast pictures so that therapists could learn.

References

Ayres, A. J. (1972). *Sensory integration and learning disorders.* Los Angeles: Western Psychological Services.

Ayres, A. J. (1976). The effect of sensory integrative therapy on learning disabled children: The final report of a research project. Los Angeles: University of Southern California.

Kimball, J. G. (1986). Prediction of methylphenidate (ritalin) responsiveness through sensory integrative testing. *American Journal of Occupational Therapy, 40,* 241–248.

Kimball J. G. (1988). Hypothesis for production of stimulant drug effectiveness utilizing sensory integrative diagnostic methods. *Journal of the American Osteopathic Association, 88,* 757–762.

Oetter, P., Richter, E., & Frick, S. (1992). *MORE integrating the mouth with sensory and postural function.* Hugo, MN: PDP Products.

Sagan, C. (1977). *Dragons of Eden.* New York: Random House.

Wilbarger, P., & Wilbarger, J. (1991). Sensory defensiveness in children 2–12. Santa Barbara, CA: Avanti Education Programs.

Williams, M. S., & Shellenberger, S. (1994). *How does your engine run?* Alburquerque, NM: TherapyWorks.

CHAPTER 9

Visual Information Analysis: Frame of Reference for Visual Perception

VALORIE RICCIARDONE TODD

Occupational therapists have long been concerned with visual perception and its contribution to task performance. In the search to formulate a sound theoretical basis for intervention strategies directed at modifying or overcoming visual perceptual problems in children, occupational therapists have been influenced by cognitive and developmental psychology (Gibson, J. J., 1966; Gibson, E. J., 1969; Piaget, 1953), neurology (Luria, 1980), education (Frostig, 1973; Kephart, 1971), and optometry (Getman, 1965). Occupational therapists have used concepts from the various disciplines to develop guidelines for intervention related to visual perceptual dysfunctions in children and adults (Abreu, 1994; Ayres, 1972; Bouska, Kauffman, & Marcus, 1985; Toglia, 1993; Warren, 1993).

In some developmental theories, especially those describing normal cognitive development or those addressing visual perceptual problems for children that are developmentally delayed or learning disabled, it has been proposed that visual perception lies between sensation and cognition (Piaget, 1952; Strauss & Lehtinen, 1947) and that it is separable from sensation and cognition. However, in this frame of reference, visual perception is conceptualized as the ability to interpret what one sees as an outcome behavior reflective of the interaction between specific visual and cognitive skills. During this interpretation, visual stimuli are related with sensory input from the other senses. Thus, visual perception relies on the individual's innate skills and his or her abilities developed through purposeful interaction with the environment.

Visual information analysis refers to cognitive skills used for extracting and organizing visual information from the environment and integrating this information with other sensory modalities, previous experiences, and higher cognitive functions (Scheiman, 1997). In this frame of reference, visual perception is not viewed as an in-between phase of processing visual information, but as a cognitive process that "changes as a function of learning, labeling and experience" (Mussen, Conger, & Kagen, 1969, p. 287).

Vision, integration of visual input, the other senses, and cognitive analysis skills influence a person's ability to interpret and act on what he or she sees. Many, if not most, children who have physical, developmental, or learning disabilities have some sort of deficit in their visual system. The most common vision disorders include strabismus, amblyopia, significant refractive errors, nystagmus, and optic atrophy (Scheiman, 1997). Visual clarity and ocular motor skills can greatly influence a child's performance. Further, vision deficits can effect a child's ability to accurately take in visual information. Neurological researchers (Chedru, Leblanc, & Lhermitte, 1973; Gianutsos, 1987), optometrists (Scheiman, 1997; Getman; 1965), and occupational therapists (Bouska & Gallaway, 1991; Erhardt, 1990; Warren, 1994) have described the direct influence that vision and ocular motor skills have on perception and motor performance. They have also substantiated the frequency of visual perceptual deficits in children with other disabilities. What sometimes appears to be a visual perceptual deficit may actually be the result of an undiagnosed visual problem or an ocular motor disturbance (Gianutsos, Ramsey, & Perlin, 1988).

It is therefore critical that occupational therapists acquire information on vision and ocular motor skills to better understand and assess the impact of vision on visual information analysis and functional performance. (For additional information see *Understanding and Managing Vision Deficits: A Guide for Occupational Therapists* by Mitchell Scheiman, 1997.)

The visual system has neural interconnections with all of the other sensory systems (Ayres, 1972). During the processing of visual information, input received through the visual system is integrated with information from the other sensory systems. The importance of this intersensory integration cannot be undervalued; however, it will not be addressed within this chapter (See Chapters 7 and 8). This frame of reference addresses those children who have adequate visual and ocular motor skills but are unable to efficiently process and utilize visual input.

THEORETICAL BASE

In order to interpret what is seen, the individual relies on his or her ability to receive visual input accurately through the visual system, combine vision with the other senses, and use his or her cognitive analysis skills. Although visual and the intersensory integration components are not addressed in this chapter, they are important to visual information analysis. The ability to accurately and efficiently receive visual input is dependent on many visual and ocular motor skills. The integration of vision with the other senses, particularly the body senses (i.e., vestibular, tactile, and proprioception) is also vitally important to visually-directed motor performance.

The focus of this chapter is the cognitive analysis skills used to extract, attend to, remember, and discriminate visual information from the environment. Problems in cognitive skills analysis can be seen with and without visual or sensory integration problems. If there are deficits in the other areas, they need to be additionally considered in the overall intervention plan.

This theoretical base is divided into four major sections. The first section summarizes the information processing model as a basis for visual information analysis. The second section defines and describes the cognitive analysis skills integral to this frame of reference: selective attention, visual memory, and visual discrimination. The third section describes four specific visual discrimination skills: recognition, matching, categorization, and detection of relationships. And finally, the fourth section discusses the influence that learning has on the development of visual information analysis.

Information Processing Model

The information processing model is a cognitive approach that explains the flow of information through the human cognitive system. It focuses on how the learner attends to, recognizes, transforms, stores, and retrieves information for later use. The flow of information begins with the *sensory input* that is present in the environment and is received by the sensory organ. *Processing* requires that the sensory input be attended to, compared with previously stored information, transformed into some mental representation, and assigned meaning or acted on. *Output* is observable behavior that reflects whether learning has occurred, or it can be mental information that is stored. *Feedback* to the system comes from output, reinforcing observable behavior, and providing new input (Miller, 1983) (Figure 9.1).

Visual input is dependent on the external stimulation as a source of the input and the capacities of its visual receptors. Visual information comes from the environmental stimuli through the visual receptors to the numerous processing centers throughout the central nervous system.

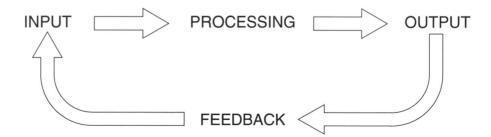

Figure 9.1   Feedback to the system comes from output, reinforcing observable behavior and providing new input.

Visual Input From Environmental Stimuli

The environment, external to the viewer, is an important consideration for the occupational therapist because it is an area that can be directly influenced (Niestadt, 1994). According to Gibson (1969), the environment consists of five types of stimuli: objects, space, events, representations, and symbols. All visual stimuli fall into one of these categories:

1. *Objects:* Three-dimensional forms present in the environment.
2. *Space:* Three-dimensional space. This is a basic level of perception of depth and distance.
3. *Events:* Happenings over time and through space.
4. *Representations:* Two-dimensional pictures or drawings of objects, space, or events.
5. *Symbols:* Coded stimuli; designed to correspond with some other set of stimuli. Language, Morse code, letters, and numerals are examples of coded stimuli.

The first three visual stimuli (i.e., object, space, and events) rely on direct input from the three-dimensional world and are supported by observation and self-generated interaction with objects, space, and events. Three-dimensional stimuli provide direct, multisensory input for learning about objects, space, and events. These stimuli enhance the integration of visual input with the other senses and can be used as strategies to improve visual attention, memory, and discrimination.

The other two visual stimuli, representations and symbols, are man-made and stand in place of objects, space, and events. Although representations look like the objects, space, and events they portray, symbols do not appear anything like the stimuli they represent. The ability to discriminate objects is quickly generalized to representations; so visual discrimination skills may be developed through the use of representations. Symbols differ from representations because they do not look anything like the stimulus they represent. Their meaning must be associated with the stimulus that they correspond to. They are also different because the information given by symbols is given in sequence. A skill such as reading is highly complex and, at the least, relies on associating the language and visual codes simultaneously. Deficits in reading may be the result of reduced language or visual coding or their combination. The term "visual stimuli" will be used throughout this chapter to include all five categories.

Sensory Input—Visual Receptors

Children obtain information about their external environment from the sensory input received through the visual receptors. Visual input is received through the structures of the eye and transmitted to the visual cortex and its association areas where it is processed for interpretation and use. The quality of the visual reception is based on the integrity of different visual receptors and their ability to communicate with each other. There are many parts of the vision apparatus that, if not functioning properly, may interfere with adequate visual reception.

The impact of diagnosed visual or ocular motor disturbance on performance and understanding the potential for change is important to consider. The following skills are believed to impact visual reception of environmental stimuli: motor components including fixation, saccades, pursuits, vergence, accommodation, and vestibular-ocular reflexes; and sensory components including retinal registration of light and movement, visual fields (central and peripheral), acuities, and perception of form, space, and the constancies (definitions are included in Appendix 9A).

Processing

Processing skills in this frame of reference are cognitive in nature and are termed "cognitive analysis skills." They develop throughout the course of a child's development and are subject to the child's genetic and neurologic capacities and his or her experiences with the environment (learning). The cognitive analysis skills include: *visual attention*, which involves the selection of visual input; *visual memory*, which involves the integration of visual information with previous experiences; and *visual discrimination*, which is the ability to detect features of stimuli for perceptual differentiation. These skills will be discussed in greater detail in the cognitive analysis skills section.

Output

The observable output skills that are dependent on visual information analysis are: *recognition, matching, categorization,* and *detection of relationships* among visual stimuli. These receptive skills develop before and form the basis for expressive perceptual-motor skills. However, there are additional cognitive, intersensory, and motor control responses that have an impact on observable output skills. *Production skills* occur at different levels of complexity and require the use of visual information analysis with other intersensory or cognitive abilities, depending on the task. For example, visual information analysis, combined with good body scheme and awareness of the body in space is important for efficient movement through the environment (Figure 9.2).

Cognitive Analysis Skills

The cognitive analysis skills of selective attention, visual memory, and visual discrimination overlap and depend on each other to function optimally. Therefore, it is believed that a deficit in any one of these skills can interfere with the development of the others and have an impact on visual information analysis. Each child's ability to develop visual information analysis skills depends on his or her inherent capacities (e.g., health, current state of the central nervous system, sensory receptor skills), age, and his or her unique experiences with human and nonhuman environments.

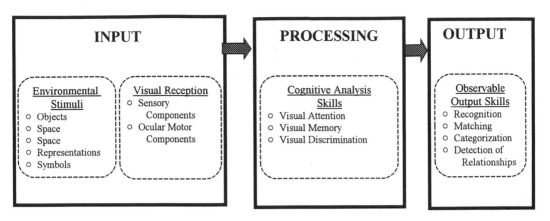

Figure 9.2 Visual Information Analysis.

As children develop visual analysis skills, they develop the abilities to process greater amounts and complexity of information with increased speed. This is accomplished through the development of improved attention abilities, improved storage and retrieval, and the improved ability of abstracting invariant features and higher order structures from visual stimuli. This frame of reference assumes that visual perceptual tasks require the use of different cognitive analysis skills and are not separate visual perceptual skills such as figure-ground, form constancy, or spatial relations.

Visual Attention

Attention, the volitional selection of visual input, is not a unitary skill and includes different components, such as alertness, selective attention, and vigilance (Posner & Rafal, 1987). It is dependent upon many neurologic processes and is influenced by the environment. Visual attention affects visual information analysis and learning.

Arousal is the transition from sleep to a waking state. *Alerting* is the transition from waking to an attentive state. An alert state is needed for active learning and adaptive behavior (Meldman, 1970). Children and adults alike alert to either novelty or a change in their environments. Conversely, they habituate, or stop attending, when the stimuli are familiar or after repeated presentations. Further, alertness may be altered by time of day, fatigue level, inner drive, emotional state, and medications (Toglia, 1993).

Because people have a limited capacity to attend, it is necessary to screen out irrelevant information. *Selective attention* is the ability to choose relevant visual information while ignoring the less relevant information. Selective attention depends on the child's ability to attach meaning to a stimulus or on his or her motivation for attending to a particular task (Levine, 1987). As familiarity and meaning increase, selective attention changes so that the child can screen out familiar or unnecessary stimuli and becomes less easily distracted. In this way, children are able to direct their attention to a stimulus in an array or to its details for further visual analysis. Dysfunctions in selective attention are a common source of problems in many of the children seen by occupational therapists.

Vigilance is the conscious mental effort to concentrate and persist at a visual task. This is the quantitative aspect of attention (attention span) that determines the length of time a child spends on a visual task and allows deeper cognitive analysis. Vigilance is affected by the child's alertness and selective attention and his or her understanding, motivation, effort, problem-solving skills, and reasoning capabilities. These can vary and may often depend on the task itself.

As children develop, their selective attention becomes less stimulus bound and more voluntarily directed. Initially, a young infants' selective attention is drawn to any stimulus that he or she detects. Any new stimulus is as equally attractive and will distract his or her attention. Over time, selective attention increasingly comes under the child's control as he or she attends more selectively and for longer periods of time to stimuli that he or she understands or enjoys. Therefore, children's attentional skills differ based on the child's age and ability to voluntarily direct his or her attention to an age appropriate task.

With age, there are developmental changes in selective attention that are subject to the development of the child's central nervous system. Disruptions to the development of the central nervous system may result in deficits in selective attention. Many of the children with known central nervous system damage (i.e., cerebral palsy, spina bifida, Down's syndrome) or delays have selective attention difficulties. Additionally, a child who is in a compromised emotional state, such as depression or anxiety, may have great difficulty visually attending (Levine, 1987). Children with attention deficits often remain stimuli bound, are frequently distracted by available stimuli, and have difficulty selecting or directing their attention to more relevant stimuli.

Visual Memory

The availability of stored information is essential to visual information analysis and learning. As visual information is received by the child, it is compared to and contrasted with previously experienced information that has been stored. *Visual memory* is defined as the ability to retain and recall visual experiences. It is highly dependent on attention because information needs to be attended to before it can be stored. Memory can be viewed in many ways, according to its duration (i.e., short-term memory or long-term memory), its specific sensory modality (i.e., visual, auditory, or kinesthetic), or its task (i.e., procedural or semantic memory). However, three processes fundamental to visual memory are registration, coding, and retrieval.

Registration. As previously stated, a child must be able to attend to information for it to be stored. This begins through control processes that determine how the information is encoded. The initial control processes include attention, recognition, and rehearsal (Biehler & Snowman, 1990) and affect whether information is lost or transferred into long-term memory.

Coding and Storage. For information to be used later, it must be coded and then stored. Although the way in which data is stored is not completely understood, encoding of information seems to depend on the child's ability to understand and structure the data. One way a child may code the information is through association, which relates new information to information already stored in long-term memory. This ability facilitates the transfer of this combined information to long-term memory. Coding for long-term storage may occur through semantic or linguistic associations or through visual imagery, categorization, and seriation strategies. *Visual imagery* involves the relation of incoming data to meaningful visual images. *Categorization* involves the grouping of data into classes and subclasses. *Seriation* requires the organization of data into a particular memorable sequence (Levine, 1987). These learned strategies may be taught to children.

Retrieval. Retrieval of information requires finding information stored in long-term memory and depends on how the child initially registered and stored the information. Recovery of information may be facilitated by using *association skills,* which link units of information together, and by *recognition skills,* which rely on cues to elicit the memory of a previously encountered stimulus. Some children may be able to recall an appropriate answer when the stimulus is present (e.g., recognizing a letter using an alphabet strip) but may not be able to retrieve it from memory. External memory cues and different strategies may be used to assist in learning to retrieve information.

As children become more capable of associating and storing new information with their knowledge base, their memories improve. As they have more information available, they develop the abilities to reconstruct memories and retrieve them (Meadows, 1993). Repeated exposure and experiences with visual stimuli assist in the development of recognition skills. Familiarity of visual stimuli is helpful in allocating appropriate attentional and discrimination skills for associating and remembering new information.

Before primary school, children show little use of strategic memory and are not aware of what they are capable of remembering. By 7 years of age, children become more aware of memory strategies and they learn how to use them to remember data. These strategies are deliberate activities used to enhance memory such as rehearsal, imagery, and verbal elaboration. Precision, speeds of recall, and ease with which children can retrieve information are significant learning skills and become increasingly important throughout the academic years (Levine, 1987).

Visual Discrimination

Visual discrimination is the ability to detect distinctive and invariant features of a visual stimulus. Visual discrimination develops though what Gibson (1969) termed "perceptual learning," which is the ability of individuals to get increasing amounts of information from their environment as a result of practice with the array of stimulation. From these experiences, children learn to differentiate stimuli through the discovery of distinctive features that distinguish one stimulus from another. Children learn that each stimulus does not have only one distinctive feature but contains many features that make it identifiable or unique. Children gradually develop the ability to extract increasing amounts of information from the same visual stimulation. They learn to detect invariant or unchanging characteristics among visual stimuli. They also learn stimulus invariance when relations and properties remain constant despite visual changes. Ultimately, children become efficient and rapidly differentiate stimuli from each other, resulting in perceptions becoming more specific and economical (Gibson, 1969).

For example, children learn to distinguish a cup from other objects in their environment through experiences with the cup and other objects. They differentiate a cup by its visual characteristics including its cylindrical shape, its opening, and its handle. They learn more about it by using it functionally and by hearing its label "cup." Through their repeated experiences with a variety of different cups, they are able to recognize a variety of cups and develop the concept of a cup. They also learn to be more specific by discriminating mommy's cup from all other cups.

When stimuli are given distinctive names, attention is drawn to the stimulus or its quality and it becomes easier for the child to perceive the features that make it the same or different from others. Therefore, the technique of *labeling* plays an important role in visual discrimination.

Young children have the tendency to overgeneralize the similarities of stimuli. All furry, four-legged animals may be grouped by their common characteristics and are all called "doggie," for example. With experience, children learn to discriminate a dog from a cat and then even to differentiate different types of dogs or different dogs of the same breed. There is an increased ability to pick up the distinctive features of a stimulus and an increase in more specific discriminations among similar stimuli. There is also a time during concept formation that children may be overly specific or concrete and identify only one dog as "a dog." In this case, they have not yet generalized the concept of a dog from one stimulus to a group of similar stimuli.

The ability to selectively attend results in improved attention to details and allows for improved abstraction of interrelationships among stimuli. Recognition, matching, categorization, and detection of relationship skills become easier and faster as children are better able to filter out the irrelevant information and detect the relevant. Attentional deficits may significantly interfere with visual discrimination.

As children mature, they progressively develop the ability to extract relevant information from the environment more effectively. They become better able to differentiate stimuli by a minimal set of features that make them recognizable. Children also become better at differentiating new or unfamiliar stimuli by abstracting invariant features and patterns among visual stimuli more readily.

Detection and matching of stimulus characteristics (e.g., size, color, and external contour [shape]) seem to precede the ability to differentiate changes in position. For example, children can identify their teddy bears no matter what position it is in or from what position they view it. Such judgment is based on the child's ability to detect the object's invariant properties, no matter its position or the child's point of view (form constancy). The object remains the same no matter its position. It is not until discrimination of symbols (letters and numbers), that position becomes an important differentiating distinctive feature.

Children begin to detect the positional difference of upside down and right-side up (inversions) before left and right (reversals) or before other spatial orientations (angles or tilt). Positional changes seem to become more easily detected and remembered as children grow older (approximately at 7 years of age). This may be one reason why reversals by children are common until the age of 7 years.

Visual Discrimination Skills (Output skills). As visual attention and memory develop, the specific visual discrimination skills of recognition, matching, categorizing, and detecting relationships are also learned. Common to the visual discrimination skills are the abilities to detect similarities and differences and group visual stimuli.

Recognition. Recognition is the ability to note key features of a stimulus and relate them to memory (Biehler & Snowman, 1990). Recognition requires that the observer selectively attend to the stimulus, detect its distinctive features, store them, and/or compare the present stimulus to the stored image. It is a form of "mental matching".

As children mature, more sophisticated visual discrimination skills allow them to recognize more subtle similarities and differences among stimuli. Gradually, they are able to immediately recognize a wide variety of stimuli. These learned skills increase a child's speed and efficiency in processing visual information for other tasks. Familiarity of certain environments or certain tasks may allow attentional skills to be reallocated to the new or pertinent information at hand.

Matching. Another visual discrimination skill is matching, which requires identification of stimuli that are exactly alike. Matching is the basis of many visual perceptual assessments and worksheets. In most matching-to-a-sample tasks a specific stimulus is given to match to one or more in the given array (Figure 9.3). Matching requires detection of the differences among the stimuli because the child will make errors if he or she only matches by similarities. This error is common at young ages and in children who have difficulty selectively detecting or attending to details.

Matching tasks require selecting stimuli that are exactly alike and can be presented on a continuum from simple-to-complex. They become more complex when the differences between the stimuli are minimal, the number of features to be discriminated are increased (Figure 9.4), or the stimuli are presented with extraneous "distracters" (Figure 9.5). Children learn strategies to increase their attention to detail and to discriminate distinctive features through matching.

Categorization. Another visual discrimination skill is categorization. Categorization requires grouping stimuli based on a common characteristic or characteristics. Although matching is dependent on discriminating all the same characteristics of the stimuli, categorizing stimuli by visual features requires extracting the invariant features among stimuli despite visual differences. This skill reflects a different and higher level of abstraction.

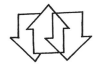

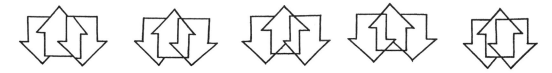

Figure 9.3   Matching task. TVPS VD1. (Reprinted with permission from Psychological and Educational Publications, Inc., Hydesville, CA.)

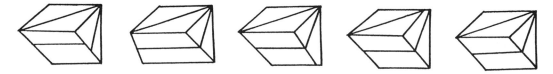

Figure 9.4   Complex matching task: differences are minimal; the number of features to be discriminated are increased. (Reprinted with permission from Psychological and Educational Publications, Inc., Hydesville, CA.)

One type of categorization task requires that the similar stimuli are grouped while stimuli that are different are excluded from the group (Figure 9.6). Unlike matching tasks, a sample item is not visually present. A child must form his or her own mental group and detect the one stimulus that does not match the group.

In another categorization task, children may be asked to find stimuli that are alike despite changes in color, size, or position (Figure 9.7). They must be able to abstract the invariant feature common to the stimuli despite the difference of one or more

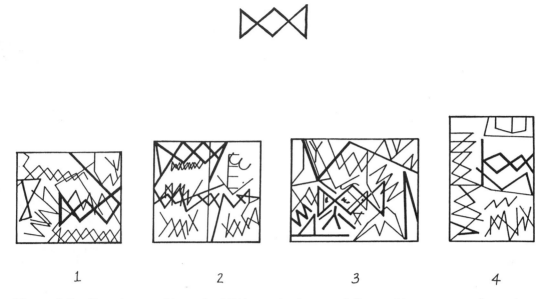

Figure 9.5 Complex matching task: child is required to match figure with extraneous distractions. (Reprinted with permission from Psychological and Educational Publications, Inc., Hydesville, CA.)

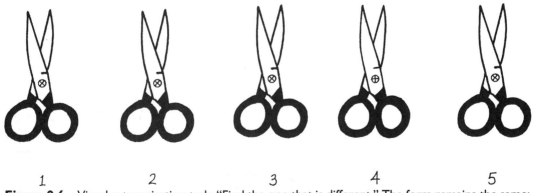

Figure 9.6 Visual categorization task: "Find the one that is different." The form remains the same; the difference is a change in position. (Reprinted with permission from Psychological and Educational Publications, Inc., Hydesville, CA.)

features. Children who have delays in concept formation may have difficulties with these types of categorization tasks. They may not yet be able to abstract the similarities because of the apparent differences in size, number, color, or position. Children learn to abstract invariant features and develop specific concepts (e.g., color, size, number, and position) from categorization tasks.

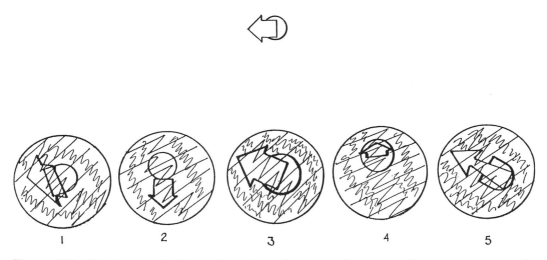

Figure 9.7   Visual categorization task: requires abstracting the invariant feature common to the stimuli despite visual differences. (Reprinted with permission from Psychological and Educational Publications, Inc., Hydesville, CA.)

Detecting relationships. A fourth visual discrimination skill is the ability to detect relationships among stimuli. This ability depends on the ability to abstract connections or associations between stimuli. Common relationships that are abstracted in visually presented stimuli are sequence and position. Serial activities (e.g., nesting cups and graduated pegs) reflect the ability to detect relationships among stimuli (Figure 9.8). The child must be able to determine size relationships among the group of objects and then organize them in a graduated series. This requires simultaneous comparisons of each item to every item in the group. The greater number of items, the more complex the task. Story sequence cards are even more abstract because interpretations about the actions and consequences in each picture must be made and then organized into a logical sequence. They are easier when they depict more familiar sequences of events than when the sequence needs to be inferred.

Many constructional tasks, in part, require the ability to determine relationships between the parts. Puzzles, block designs, and graphic copying (Figure 9.9) depend on this ability in combination with other skills. Although visual motor in response, these tasks rely on the cognitive abstraction of positional relations between the parts; constructional tasks are sequential and require judgment and problem-solving.

Learning

This frame of reference is based on the belief that the development of visual information analysis is based on learning. Learning is an unseen process and can only be observed though a change in the child's verbal or non-verbal behavior (Gibson,

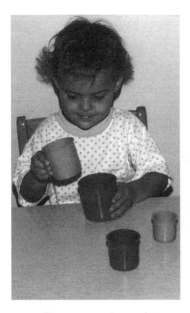

Figure 9.8 Child nesting cups. Detecting relationships among stimuli: size sequencing.

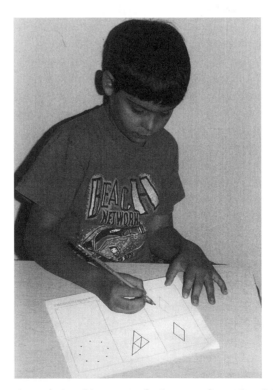

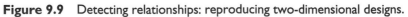

Figure 9.9 Detecting relationships: reproducing two-dimensional designs.

1969). Although therapists may create environments where learning is facilitated, it is the child who engages with the environment who actually learns (Mosey, 1986).

Learning occurs through the integration of the child's developmental abilities and his or her interactions with the human and non-human environment. It changes over time through the child's repeated experiences with the visual world (Gibson, 1969). The child uses his or her visual and cognitive skills to actively explore the visual environment; he or she is not passive in his or her visual reception. He or she searches out visual stimuli that are novel and interesting, interacts with them, and learns from them. With repeated exposure and developmental growth in cognitive skills, he or she learns to abstract meaning from the visual world.

Visual information analysis is based on a child's visual skills, the integration of vision with his or her other senses, and his or her cognitive analysis skills. Visual information analysis skills are learned and can be influenced directly by the teaching-learning process. Learning results in the abilities to differentiate stimuli and sequence, categorize, form concepts, perform intellectual operations in space, problem-solve, and generalize. It is assumed that for visual stimuli to be understood and used, information from the visual system must be processed mentally and learning must take place. This mental processing involves the integration of visual information through the cognitive realm of understanding. This includes the mental processes of thinking, understanding, knowing, and judging.

The therapist's role in this teaching learning process is to choose appropriate goals and then provide environmental and task modifications or strategies that facilitate learning. The skills that are taught are intended to generalize to a variety of tasks or, if not possible, to at least assist in functional daily performance.

FUNCTION/DYSFUNCTION CONTINUA

Function/dysfunction continua provide therapists with descriptions of observable behaviors that are clinically relevant and that identify function and dysfunction in children.

VISUAL ATTENTION

Visual attention allows a child to take in information from his or her physical environment and learn from it. To be ready to receive visual information, the child must be in a balanced state of arousal. Selective attention assists in choosing which of the available stimuli are most likely to be useful. Vigilance to visual stimuli allows greater precision in the exploration of distinctive features and supports prolonged processing of visually presented materials.

Although not directly addressed by this frame of reference, it is important to consider a child's visual attention. If a child has difficulty with visual attention, then visual processing skills may be affected. Attentional problems may be seen in alertness, selective attention, and/or vigilance. The child may be overaroused by sensory input received through the visual system. He or she may not be able to select the features that require further attention or analysis. If he or she is unable to persist in an activity because of a short attention span, he or she may miss important details or overgeneralize his or her visual interpretations. He or she may not attend long enough to store information in his or her memory. Children with problems with alertness may demonstrate the following: be easily distracted by environmental stimuli or be difficult to arouse, have difficulty sustaining visual gaze, have erratic sleep and wake cycles, have high or low activity levels, or fatigue easily. Although these areas of dysfunction are not directly addressed in this frame of reference, they must be addressed simultaneously or sequentially using another frame of reference.

Selective Attention

Selective attention assists in choosing which of the available stimuli are most likely to be useful.

Indicators of Function and Dysfunction

At the functional end of the continua, selective attention to visual stimuli is the ability to attend to relevant visual information while ignoring the irrelevant. This includes the ability to select relevant information, explore stimuli for relevant information, and screen out competing stimuli. Problems in this area are evident when a child has difficulty screening out unimportant information, is easily distracted by unimportant or extraneous stimuli, and tends to focus on irrelevant or unimportant stimuli (Chart 9.1).

Vigilance

Vigilance to visual stimuli allows greater precision in the exploration of distinctive features and supports prolonged processing of visually presented material.

Chart 9.1   Indicators of Function and Dysfunction for Selective Attention.

Selectively Attends to Visual Stimuli	Reduced Ability to Attend to Visual Stimuli
FUNCTION: Ability to attend to relevant visual information while ignoring the irrelevant	DYSFUNCTION: Difficulty in selecting relevant visual information; Difficulty-ignoring the irrelevant
INDICATORS OF FUNCTION	**INDICATORS OF DYSFUNCTION**
Selects relevant information	Difficulty screening out unimportant information
Explores stimulus for relevant information	Easily distracted by unimportant or extraneous stimuli
Screens out competing stimuli	Tends to focus on irrelevant or unimportant stimuli

Indicators of Function and Dysfunction

Functionally, vigilance is the ability to concentrate on and persist in a visual task for the appropriate length of time to complete the task. Problems with vigilance are evident when a child is unable to concentrate on or persist in a visual task. The child may have difficulty identifying visual details or may not be able to maintain selective attention for an appropriate length of time to allow for adequate performance (short attention span) (Chart 9.2).

Visual Memory

Children who exhibit functional memory skills can store and retrieve previously presented stimuli. They are able to attend to the stimulus long enough to encode it for later retrieval.

Indicators of Function and Dysfunction

Children with adequate visual memory are able to store and retrieve visual information, which are indicators of function. They are able to recognize previously presented visual information, recall information from their own memory on demand, and use mnemonic strategies to improve their own memory stores.

At the dysfunctional end of the continuum, children who have difficulty attending to or associating new input with stored information may have difficulty remembering stimuli that have been presented many times and over long periods of time. They often require concrete cues to assist in the recall of information, have difficulty retrieving information, and have difficulty using mnemonic strategies. Visual memory deficits are usually noted by poor recognition of objects, representations, and symbols and reduced memory about space and events. Poor recognition is seen in the inability to use or name objects, representations, or symbols appropriately. Some children with memory deficits have difficulty remembering spatial cues from the environment or the actions of a previously experienced event (Chart 9.3).

Chart 9.2   Indicators of Function and Dysfunction for Vigilance.

Concentration on and Persistence at a Visual Task	Reduced Persistence at a Visual Task
FUNCTION: Ability to concentrate on and persist at a visual task	DYSFUNCTION: Unable to concentrate on or persist at a visual task
INDICATORS OF FUNCTION	**INDICATORS OF DYSFUNCTION**
Visually attends to tasks for appropriate length of time for task completion	Cursory examination of visual stimuli; is not vigilant enough to allow for identifying visual details Cannot maintain visual attention for an appropriate length of time to allow for adequate performance (short attention span)

Chart 9.3 Indicators of Function and Dysfunction for Visual Memory	
Adequate Visual Memory Skills	**Poor Visual Memory Skills**
FUNCTION: Ability to adequately store and retrieve visual information	DYSFUNCTION: Poor or reduced ability to store and retrieve visual information
INDICATORS OF FUNCTION	**INDICATORS OF DYSFUNCTION**
Recognizes previously presented visual information	Fails to recognize previously presented visual stimuli
Recognizes given information appropriately needed for the situation	Requires concrete cues to assist in recall of information
Recalls information from own memory on demand	Fails to retrieve information; inconsistent recall
Uses mnemonic strategies to improve own memory stores	Fails to use mnemonic strategies; fails to relate information to prior knowledge
	Response time may be prolonged as memory is explored

Visual Discrimination Skills

As children develop the ability to detect distinctive and invariant features that make visual stimuli identifiable, they develop the ability to recognize, match, categorize, and determine relationships. Physical properties of visual stimuli that are commonly discriminated are shape, size, color, number, position, and internal details.

Indicators of Function and Dysfunction

Visual discrimination skills include the ability to visually recognize, match, categorize, and detect relationships. Children with adequate skills are able to recognize previously experienced visual stimuli, match exact visual stimuli despite subtle differences or competing backgrounds, categorize visual stimuli despite apparent differences in presentation, detect and reproduce positional relationships among visual stimuli, and detect and reproduce sequential relationships among visual stimuli.

Children who have problems with visual discrimination skills are unable to identify objects from their visual features. They may have difficulty detecting the distinctive features of a stimulus or the similarities and differences between stimuli. Because of these deficits, these children have difficulties with recognition tasks. Recognition deficits can be quite significant.

Other children demonstrate poor visual discrimination in their difficulty with matching tasks. They may match one general feature and are unable to attend to the other distinguishing characteristics of the stimulus. Some children demonstrate poor categorization when they are unable to determine a category for a group of presented stimuli. They have difficulty in sorting tasks when given a group of related stimuli and asked to put things together that go together. They may have difficulty discriminating similarities among related stimuli when they vary by more than one parameter (Figure 9.10). Deficits in categorization can be associated with poor concept formation.

Deficits in the ability to detect relationships may contribute to difficulties in performing visual motor tasks. They may have difficulty detecting positional or se-

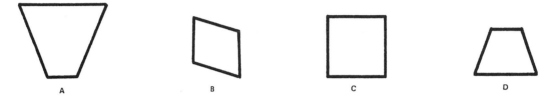

Figure 9.10   Detecting invariant features that vary by more than one property is more difficult than when the stimulus only varies by one difference. (Reprinted with permission from Academic Therapy, Novato, CA.)

quential relationships, which is essential for copying and other constructional tasks. These tasks usually require a motor response based on the ability to detect and then produce a copy based on the appreciation of the relationships between parts of the stimuli. Sequential relationships are also used in most constructional tasks, as the ability to know where to begin and how best to proceed is inferred in the process. Children with visual discrimination deficits are usually unable to make quick, reliable, and refined interpretations of visual information (Chart 9.4).

GUIDE TO EVALUATION

Children who are referred to occupational therapy are usually exhibiting a performance deficit. Presenting problems often include motor clumsiness, difficulty with scissors or pencil control, or poor handwriting. Assessment of visual information analysis may be included in an overall occupational therapy evaluation to analyze its potential effects on motor performance. The tasks chosen to evaluate visual information processing should elicit behaviors in each cognitive analysis area. The stimuli may vary according to the child's presenting problem.

It is important for an occupational therapist to know about the child's vision and ocular motor skills before assessing visual information analysis skills. Although occupational therapists are not expected to perform vision evaluations, they may screen children for certain visual receptor disorders and make referrals to appropriate vision professionals. A checklist (Figure 9.11) is useful in documenting and reporting visual

Chart 9.4 Indicators of Function and Dysfunction for Visual Discrimination Skills.

Adequate Visual Discrimination Skills	Inadequate Visual Discrimination Skills
FUNCTION: Ability to detect distinctive features and invariant relationships	DYSFUNCTION: Inadequate ability to detect distinctive features and invariant relationships
INDICATORS OF FUNCTION	**INDICATORS OF DYSFUNCTION**
Recognizes previously experienced visual stimuli	Poor recognition skills despite numerous presentations
Matches exact visual stimuli despite subtle differences or competing background	Difficulty matching visual stimuli; matches by general features; does not perceive subtle differences among stimuli (e.g., confuses similar shapes: b/d; n/u; E/F; g/p/q)
	Difficulty matching a form within a competing background
Categorizes visual stimuli despite apparent differences in presentation	Poor categorization skills; unable to discriminate invariant features among similar stimuli
	Poor grouping skills of a number of visually similar stimuli
Detects and reproduces positional relationships among visual stimuli	Fails to determine which stimulus is different when presented with visually similar group of stimuli
	Difficulty with puzzles, block designs, and other constructional tasks
Detects and reproduces sequential relationships among visual stimuli	Difficulty with size seriation tasks (e.g., nesting cups, graduated pegs)
	Difficulty with sequence cards

behaviors that may alert parents and teachers to the possibility of a vision problem and help the vision professional address the visual concerns of the child.

A vision examination should include more than just visual acuity. An ocular motor screening is usually informative. Knowing that there is a visual or ocular motor deficit can help to understand a child's behaviors. The knowledge that a visual deficit is present may help reduce misunderstanding of the child's behavior.

Evaluation of Visual Attention Skills

Visual attention is often related to a child's general attentional abilities. Prior information about the child's attention is helpful in designing the environment and tasks. Children with general attentional deficits may require more careful preparation of the environment and the sequence and choice of tasks used for evaluation. Although their attentional deficits may be known, eliciting their optimal attention provides information about their strengths and allows improved discrimination of their abilities in other areas being assessed.

Direct observation of a child's selective attention while performing the selected evaluation tasks continues throughout the evaluation session. In a solitary occupational therapy evaluation session, direct observation of attentional skills is limited by the time spent with the child and is influenced by the one-to-one interaction, novelty of the examiner, and the particular tasks presented. Often, this type of session may yield the child's best (or worst) attentional capabilities. That is why it is important to have information about the child's attention skills in other situations. Questionnaires and interviews are good ways of gathering that information.

If there are concerns regarding the child's alertness or activity level, a sensory

Observations of Visual Function in Children

Behaviors	Frequent	Seldom	Never
Turns head, tilts head, thrusts head forward			
Shuts or covers one eye			
Rubs eyes			
Excessive head movement			
Excessive blinking			
Excessive distractibility			
Excessive squinting or frowning			
Irritability after sustained visual work			
Fatigue after sustained visual work			
Limited attention span for visual tasks			
Holds objects close to eyes			
"Misses the mark" when starting to cut a line or string a bead			
Unable to see distant objects clearing			
Loses place when reading			
Skips or repeats words or lines when reading			
Skips or repeats letters, words or lines when copying			
Appearance			
Eyes cross or diverge			
Eyes are inflammed or watery			
Eyes are red-rimmed, crusty, or swollen			
Nystagmus			
Complaints			
Blurry Vision			
Double Vision			
Headache, nausea, dizziness following close work			
Itchy, burning, scratching feeling in eyes			

Kathleen Tsurumi, O.T.R.

Figure 9.11   Checklist for teachers and parents. (Courtesy of Kathleen Tsurumi, OTR.)

history (Dunn & Westman, 1997) may help in examining the child's sensory processing, which may be impacting the child's overall attentional abilities. Questionnaires designed to examine Attention Deficit Disorders (ADD) and Attention Deficit and Hyperactivity Disorder (ADHD) (Conners Teacher Rating Scale, 1969; McCarney, 1989) may also be helpful in getting information about their selective attention and vigilance and how their attention deficits may be impacting on everyday performances.

The following is a list of questions that may be helpful to the therapist in assessing selective attention. These questions may be asked of the parent, teacher, or evaluator as he or she presents different tasks during the assessment. This information may be viewed in relation to child's attentional capabilities across contexts and can be used to find his or her strengths when planning for intervention.

- What types of visual activities does the child enjoy? What types does he or she not like? Are three-dimensional objects more alluring than pictures, or are pictures more alluring than symbols?

- Does the child use vision effectively when moving through the environment? Or, is the child inattentive and impulsive?

- Does the child "tune out" visually? Or, does he or she demonstrate incessant visual searching?

- How much structure is necessary to gain the child's selective attention? Are additional sensory cues necessary, such as auditory or tactile cues? Can the child's distraction level be decreased by restructuring the environment?

- Does the child notice unimportant, incidental information rather than what is important or typically attended to?

- How easily can the child be redirected back to a visual task?

- How long can the child attend to age appropriate visual tasks? Does he or she become fatigued during tasks that require sustained selective attention?

- Can the child sustain effort on a visually demanding task?

Poor selective attention and impulsivity may interfere with the child's test taking skills. Alternative strategies may assist the therapist in determining the child's "true" abilities. When giving standardized tests of visual discrimination, visually isolating each choice from the others and asking "Do they match?" may provide information about their ability to detect similarities and differences in a simpler presentation. If they impulsively point to the first one they look at, encourage them to "look at all the choices" before you answer. A therapist may even need to help children look at each one to assist them in their attention. When a child automatically corrects a mistake, the therapist may advise the child to slow down before he or she answers and then make note that the child is able to self correct that item. Of course if adaptations are made, the standardized scores cannot be used. However, information has been gained about the child's discrimination skills, despite his or her attentional problems and information regarding the effects of visual task modifications that can be used when planning intervention strategies.

Evaluation of Visual Memory

Again, reports from parents and teachers regarding a child's memory may be helpful. These reports are especially valuable in gaining data about a child's long-term memory. Some questions to guide assessment in this area are:

- What types of information does the child remember? What kinds of things does he or she have difficulty remembering? Is the child better at remembering experiences that are multisensory, autobiographical, or auditory versus visual?
- Is the child consistent in his or her ability to recognize and name objects, pictures, or symbols? Does the child recognize and name only in one area?
- How often does information have to be repeated for the child to remember it?
- Is the child's memory erratic? Does he or she sometimes remember information on one day and forget it the next?

There are several standardized visual perceptual assessments that contain short–term visual memory subtests such as the *Test of Visual Perceptual Skills* (Gardner, 1988) and the *Motor Free Test of Visual Perception* (Callarusso & Hammill, 1972). Performance on these tests gives an idea of how well a child attends to and retrieves visual information that has been presented briefly. Observations during the test may include observations about selective attention and encoding strategies used (e.g., subvocalizing, tracing) to retain the visual information.

- Does the child visually attend for the allotted time, or does the child tell you that he or she is "ready" after only a brief glance?
- Does the child scan all the items or does he or she impulsively point to one?
- To gain some information about the child's strategies for coding visual information, a therapist can question the child about how he or she remembered the stimulus.
- Did the child name the figure (semantic coding)? Did he or she rely on immediate revisualization only (eidetic memory)? Did he or she only look at one part, details only, or did he or she take in the gestalt?

The therapist needs to consider the effectiveness of the child's strategies. To collect additional information, a therapist may suggest an alternative strategy and see if the child is able to use it. In this way, information can be obtained about the child's ability to learn how to encode visual information. Error analysis of test items may reveal that a child is having difficulty discriminating between similar stimuli or if the child is only attending to a certain side of the page.

Evaluation of Visual Discrimination Skills

A child's basic visual discrimination skills have been acquired through active visual exploration, the abstraction of distinctive features, and invariance among visual stimuli. The ability to discriminate is a basic skill to understanding the world. Discrimination skills are applied to all forms of stimuli, which are objects, space, events, representations, and symbols. However, there is no one instrument for assessing the processing of each of these stimuli. It is up to the therapist to design an evaluation based on the child's presenting problems. It is important to choose the appropriate stimuli that will allow observation of the child's functional and dysfunctional skills.

- Is there a problem with discriminating objects? Does the child have difficulty understanding and acting in three-dimensional space? Can he or she interpret pictorial representations or only objects in the symbolic area?
- Can the child match stimuli? Does he or she discriminate subtle differences?
- Can the child categorize visually similar stimuli? What kinds of stimuli can he or she categorize?

Discrimination tasks using objects are helpful when assessing young children. Functional use of objects is one measure of recognition of familiar stimuli. Early language that the child uses to label objects can assist in determining what objects are being differentiated. As the child's object recognition expands, the child sees and attends to new and different properties of objects such as size, color, shape, and internal details. Form boards and single piece puzzles are ways to evaluate early discrimination of shapes. Single piece puzzles may use simple, familiar shapes or more complex contours. Pictured details may not be helpful to the discrimination of shape. Unicolored objects can be used to assess color matching or categorizing. Graduated cylinders or pegs and nesting cups or rings can be used to assess sequencing by size. Simple picture books can be used to assess skills to attend to representational stimuli or identify objects or their characteristics.

There are many standardized tests of visual perception including the *Motor Free Test of Visual Perception* (Callarusso & Hammill, 1972), *Developmental Test of Visual Perception-2* (Hammill, Pearson, & Voress, 1993), and *Test of Visual Perceptual Skills* (Gardner, 1988) that propose that there are different visual perceptual skills that develop relatively independently of each other. Three such skills are figure-ground, form constancy, and spatial relations (Frostig, 1973).

In this frame of reference it is assumed that visual perceptual tasks, typically seen in visual perceptual tests and worksheets, require the use of different cognitive analysis skills and are not dependent on separate visual perceptual skills such as figure-ground, form constancy, or spatial relations. Thus, when standardized tests of visual perception are used in this frame of reference, they are used to assess the cognitive analysis skills of visual attention, visual memory, and visual discrimination of representational stimuli. When standardized visual perceptual tests are used, different levels of cognitive analysis skills are needed, based on how the visual stimuli are presented. The visual stimuli in these tests are typically presented on a continuum of simple-to-complex, which gives them their developmental nature. It is the development of cognitive analysis abilities that enable the interpretation of the visual stimuli that are presented in a more complex, developmentally demanding way.

According to this frame of reference, these visual perceptual tests primarily assess the visual discrimination skills of matching and categorizing of black and white representational stimuli, which is only one form of visual stimuli. A child's performance on these tasks may not match his or her ability to discriminate other forms of stimuli. Thus, a therapist should be careful when interpreting the significance of a child's performance on specific subtests, to performance on other visual tasks.

An additional point about standardized perceptual tests is the names that the authors use to subcategorize perceptual skills. These various labels can be confusing because the subjects do not represent the skills they were named after, nor do all the similarly named tests assess the same skill. For example, the spatial relations subtest on the *Test of Visual Perceptual Skills* (Gardner, 1988) (Figure 9.6) requires that the child find the one that is different. The items are exactly the same except for one, whose only difference is position. On the *Developmental Test of Visual Perception* (Hammil et al., 1993) (Figure 9.12), the spatial relations subtest requires copying designs on dot grids. This task is in the visual motor section and requires motor control and the ability to determine the positional relationships between the lines. Both tasks are named "spatial relations" yet neither requires discrimination of three-dimensional space and each one requires quite different responses. Difficulties with perception of space may have nothing to do with poor performance on these subtests but may be related to the poor ability to categorize in one case or poor motor control in another.

Another subtest is "figure-ground," which is a term initially defined as an innate skill by which a child detects a figure while the rest of the visual field becomes background. Accuracy on this task is based on the ability to selectively attend to and match the given stimulus while ignoring the distracters (Figure 9.13). This ability may be more related to selective attention abilities. Complexity on figure-ground tests is increased by the amount of distracters surrounding the stimulus. There are items in other subtests that require this same ability, but they are included in a different category under a different subskill name (Figure 9.14).

There are other visual perceptual evaluation tasks, like copying block designs, that rely on motor output and also rely on visual discrimination skills, especially the ability to detect relationships. These expressive tasks are included in many developmental assessments such as the *Miller Assessment for Preschoolers* (Miller, 1982) and the *Peabody Developmental Motor Scales* (Folio & Fewell, 1983) and usually are located in the fine motor or adaptive skills sections of these tests.

The ability to copy graphic designs is standardized in assessments such as *Developmental Test of Visual Motor Integration* (Beery, 1989), *Developmental Test of Visual Percep-*

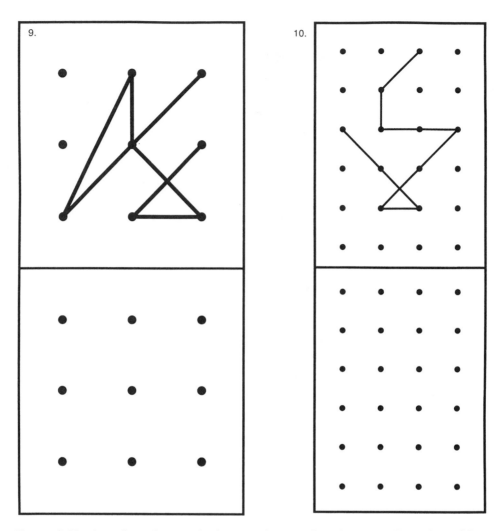

Figure 9.12   Item from the spatial relations subtest on Developmental Test of Visual Perception-2. (Reprinted with permission from Pro-ed, Austin, TX.)

tion-2 (Hammill, Pearson, & Voress, 1993), and *The Test of Visual Motor Skills* (Gardner, 1988). These assessments require that the child detect relationships and then reproduce them. These tasks are not used to assess the quality of motor output, but rather the ability to analyze a visually presented stimulus, break it down into its components, and reorganize the components into an accurate copy. The child's motor control may be looked at separately. These tests may not be appropriate if a child has a motor deficit.

Beyond analyzing the errors that a child makes when performing a motor task, a therapist can find out additional information about how a child visually analyzes in-

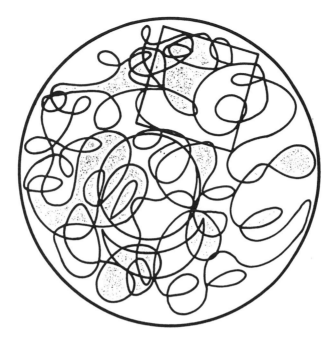

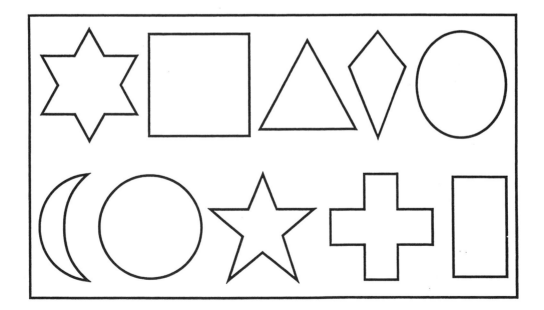

Figure 9.13   Figure-ground task: demonstrating complexity by the increased amount of distracters surrounding the stimulus to be detected. (Reprinted with permission from Pro-ed, Austin, TX.)

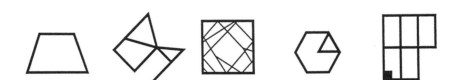

Figure 9.14 "Form constancy" task that also requires finding the "figure" in an embedded "background." (Reprinted with permission from Pro-ed, Austin, TX.)

formation by talking with him or her. Specifically, a therapist can ask a child if he or she thinks his or her reproduction matches the stimulus. Can the child identify his or her errors? Can the child correct his or her errors? Can the child describe why he or she made the error? ("My hand did not do what I wanted it to"). Whenever a therapist asks a child to describe what he or she is doing or why, the therapist should be sensitive to the child's ability to admit his or her own errors and then take this factor into consideration.

Summary

A child is usually referred for an occupational therapy evaluation because of an observable performance deficit. In this frame of reference, problems of concern are caused by inefficient cognitive analysis skills. This determination must be made within the context of the child's overall level of functioning. Additional information may be obtained by reviewing other records, such as psychological or speech and language reports. When analyzing visual information analysis, it *must be* viewed within the context of other cortical skills. Often visual information analysis problems are seen with other cortically-based problems, especially language deficits. It is important not to look at the visual perceptual deficits isolated from these other problems.

When the occupational therapy evaluation is completed, the information about visual information analysis must be analyzed and interpreted within the broader context of the child's other capabilities, which may include visual receptor skills, sensory motor processing, and other cognitively-based processes (e.g., language, reasoning and problem-solving). Based on this frame of reference, analysis of evaluation findings determines whether the poor performance on the visual information analysis part of the evaluation is primarily caused by deficiencies in the selective attention, memory, or discrimination skills.

POSTULATES REGARDING CHANGE

When the evaluation results indicate a dysfunction in visual information analysis, the therapist must address the components that interfere with function. The postulates regarding change can be used to formulate intervention strategies and select activities and to choose materials.

There is one general postulate regarding change based on this frame of reference:

1. Visual attention, visual memory, and visual discrimination are facilitated through teaching learning principles (Table 9.1).

Four postulates regarding change are related to visual attention:

2. Visual attention is facilitated when a child is in the appropriate state of physical, mental, and emotional preparedness.
3. Selective attention is enhanced when relevant stimuli are emphasized and less relevant stimuli are at a minimum.
4. Selective attention is supported by visual exploration.
5. Concentration and persistence in visual tasks increase if motivation, comprehension, and intrinsic interest are present.

Six postulates regarding change are related to visual memory:

6. Registration in visual memory is enhanced when selective attention, motivation, and comprehension are present.
7. Storage in visual memory is enhanced when a visual stimulus is combined with additional sensory input. Thus, sensory input may include tactile, proprioceptive, or auditory input. When the input is of an auditory nature, it is called labeling.
8. Storage in visual memory is enhanced though repeated presentations, routine, and predictability.
9. Storage in visual memory is enhanced through associations with previous knowledge.

Table 9.1 Teaching Learning Principles

The teaching-learning process has been a tool of occupational therapy since its inception (Mosey, 1986). These teaching-learning principles are based on current knowledge about learning. They are applied by the therapist according to what he or she assumes will best help the child learn. They are a guide to how the environment, tasks, and human interactions can be deliberately structured to facilitate change.

Learning is influenced by the individual's inherent capacities, current assets and limitations, age, sex, interest, and past and present culture group membership.

Learning goals set by the individual are more likely to be attained than goals set by someone else.

Learning is enhanced when the individual understands what is to be learned and the reason for learning.

Learning is increased when it begins at the individual's current level and proceeds at a rate that is comfortable for the individual.

Learning can be enhanced through trial and error, shaping, and imitation of models.

Frequent repetition or practice facilitates learning.

The environment in which learning takes place is an important factor.

Conflicts and frustrations inevitably present in the learning situation must be recognized and provisions made for their resolution or accommodation.

Reinforcement and feedback are important parts of the learning experience.

There needs to be continuity between the learning situation and the experiences for which the learning constitutes preparation.

10. Visual memory is enhanced through mnemonic strategies (e.g., elaboration, seriation, imagery, categorization).
11. Visual memory is enhanced through external devices designed to elicit retrieval.

There are three postulates regarding change related to visual discrimination:

12. Visual discrimination skills are facilitated through simplified visual presentations, few stimuli, non-competing background, structured organization, exaggerated distinctive features, and reduced irrelevant stimuli.
13. Visual discrimination is enhanced by attention to the distinctive and invariant features of a stimulus. Attention to these features denotes the detection of difference.
14. Visual discrimination is enhanced through attention, memory, sensory motor experience, and labeling.

APPLICATION TO PRACTICE

Goals are set once the evaluation is completed and information is obtained regarding the child's functional performance deficits that will be addressed by occupational therapy. Based on the goals and the child's strengths and needs, the therapist selects the appropriate postulates regarding change that address the deficit area(s) contributing to poor skill development. The postulates regarding change guide the therapist in designing activities, selecting materials, and establishing interpersonal interactions with the child

This frame of reference is based on the belief that visual information analysis is a learned process. The occupational therapist who uses this frame of reference is concerned with how a child learns to make sense of out what he or she sees. An essential aspect of intervention is to facilitate the child's learning through environmental and teaching/learning strategies. Teaching strategies are used by a therapist to help a child process visual stimuli in a meaningful way (Table 9.1). Learning strategies require a child to change his or her knowledge about specific stimuli through repeated experiences. A therapist assists in this learning process by utilizing environment strategies that encourage a positive change in the child's behavior.

In this frame of reference, occupational therapists change the environment in certain ways to enable learning. Yet, it is only the child who can change himself or herself. Internal awareness and motivation to engage in mutually decided goals will facilitate optimal changes for that child. The eventual goal is that the child is aware of his or her own difficulties and is willing and able to engage in self-monitoring and self-correction strategies.

Environmental and teaching/learning strategies can be useful and are necessary, especially at young ages. Together both types of strategies enable children to take in and learn as much as possible, despite their deficits. Planning for the transfer of skills across a variety of tasks is another important consideration in selecting specific postulates and activities. Intervention related to difficulties in visual information analysis requires that a child learn to use cognitive analysis skills to attend, remember, and discriminate all forms of visual stimuli.

Visual Attention

To improve a child's visual attention, a therapist needs to consider the following three components: arousal/alerting, selective attention, and vigilance. The intervention plan needs to consider how to facilitate improved attentional skills so that those skills can be learned. Attentional deficits may be identified as a limiting factor to skill acquisition. The therapist needs to select activities and materials that will gain the child's active involvement in the activity. A therapist needs to consider the child's developmental level, age, sex, and interests. Young children may like brightly colored toys that can be handled, that move, and make sounds. Primary school children may enjoy objects that can be manipulated and that relate to an interest, such as the latest cartoon characters. There has been much discussion on the importance and need for activity modification (Mosey, 1986; Pedretti, 1996). Aspects of activity modification include changing the sequence of the tasks; changing the size, shape, weight, or texture of the materials; changing the procedures used in the task; and changing the nature and degree of personal contact (Hinojosa, Sabari, & Pedretti, 1993). Using environmental strategies to structure the external characteristics of a visually presented task can be used to facilitate visual analysis. Teaching/learning strategies will assist the child in transferring this cognitive analysis skill from one task to a different task (Toglia, 1992).

Arousal/alerting

One component of visual attention is arousal/alerting. The occupational therapist may choose among various environmental and teaching/learning strategies to improve a child's arousal/alerting problems.

Environmental Strategies. Arousal/alerting is facilitated when a child is in the appropriate state of physical, mental, and emotional preparedness. A child's alertness level may vary depending on variables such as time of day, physiological state, medications, or amount of sleep. The therapist's awareness of the child's alertness level is important so that the environment and tasks can be appropriately presented or changed in a way to maintain optimal selective attention.

General sensory stimulation or inhibition may need to be performed before or during visual activities. Often, activities based on the sensory integration frame of reference (see Chapters 7 and 8) may be effective in assisting the child to an appropriate state of preparedness. Visual stimuli that commonly attract attention and increase alertness are objects, people, events, and tasks that provide novelty, complexity, conflict, surprise, and uncertainty (DeGangi & Porges, 1990). Other characteristics of visual stimuli that elicit alertness are light, movement, and stimuli of high contrast and contour. Materials may include those that contain light, movement, or brightness such as shiny or neon objects. Tactile input, proprioception, sounds, and verbal cues are also helpful in maintaining an alert state (Figure 9.15). Activities that incorporate movement often help the child maintain visual alertness. For example, an activity requiring discrimination of a specific visual stimulus can be done on a scooter board, net swing, or by throwing a beanbag to it. Another child may be able to maintain his or her alertness if motor tasks are alternated with more sedentary ones.

For another child, the environment and tasks may need to have reduced extraneous input so that the selected task can be attended to. This place may need to be free from distractions and be a visually and auditorily "quiet" place. Auditory stimuli should also be carefully monitored with children who have difficulties with arousal levels. Variables to consider are ambient noise and the therapist's own voice. Elimi-

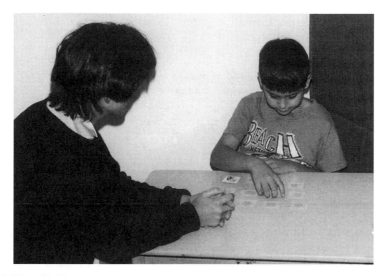

Figure 9.15   Child is in a low stimulus environment with few visual distractions, clear physical boundaries, and one-to-one adult attention to assist with attentional skills.

nating distracting noises may be done with background music or headphones. Changing the volume of a voice, higher or lower, can be alerting. Making sounds associated with the stimuli may help the child sustain his or her attention.

Teaching/Learning Strategies. The child can learn to assess his or her own arousal/alerting levels and develop and utilize a repertoire of techniques to effect necessary changes in alertness. The Alert Program (Williams & Shellenberger, 1992) is one model for teaching self-regulation awareness. According to Williams and Shellenberger (1992), children learn to monitor their levels of alertness through the Alert Program, and they also improve their self-esteem, self-confidence, and self-monitoring skills.

Selective attention

Selective attention is a second component of visual attention. The occupational therapist may choose among various environmental strategies and teaching/learning strategies to improve a child's selective attention difficulties.

Environmental Strategies. Selective attention of visual stimuli includes focusing on one aspect of the visual environment and attending well enough to explore its details or features. Selective attention to objects, space, and events is fundamental to efficient mobility through the environment and visual discrimination. Selective attention to pictures and representations provides another way of attending to and discriminating visual information. Visual symbols require selective attention to the distinctive features of letters and their sequence, patterns, and grouping. Attention is an important foundational skill that the child ultimately needs to take responsibility for. A child may need to be given feedback about his or her difficulties with accompanying techniques for monitoring and modifying his or her own attentional behaviors.

In visual tasks, children who have difficulty with selective attention may have difficulty discerning the salient features of a stimulus and/or may have difficulty screening out the irrelevant features. The environment can greatly influence the children's ability to selectively attend and may be very distracting or overwhelming for them. They may benefit from some of the same environmental strategies as a child with increased arousal levels.

A clearly organized environment with appropriate amounts and types of visual stimuli can help a child attend to the relevant cues. Visual stimuli should be available but not be overwhelming. The child who can function within that environment is the only one who can determine what is overwhelming. The therapist needs to be aware of cues from the child that he or she is feeling overwhelmed. Such cues include increased levels of distractibility, inattention, increased motor activity, or shut-down behaviors such as yawning and closing eyes. Visual stimuli that are familiar to the child tend to be inhibited more easily; novel stimuli tend to gain attention. New changes to the environment should be introduced with adequate time allowed for the child to explore them before selective attention is expected. Children with poor selective attention benefit from increased emphasis on the distinctive features to be detected and through reduction of unimportant visual detail. Increasing awareness of the distinctive feature to be detected may be done through highlighting the stimulus or feature by touching it, tracing it, or providing visual stimuli that exaggerate it.

Teaching/Learning Strategies. To assist the child in attending to salient features, the occupational therapist may provide simplified visual presentations that emphasize the feature to which the child must attend, thus minimizing the irrelevant (Figure 9.16).

Reduction of unimportant information may be through occluding unnecessary visual information (study carrels, masking) (Figure 9.17) or through presenting a reduced number of stimuli or stimulus features. Worksheets may be difficult for these children as they often include extraneous decorations and often there is too much on the page. They have difficulty discerning the important features or are distracted by the extraneous. Dividing worksheets by color coding or grid lines may assist the children in attending to separate groups of information. Modifications may include removal of extraneous information, folding the paper in half to reduce the amount of stimulation, or choosing a worksheet with less on the page (Figure 9.18).

Selective attention to objects can also be facilitated by supporting visual exploration with touching, moving, and functionally using the objects. Characteristics to be abstracted can be pointed out and labeled for increased emphasis. Motor activities that require self-directed movements through space, such as placing or stacking objects or moving the total body through space (walking, running, stair climbing), can be structured to encourage a child to attend visually to spatial features (Figure 9.19).

Using pointing and simple appropriate labeling may assist in selective attention to the salient features of a stimulus. A therapist may point out the important visual

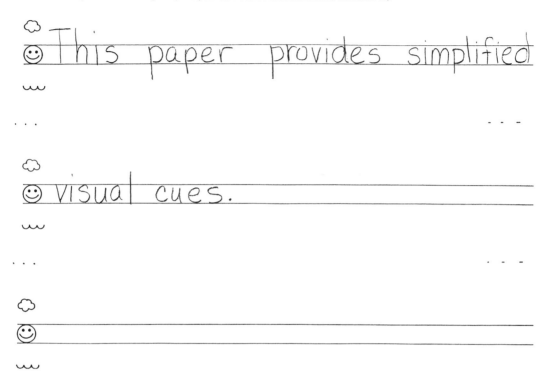

Note: For students who need extra help in printing lower case letters, use these lower case sentence strips. You will demonstrate letter by letter on your strip, using the cloud and wave image to emphasize placement. The student imitates on his own lower case sentence strip.

Figure 9.16 This handwriting paper simplifies teaching letter formation by reducing extraneous stimuli and training how to write letters between two lines. A consistent visual cue is provided to teach left to right, and the enlarged spaces between lines are exaggerated to teach spacing between lines. (Reprinted with permission from Handwriting Without Tears courtesy of Jan Z. Olsen, OTR.)

information with his or her finger or the child's finger. When a child uses his or her own finger to trace or point, it can be a strong stimulus to increase his or her selective attention (Figure 9.20).

A therapist must be careful about the type and amount of verbalization he or she uses during an activity because sometimes it becomes too distracting. A therapist should redirect attention with positive comments such as, "Look at the paper" rather than "Don't look over there." If a therapist concludes that his or her verbalizations are overwhelming or distracting, he or she should keep them brief and simple, drawing attention to one feature at time, or by using nonverbal cues.

Vigilance

The third component of visual attention is vigilance. The occupational therapist may choose among various environmental strategies and teaching/learning strategies to improve a child's vigilance problems.

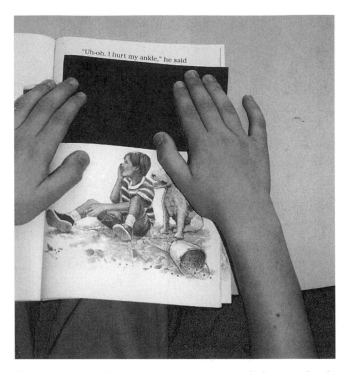

Figure 9.17 Mask can be used to cover extraneous stimuli that may be distracting or assist the eyes in moving across the page.

Environmental Strategies. Maintaining sustained selective attention to a task is a frequent problem for children with attentional deficits. These children are able to attend longer when tasks are self-directed and interesting to them. Interest may depend on their ability to understand the task and their motivation for engaging in the task. Visual stimuli that elicit prolonged selective attention may involve objects and space more than representations or symbols. Using a variety of visual stimuli that address the same goal may assist in engaging and maintaining the children's selective attention for learning.

If a child is involved in planning the treatment session and has some choices of tasks or materials, he or she may be more motivated to attend and participate. A child often attends better when he or she knows what is coming next, what constitutes task completion, and when the task is going to end. Listing the activities together by pictures or words can give a predictable structure to the session. It is important to include "clean up time" within the structure of the treatment session because it helps a child attend to a designated structure, know the end of the activity or session, and develop good organizational work habits.

Teaching/Learning Strategies. Depending on the child, familiar or novel activities may stimulate prolonged selective attention. A therapist should consider how to use

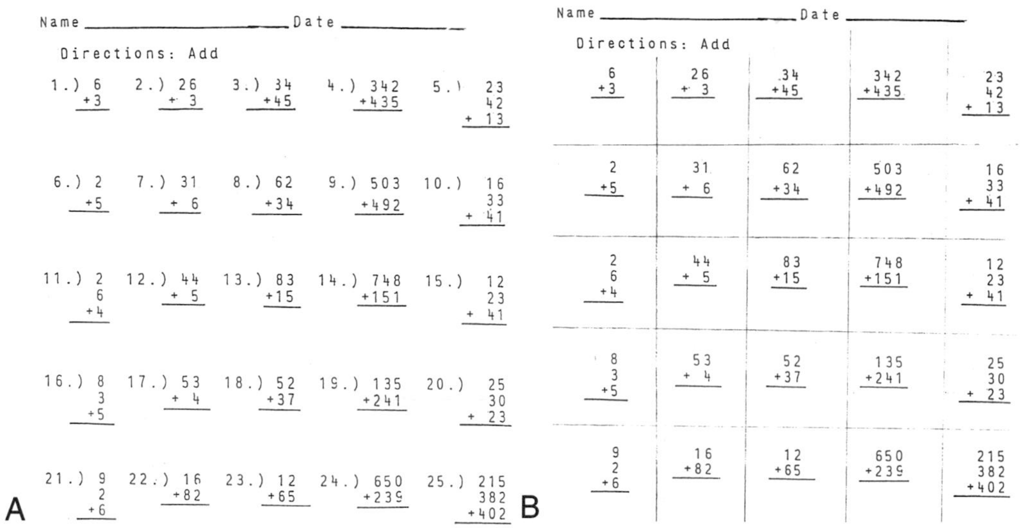

Name _____ Date _____

Directions: Add

```
1.) 6    2.) 26   3.) 34   4.) 342   5.)  23
   +3       + 3     +45      +435         42
                                      + 13

6.) 2    7.) 31   8.) 62   9.) 503  10.)  16
   +5       + 6     +34      +492         33
                                      + 41

11.) 2  12.) 44  13.) 83  14.) 748  15.)  12
     6      + 5     +15      +151         23
    +4                                + 41

16.) 8  17.) 53  18.) 52  19.) 135  20.)  25
     3      + 4     +37      +241         30
    +5                                + 23

21.) 9  22.) 16  23.) 12  24.) 650  25.) 215
     2      +82     +65      +239        382
    +6                               +402
```

A

Name _____ Date _____

Directions: Add

```
  6      26      34     342        23
 +3     + 3     +45    +435        42
                               + 13

  2      31      62     503        16
 +5     + 6     +34    +492        33
                               + 41

  2      44      83     748        12
  6     + 5     +15    +151        23
 +4                            + 41

  8      53      52     135        25
  3     + 4     +37    +241        30
 +5                            + 23

  9      16      12     650       215
  2     +82     +65    +239       382
 +6                              +402
```

B

Figure 9.18 Worksheets (A) may be modified (B) to reduce unnecessary stimuli and provide clear boundaries for independent task completion.

familiar and novel activities because children need to learn to attend to both in order to learn. This is especially true in academic learning because it can seem repetitive and familiar yet unlearned. Familiar activities may allow a child to recapitulate positive experiences or may be adapted to teach different skills. However if a child will only attend to familiar, known activities (perseveration), adaptation and variation of the activity will be required.

Novel materials or activities encourage a child to engage in new and different tasks, and they also encourage the generalization of learned skills. Some children seek novelty and easily tune out to the familiar. This may be one reason why computer programs are so successful with these children. Computers include lots of novelty, color, movement, and immediate reinforcement. However these children may also need to learn how to attend to a less novel presentation of information. These are the children who may be more motivated to attend when tasks can be completed within a short period of time. These children benefit when large projects are broken down into short-term pieces that then successfully conclude with a larger final product.

The pacing of a treatment session can help the child increase his or her selective attention. If a child has a very short attention span, numerous activities may need to be available that will get and maintain his or her goal-oriented attention. Initially, the therapist assists in prolonging attention to the task through modeling, turn taking, and other strategies he or she knows will engage the child with that task for longer periods of time. When focusing on prolonging attention to a task, a therapist needs to know how long a child is able to attend to the activity and devise a means

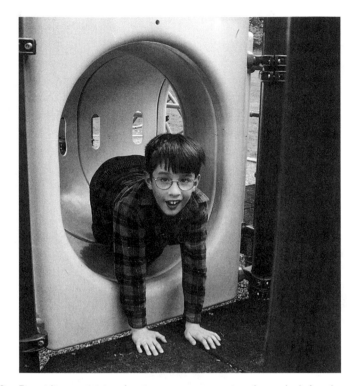

Figure 9.19 Providing activities that incorporate moving through defined space assist the child in visually attending to space and events.

to increase his or her attention to it, elaborating or repeating as needed. High degrees of external motivation and positive reinforcement may need to be employed to facilitate vigilance. Sustained vigilance and effort eventually need to develop internally from the child. However, it may need to begin with lots of external motivation, reinforcement, and success.

Challenging the child in a positive way to complete more repetitions of a task can motivate some children to sustain selective attention. For example, a therapist may say, "See if you can beat your record" or "I bet you can (can't)" for another child. The use of a timer can be beneficial in keeping the child sustaining his or her attention to the task. In this case, a therapist may say, "Let's see if you can finish this design in 2 minutes instead of 5" or "you worked for 10 whole minutes before you got tired or wanted to change activities." The therapist should be sensitive to a child's fatigue level and give him or her "break time" when appropriate. It is also important to positively reinforce "on task" behaviors or task completion for the child who may receive a lot of negative comments about his or her inability to attend.

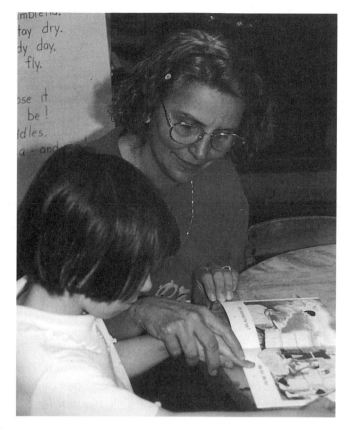

Figure 9.20   Pointing to visual stimuli can assist in gaining selective attention.

Visual memory

Visual stimuli are omnipresent. For something to be remembered, it usually has some meaning to the observer. Meaningfulness depends on the observer's previous knowledge, his or her ability to associate new information with old, and his or her motivation for remembering it. Difficulties in visual memory may be the result of deficits in one or more of the three fundamental processes of visual memory (i.e., registration, coding, and retrieval). Knowing the extent of the memory deficit and how it impacts on function will assist in setting goals and choosing the stimuli that are the most important to remember and learn. When a child has a memory deficit, meaningful stimuli need to be selected for him or her to learn about and store in his or her memory. Choosing appropriate visual stimuli that need to be remembered is based on the child's age and the visual stimuli that are needed for functional performance. Commonly used objects are most important with young children; representations of objects, events, or their characteristics may be used for preschool and school age children. Symbols are most important during academic learning, and letters and numbers should be used repeatedly in activities for children who need to code and remember them. Conversely, choosing visual recognition of community signs may be more appropriate for individuals whose reading is slow to develop or not a goal.

Registration

The first fundamental process of visual memory is registration, which is comprised of three initial control processes (i.e., attention, recognition, and rehearsal). The occupational therapist may choose among various environmental strategies and teaching/learning strategies to improve a child's registration difficulties.

Environmental Strategies. To improve the registration aspect of visual memory, the occupational therapist may need to select visual stimuli that will encourage the child's attention, motivation, and comprehension. Registration deficits can severely limit visual memory. Many of the techniques used to address selective attention can be used for registration in visual memory. Using concrete visual stimuli that can be explored through visual and other senses is a primary means of gaining attention for registration into visual memory. Motivation to register visual stimuli may be based on the meaning of the stimulus to the child and will influence the choice of stimuli to present.

Visual experiences can be associated with multisensory input to heighten registration; using multiple sensory pathways may assist in improving each of the three control processes of registration. An object may be combined with another visual stimulus to improve a child's attention. If a child attends to certain colors more readily, the occupational therapist may combine new visual stimuli with the child's preferred color. A black and white bull's eye or checkerboard pattern, which is fascinating to an infant, can be used to introduce color to the baby. Children may pay more attention to moving objects than stationary objects and react to the finish of objects. A shiny, flashy surface that reflects light may be more stimulating to a child than a toy with a flat finish. Visual stimuli can also be linked with other sensory stimuli. A specific song may help a toddler attend to mealtime, and bubblegum flavored toothpaste often makes oral care more efficient and effective.

Repeated experiences with specific visual stimuli increase the opportunities for a child to recognize and remember them. Presentations may be repeated in exactly the same way or in varied ways. The occupational therapist may use the same stimulus for a child who has difficulty generalizing or may use a variety of materials to help the child to associate and remember the stimulus for generalization.

Teaching/Learning Strategies. For visual memory, comprehension of the visual stimulus is important. It is important to know what a child understands in selecting stimuli to remember so that new information can be associated to what is known. Recognition of stimuli may be easier in the context where it is used, such as hand soap by the sink.

To compensate for poor visual memory, the occupational therapist may select compensatory techniques that include visual aids like lists and signs. Children with poor memory skills may need visual reminders of what they need to do. Encouraging a child to follow a set of visual cues to perform a functional task can help that child remember how to do an activity. The visual cues can be placed near the location for the activity, whether it is at home getting ready for school, or at school preparing for the day. Classrooms often display alphabet strips and number lines that may assist in recalling names or helping in letter formation. Some children need to be taught how to use these devices and be reinforced for using them.

Coding

Coding and storage of information, a second fundamental process of visual memory, involves visual imagery, categorization, and seriation skills. To improve a child's coding and storing difficulties, the occupational therapist may choose among various environmental strategies and teaching/learning strategies.

Environmental Strategies. Environmental structuring and routines are effective in improving a child's visual memory and in anticipation of the sequence of events. Visual cues can be used to elicit memories so that predictability is possible. Devising and posting schedules or pictures of routines may help a child remember what is next. Although these strategies are helpful for memory deficits, some children who have difficulty with flexibility may need additional considerations for some of these suggestions because they may become too rigidly dependent on these routines.

Teaching/Learning Strategies. Some children use visual imagery to relate incoming information into meaningful images. A therapist may model this technique saying "I'm going to remember that a 'U' can catch rain like a cup, so imagine drinking water from a cup." A child may have to invent his or her own memory hooks to make things more meaningful. Using humor often makes them more memorable. Other common strategies include rhymes, songs, and acronyms.

Presenting stimuli that go together is a way of categorization, which is the process of analyzing and placing information into subcategories and understanding interrelationships. Children may be able to remember how to use objects when they are presented in context for their use or with their associated stimulus. This is especially true in self care tasks. Presenting all the items for a task, such as in tooth brushing, may facilitate the recognition and use of the stimuli. Learning color names can be accomplished through association (e.g., "It's the same color as grass"). Associating pictures for sound and symbols (e.g., "c as in cat") is a common association strategy used in school. Associating letters that begin friends' names may be more meaningful to certain children and can be used for letter recall (e.g., "M for Michael"). Shared common experiences often give adults ways of helping the child retrieve information through associations (e.g., "Remember what happened when we . . . ."). Labeling the stimulus or characteristic assists in drawing attention to its distinction from other stimuli. Using consistent names helps to code the stimuli for storage and retrieval.

Seriation requires that information be organized in a particular sequence. Because there is a tendency to remember items better at the beginning and end of a series, short lists often eliminate the difficulty to remember the middle area. Also, remembering series placed in alphabetical or numerical order assists in organization and memory. Spelling often relies on memory of a series or pattern of letters and is not always based on phonetic sounds.

Retrieval

The third fundamental process of visual memory is retrieval. A child can retrieve information that has been initially registered, coded, and stored by using association and recognition skills. The occupational therapist may use one or more environmental strategies and teaching/learning strategies to improve a child's retrieval difficulties.

Environmental Strategies. If visual experiences were associated with multisensory input during registration and coding, then multiple sensory pathways may be used to assist in retrieving visual information. Visual stimuli, such as objects, are rich with multisensory potential and can be used to enhance visual memory.

Teaching/Learning Strategies. Mnemonic devices are memory-directed tactics that help transform and organize information to enhance its retrievability (Biehler & Snowman, 1990). These memory enhancing techniques, which rely heavily on semantic coding, are not commonly used until a child is 7 years old. One example of a mnemonic device is organizing information into smaller chunks, which may help simplify a complex task. Chunking can be used when a child is copying a word. A child looks at the word and, instead of copying one letter at a time, chunks it into syllables of two to three letters at a time.

Rehearsal techniques can be helpful for storing information. Maintenance rehearsal (repetition) holds information in short-term memory for immediate use, such as remembering a telephone number that one is about to call; however, a maintenance rehearsal has no effect on long-term storage. Elaborative rehearsals (association) consciously relate new information to knowledge already stored in long-term memory. Grouping information in ways that provide retrieval cues can help a child remember interrelated data. The combination of visual and semantic coding becomes especially important for academic performance.

Visual Discrimination

Visual discrimination of stimuli requires the ability to detect distinctive and invariant features. This develops through observations and experiences with objects, space, events, representations, and symbols. Through observation and comparison of stimuli, increasing information about the stimuli is extracted and similarities and differences are noted. Objects are recognized, matched, and categorized. Concepts are formed and language develops.

Developmentally, identification of distinctive features becomes increasingly specific and detection of properties and relationships can be abstracted from stimuli. A child begins to abstract color, size, shape, number, and internal details among visual stimuli. He or she begins to make other relative comparisons (e.g., bigger/smaller) and begins to detect positional relationships (e.g., on top/under, in front/behind) among objects or their parts. As visual discrimination continues to develop, specific visual stimuli are more easily differentiated from others. General and specific features can be abstracted quickly and efficiently. Extraneous information is ignored, and discrimination is possible across a variety of visual presentations.

To discriminate among visual stimuli, distinctive features and invariant relations need to be detected and abstracted. Tasks that incorporate recognition, matching, categorizing, and detecting relationships can be used to apply this postulate for visual discrimination.

Recognition

One visual discrimination skill is recognition. The occupational therapist may select among many environmental strategies and teaching/learning strategies to improve a child's recognition skills.

Environmental Strategies. The choice of visual stimuli may depend on the distinctive feature that needs to be detected. Objects or representations are good visual stimuli for detecting the properties of shape, size, color, number, and position. Attending to the distinctive features of space and events is stimulated by observations of movements and self-generated movement through space. Discrimination of the distinctive features of letters and numbers assists in symbol recognition (although this is only one piece of symbolic coding necessary for reading and writing).

Teaching/Learning Strategies. When focusing on discrimination of certain features, the therapist provides simple visual presentations of the stimulus. Color or increased details may act as distracters for young children or children with attentional deficits. Irrelevant information should be reduced as much as possible for the child to attend to and abstract the distinctive or invariant features. As familiarity with the stimulus increases, then tasks may be presented with varying amounts of extraneous information that may act as distracters. It is important to consider that some children may attend better when the presentation is complex.

Other ways of enhancing visual discrimination are by presenting only a few stimuli at a time and providing a visual presentation that is organized and has a clearly differentiated background. Early children's books utilize this principle quite often. Representations that isolate or exaggerate features can also be helpful (Figure 9.21).

Matching

Matching is another visual discrimination skill. The occupational therapist may choose from many environmental strategies and teaching/learning strategies to enhance a child's matching skills.

Environmental Strategies. The ability to differentiate similar stimuli or their fea-

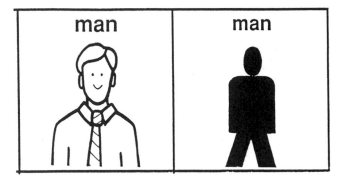

Figure 9.21 Communication symbols demonstrate reduction of a visual stimulus to its most distinctive features. The first presentation is a simple black and white line drawing with few distracting details. The second version contains color and more details. These additional features may help a child develop recognition skills. (Mayer Johnson Symbols)

tures is relative to the other stimuli that are visually presented. Presenting visual stimuli may be graded on a continuum from simple to complex. Matching is easier when stimuli are presented in a simple way with extraneous information kept at a minimum. Simple presentations include presenting the stimuli in a visually non-competing background so that it can be attended to and matched, presenting the stimulus to be matched with only a few other stimuli, presenting the stimulus in a structured organization that will facilitate matching, exaggerating the stimuli's distinctive features to be matched, and reducing irrelevant stimuli. Complex presentations are the opposite and require greater amounts of visual discrimination. Complex presentations contain many stimuli, are poorly structured for easy visual scanning and differentiation, and contain lots of extraneous visual "noise."

Teaching/Learning Strategies. Matching and categorization tasks can be designed to facilitate the detection of "same" while providing contrasts of "difference." The difference in choices may vary from gross to subtle. It is easier to detect similarity when there are gross differences among the choices, and it is more difficult when the differences are subtle. Matching can also be used for learning attention to details and self-correction techniques as the child's needs to match his or her self-generated responses to the correct answers.

If a young child is sorting a collection of objects by color, the objects may all be identical except for the color. Different colors are provided, and the therapist may ask to group all the items that are red. The number of different colors may begin with two (red and not red) and then include others as the discrimination of color is abstracted and color concepts are formed. Then, nonidentical objects may be given to sort by color. The distinctive feature of shape can be similarly accomplished by matching or sorting tasks that use shapes that are clearly dissimilar (circle, squares) and then move to more similar shapes (squares, rectangles; different triangles). In many matching worksheets, grossly different stimuli usually have different general contours or shapes whereas subtly different stimuli usually have the same external configuration but the internal features vary.

Categorization

A third visual discrimination skill is categorization. The occupational therapist may select among many environmental strategies and teaching/learning strategies to improve a child's categorization skills.

Environmental Strategies. To be abstracted, important common categories to readiness skills are shape and position. If discrimination of shape is required, shapes may differ by size, color, position, or internal features. Discrimination becomes more complex when a stimulus is different by more than one dimension, such as size and position or if there are many internal features, which can all serve as distracters.

Teaching/Learning Strategies. Categorization activities can also be used to facilitate the detection of distinctive features. In categorization tasks, stimuli are presented that need to be grouped together by some common property. The same items may be used to form different categories. In one task, the child must abstract the characteristic from the array and then determine which fits the group and which does not (Figure 9.6). In another categorization task, the feature to be abstracted may not be an exact visual match to the other stimuli; it may be an invariant, unchanging characteristic common to the stimuli that must be abstracted. In another task, the items may be categorized in the following variety of ways: color, size, or thickness, etc. (Figure 9.22). These types of categorization activities are frequently used to facilitate

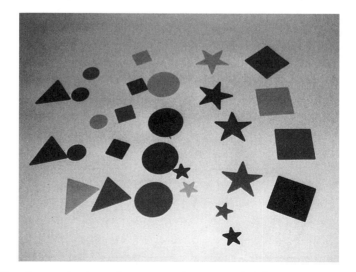

Figure 9.22 Categorization: objects may be grouped differently by shape, size, and thickness.

concept formation. The concept being taught is presented in a variety of ways so that the common feature can be detected, despite visual differences. Typical "sorting" activities use categorization skills; yet it becomes a matching task once the categories are determined.

Detection of Relationships

Detection of relationships is a fourth visual discrimination skill. The occupational therapist may choose from many environmental strategies and teaching/learning strategies to enhance a child's detection of relationships skills.

Environmental Strategies. The items in the group should vary only by their position if position is the feature to be discriminated (Figure 9.23). The ability to detect position and sequence relationships is needed to perform most visual motor tasks. Constructional tasks can be used as a strategy to encourage this ability. Using objects for construction combines visual input with the other senses as they are manipulated and moved through space. The child can monitor the changes in appearance as he or she moves the object. The child can also see and touch all the parts that may help focus his or her attention on how they relate to the entire design. For example, a child can manipulate take-apart toys such as cars and puzzles, which encourage the child to attend to its parts and then synthesize parts back into a whole (Figure 9.24). Limiting the number of stimuli or the possible ways they fit together assists in successful task completion.

Teaching/Learning Strategies. Cut and paste activities and sticker books are good constructional tasks that combine detecting distinctive features of the shape that needs to be matched to the background space. Sticker activities may require ignoring the internal details on the sticker to match its outline, focusing on the detection of contour. Cutting may provide sensory motor feedback about the shape. Rotating for positional matching of the piece is also necessary.

Other constructional materials include blocks, legos, and tinkertoys and parquetry, bead, and geoboard designs. They may be simple-to-complex, and typically have limitless ways in which the parts can be combined. At first, the child may explore how the parts work together. They may then imitate the therapist by copying the design piece by piece. Along the way, the therapist may point out and label positional and sequential relationships (e.g., "I'm going to begin here," "put this block

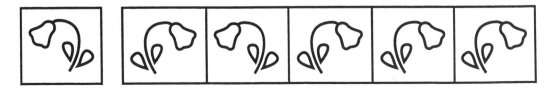

Figure 9.23 Visual discrimination: difference in position is to be detected. (Reprinted with permission from Pro-ed, Austin, TX.)

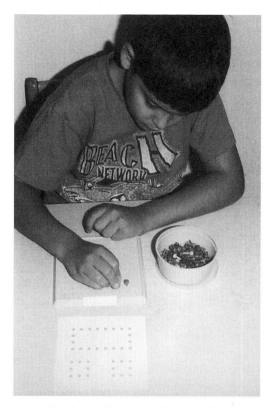

Figure 9.24   Constructional tasks can be used to facilitate the ability to detect relationships.

on top of"). They can be more complex when the child must follow pictorial directions, copy from a completed model, or direct the therapist in how to complete the design. Designs become more complex when an increased number of stimuli are required and when there are an increasing number of relationships between the parts of a design. Diagonal and empty spaces are later used to detect and develop more complex relationships; the use of these spaces seems to rely on higher level skills.

Spatial concepts are subject to the child's concept development. Children who demonstrate difficulties in constructional tasks may have conceptual and/or language delays. Constructional tasks can be used to learn spatial concepts. It is often beneficial to teach these concepts because the child may learn to use these concepts and their verbal labels to follow directions or to cue himself or herself verbally.

There are many computer programs that incorporate recognition, matching, and categorization skills and the detection of positional and sequential relationships among stimuli. Computer programs may be analyzed and used based on how they match the needs of the child. Factors to consider include choice of stimuli (representations or symbols) and familiarity and simplicity or complexity of the visual presentation styles. Computer programs have an advantage through use of color and movement and their quickness to respond to or reinforce a child's answer. Movement is a characteristic of programs that can increase selective attention and visual discrimination unlike statically presented paper and pencil tasks. Computer programs frequently combine vision with auditory and motor input. These factors may often assist in gaining or sustaining selective attention; however, they may need to be monitored because the visual presentation styles can be overstimulating and have the opposite overwhelming effect.

Overlapping Cognitive Analysis Skill Deficits

A deficit in selective attention or visual memory can significantly impact a child's ability to differentiate, recognize, and use visual information. Discrimination is reduced and erroneous judgments are made if there is a quick or cursory search for or memory of distinctive features. The child may need to repeat experiences that reemphasize distinctive features or slow down his or her impulsive responses. Some children who continue to make erroneous judgments may have stored information incorrectly or may not take the time for adequate retrieval. Any of these factors can interfere with discrimination tasks (e.g., letter recognition) and may contribute to difficulties with reversals. Many types of visual motor activities can be used to incorporate detection of distinctive features such as pointing to them, tracing them with the hand or pencil, coloring them, or reconstructing them. Labeling and repeated experiences with stimuli that assist in coding the information for storage and retrieval also assists in visual discrimination.

Summary

Visual information analysis refers to a group of cognitive skills used for extracting and organizing visual information from the environment and integrating this information with other sensory modalities, previous experiences, and higher cognitive functions. Visual information analysis occurs as a result of the interaction of environmental input received through the visual system that is integration with the other senses and the cognitive analysis skills. The information processing model is one way to explain the cognitive analysis skills used for visual learning.

The theoretical base of this frame of reference includes three major assumptions. First, visual information analysis is learned and is dependent on the child's inherent capacities and his or her interactions with the human and nonhuman environments. Next, the cognitive analysis skills of visual attention, memory, and discrimination develop in their own sequences; however, the development of each skill affects the acquisition of the others. And finally, by varying the types and presentation formats of visual stimuli, different visual, intersensory, and cognitive analysis skills are used. The types of visual stimuli available are objects, space, events, representations, and symbols. The visual presentation formats may be graded on a continuum from simple to complex.

This frame of reference contains function/dysfunction continua, which include visual attention, visual memory, and visual discrimination skills. The function/dysfunction continua describes behaviors that are observed clinically and that may indicate that the child is having difficulty processing visual information. In this frame of reference, the 15 postulates regarding change, which draw heavily on learning theory, concentrate on structuring the visual environment so the child can learn to attend to, remember, and discriminate visual information in ways that are increasingly complex.

Application of the visual information analysis frame of reference is based on the teaching/learning process. Activities are chosen that will facilitate learning through the presentation of comprehensible visual stimuli and the active involvement of the child. In this frame of reference, the therapist plays a major role in providing environmental strategies and teaching/learning strategies so the child is able to analyze and understand visual information.

References

Abreu, B. (1994). Perceptual Motor Skills. *AOTA self study series: Cognitive rehabilitation.* Rockville, MD: American Occupational Therapy Association.

Ayres, A. J. (1972). *Sensory integration and learning disorders.* Los Angeles, CA: Western Psychological Services.

Beery, K. E. (1989). *Developmental test of visual motor integration* (3rd revision).Cleveland, OH: Modern Curriculum Press.

Biehler, R. F., & Snowman, J. (1990). *Psychology applied to teaching.* Boston, MA: Houghton Mifflin.

Bouska, J. J., Kauffman, N. A., & Marcus, S. (1985). Disorders of the visual perceptual system. In D. Umphred (Ed.). *Neurological rehabilitation* (pp. 552–585). Philadelphia: F.A. Davis.

Bouska, M. J., & Galloway, M. (1991). Primary visual deficit in adults with brain damage: management in occupational therapy. *Occupational Therapy Practice, 3(1),* 1–11.

Callarusso, R., & Hammill, D. (1972). *The motor free test of visual perception.* Novato, CA: Academic Therapy.

Chedru, F., Leblanc, M., & Lhermitte, F. (1973). Visual searching in normal and brain damaged subjects. *Cortex, 9,* 94–111.

DeGangi, G., & Porges, S. (1991). Attention/alertness/arousal. In C. Royeen (Ed.). *AOTA self study series: Neuroscience foundations of human performance.* Rockville, MD: American Occupational Therapy Association.

Dunn, W., & Westman, K. (1997). The sensory profile: The performance of a national sample of children with disabilities. *American Journal of Occupational Therapy, 51,* 25–34.

Erhardt, R. P. (1990). *Developmental visual dysfunction: models for assessment and management.* San Antonio, TX: Therapy Skill Builders.

Folio, M. R., & Fewell, R. R. (1983). *Peabody developmental motor scales and activity cards.* Allen, TX: DIM Teaching Resources.

Frostig, M., & Horne, D. (1973). *The Frostig program for the development of visual perception.* Chicago: Follett.

Gardner, M. (1988). *Test of visual perceptual skills.* San Francisco: Health Publishing.

Gardner, M. (1986). *Test of Visual Motor Skills.* San Franscisco: Children's Hospital of San Francisco Publications Department.

Getman, G. N. (1965). The visuomotor complex in the acquisition of learning skills. In J. Helmuth (Ed.). *Learning disorders.* Washington, D.C.: Special Child Publications.

Gianutsos, R., & Matheson, P. (1987). The rehabilitation of visual perceptual disorders attributable to brain injury. In M. J. Meier, A. L. Benton, & L. Diller (Eds.). *Neuropsychological rehabilitation* (pp. 202–241). New York: Guilford Press.

Gianutsos, R., Ramsey, G., & Perlin, R. (1988). Rehabilitative optometric services. *Archives of Physical Medicine Rehabilitation, 69,* 573–578.

Gibson, E. J. (1969). *Principles of perceptual learning and development.* New York: Appleton, Century, Crofts.

Gibson, J. J. (1966). *The senses considered as perceptual systems.* Boston: Houghton Mifflin.

Hammill, D. D., Pearson, N. A., & Voress, J. K. (1993). *Developmental Test of Visual Perception* (2nd ed). Autsin, TX: Pro-ed.

Hinojosa, J., Sabari, J., & Pedretti, L. (1993). Position paper: Purposeful activity. *American Journal of Occupational Therapy, 47,* 1081–1082.

Kephart, N. C. (1971). *The slow learner in the classroom* (2nd ed.). Columbus, OH: Charles C. Merrill.

Levine, M. (1974). A transfer hypothesis whereby learning-to-learn, einstellung, the PREE, reversal/nonreversal shifts, and other curiosities are elucidated. In R. L. Solso (Ed.) *Theories in cognitive psychology* (pp. 289–303). Potomac, MD: Lawrence Erlbaum Associates.

Luria, A. R. (1980). *Higher cortical functions in man.* New York: Basic Books.

McCarney, S. B. (1989). *Attention deficit disorders evaluation scale.* Columbia, MO: Hawthorne Educational Services.

Meadow, S. (1993). *The child as thinker: the development and acquisition of cognition in childhood.* New York: Routledge.

Meldman, M. J. (1970). *Diseases of attention and perception.* Oxford, England: Pergamon Press.

Miller, L. J. (1982). *Miller assessment for preschoolers.* San Antonio, TX: Psychological Corporation.

Mosey, A. C. (1986). *Psychosocial components of occupational therapy.* New York: Raven Press.

Mussen, P. H., Conger, J. J., & Kagan, J. (1969). *Child development and personality* (3rd ed.). New York: Harper Row.

Niestadt, M. E. (1994). The neurobiology of learning: Implications for treatment of adults with brain injury. *American Journal of Occupational Therapy, 48,* 421–430.

Pedretti, L. W. (1996). *Occupational therapy practice skills for physical dysfunction* (4th ed.). St. Louis, MO: Mosby.

Piaget, J. (1952). *The origins of intelligence in children;* translated by Margaret Cook. New York: International Universities Press.

Posner, M. I., & Rafal, R. (1987). Cognitive theories of attention and the rehabilitation of attentional deficits. In M. J. Meier, A. L. Benton, & L. Diller (Eds.). *Neuropsychological rehabilitation.* New York: Guilford Press.

Scheiman, M. (1997). *Understanding and managing vision deficits: A guide for occupational therapists.* Thorofare, NJ: Slack.

Strauss, A. A., & Lehtinen, L. E. (1947). *Psychopathology and education of the brain injured child.* New York: Grune & Stratton.

Toglia, J. (1992). Cognitive perceptual rehabilitation: A dynamic interactional approach. Workshop notes.

Toglia, J. (1993). Attention and memory. In C.B. Royeen (Ed.). *AOTA self study series: Cognitive rehabilitation.* Rockville, MD: American Occupational Therapy Association.

Warren, M. (1993). A hierarchical model for evaluation and treatment of visual perceptual dysfunction in adult acquired brain injury. *American Journal of Occupational Therapy, 47,* 42–45.

Warren, M. (1994). Visuospatial skills: Assessment and intervention strategies. *AOTA self study series: Cognitive rehabilitation.* Rockville, MD: American Occupational Therapy Association.

Williams, M. S., & Shellenberger, S. (1994). *How does your engine run?* Alburquerque, NM: TherapyWorks.

Definition of Terms Related to Vision.

SENSORY ASPECTS OF VISION

Central vision (focal vision) is vision that occurs in the central field (i.e., resulting from stimulation of the fovea centralis).

Peripheral vision (ambient vision) is vision that occurs in the peripheral visual fields (i.e., resulting from retinal stimulation beyond the macula).

Recognition acuity refers to the task of recognizing target stimuli at specific distances (e.g., the letters of the Snellen eye chart).

Contrast sensitivity refers to the task of resolving discrete elements of a pattern across a range of spatial frequencies and levels of contrast.

THE MOTOR ASPECTS OF VISION

Fixation is the process or condition of directing the gaze toward an object of regard so the image of the object falls on that area of the retina, the fovea centralis, where the most acute vision occurs.

Saccades are rapid eye movements that refixate the eyes from one point of fixation in the visual field to another.

Ocular pursuits are the continued fixation of the eyes on a moving target. Often referred to as tracking.

Ocular vergence is the coordinated movement of the eyes that allows both eyes to fixate on the same visual target from a near point to infinity. Convergence of the eyes allows fixation on a near target. Divergence of the eyes to a parallel position allows fixation on a distant target.

Lens accommodation is the act or state of changes in the curvature in the lens of the eye when focusing at various distances. These changes are brought about by the elasticity of the lens and by contraction of the ciliary muscles.

Vestibular ocular reflex movements are compensatory reflexive eye movements that serve to stabilize the visual image on the retina and maintain the visual field in normal orientation in relation to gravity as much as possible during changes in head position or during body movement.

Appendix 9 was compiled by K. Tsurumi, 1994.

CHAPTER 10

Biomechanical Frame of Reference

CHERYL ANN COLANGELO

The biomechanical frame of reference is applied when a person cannot maintain posture through appropriate automatic muscle activity because of neuromuscular or musculoskeletal dysfunction. Consequently, artificial supports are provided, temporarily or permanently, to substitute for lack of postural control and to provide the most efficient positions of the body for functional activity.

Every time a person moves in relation to another person or object, the person must first move in relation to a greater force (i.e., gravity). This movement is done in a subtle way. Each time a person eats a sandwich, embraces a child, or reaches for a book, he or she must always relate first to the earth's gravitational pull. For controlled movement, the human body must provide a stable center from which the head and limbs can move. Every peripheral movement creates a shift in the center of gravity that requires a compensatory postural reaction (Figure 10.1) to prevent falling in the direction of the movement.

Gravity affects the human body on physical, mechanical, and physiological levels. Physically, gravity pulls the body toward the earth. It makes a person tend to fall down. It also makes the movement of limbs away from the earth's surface more difficult to execute. Mechanically, each time a person extends a limb away from the center of the body (e.g., when reaching), a lever arm is created that tends to topple the body by pulling the trunk in the direction of the limb. Fortunately, there are physiological mechanisms that help the body to adapt to the forces of gravity. Receptors, triggered by changes in speed, direction, and joint position, stimulate an equilibrium reaction that allows the body to remain upright or balanced. Through interaction of these receptors with a healthy nervous system and responsive muscles, the human body reacts to the forces of gravity in a predictable and functional way. Thus the term "biomechanical," which is the interaction of physical forces with the responses of a living being.

The general goals of the biomechanical frame of reference are twofold. The first goal is to enhance the development of postural reactions by reducing the demands

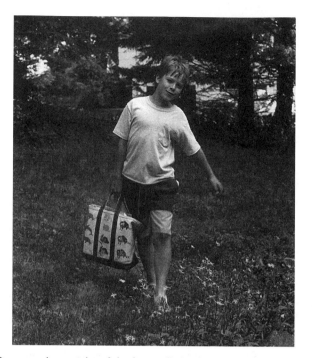

Figure 10.1 Because the weight of the bag pulls his body to his right, the child regains his center of gravity by flexing his trunk to the left and abducting his left arm.

of gravity and by aligning the body. The second goal is to improve distal function and skilled activity by reducing the need for and the demands on postural reactions by providing external support.

The biomechanical frame of reference frequently is used as a primary approach with children who exhibit severe physical disabilities. In addition, this frame of reference is used in combination with other frames of reference. For example, often it is used in conjunction with dynamic therapeutic handling (e.g., NeuroDevelopmental Treatment, Brunnstrom, or proprioceptive neuromuscular facilitation). When applied in this way, it allows for a carryover of goals throughout the day in the absence of constant physical handling.

THEORETICAL BASE

The biomechanical frame of reference draws from theories in physics and physiology. It addresses the implications of physical and physiological principles on motor development. Two assumptions are accepted by the biomechanical frame of reference in terms of normal development: (1) motor patterns develop from sensory stimulation and (2) automatic motor responses, which maintain posture, develop in a predictable way. This frame of reference also contains the assumption that dysfunction of or damage to the musculoskeletal or neuromuscular systems can interfere with effective postural reactions.

Motor Patterns Develop from Sensory Stimulation

Motor behaviors most often are reflexive in infancy. Reflexes are stereotypical reactions that occur in response to specific stimuli that generally are tactile, proprioceptive, or vestibular in nature. These motor patterns, once executed, provide additional sensory input, which contributes to the modification of reflexes and development of motor control. One example of a stereotypical reflexive reaction is the asymmetrical tonic neck reflex. The asymmetrical tonic neck reflex is elicited by turning the head, producing extension and abduction of the arm on the face side with flexion and adduction of the arm on the skull side. When a baby extends an arm as part of this reflex and comes in contact with an object, then the baby receives simultaneous sensations from proprioceptors in the shoulder related to reaching, tactile receptors in the hand, and visual awareness of the hand and object. The baby ultimately associates these sensations with the experience of touching an object, and, by reproducing the "feeling" of shoulder and arm movements, may reach successfully and touch the object again. The implication is that motor patterns are elicited by and develop from sensation.

Automatic Motor Responses That Maintain Posture Develop Predictably

The most sophisticated postural responses, righting and equilibrium reactions, are well developed by the second year of life. Righting reactions are movements that maintain alignment of the head in space and of the trunk in relation to the head. For example, if a seated child leans forward to rest his or her arms on a desk, neck extension is the righting reaction used to maintain his or her head in an upright position despite the forward tilt of his or her trunk. Equilibrium reactions are movements that help to maintain balance when the child's center of gravity is disturbed by an external force. Examples of external forces that provoke equilibrium reactions are when a child is pushed and when a child is carrying or manipulating a heavy object. Equilibrium reactions are manifested by movements of the trunk and extremities in the direction opposite to the displacing force to reestablish the center of gravity. If a seated child is pushed backward, his or her trunk curves forward, accompanied by forward thrusting movements of the limbs. This may involve shoulder flexion with elbow extension or hip flexion with knee extension. If the child is pushed toward the left, the equilibrium reaction is demonstrated when the child's trunk curves against the force to the right. This reaction may also involve abduction and extension of the right arm and leg.

Equilibrium reactions often are accompanied by protective reactions. Protective reactions are limb movements that occur in the same direction as the displacing force. The primary purpose of these reactions is to protect the body from harm by breaking a potential fall. When the seated child is pushed to the left, the equilibrium response causes the right limbs to extend to regain the center of gravity. Concurrently, the left limbs may extend and abduct protectively. Equilibrium reactions also may be seen alone. This occurs more frequently with slow or gentle displacement. Equilibrium reactions may be replaced entirely by protective reactions when the displacement is more vigorous. In the previous example, if the seated child had been pushed hard to the left, then the left limbs would have extended and abducted to protect against a possible fall.

Righting and equilibrium reactions form the foundation for movements from one position to another. They assist in the maintenance of body position when the center of gravity is changed by moving or by engaging the limbs with objects. Before these reactions can develop, the child must integrate specific lower level reflexive responses, which are primarily for survival, such as flexor withdrawal or rooting (e.g., turning the head in the direction of a stimulus to the mouth or cheek). Higher level reflexive responses, such as the asymmetrical tonic neck reflex and positive supporting reactions, which provide movement and proprioceptive input, must also be integrated into functional movement. Development is overlapping, so that as one level approaches completion, the next has already begun to develop. These levels continue to develop sequentially, within the body in a cephalocaudal fashion and in space from a horizontal to vertical position.

Another developmental sequence that is relevant to the biomechanical frame of reference has been described as motor patterns, which were investigated by Margaret Rood (Stockmeyer, 1967). Along with cephalocaudal and horizontal-vertical sequences, postural reactions can be viewed within this third category.

Motor patterns include sequences of motor development that go from unorganized movement to skilled movement (skilled movement includes the maintaining of posture and the ability to reestablish a center of gravity). Skilled motor patterns depend on the ability to bear weight without collapsing and the ability to shift weight from one part of the body to another.

The process of motor development begins with mobility during infancy. Initially there is a good deal of phasic movement, the lowest level of muscular control, which consists of large undirected movements (e.g., spontaneous kicking, waving, and banging). Muscles that primarily perform phasic movements tend to be superficial and distal members of the flexor group and often cross over more than one joint. They are used more for "light" work (i.e., movement of distal parts) than for "heavy" work (i.e., prolonged contractions needed for posture). Later in development, phasic movements are under more voluntary control and therefore are incorporated into skilled movements.

After the child has acquired mobility, he or she begins to develop stability. Stability refers to the child's ability to maintain a weightbearing position by the cocontraction of agonist and antagonist muscles around a joint. Muscles that primarily perform tonic contractions tend to lie more deeply and proximally and generally are extensors that cross over only one joint. They are responsible for sustained tonic contractions around a joint. These muscles are under greater reflex control than phasic muscles.

Once a child has developed stability, he or she is able to bear weight (i.e., to maintain a posture). From there, he or she begins to play with movement in that position. For example, take the prone-on-elbows position. At first the child supports himself or herself on his or her arms, but if the child begins to move, he or she may collapse. Soon the child can rock from side to side without falling over. This grading of movement indicates that the child can create movement (mobility) in a joint without losing the joint's capacity to support (stability); this is referred to as mobility superimposed on stability. Functionally, this appears as weightshifting (i.e., the ability to transfer some or all of the weightbearing load to another joint or to maintain support in one joint as the body's center of gravity changes slightly). When the baby rocks laterally in a prone position, the weight is partially shifted back and forth between the two shoulders. A complete shift of weight to one shoulder frees the other side for reaching. Even then, the weightbearing shoulder must engage in weightshifting activity because movements of the freed arm cause the body's weight to move slightly over the weightbearing shoulder.

The ability to superimpose mobility on stability can be demonstrated in two ways when a baby in the prone position is observed while propped on a bed. (1) If an adult sits alongside the baby, the adult's weight depresses the mattress; the baby must shift weight away from the mattress depression to avoid rolling over; (2) When this same baby reaches for a toy in the prone position, he or she must readjust his or her center of gravity toward one shoulder for weightbearing. These movements free the baby's other arm to reach for the toy (Figure 10.2).

This reaching out action demonstrates the baby's transition to another level of motor development (i.e., the acquisition of skilled movement). Skill is the highest level of motor function. In the previous example, the distal portion of the baby's arm is free, and this serves as the basis for volitional, coordinated movement. The shoulder's ability to hold the arm out in space and yet direct placement of the hand reflects the development of stability on mobility. Phasic movements have been refined into skill through their interaction with tonic movement, weightbearing, and weightshifting.

Components of Postural Control and Skill Development in Developmental Positions

The biomechanical frame of reference focuses on function within a relatively static position rather than on transitional movements. It is essential, therefore, to examine the developmental sequence of motor behaviors characteristic of various positions.

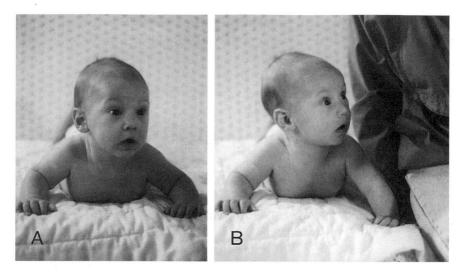

Figure 10.2   The infant weight shifts toward his right side (A) to keep from rolling into the depression created when his mother sits on the bed (B).

Children with neuromuscular dysfunction often have immature motor patterns; an understanding of this sequence contributes to a therapist's ability to facilitate change.

Supine Position

Although flexor tone predominates in the newborn, it is modified by the influence of the tonic labyrinthine reflex, which causes an increase of extensor tone in the supine position. Gravity also strongly influences the movements of the newborn; the head is held to the side and the scapulae are retracted and accompanied by shoulder elevation and external rotation. Despite increased extensor tone in the supine position, the hips are flexed. Yet, gravity pulls them into abduction and external rotation. Because of the influence of the asymmetrical tonic neck reflex, the newborn experiences more extensor tone on the face side and more flexor tone on the skull side of the body. The flexor pattern on the skull side causes shoulder retraction and lateral trunk flexion, which moves the infant's center of gravity over to the extended face side. This provides the initial sensation of weightshifting and weightbearing on the extended side. Each time the infant turns his or her head, he or she shifts weight slightly to the other side.

Flexor activity contributes to emerging midline control as the baby manages to center his or her head. Eventually, the baby is able to flex his or her neck against gravity enough to achieve a chin tuck, at which point the chin comes in contact with the chest. Later, this controlled flexion, when combined with neck extension, provides head control in an upright posture.

In the supine position, the infant develops the ability to bring his or her hands to the chest and then reach upward by using a succession of movements. This is first accomplished using internal rotation, then shoulder flexion, and, finally, protraction against gravity (Figure 10.3). *The ability to reach out in the supine position in a directed and controlled fashion, which is a skilled movement, begins at the same time that the infant masters weightbearing in the prone-on-elbows position* (i.e., mastery of mobility superimposed on stability in the shoulders). As the infant reaches upward and outward, a stable base of support is needed to keep from flipping over. Initially, abdominal support is low, and the legs are held off the floor because of the flexed, abducted, and externally rotated hips. The development of the abdominal musculature in conjunction with a decrease in hip flexor tone allows the infant to plant the soles of his or her feet firmly on the supporting surface, contributing to trunk stability during reaching. It is important to be aware that directed reaching in the supine position can be mastered with limited demands on head and trunk control because the child is supported fully, whereas reaching in the upright position requires additional control of the head and trunk to maintain a vertical position.

During infancy, eye movements are not separated from head movements. Visual fixation and tracking are influenced by the development of head control. Oral-motor control is influenced by the force of gravity on the jaw and tongue and the development of postural tone. Initially, in the supine position, the infant's tongue goes toward the back of his or her mouth, and the lips and jaw are slightly open. As the ability to flex against gravity develops in the neck, a similar development occurs orally:

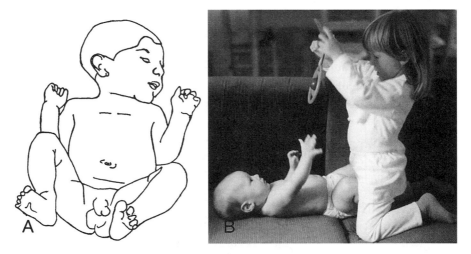

Figure 10.3   In the newborn, the head is held to the side, scapulae are retracted, and the hips are flexed, abducted, and externally rotated (A). As he develops, the infant gains the ability to reach upward by using shoulder flexion (B). He will later develop protraction against gravity.

the jaw closes, the lips come together more easily, and the tongue can come forward. A more mature sucking pattern is now possible.

Prone Position

Following several crowded months of flexion in the womb with resulting physiological flexor hypertonus, the effects of the tonic labyrinthine reflex in the prone position increase flexor tone even further in the newborn. This results in a little ball of a person in the prone position. Hip flexion places the buttocks high in the air, so that body weight is distributed over the chest and face area. The newborn's head is turned to the side for breathing. The infant must hyperextend his or her neck to raise the head or turn it from side to side because the spine is descending from the pelvis toward the neck. Maintaining the head in a righted position using hyperextension requires a great deal of energy. *Head righting in the prone position does not develop until the hips begin to extend, the pelvis approaches the supporting surface, and the spine becomes more horizontal with weight distributed along the trunk and pelvis.* This postural change decreases the amount of neck extension needed to right the head. At first, headrighting is accompanied by unopposed extension of the upper trunk. This prepares the neck and back extensors for additional heavy work in any upright position.

When infants prop on their arms, flexor muscles work in conjunction with extensor muscles. The chest muscles bring the arms forward and down, so that elbows that were previously behind the shoulders now come directly beneath the shoulders in a tonic, weightbearing position. Once the upper trunk can be supported on the forearms and back extension is modulated by interaction with flexors, graded movements of the neck can be accomplished by the interplay of flexion and extension (Figure 10.4). This provides for ease of volitional head movement. From this maturational base of neck mobility and stability, directed head movements and skilled eye and oral movements can develop in upright positions.

Once the infant has developed stability in the shoulders, he or she begins to weightshift. Weightshifting requires the infant to move his or her chest over the weightbearing arm to change his or her center of gravity. This allows the infant to maintain balance on an unstable surface or to reach out with the opposite arm. This action curves the spine, elongating the weightbearing side of the body and shortening the nonweightbearing side. *The pattern of extension on the weightbearing side and flexion on the mobile side can be seen during weightshifting activities in all positions as the child matures.*

Although the focus of this section for the most part has been on movements of the head and upper extremities because of their relevance to functional activity in a static posture, the biomechanical frame of reference also recognizes the critical role of the pelvis in the maintenance of stability. This is different from the frequent concentration on the development of pelvic movements in relation to end-goal ambulation.

Lower trunk and pelvic stability in the supine position allows for controlled head and arm movements, preventing the child's body from rolling whenever the head is

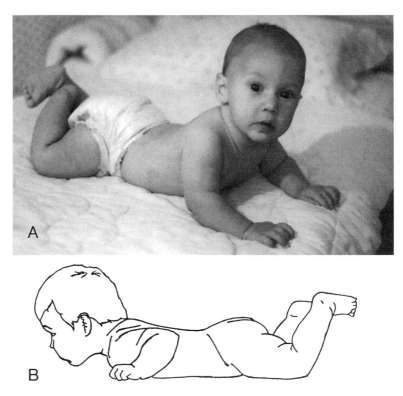

Figure 10.4 Before protraction develops in the prone position (A), elbows are behind shoulders, trunk is horizontal, and neck hyperextension is necessary to right the head (B).

turned or an arm reaches out. In the prone position, balanced interaction of neck flexion, extension for head control, and placement of shoulders and elbows for weight-bearing, depends on the position of the pelvis and legs.

Sidelying Position

The tonic labyrinthine reflex has no influence in the sidelying position; therefore, asymmetrical movements can be executed more easily. Sidelying provides dramatically different sensory input to either side of the baby's body to help develop a sense of laterality or the awareness and control of the separate sides of the body (Figure 10.5).

In the prone and supine positions, the infant coordinates dorsal extensors with ventral flexors for trunk stability. Sidelying requires more sophisticated control because the flexors and extensors on one side of the body must work together and in opposition to the coordination of flexors and extensors on the other side. Lateral headrighting in sidelying is a good example: the neck flexes to the up-side through the activation of up-side flexors and extensors against relaxation of the corresponding muscles on the down-side.

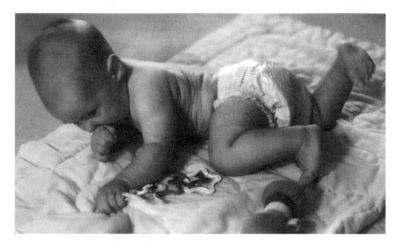

Figure 10.5   In sidelying, the weightbearing side is extended and supporting and the non-weightbearing side is flexed and mobile.

The lateral neck flexion against gravity that develops in sidelying as the child rights his or her head contributes to neck stability and head control in the upright posture. For example, in sitting or standing, every shift in weight to one side of the body necessitates lateral neck flexion to maintain the head in a righted position. The repeated movement of the head against gravity in the sidelying position helps this movement become effortless in the upright position. The same principle applies to the lateral trunk flexion that appears later in sidelying as the child begins to prop on one arm.

The interaction between dorsal trunk extensors and ventral flexors bilaterally is also essential in sidelying. Too much extension pulls the child onto his or her back; too much flexion causes him or her to roll forward. This interaction is particularly important as the infant experiments with head and arm movements because each of these movements shifts the infant's center of gravity.

Once stable in sidelying, the infant has an excellent opportunity to try out skilled arm and hand movements of the up-side arm. *This horizontal position demands less trunk control than sitting, reducing the stress of controlling posture and skilled movements simultaneously.* No weightbearing demands are made on the shoulder of the arm that is not reaching (as opposed to the prone position) nor does the infant have to work against gravity to use his or her hand in front of his or her face, as in the supine position. When the infant reaches out toward an object on the floor with his or her up-side hand, it naturally falls toward the midline and into the visual field.

Sitting Position

Sitting is the infant's first independent upright position. Head and shoulders have become stable in the horizontal positions, and, although the demands of gravity on neck extension decrease when upright, the infant still must master the interaction of muscle groups in the neck to produce controlled head movements in the new position. Until that point, the infant often uses elevated shoulders to nestle the head to help steady it. *This shoulder elevation frequently limits arm mobility.*

Infants use ring sitting (i.e., hips abducted and externally rotated, knees flexed), which provides a wide base of support and a low center of gravity. The back is rounded, and lower back extension has yet to develop (Figure 10.6). The shoulders and arms provide postural stability in one of two ways: (1) shoulders can be retracted to assist upper back extension to compensate for the rounded lower back, or (2) arms can be extended and used as props in front of the infant to keep him or her from tumbling forward. In the latter sitting posture, known as tripod sitting, neck hyperextension is required to right the head and often is accompanied by an open jaw. In either scenario, the hands are not free to engage in play. As head and trunk control develop, the back straightens and shoulders, which had been elevated and retracted, come down and forward. As the pelvis becomes stable, the wide base is no longer necessary and long sitting is possible. In long sitting, the legs come together, putting the hip joints in a more neutral position than in ring sit. This makes weightshifting to the side easier because one hip can move into extension and external rotation, while the other flexes and rotates internally.

The ability to weightshift over the hips has implications for midline crossing with the arms, allowing for more functional activity with the arms. As the child rotates the trunk and reaches toward the contralateral side, he must weightshift over

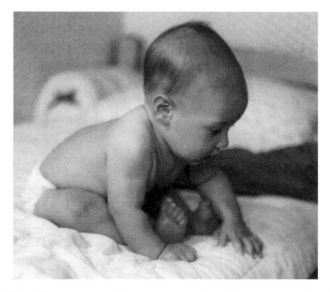

Figure 10.6 The infant must use his arms to prop in early unsupported sitting. His hands are not free for exploration, and the pelvis is forward for stability.

the contralateral side. The mature sitter can reach with a fully extended arm in all planes and still maintain posture and equilibrium.

Standing Position

In the biomechanical frame of reference, standing is viewed as an alternate postural base for skilled movements of the head and arms rather than as a dynamic prerequisite for walking. It is particularly important for those children who are least likely to stand or walk independently.

The standing position is unique because of the amount of extensor activity required to maintain the posture. As in sitting, when the child begins to stand, he or she uses scapular retraction to assist with upper back extension and to compensate for the lordosis created as the lower back is pulled forward by the weight of the abdominal cavity. As abdominal control develops, the pelvis tilts posteriorly into a neutral position, the spine becomes straighter, and the arms are liberated for skilled use.

When the standing posture is fully developed, a child can maintain a resting position of erect spine, neutral or slightly posterior pelvic tilt, and hips extended with neutral rotation. The knees are extended but not hyperextended. "Locking" of the knees may be used in the absence of muscular stability to provide mechanical stability. Ankles are at 90° of flexion and in neutral alignment laterally. If irregularities occur in the distal parts of the lower extremities during standing, proximal stability is influenced.

It should be noted that mobility in and out of positions has not been discussed. Although an understanding of these concepts is critical to the knowledge base of the occupational therapist, these concepts are not used in the biomechanical frame of reference. In this frame of reference, posture is looked at in a relatively static way, emphasizing those components that contribute to a stable, relatively immobile trunk as a basis for distal movements.

Interference with Postural Reactions That Result from Damage or Dysfunction

Dysfunction of the musculoskeletal system has serious implications for postural control. As discussed in the previous section, mobility of all major joints is essential to weightshifting and equilibrium reactions. Fixed bony deformities and muscle contractures clearly would interfere with this freedom of movement. Lack of proper bone formation similarly can affect the balanced interaction of the movements needed for a child to keep himself or herself righted in space. For example, incomplete development of the spinous processes on one side can result in a fixed lateral flexion of the spine. The fixed lateral flexion of the spine interferes with weightshifting onto the affected side in sitting. Without lateral movements to the opposite side, the child is unable to reestablish his or her center of gravity and is likely to fall to the affected side.

A compensatory movement or posture is the body's attempt to correct an error.

In the previous example with fixed lateral flexion of the spine, compensatory positions are necessary in the neck and hips. Two possible compensations are (1) the child flexes the neck or nonaffected part of the spine in the opposite direction, creating an S-curve while keeping himself or herself upright; or (2) the child uses one arm as a prop to support the tipping trunk. In the first situation, neck mobility is limited, with possible negative effects on visual and oral-motor function and soft tissue shortening. In the second situation, bimanual activity is impossible. Compensations often decrease mobility in joints that are not affected directly by the initial deforming process because the compensatory positions must be maintained to provide a stable posture. They may occur in the presence of bony deformities and in any situation in which normal movement patterns are compromised.

Motor problems that result from the neuromuscular dysfunction caused by central nervous system (CNS) deficits (e.g., cerebral palsy or static encephalopathy) may be more diverse and complex. Motor problems may be more diverse because such neuromuscular dysfunction is more global and is rarely isolated to one specific site in the body. Similarly, motor dysfunctions may be more complex because the manifestations of these deficits can fluctuate in relation to many factors, including changes in the child's position in space, effort in activities, affect, and stimulation in the environment.

Neuromuscular dysfunction often affects muscle tone. Within this frame of reference, muscle tone refers to the muscle's responsiveness to stretch. A common error is to confuse high tone with strength and low tone with weakness. Normal tone gives muscles the ability to contract on command and to maintain or cease activation as necessary. Normal tone depends on the integrity of motor neurons and muscle fibers, and the ability of CNS to receive and respond to proprioceptive cues with the simultaneous excitation of certain muscles and inhibition of others. Normal muscle tone allows the muscle to react immediately with enough tension for weightshifting and support yet still have enough "give" to allow for quick changes in movement (Scherzer & Tscharnuter, 1982; 1990).

Muscles characterized by low tone, or hypotonia, produce delayed responses. Children who have hypotonic musculature are "floppy" and tend to succumb to gravity. Their shoulders and backs often are rounded and their hips generally are abducted and externally rotated. Their joints are very mobile. However, they may develop compensations for inadequate antigravity responses in the upright position (e.g., shoulder retraction and lumbar hyperextension). Despite low muscle tone, the compensatory muscle groups may be shortened or contracted because they often are used to maintain posture. Prolonged shortening or contraction of the muscle groups because of such compensation may result in decreased range of motion and deformity.

Muscles that exhibit high tone or hypertonus often are described as spastic. They exhibit a hyperactive stretch reflex. Clinically, this means that the muscle shows increased resistance to passive stretch. Functionally, these muscles generally respond to activation with full, rapid contractions. Antagonist muscles may be relatively inactive or they may co-contract with less force. This results in ungraded movements that are maintained with the muscle in a shortened state and decreased joint mobility.

Hypertonicity appears primarily in antigravity muscle groups; however, all muscles in the group may not be hypertonic, even though it may appear otherwise. When the muscles work together as a group, the hypertonic muscles influence those muscles that have normal tone to produce atypical postural patterns. Two atypical postural patterns are (1) a flexion pattern of flexion, abduction, and external rotation in the upper extremities; and (2) an extension pattern of extension, internal rotation, and adduction in the lower extremities. Children who show hypertonicity resist gravity and do not succumb to its force. They also have limited ranges of motion because of the overactivity of certain muscle groups. In addition, it is important to note that muscles that may not be hypertonic can become shortened because they are part of a pattern of movement initiated and maintained by hypertonic muscles.

It is also possible to have fluctuating muscle tone. This condition is commonly referred to as athetosis. In this case, antagonistic muscle groups contract and reflex almost in turn rather than interactively. This causes exaggerated movements with little control in the midranges.

In addition to muscle tone, it is important to consider the effects of the action of the muscles on the joints. One example of this is the multiarthrodial muscles (i.e., those muscles that cross over more than one joint). The control of such joints may be particularly affected when children have high tone or shortening, and this has implications for postural control. For example, the hamstrings, which run across both hips and knees, often are shortened in children who have tone irregularities. It is difficult for these children to elongate those muscles over both joints simultaneously, making it difficult for them to combine hip flexion with knee extension. It is hard for these children to sit for long periods of time because hip flexion often is compromised and the pelvis is pulled into a posterior tilt. To stay upright, these children develop a compensatory forward curve of the trunk.

When children have intact central nervous systems, their movements and postures are effected by touch, proprioception, sight, sound, smell, health, and attitude. The influences of these factors are exaggerated in children who have tone problems. Postural stability in children who have CNS dysfunction may be influenced by movement, position in space, position of the head, tactile stimulation, stress or effort, temperature, surface support, intensity of environmental stimulation, and affect.

Movement includes active and passive movement and movement of individual joints or of the body through space. Rapid passive movement of a joint in a hypertonic child may increase tone, as may efforts to initiate active movement. Rapid changes in speed can increase tone, particularly when unexpected. Slow, gentle rocking often decreases tone.

Position in space refers to changes in position of the body (e.g., upright, supine, tipped back). These positions are registered through vestibular, proprioceptive, and tactile receptors that stimulate reflexive responses. Mature, functional responses include righting and equilibrium reactions. In children who have CNS dysfunction, reflex activity (i.e., involuntary, stereotypical movements in response to specific stimuli) often is primitive or pathological. A primitive reflex is one that normally occurs before the development of righting and equilibrium reactions and, therefore, should not recur after the first year of life. Such reflexes sometimes continue to happen in children who have CNS dysfunction and who have not developed normal postural reactions. A reflex is pathological when it occurs with greater persistence and when the child cannot willfully move out of the stereotypical pattern. An example of a primitive reflex influenced by the body's position in space is the tonic labyrinthine reflex, which is triggered by increased flexor tone in the prone position and extensor tone in the supine position. A pathological manifestation of this reflex may be a total extension pattern in the supine position, with the child unable to tuck his or her chin, close his or her jaw, or bring his or her hands together or up to his or her mouth.

Position of the head in relation to the body may affect reflex activity. Examples include asymmetrical tonic neck reflex and the symmetrical tonic neck reflex, each of which creates different movement patterns, depending on whether the neck is rotated, flexed, or extended. The asymmetrical tonic neck reflex interferes with midline activity, whereas the symmetrical tonic neck reflex interferes with freedom of arm movements and pelvic stability for sitting. In addition, changes in head position can produce stereotypical, whole-body reactions in the presence of neuromuscular dysfunction. For example, head extension in a hypertonic child can create a strong, total extension pattern with shoulder retraction, arched back, and extended hips. Conversely, when that child's neck is flexed passively, then the entire body relaxes.

Tactile stimulation includes light touch and deep pressure. Light touch often elicits phasic movements, which are undesirable in maintaining posture. Reflexes such as rooting and the Gallant are elicited by light touch and affect head or body position. The rooting reflex response takes the head out of the midline and may also elicit an asymmetrical tonic neck reflex, causing the entire body to be asymmetrical. The Gallant reflex causes trunk incurvation toward a source of touch on the lateral trunk, creating a temporary asymmetry of the spine.

The amount of stress or effort that an activity requires influences a child's movement and posture. An isolated movement that is difficult to execute may be accompanied by a total body reaction. For example, a child who easily is able to right his or her head when tipped forward 5° may have more difficulty when his or her head is tipped forward 20°. When the head is tipped forward 20°, the child may respond with total body extension because of the effort needed to meet the increased demands on neck extension. Furthermore, strenuous activity or emotional stress also may exacerbate associated reactions. An associated reaction, such as tongue protrusion when a typical child concentrates on a fine motor task, may be more pronounced in a child who has neuromuscular difficulties. For example, when a child with neurological impairment engages in a writing task with the dominant arm, exaggerated mirror movements may occur in the other arm. In the extreme case, the associated reaction may result in the nondominant upper extremity retracting and flexing, accompanied by fisting of the hand. This asymmetrical posture would interfere with bilateral use of hands, such as holding down the paper as the child writes.

The temperature of the environment also may influence movement and posture. Cool temperatures can increase muscle tone. Neutral warmth that approximates body temperature (provided by warm clothing or ambient temperature) tends to reduce muscle tone.

Surface support refers to the surface on which a child is placed. Hard surfaces tend to be alerting and, therefore, may increase muscle tone. Hypertonic children may relax on well-cushioned but firm surfaces, whereas children who have lower tone may sink into the embrace of heavily upholstered surfaces and respond with more active postural control to a harder surface.

Frequent changes and high intensity of environmental stimulation increase tone, whereas monotony and low levels of intensity have lulling effects and generally are associated with a reduction of muscle tone.

Affect also may influence posture and movement. Affect refers to the child's state of mind and his or her emotional responses to events that occur in the environment. Strong affectual responses increase tone, regardless of their positive or negative associations. The strong positive emotions associated with motivation, and particularly well-being, obviously should not be discouraged for the sake of modifying hypertonus.

The last major assumption related to the effects of neuromuscular dysfunction on postural reactions and function applies to Rood's concept of phasic and tonic muscles and their appropriate purposes (Stockmeyer, 1967). Tonic muscle groups are best suited to postural maintenance and are located more proximally. Physiologically, these muscle groups are better suited for sustained contractions. When these muscles are unable to perform their tasks adequately, the phasic muscles act as substitutes. Because the primary functions of phasic muscle groups are mobility and skill, they are ineffective in postural maintenance. For example, children who have CNS dysfunction may use their shoulders and arms to "hold themselves up" because of inefficient tonic muscle groups that cause poor postural tone. The result is fatigue and a lack of development in volitional skills for the extremities. Fatigue occurs because the phasic muscles are not well equipped for sustained contraction. Volitional skills do not develop because the extremities are used to maintain posture and are not free to engage in skilled activities.

The fundamental goal of the biomechanical frame of reference is to provide an artificial posture base from which the child can attend freely to his or her environment. An additional goal is to liberate the distal extremities so that the child can use them to interact with the environment. For one child, this may mean providing enough head control to make and maintain eye contact with a care provider or enough tone reduction to breathe deeply and easily. For another, it may mean the physical capacity to manipulate toys. This approach assumes that all children need consistent, effective postural responses for optimal manipulation of and interaction with their environments. When children are unable to do this effectively, therapists who use the biomechanical frame of reference can help the child develop those postural responses or can provide external substitutions for them.

Review of Assumptions

As previously discussed, the biomechanical frame of reference maintains the following five major assumptions:

1. The biomechanical frame of reference contributes to independence by providing external supports to substitute for inadequate or abnormal postural reactions and therefore
   a. It facilitates the development of some postural control by reducing the effects of gravity, or,
   b. It provides a permanent support when potential to improve seems negligible.
2. Children learn to move effectively through sensory feedback, especially through the proprioceptive, vestibular, tactile, and visual systems. They repeat successful movements based on the sensory cues that the movements provide.
3. Normal motor development is predictable and sequential. The development of motor abilities depends on a stable base of support and on the righting and equilibrium reactions that allow a person to respond unconsciously to the forces of gravity.
   a. Posture depends on the body's response to gravity.
   b. Postural reactions develop sequentially. Each new skill is based on a previously developed skill.
4. Dysfunction or abnormalities of muscle, bone, or CNS may impair the development of normal postural reactions.
   a. Tone affects posture; tone is influenced by many internal and external factors, all of which can be modified.
   b. If normal postural reactions have not developed, the body compensates by using substitute movements, more effort, and more conscious attention. All of these things may interfere with function.
5. Occupational therapists must determine the level of postural dysfunction and the external factors that may affect performance. Treatment needs to provide substitutes for absent skills yet still make demands on the child's existing capacity to function.

FUNCTION/DYSFUNCTION CONTINUA

There can be many causes of delays or dysfunction in a child's ability to interact with his or her environment. Only those things related to compromised postural reactions that interfere with skill development are appropriate targets for the biomechanical frame of reference. For example, the inability to use both hands at midline may be related to delayed sitting skills, which may result in retracted shoulders or the need to always prop on one arm for support. Conversely, that same inability may be the result of perceptual processes such as poor bilateral integration or tactile defensiveness and may exist regardless of postural competence. On the one hand, lack of fine motor control in ocular, oral, or hand skills may be related to head and shoulder instability. Conversely, the problem may be specific to isolated distal muscles, or it may come from a lack of organizational skills unrelated to posture. If postural reactions are delayed, weak, exaggerated, or performed by improper muscle groups, then the biomechanical frame of reference should be considered.

Indicators of Function and Dysfunction: Range of Motion

Range of motion is the ability to passively move a child's head and extremities through their full span of movement. Problems in this area are evident when a child has limitations in range of motion or contractures (Chart 10.1).

Indicators of Function and Dysfunction: Head Control

In this continuum, function is represented by the child who can maintain his or her head in a righted position, when moving, and who can direct head movements as desired. This provides stability for ocular tasks such as eye control and visual fixation and for oral-motor control and mobility for turning the head toward a source of stimulation. Dysfunction is represented by limited mobility or stability. This may occur primarily through inadequate muscular control or secondary to compensatory movements, such as stabilizing the head through use of shoulder elevation, which limits active range in the neck and shoulders (Chart 10.2).

Indicators of Function and Dysfunction: Trunk Control

Function is represented by the child who demonstrates equilibrium reactions in the trunk in an upright position and who has full thoracic range for inspirations and expirations. Here, respiration is only considered related to tone and position of the trunk. With less trunk control, dysfunction appears as (1) an inability to remain upright once distal limb movements are initiated or (2) an inability to maintain any upright position at all. Abnormal muscle tone in the trunk can compromise respiratory capacity. Trunk deformities may occur from the force of gravity curving the trunk or from constant use of compensatory movements. Lateral or forward curvature of the

---

Chart 10.1   Indicators of Function and Dysfunction for Range of Motion.

Full Passive Range of Motion	Contractures, Deformities
FUNCTION: Full Range of motion	DYSFUNCTION: Limitations in range of motion or contractures
INDICATORS OF FUNCTION	**INDICATORS OF DYSFUNCTION**
Full, active range of motion	Functional limits of range of motion Fixed contractures

Chart 10.2 **Indicators of Function and Dysfunction for Head Control.**	
Good Head Control	**Poor Head Control**
FUNCTION: Normal head control and mobility **INDICATORS OF FUNCTION**	DYSFUNCTION: Poor head control and mobility **INDICATORS OF DYSFUNCTION**
Head is righted and mobile in all planes	Child can maintain head in an upright position but loses head control when initiating a movement Child is unable to right head or control any head movements

spine (e.g., scoliosis and anterior kyphosis) reduces the thoracic space and may impair respiration with detriment to health, energy, and phonation (Chart 10.3).

Indicators of Function and Dysfunction: Control of Arm Movements

The child who can reach in all planes, regardless of position, and who can maintain his or her hands where he or she would like them is at the functional end of the continuum. Dysfunction is represented by an inability to direct the hands because shoulders are involved in supporting the trunk (as a result of tone in the arms being abnormal) or because arm movements against gravity are difficult to execute. Providing trunk support or changing the child's position in space can enhance function (Chart 10.4).

Indicators of Function and Dysfunction: Mobility

The ability to move through space to attain a goal, explore an environment, or experience movement in many planes is at the functional end of the continuum. Mobility that is stressful or slow is dysfunctional because the child often may feel that the effort is not worth the goal or the child may be too fatigued to interact with the person or object once he or she attains his or her goal. Lack of mobility is also dysfunctional in that the child is deprived of essential sensory experiences, particularly vestibular and proprioceptive, which are provided by movement through space (Chart 10.5).

Function and Dysfunction Continua Related to Functional Performance Behaviors

The functional goal of the biomechanical frame of reference is to provide a secure postural base through positioning or with the assistance of external support. With a secure postural base, the child can engage in functional activities. Other function/

Chart 10.3   Indicators of Function and Dysfunction for Trunk Control.

Good Trunk Control	Poor Trunk Control
FUNCTION: Good trunk control	DYSFUNCTION: Poor trunk control
INDICATORS OF FUNCTION	**INDICATORS OF DYSFUNCTION**
Child's trunk is righted and stable in an upright position and is symmetrical when the child is seated or standing on a horizontal surface	Child's trunk is righted but unstable when limb movements are initiated
Child can take advantage of normal respiratory capacity	Child's trunk is not righted; child is unable to remain upright or remains upright with asymmetry
	Child's respiratory capacity is compromised by decreased size of thoracic cavity because of trunk and shoulder position
	Child's respiratory capacity is decreased because of abnormal muscle tone on respiratory muscles, such as the intercostals

---

Chart 10.4   Indicators of Function and Dysfunction for Control of Arm Movements.

Good Control of Arm Movements	Poor Control of Arm Movements
FUNCTION: Ability to reach in all planes	DYSFUNCTION: Inability to reach in all planes
INDICATORS OF FUNCTION	**INDICATORS OF DYSFUNCTION**
Child can place, maintain, and control his or her hands where he or she pleases when in an upright position	Child's arms are not liberated in an upright position; either they are needed for propping, or shoulders are retracted to aid in upper trunk stability, bringing the hands back with them
	Child cannot move his or her arms in gravity (resisted planes of movement) and therefore cannot place or maintain his or her hands where he or she wants them

---

Chart 10.5   Indicators of Function and Dysfunction for Mobility.

Mobility	Immobility
FUNCTION: Mobility through space	DYSFUNCTION: Slow, effortful mobility, or immobility
INDICATORS OF FUNCTION	**INDICATORS OF DYSFUNCTION**
Child is mobile through space in all planes (walking; climbing in, out of, and over obstacles)	Child can only locomote by rolling
Child can locomote in a horizontal position (crawling or creeping) on a flat surface	Child cannot move his or her body through space

---

dysfunction continua are directed toward providing a secure postural base. Eating and accessing switches for technological aides, which are examples of function/dysfunction continua, are important examples of functional performance behaviors.

Indicators of Function and Dysfunction: Eating

The functional end of this continuum includes adequate oral-motor control to ingest food safely in an average amount of time without choking. Although feeding difficulties may exist despite the development of postural control, the absence of good head and trunk control exacerbates oral-motor dysfunction. Dysfunctional eating patterns (e.g., lack of jaw stability; poor tongue, cheek, and lip control; and disorganized swallowing) are affected by an unstable neck, compensatory movements in the shoulder girdle, impaired respiration, and abnormal tone associated with certain postures (Chart 10.6).

Indicators of Function and Dysfunction: Toileting

Function in toileting includes the ability to sit independently on a toilet or commode and the ability to void. Dysfunction, with its concomitant lack of comfort and dignity, is represented by a lack of awareness or control of the voiding process or the inability to relax enough to void when sitting unsupported on a toilet. Awareness and control may be affected by abnormal tone, and postural control has a direct effect on the ability to relax when sitting independently (Chart 10.7).

Indicators of Function and Dysfunction: Accessing Switch for Technological Aides

The child who can make and maintain contact with a switch, button, or joystick and release it at will, is at the functional end of this continuum. The section of switches to control augmentative communication devices and power wheelchairs, environmental controls, and other technological devices is extensive. The highest level of function consists of controlling the switch rapidly and efficiently without

---

Chart 10.6   Indicators of Function and Dysfunction for Eating.

Safe Eating	Unsafe Eating
FUNCTION: Safe, efficient eating **INDICATORS OF FUNCTION**	DYSFUNCTION: Difficulty with chewing and swallowing **INDICATORS OF DYSFUNCTION**
Child can chew and swallow food successfully without aspirating	Child is unable to grade jaw movements or control lips and tongue when eating Child frequently aspirates food

---

Chart 10.7   Indicators of Function and Dysfunction for Toileting.

Continence	Incontinence
FUNCTION: Independence on toilet **INDICATORS OF FUNCTION**	DYSFUNCTION: Inability to void in toilet **INDICATORS OF DYSFUNCTION**
Child can empty bowel and bladder when seated on toilet	Child can only void intentionally when lying down Child cannot maintain sitting balance on a toilet Child can maintain sitting balance on a toilet but cannot direct the flow of urine into the bowl Child has no conscious bowel and bladder control

fatigue. Ideally, this would be accomplished through controlled arm and hand movements. However, movement in virtually any part of the body can be harnessed to drive a device. Switches may be controlled, for example, by inspiration/expiration or movements of head, neck, eyelids, shoulders, or feet. Function is decreased if, by harnessing one of these movements, another skill related to that movement is impaired. For example, does a breath-driven device interfere with speech or create excessive drooling? Or does the child use a shoulder movement at the expense of postural symmetry or with compensatory movements that eventually impair posture or mobility (Chart 10.8)?

Each of these functions depends on the interaction of numerous factors. Cognition, perception, and behavior, as well as fine motor and organization abilities, contribute to these skills. Evaluation of the postural components necessary for function will determine whether and, specifically, which biomechanical assists are appropriate.

GUIDE TO EVALUATION

The purpose of the evaluation is to assess the postural components of a given dysfunction to plan intervention. This can be done by using the function/dysfunction continua.

Within the biomechanical frame of reference, the child's potential for change in the area of postural reactions is a major concern. This requires the use of professional judgment and may require ongoing assessment over a period of months. The child's potential for change is an important factor because it helps determine what type of postural aides should be used and how they will be most effective.

At times, the assessment of a child's needs within this frame of reference may be done by a therapist who has particular expertise in this area or through a clinic. The therapist who treats the child should be actively involved in equipment decisions because of his or her long-term interaction with the child and understanding of the child's potential for change.

Chart 10.8   Indicators of Function and Dysfunction for Accessing Switch for Technological Aides.

Switch Access	Lack of Switch Access
FUNCTION: Ability to independently use technological aides	DYSFUNCTION: Inability to independently use technological aides
INDICATORS OF FUNCTION	**INDICATORS OF DYSFUNCTION**
Child can approach, contact, and release switch with adequate speed and control using hand	Child cannot approach, switch, or maintain contact and control release
	Child cannot sustain approach or release sequence for duration of activity
Child can approach, contact, and release switch using body part other than hand	Child can approach, contact, and release switch with a body part, but the action impedes another function

The assessment of the child begins by considering age, therapeutic history, physical status, prognosis, and environment because they all contribute to the child's potential for change. Age is an important consideration because of the plasticity of CNS. Therapeutic history is important because it indicates the types and focus of the child's previous contact with therapy and the child's responsiveness to intervention. Physical status indicates the child's general health, medication regime, and surgical history. Prognosis indicates the sequelae of the child's diagnosis. The environment influences the child's potential for growth and motivation.

When a child is evaluated for positioning options, the therapist needs to observe carefully any sequence of specific elements of postural control. The outline in this section is intended to assist with this process.

- Can child move all body parts through full range against gravity?
- Can child right his or her head and is it mobile in all planes?
- Can child right his or her trunk and maintain stability?
- Can child place, maintain, and control position of his or her hands?
- Is child mobile through space in all planes?
- Can child chew and swallow food successfully without aspirating?
- Can child void when seated on a toilet or potty?
- Can the child access a switch to activate a technological device?

It is important during this scrutiny to remember, however, that all elements of movement are interrelated, and that the therapist must step back and view the child's body as a whole. To take this further, it is imperative to apply the evaluation and intervention process to the child's life—*the end goal is not that the child look good posturally in the therapist's eye but that the child can do something that is important to him or her.*

The assessment of the child should be done with the child involved in activities. This provides the therapist with an opportunity to analyze movement as it relates to posture and gravity. It is important to look at the child's ability to make rapid, unconscious, postural changes within the context of an activity. References and charts are available to assist in this evaluation of the sequential development of motor skills (Bly, 1994; Fiorentino, 1981; Green, Mulcahy, & Pountney, 1995; Richardson, 1996). In addition, wheelchair assessment forms are available from wheelchair manufacturers and are found in textbooks (Barnes, 1991; Bergen & Colangelo, 1985). Concentration is on those central postural skills needed to support movement of the head and limbs to manipulate the environment.

The following questions provide some guidelines for evaluating motor development in terms of functional posture, as derived from the function/dysfunction continua. In all cases, it is important to determine if dysfunctional movement is delayed (slow to develop) or pathological (influenced by abnormal tone or reflexes). Each of the following questions is directed toward the functional end of the continuum.

Can child move all body parts through full range against gravity?

This involves the assessment of the child's passive range of motion and the presence of fixed or dynamic contractures. Just as important as passive range of motion are the effects of movement and changes in position on functional range of motion. Is muscle tone high, low, or fluctuating? What kinds of stimuli increase pathological tone and, possibly, interfere with active range of motion? Does the effect of gravity prevent certain ranges of movement mechanically or physiologically, and can movement be enhanced by changing position to decrease the effects of gravity or by using gravity to assist movement? What movements or positions elicit reflexes that compromise full range?

If functional range is influenced by position, then the therapist needs to know how much of each day the child spends in different positions. A positioning log can be completed with the help of parents, care providers, and educators. How is the child fed, transported, toileted, and positioned for rest, recreation, and school? Which positions have been selected with function in mind, which can be modified to enhance movement, and which are selected to reduce stress on the family or care providers? In addition to the time spent in school chairs, high chairs, and wheelchairs, the child's time in backpacks, baby swings, car seats, and beanbag chairs and on the floor and bed should also be assessed. From the positioning log, the therapist can make modifications or suggestions to promote independent movement for the child and ease caretaking for his or her family and school staff.

Can child right his or her head and is it mobile in all planes?

In the supine position, can the child maintain his or her head in midline, turn it to either side, and tuck his or her chin to observe people, body parts, and what may be in the child's hands? Is development delayed yet following a normal sequence, or is pathology present (Figure 10.7)? Is difficulty with movement caused by low-tone struggle against gravity, or is immobility caused by high tone? Is there increased extension in this position because of the influence of the tonic labyrinthine reflex? This may include neck hyperextension, an open jaw, retracted lips, or upward gaze. Does the rooting reflex cause the child to press one side of his or her face against the floor? Does the inability to maintain the head in midline elicit an asymmetric tonic neck reflex? When attempting to lift his or her head from the supine position, does the child use peripheral, phasic musculature (e.g., the sternocleidomastoids) to substitute for deep tonic work?

In the prone position, can the head be lifted to 90°, or can it be turned freely to either side and be isolated from body movements so that the child does not flip over when he or she turns his or her head? Can the child raise and lower his or her head with graded movements? Functionally, can the child turn his or her head to examine

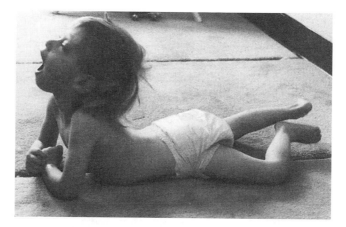

Figure 10.7   The child's head is thrown back for stability. Note the position of the mouth because of hyperextension.

the world visually, and can the child control his or her mouth for age-appropriate speaking and swallowing in this position? If delay or pathology is present, is neck hyperextension necessary to keep the head upright? If so, is it accompanied by extension throughout the body? Can the child close his or her mouth when the head is righted, or is the jaw pulled into extension? Does the child simply collapse to lower his or her head?

In sidelying, where the effects of gravity on the head are minimized, can the child look up and to the side without flipping into a prone or supine position? Can the child use lateral neck flexion against gravity to right his or her head or initiate movements of his or her body?

In the upright position (either sitting or supported standing), is the child's head aligned in space? Is it aligned with the child's body? It should be noted that the head may be righted but the neck may be flexed laterally or hyperextended to compensate for poor trunk position (e.g., in patients with scoliosis or kyphosis). If head control is poor, is shoulder elevation used to "nestle" the head for stability, thereby limiting neck mobility? Or, is the head generally thrown back or flopping forward? What is the controlled range of head movements? Can the child flex his or her neck forward 5° and right it again but loses control if he or she flexes 10° or more? If head control is inadequate, does tipping the trunk slightly forward or backward activate righting reactions or change muscle tone so that head stability is enhanced? If head control is minimal, how far back must the therapist tip the child's seat or stander until the child's head rests on a supporting backpiece without flopping forward? If the therapist supports the head by tipping the seat back in space, is this a functional position for viewing the world and a safe position for swallowing?

Can child right his or her trunk and maintain stability?

In this context, the trunk is seen not in terms of mobility but as a stable base of support for the head and arms (i.e., the primary parts of the body for seeking stimuli and manipulating the world). This is not meant to minimize the importance of the whole body in learning but to establish priorities for someone who is limited in functional movement. The therapist, therefore, looks at the trunk's capacity to stay upright in response to displacement and its ability to support the head and arms as they change position in relation to the trunk (Figure 10.8). The roles of the pelvis, legs, and feet are observed in conjunction with the trunk as part of the support basis for the body rather than in their roles of providing mobility through space.

A functional trunk also provides the base for good respiration; the rib cage is mobile and no fixed or functional contractures exist to reduce the thoracic space in which the lungs expand. For example, a fixed scoliosis may reduce the capacity of the lung on the flexed side.

Although the ultimate goal is a trunk that works well in an upright position, that capacity is based on postural skills that have developed first in a horizontal position. Attention to this area is particularly important in a dynamic approach when goals include improving motor skills in a developmental continuum.

In the supine position, is the trunk free from the influences of abnormal tone or pathological reflexes? Is the back hyperextended or asymmetrical? Are the legs stuck in a froglike position or extended and abducted? Can the trunk maintain the body's position when the head turns and the arms reach away from midline, or does the

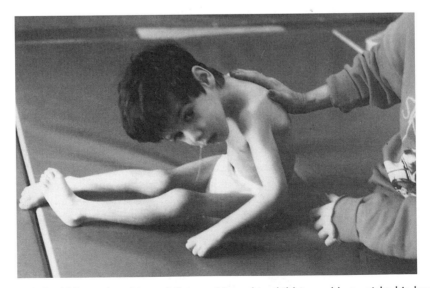

Figure 10.8 When placed in a sitting position, this child is unable to right his head or trunk. Protective extension is absent.

child inadvertently roll over during head/arm movement? Is the pelvis mobile enough to allow the child to play with his or her feet? Or is it tilted anteriorly as part of an extension pattern so that there is a space between the lumbar spine and the floor? If the child needs extra stability, can the child plant his or her feet on the floor?

In the prone position, is the child trapped by increased flexor tone or by the inability to extend against gravity? Is the pelvis flat on the floor, or does hip flexion push the center of gravity toward the chest so that it is difficult to raise the chest off the floor? Likewise, do exaggerated hip abduction and external rotation tip the pelvis in the anterior direction? Do the arms help support the chest, or does the child need to use back hyperextension to raise the chest and reach out? When lifting the head and chest, is there associated hyperextension in the neck, lower back, and legs? When reaching upward, is there adequate abdominal activity to keep the child from rolling onto his or her back?

In the sidelying position, can the child maintain the position without bracing himself or herself with arms or legs forward to keep from rolling? Can the child look and reach in all planes and still maintain the position? Does an increase in extensor tone create arching and flipping back? Are there any trunk asymmetries that are exaggerated when lying on one side (Figure 10.9)?

In an upright position (i.e., seated or standing at rest), is the trunk righted, stable, and symmetrical? Are adequate space and mobility evident in the chest for effective respiration? Can the child sit in various positions, or is the child limited to one

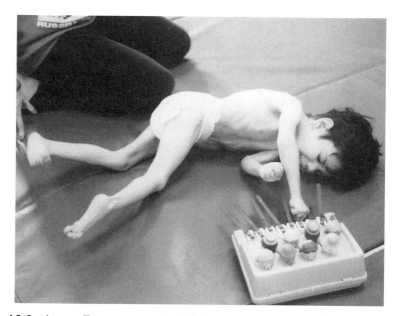

Figure 10.9 In an effort to maintain sidelying, tone is increased. The lower extremities are not available for stabilization, and the hands are fisted.

because of the stability it provides, (e.g., ring sitting or "W" sitting)? Are equilibrium reactions fully effective or only within a limited range of displacement? Are arms liberated; can the child reach in any plane without losing balance, or is activity in the shoulder girdle or arms necessary to maintain an upright trunk? For example, retracted shoulders may assist upper back extension, or there may be a need to prop on one or both arms. Can the trunk support the head and itself but not the weight of the arms? This can be determined if the child can sit erect only when resting, not when leaning, with his or her arms placed lightly on a tabletop.

How do the positions of the pelvis and legs affect the trunk? Is weight distributed equally to both sides of the pelvis? Is the pelvis relatively neutral or tilted in the anterior or posterior direction? Is the pelvis too far forward, requiring compensatory lumbar hyperextension or shoulder retraction to remain upright? Does a pelvis tilted toward the posterior create a rounded back, possibly with protracted shoulders and a hyperextended neck?

In the sitting position, does hip extension cause the child's back to press against the back of the chair, sliding him or her toward or off the front edge of the chair? Are the hips abducted in such a way that the child has no lateral stability, or abducted in such a way that he or she has little anterior stability? Can hips, knees, and ankles be maintained in a position that allows feet to be planted firmly on the floor? Does the child seem to be more functional in a standing or sitting position?

Can child place, maintain, and control position of his or her hands?

In this area, the therapist's concern is not fine motor skill but the ability to get the hands where they need to be, keep them there as long as necessary, and change their position through controlled movements of the shoulders and arms from a stable base. Improving function in this area may have secondary effects on fine motor skills in two ways. First, modification of muscle tone in the trunk and shoulders often improves tone in the extremities. Second, control of hand placement provides more opportunity for manipulation and the sensory experiences that contribute to fine motor control.

As with previous areas, the clinician must look at the quality of muscle tone. How can gravity impede or improve movement mechanically and physiologically? Mechanically, the concern is how gravity weighs limbs down in various positions. Physiologically, the concern is how it elicits righting or reflex activity in various positions. Also, what compensatory movements or associated reactions interfere with function?

In the supine position, can the child reach in all planes against gravity and maintain his or her hands away from his or her body without the need to stabilize by grasping an external object? For example, can the child reach up and touch a mobile or does the child need to hold onto it to keep his or her hand in that position in space? Can the child bring his or her hands to the midline or does gravity or the activity of an asymmetrical tonic neck reflex or tonic labyrinthine reflex prevent this (Figure 10.10)? Can the child get his or her scapulae off the floor by protracting for an upward reach? Can the child look at and reach his or her tummy, knees, or toes, or must the child look up and initiate a symmetrical tonic neck reflex to reach down?

In the prone position, can the child lift his or her chest off the floor by using interaction of his or her flexors and protractors to bring arms forward as supports or with extensors to bring the child's head and back up so that his or her elbows are beneath the shoulders (Figure 10.11)? In the absence of flexor activity, is the chest raised by back extensors with little or no weightbearing on the forearms? Can the

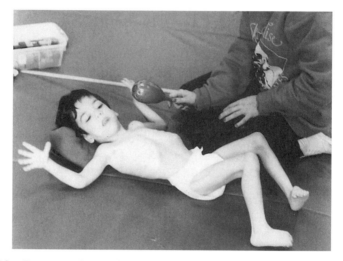

Figure 10.10 Because of the influence of the tonic labyrinthine reflex, this child is rendered dysfunctional by extensor tone.

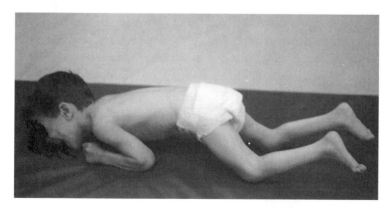

Figure 10.11 Hip flexion causes the center of gravity to shift toward the child's chest. He is unable to bring his arms forward to prop.

child shift weight onto one arm to reach out with the other? Does the child collapse onto his or her chest when attempting to reach out, or compensate with neck and back hyperextension to keep from collapsing? Is shoulder stability adequate for sustained play in this position?

In the sidelying position, is the upper arm fully mobile in the sagittal plane? Can the child reach up from the floor against gravity? Are shoulder movements isolated, or does the child need to initiate them with changes in the position of his or her head? Is the child's shoulder trapped in an internally rotated position by the effects of gravity in this position?

In an upright position, are the shoulders and arms free to move in all planes? Are there compensatory movements such as elevation, retraction, and external rotation or protraction and internal rotation to assist an ineffective head or trunk? Is the shoulder girdle mobile enough for full range but stable enough to maintain a position against gravity? Can the child use his or her arms only when supported by a table-top? How does the position of the shoulder girdle affect mobility of the humeri and forearms? For example, protraction often is accompanied by internal rotation, adduction, extension, and pronation in children who have tone problems. How do the positions of the trunk and pelvis affect the position of the shoulders?

Is child mobile through space in all planes?

In this area, the concern of the therapist who uses the biomechanical frame of reference is not ambulation but mobility through space for two purposes. (1) Can the child move to attain a goal such as a toy, person, or food? (2) Can the child move to provide proprioceptive and vestibular input to enhance the development of body schema and spatial awareness? The clinician looks at how the child moves independently through space and if mechanical assistance would be beneficial.

Can the child get to a desired goal by walking, creeping, crawling, or rolling? If so, does this process require pathological movements? Is the amount of time needed for the movement too extreme, or is the effort too exhausting? What alternatives for goal-oriented movement are realistic? Does the child have the potential to propel a wheelchair (either mechanical or powered), tricycle, or scooter board based on what the therapist knows about his or her functional range, postural reactions, and ability to maintain and control his or her hands? If the child has independent but not optimal locomotion, is the potential improvement gained through a piece of equipment worth the extra training required for the child, family, and care providers? Further, the therapist should explore with the child, family, and care providers their feeling about the use of this hardware and their ability to follow through with its use. Finally, the therapist should consider the expense of the equipment in relation to its need and the potential for reimbursement. If the child has no independent movement through space, which one of several methods is most appropriate for his or her physical and emotional growth and his or her life style? In addition to goal-directed movement through space, what kinds of passive movement through space can be provided? How can the child's position be modified so that he or she feels comfortable and secure?

Can child chew and swallow food successfully without aspirating?

Feeding skills are assessed by the impact of posture on oral-motor function. The assessment of hand placement and control, as previously discussed, should yield similar information in relation to self-feeding skills. Although assessment of posture is critical to effective feeding intervention, it is only one part of a sophisticated evaluation of sensory, fine motor, cognitive, and behavioral skills that goes beyond the scope of this chapter.

Without describing an in-depth feeding evaluation, the following explanation gives examples of how posture and tone are incorporated into oral-motor assessment. Are the trunk and neck stable to provide a base for movements and stability of the jaw? Can the head be maintained in a neutral or slightly flexed position? Is the neck extended so that the airway is open and aspiration of food is more likely, or is it flexed in such a way that swallowing is difficult? Is the trunk in an optimal position for respiration so that the coordination of swallowing and breathing is enhanced?

Does the presence of hypertonicity contribute to such oral reflexes as rooting or the bite reflex? Does it prevent isolated movements, such as separation of the tongue from the jaw? Are the tongue and lips retracted in association with extensor tone so that the tongue cannot come forward and the lips cannot come together?

Is gradation of oral movements affected? Does the jaw just open and snap shut when food is presented? Can support of the head and trunk or changes in body position in space modify high tone so that oral control is enhanced? How does gravity affect oral-motor control in the presence of hypotonicity?

Does the child bite on the spoon because of ungraded jaw movements or because he or she is trying to keep his or her head from wobbling? Do the tongue and lips fall backward in a passively retracted position when the head is tipped back and forward when the neck is flexed? Can the child create enough lip pressure to keep food from falling out of his or her mouth? Is there enough activity in the cheeks to keep food from spilling over the teeth and pocketing in the cheeks? Does the child manage better in supported standing or reclined sitting positions? Does a change in position increase postural tone, or is extra support needed to accommodate for lack of tone?

Can child void when seated on a toilet or potty?

As with feeding, the biomechanical frame of reference is part of a complex evaluation of independent toileting. Information about the child's levels of cognition and sensory awareness is essential. Furthermore, it would be helpful for the therapist to know about the child's diet and behavior patterns.

The postural component addresses comfort, trunk stability, and the ability to relax hip extensors and abductors that otherwise may interfere mechanically with controlled elimination. The assessment is the same, then, as an evaluation of the child's capacity to sit in a stable, comfortable position with hips flexed and slightly abducted. In addition, the child should be assessed for the ability to direct the flow of urine into the toilet rather than onto the floor. This can be an issue with boys and girls alike and often is related to pelvic position.

An additional, extremely important component of the assessment is consideration of the family's or care provider's acceptance of any toileting aid or device in terms of size, management, and cosmesis.

Can the child access a switch to activate a technological device?

Again, the components of this task from a biomechanical frame of reference refer to the capacity to control the head, trunk, and arms. Regardless of their complexity, most devices can be driven by either an intermittent or sustained contact with a switch. However, the fewer demands on motor output when accessing a switch, the greater the cognitive/perceptual demands when using a complex device (such as augmentative communication or powered wheelchairs), where one action must be performed in a specific sequence. The process of selecting the best child/switch match is dependent upon skilled team assessment of a multitude of performance components.

Physical components to be considered include the following:

- Does the child need additional postural supports while mastering the fine control necessary for this skill?
- Where in space can the switch be placed to maximize control? (This is referred to as the "sweet spot"). If using the hand, is the most successful placement for learning to activate the switch at midline or to the side? If using movement of another body part, in what position does switch activation require the least energy and minimize compensatory movements?
- Can the necessary movements for activation be performed against gravity, or does the switch need to be placed where movements are performed in a gravity-eliminated position?
- Can the child produce adequate force to depress the switch that is selected?
- Can the child release the switch in a timely manner?
- Does the child have a variety of movements available to activate the device (e.g., keyboard, joystick) or must the child relay on one movement to activate a switch in a coded fashion?
- Does the best switch/child match consist of a switch that requires a contact to stop or a contact which produces a timed cycle response?

When providing a technological aid to assist the child to interact with his or her physical environment, one must also weigh the impact of the device's size, placement, and cosmesis on the child's ability to interact with his or her human environment.

POSTULATES REGARDING CHANGE

The biomechanical frame of reference uses external devices to promote the child's functioning. Based on the evaluation data, the occupational therapist establishes functional goals for the child that may be developmental or task specific. For example, a functional developmental goal may be to provide the child with a device to facilitate weightbearing on the forearms in preparation for controlled mobility. Another task-specific goal may be to provide the child with a switch plate to activate his or her communication device.

Postulates regarding change define relationships between concepts that structure the environment for change. These postulates help the therapist determine how and when to use adaptive equipment. In the biomechanical frame of reference, specific guidelines for the design, fabrication, and fitting of special devices are found in the application to practice section.

1. If practice time for a skill is increased, then the skill is developed more rapidly.

   During therapy sessions, the therapist often handles a child so that he or she is better able to perform a task. A great increase in therapeutic handling time generally is as impractical for the staff as it is intrusive for the child. Adapted equipment can help the child practice certain skills because equipment "reproduces" the therapist's hands, albeit in a static fashion, to enhance function.

   Regarding this postulate—that an increase in practice results in an increase in skill—the therapist must remember that there is a point of diminishing return. Judgment must be exercised in determining how often the child uses equipment and at what point its use causes stress. Without moderation, a good tool can become counterproductive.

2. If the therapist combines knowledge of the developmental progress of postural skills along with an awareness of the effects of gravity and sensory stimulation on normal and dysfunctional movement, then the therapist can determine appropriate positions to enhance a child's function.

   The therapist needs to determine at what point dysfunction occurs in the development of the child's postural skills and then how this dysfunction affects goal achievement. Another important consideration for the therapist is to explore which positioning options are most effective for a specific child.

3. If the therapist handles the child in a variety of ways, the therapist can determine how best to enhance normal postural responses in any one position.

   Once the therapist determines an appropriate position, the therapist often finds that the child cannot maintain the position independently without using compensatory movements. Because compensations defeat the purpose of using a position to enhance function, the therapist must identify the best way to help the child maintain a position correctly and still engage in as much normal postural activity as possible. This should be done by providing as much support as the child needs, but no more.

The process of determining an effective way to correct a child's position includes a combination of handling and manipulation of the child, an understanding of theoretical information, and trial and error. The understanding of theoretical information helps the therapist gain insight into what may be happening as a child moves or is moved; the therapist should not depend exclusively on that insight, however, to predict what will happen. Objective observation is essential so that the therapist sees and responds to what is happening, not what is expected to happen. This is the point at which trial and error become important: the therapist makes an adjustment in the child's position based on theoretical principles and then evaluates the child's response. If the response is not a desired one, the therapist continues to experiment and evaluate until the desired response is attained. Although the many principles for correct positioning are discussed in the application section, no rules should be accepted without question.

What follows are postulates that may be helpful when handling a child to determine how to facilitate an effective position:

4. If the therapist first provides control centrally, then the distal parts of the body may be freed from the task of assisting the trunk or from the influence of associated reactions.

    For example, if a child cannot prop in the prone position, it may be because his or her body weight is shifted onto his or her chest. Before supporting him or her under the chest, the therapist should extend the child's hips fully by pressing down on his or her buttocks. With weightshifting back over the hips, the child may now be able to bear weight on the forearms.

5. If the therapist uses the effects of gravity to the child's benefit, then the therapist may reduce the need for more intrusive pieces of equipment.

    For example, a child in a prone stander may have poor head control. A prone stander provides full support to the child's ventral body surface, with a slightly forward tipping. When the child attempts to right his or her head, a full extension pattern appears so that his or her neck becomes hyperextended, his or her arms retract actively, and his or her back arches. With a supine stander, the child can use slight neck flexion to right his or her head and lean back against the head support when fatigued, thus eliminating the need for the additional head and back controls in the prone stander. A supine stander provides support to the child's dorsal surface with the body tipped back slightly.

6. If the therapist modifies the child's sensory environment, the therapist may enhance the positive effects of adapted equipment.

    If the therapist observes how the child responds to factors (e.g., ambient noise and light, temperature, and the texture or firmness of a supporting surface), the therapist should make changes in the environment to complement the postural device. For example, a child who responds to being placed on a cold plastic chair with a startle reaction and accompanying increase in extensor tone may be more posturally competent with a lightly padded surface. A child who becomes lethargic in the presence of soft, slow music may maintain an upright position more easily with an increase in the volume and tempo of the music.

7. If the therapist can identify an effective position through handling, the therapist can reproduce that position by using an adapted device.

   The therapist can "translate" a position from handling to a durable piece of equipment by recording what supports the therapist provides with his or her hands or body and at exactly which points the supports contact the child's body. This record provides a blueprint for constructing or ordering equipment. Although specifications for measuring are included in the following section, some general principles that apply to all positioning devices include the following:

   - The surface of support units should be solid and stable so that it does not "give" or change with the child's movements. Flexible surfaces such as beanbags or sling seats on wheelchairs accommodate to the child's weightshifting and can exacerbate asymmetries or dysfunctional postures.
   - Ancillary supports, such as lateral trunk supports, leg abductors, or humeral "wings," should be large enough to distribute pressure over the surface of the body part. In this way, the controlling support does not dig in and cause discomfort or, in some cases, active resistance. Whenever possible, blocks rather than straps should be used to control.
   - The positioning devices should be fitted to the child; the child should not be fitted to the device. It may be tempting to place a child in a piece of equipment, to see how it "fits." Once in the equipment, ill-fitting parts may be difficult to observe.

8. If the therapist considers the needs of the child's care providers, the therapist may provide equipment that is more likely to be used effectively.

   Factors that influence care providers' attitudes include cosmesis, how much space the equipment fills, how difficult it may be to place the child in and out of the equipment, how the device enhances or interferes with social interaction, and its cost in relation to its effectiveness. For example, does the adapted commode fit in the bathroom at home? Or, does the chrome and plastic standing device look too industrial? If the equipment is offensive to those persons expected to use it, it is less likely to be used.

9. If the occupational therapist engages in team decision making, then the child's equipment program will be more effective.

   Working with family members, physical therapists, speech pathologists, teachers, physicians, and equipment vendors as a team provides more information about the child and makes the problem easier to solve. Each member of the team has a unique area of expertise and concern for the child. Accordingly, each team member provides distinctive input. All team members, including the family, should participate whenever appropriate in goal setting and problem solving.

APPLICATION TO PRACTICE

Application to practice is divided into two sections. The first section discusses common positions in which central stability can be provided artificially. The second section deals with postural components or pieces of equipment as they relate to functional skills.

Central Stability

Intervention related to central stability covers the function and dysfunction continua of range of motion, head control, and trunk control. In these interventions, the therapist determines the appropriate position and equipment. Any one position may be appropriate for a variety of goals, depending on where supports are provided and how the equipment and, therefore, the child's body is oriented in space. Is the equipment perpendicular or parallel to the floor or tilted, and how does this affect the child? The following section provides an outline of what general goals may be approached in various positions, and how to fit equipment to the child. Each section contains a brief review of expected skill development in each position, along with the therapeutic advantages of the position.

Supine Position

- Flexor activity develops
- Head control: midline control and chin tuck
- Shoulder protraction and flexion against gravity
- Hands to midline
- Reduced demands on trunk; more effort can be given to head, oral, ocular, and shoulder control

Although not normally functional beyond infancy, practicing some movements in a restful supine position may be beneficial for a child who has physical impairments. Keeping in mind how gravity affects the child who has low tone and how reflex activity may increase hypertonicity in the supine position, the therapist may alleviate these effects by providing passive flexion. A pillow may be placed beneath the head and shoulders of a child so that it enhances neck flexion, supports the head laterally, and protracts the shoulders passively. A roll beneath the thighs can place the hips in a flexed position and yet allow the soles of the feet to be in contact with the floor.

Prone Position

- Headrighting in a horizontal plane
- Interaction of dorsal extensors and ventral flexors for propping on forearms

- Shoulder stability during weightbearing (propping) and mobility-on-stability during weightshift
- Increased range of shoulder flexion when reaching from horizontal position
- Decreased effects of gravity on lateral asymmetries
- Hands more likely to be in visual field by nature of shoulder position when propping

A wedge provides the basic support unit to enhance prone positioning for a child who cannot prop independently. The wedge should be wide enough so that it does not tip if the child starts to roll over. The length of the wedge is determined by the point of support at the chest and hips. The lower the contact of the wedge on the chest, the greater the demands on the shoulder girdle for weightbearing. If the front edge is too far back, the child may flex his or her trunk and curl over it. The front edge of the wedge, where it contacts the child's chest, may also affect respiration (Figure 10.12).

If a child tends to be kyphotic in the upright position but has a mobile spine, then the lumbar spine can be extended passively by having the back edge of the wedge end at the child's waist. Conversely, a lordotic child who lies in the prone position with an anteriorly tipped pelvis should be provided with a wedge that extends well beyond the hips so that the lumbar curve is not exaggerated. The pelvis can be flattened further by strapping an "X" across the buttocks, each strap beginning at the iliac crest and crossing down to the opposite hip. This pelvic position, assisted by the straps, keeps the center of gravity at the hips. The straps also can prevent the child from pulling himself or herself forward over the front edge of the wedge. It should be noted that the use of a single strap often results in the strap sliding up to the lumbar area, causing an increase in lumbar extension and pelvic tilt (Figure 10.13).

The distance of the front edge of the wedge from the floor determines the demands placed on the shoulder girdle. A very low wedge provides support to the chest as the child fatigues but places high demands for weightbearing on the arms and allows more upper trunk mobility for weightshifting. A higher wedge that fully supports the chest but is low enough so that the forearms contact the floor reduces stress on the shoulders, provides proprioceptive feedback, and allows the less stable child to reach out without collapsing. A very high wedge may be used to eliminate demands on upper extremity weightbearing. In this position, a child's arms may dangle downwards, in the same direction as the force of gravity. As the influence of gravity is minimized on the arms by the position, when the child makes a slight shoulder movement it results in a larger movement of his or her hands in his or her visual field. It is important to remember that the activity provided and the height of the activity relative to the child determine how the child uses his or her arms. For example, the child may play with small figures when weightbearing on both elbows but must weightshift to place rings on a stackpole.

When used in conjunction with hip straps, lateral supports to the trunk can help

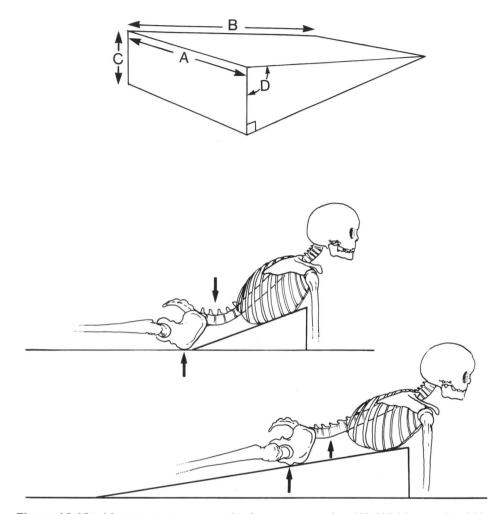

Figure 10.12 Measurements to consider for a prone wedge. (A), Width: unit should be wide enough so that it will not tip over if the child rolls over when strapped to it. (B), Length: Contact of the front edge with the chest will determine how much shoulder stability is needed; the lower on the chest, the more the child is taxed. Lumbar curve and pelvic tilt are determined where the back edge ends in relation to the child's trunk or legs. (C), Height of wedge will determine if weight is borne on forearms or extended arms. (D), Depending on which side of the wedge is chosen as the top surface, shoulders will be placed in either 90° flexion or a lesser degree of flexion.

align the spine in the prone position. With some children, head raising in a prone position is accompanied by associated extensor patterns in the lower extremities, including hip adduction and ankle plantar flexion. This pattern can be modified by placing an abductor between the knees, distributing pressure along the inner legs.

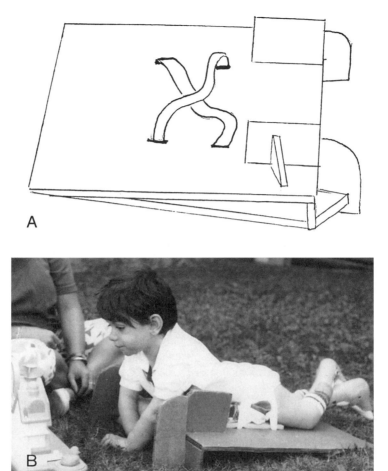

Figure 10.13   The prone lyer (A) provides hip control, lateral controls, and wings to prevent shoulder abduction and extension, keeping the arms forward of the shoulders (B).

Too much abduction creates an anterior pelvic tilt. A small roll beneath the ankle supports the instep so that the ankles are not stretched passively into plantar flexion.

Maintaining the head upright when in a horizontal position can be stressful. The therapist must monitor carefully the amount of time a child is required to be in this position.

Sidelying Position

- Lateral headrighting (a component of neck stability in the upright position)
- Differentiation of two sides of the body (bottom side weightbearing, top side mobile)

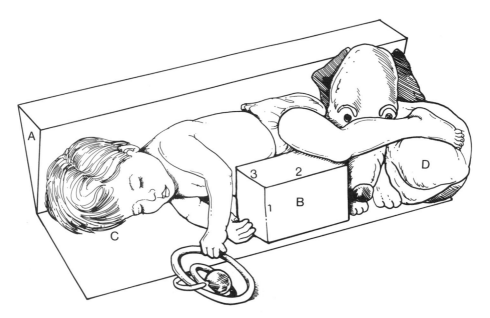

Figure 10.14 Possible components of a sidelyer: (A), Wedged back tips child forward and assists in passive protraction. (B), Chest block/ leg support. (1) Height determines the position of the upper hip (adduction/abduction; internal/external rotation). (2) Length determines if chest alone is supported or if hip, leg, and foot of upper leg are supported while lower leg is held in extension. (3) Depth is an issue only if the block also is used to maintain the position of the lower arm in shoulder flexion and elbow extension. (C), Surface is padded beneath this child's head, but no pillow is used because his head is proportionately large in relation to his body. A pillow would flex his neck laterally. (D), Stuffed animal acts as a leg block to extend the lower leg while supporting the upper leg in flexion. A longer chest block/leg support could have been used.

- Hands easily placed in visual field
- Hypertonicity reduced; tonic labyrinthine reflexes inhibited
- Effects of gravity on shoulder flexion/extension reduced

The child who cannot maintain the sidelying position independently requires front or back supports to prevent inadvertent rolling (Figure 10.14). The back support can be a wall or a board perpendicular to the floor. The front support can be a block that contacts the trunk but allows movement of the shoulders and hips. This block is preferred to straps because it distributes pressure more evenly.

The child's head should be supported by a pillow or padded block that keeps the head and neck aligned laterally with the spine to prevent asymmetry and to facilitate lateral headrighting. This also helps relieve pressure on the downside shoulder. It is important to make the pillow deep enough so that the child's head does not fall when the child flexes his or her neck. If the child tends to extend his or her neck, slight padding can be attached to the back support behind his or her head to encourage a neutral anterior/posterior neck position.

If the child tends to retract his or her shoulders, the therapist can use gravity to facilitate protraction by rolling him or her slightly forward. This can be done by angling the back support slightly forward. As the child's upper arm falls toward the floor, the shoulder tends to adduct horizontally and rotate internally. If this is not a desirable position, the top of the trunk support block can be used as an armrest. This does, however, eliminate functional hand use in this position.

The downside leg generally is extended and the upside leg is flexed. If necessary, the weightbearing leg can be extended by blocking the knee, distributing pressure along the thigh and skin. The child who has lower tone generally does not need this blocking at the knee because the upside leg can be flexed easily, adducted, and rotated internally. This is important because the child who has low tone tends to position his or her hips in abduction and external rotation. When placing the child who shows extensor hypertonicity in sidelying, his or her hips generally are positioned more appropriately in neutral abduction/adduction and neutral rotation. This is accomplished by supporting the knee, lower leg, ankle, and foot with a long block to position the hip properly and, simultaneously, to prevent the tibial torsion and ankle inversion/plantar flexion caused by lack of support to the foot.

It is important that the child be positioned in sidelying on both sides equally in most cases. A sidelyer can be provided with detachable parts so that head and leg supports switch, allowing the child to be placed on either side. One exception is the child who has a functional scoliosis; generally the scoliosis is reduced when the "C" curve faces down and is exaggerated when the "C" faces up. Another consideration for determining on which side to place a child is hand use: the upside arm is more liberated and most likely to be used.

Sitting Position

- Anterior/posterior and lateral stability of neck and trunk
- Weightshift on hips; hips in a slight anterior tilt
- Arms liberated; shoulder position independent of trunk
- Shoulders provide stable base for arm movements

The child who is unable to sit independently basically needs stability in the pelvis and lower body to use the upper trunk, arms, and the head actively (Blair, Ballantyne, Horseman, & Chauvel, 1995; Myhr, Von-Wendt, Norrlin, & Randell, 1995; Colbert, Doyle, & Webb, 1986) (Figure 10.15). Compensatory movements often occur in response to an inadequate central base of support. The therapist must first correct or support any inadequacies in the base, especially at the pelvis, hips, or legs. This may decrease compensatory movements or associated reactions elicited by stress, giving

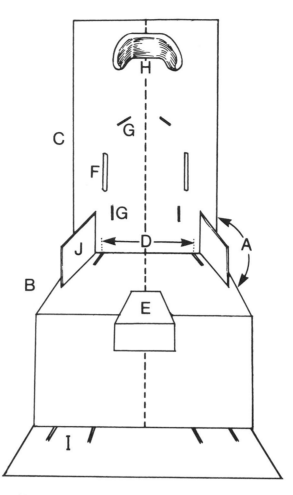

Figure 10.15 Possible components of an adapted chair: (A), Hip angle is commonly 90°, open more if hamstrings are very tight; close angle slightly if it helps to reduce extensor hypertonus. (B), Seat depth should support thighs fully without digging into calf behind knee. (C), Seat height is determined by need for trunk/head support. (D), Hip straps generally come from seat bottom to hold bottom of pelvis back. Slots or attachments should be placed directly alongside the body to prevent lateral shifting of pelvis. (E), Abductor serves to keep legs centered; amount of abduction is determined once pelvis is secured in seating unit. Abductor starts at midthigh, distributing pressure out to the front of the knees, beyond the front edge of the seat. (F), Lateral trunk supports are placed only as high as necessary to assist with trunk control. Lateral trunk supports should not interfere with humeral mobility because of height or thickness. (G), Slots or attachments for harness come in contact with shoulders without digging into the child's neck, and lower placement should be below the rib cage to allow for thoracic expansion during respiration. (H), Placement and angle of head support should be determined after hip and trunk controls are provided with decisions regarding tilt in space. (I), Footstraps may be needed if knee extension keeps feet from providing a base of support. (J), Hip guides may be necessary to keep pelvis centered and may help keep pelvic weightbearing symmetrical.

the therapist a better idea of what corrections need to be made in the more mobile, upper parts of the body. It is important to provide the least amount of artificial supports necessary, providing flexibility for the development of dynamic movement (Brogren, Hadders-Algra, & Forsoberg, 1996; Myhr et al, 1995).

Another way to modify tone to enhance the child's function is to consider the padding on the support unit. Sitting on a hard support tends to increase arousal level. Adding a medium density foam to create a softer support, which conforms to and supports the curves of the child's body, tends to reduce postural stress and hypertonicity.

The child's pelvis should be supported on a solid surface, padded if necessary, that extends to just behind the knees to support the thighs. Careful measurements must be taken when designing and ordering seating equipment. A seat that is too deep causes the edge to dig in behind the child's knees, pushing the legs and the bottom of the pelvis forward. A seat that is too shallow does not support the child's thighs, and the weight of his or her legs pulls his or her thighs downward and the bottom of his or her pelvis forward (Figure 10.16).

The back support should be no higher than necessary to discourage postural dependency. Some children do better with a back support that stops at the level of the pelvic crests or with no back support at all. If a full back that also supports the head is necessary, attention should be given to the shape of the child's head. Young children and those with hydrocephalus often have large occipital regions. The high back support may push a large head forward, causing compensatory curve in the neck. In such cases, recessing the head support allows for correct cervical alignment.

The position of the child's pelvis also is controlled by the angle of seat-to-back (the angle of hip flexion) and the angle of the seating unit in space (amount that it

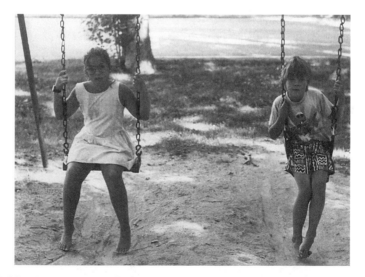

Figure 10.16 A solid seat (left) allows the hips to assume a relatively neutral position. The sling seat (right) forces the hips into adduction and internal rotation.

tilts backward). These two factors should be explored simultaneously. The hip angle generally is most effective at 90°. Increasing hip flexion or decreasing the angle of seat-to-back may reduce severe extension hypertonicity. Once high tone is reduced, however, minimal postural tone may remain in the trunk. In another situation, when a child has very tight hamstrings, extending the hips slightly (5°–10°) may reduce the posterior pelvic tilt caused by the pull of his or her hamstrings. Opening the seat angle also can be effective with a low-tone child if the back is perpendicular to the floor and the seat slopes down from the back. The increased proprioceptive input to the feet may facilitate postural alertness (Figure 10.17).

To secure the child's pelvis, a seat belt is used. Coming up from the point at which the seat meets the chairback, the belt is at a 45° angle to the hips and holds the pelvis in place. Rather than coming from the outside edge of the seat, it should be attached alongside the hips to keep the child's pelvis centered. If the belt comes from the back support parallel to the floor, it holds back the top of the child's pelvis. This is helpful when an exaggerated anterior pelvic tilt exists but, in most cases, it is contraindi-

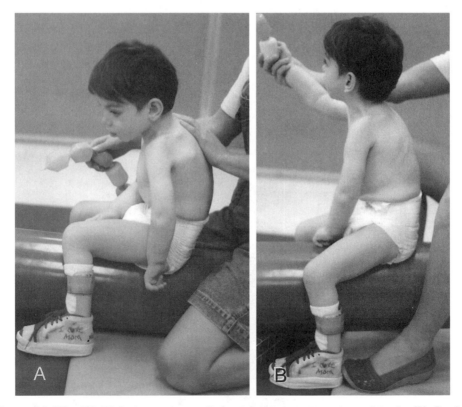

Figure 10.17   (A), Tight hamstrings pull the pelvis into a posterior pelvic tilt. (B), By decreasing the angle of hip flexion on an elevated roll, the pelvis assumes a neutral position, enhancing a sitting posture.

cated. A strap that comes from the seat perpendicular to the floor holds the pelvis back well but may cause more hip adduction than desired. The belt itself should be wide enough so that it does not dig into the child's flesh but narrow enough so that it places control only where desired. A too-wide strap placed at a 45° angle causes a posterior pelvic tilt by pulling the top of the child's pelvis backward.

If the child's pelvis tends to move laterally on the seat despite the seat belt, pelvic blocks can be used for centering. These blocks angle slightly out from the seat back to nestle the child's pelvis in place.

Depending on the degree to which it is done, tilting the seat unit slightly backward may increase or decrease postural demands. The stress and extensor tone that accompany an upright position can be decreased with a backward tilt. This provides the child with a back support on which he or she can lean intermittently. The same position may encourage activity in the neck or trunk flexors when the child comes forward into an upright position from a partial recline (Figure 10.18). When a re-

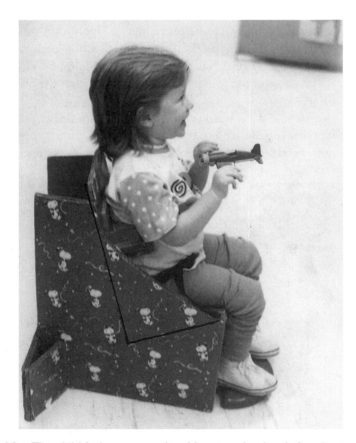

Figure 10.18   This child feels secure and is able to use her hands for play in a slightly reclined seat. Note that lines on the chair indicate seat angles.

clining position is used to reduce the effects of gravity on the trunk and the child is incapable of flexing his or her neck or trunk forward into a righted position, it is important to support his or her head so that it is upright. This allows him or her to look forward rather than at the ceiling (Nwaobi, 1987).

The child's thighs contribute to his or her base of support. Too much abduction reduces anterior/posterior stability. Too much adduction reduces lateral stability and contributes to a pattern of extensor hypertonicity. Supports that run laterally along the child's thighs reduce abduction (Figure 10.19). In general, the child's hips should be in neutral abduction/adduction. For some children, moderate hip abduction may be used to provide a wider base of support or to help reduce extensor tone in the hips or facilitate an anterior pelvic tilt (Reid, 1996). A rhombus-shaped wedge can be used to abduct the child's hips. When used, it should start at the middle of the child's thighs and extend to his or her knees, beyond the edge of the seat, to distribute pressure. A rhombus-shaped wedge also may be needed to keep the child's thighs symmetrical if one hip tends to abduct or to rotate externally while the other adducts or rotates internally (Figure 10.20).

Care must be taken that the seat is not too high from the floor so that the child's feet can be placed firmly on the floor or on the foot support. Having knees and ankles at 90° is a good guideline. Foot orthotics should be considered to correct ankles that are unstable or pathologically positioned so that the child's feet can contribute to stability.

Once the child has been positioned so that his or her pelvis is aligned properly, the therapist is better able to determine the positioning needs of the trunk, shoulders, and head. Trunk supports provide lateral stability and some shoulder correc-

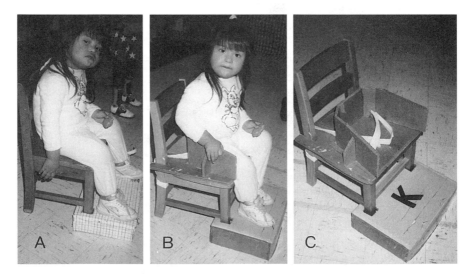

Figure 10.19   By providing support to the lower back (A) and adducting the thighs (B), this positioning device enhances an upright posture (C).

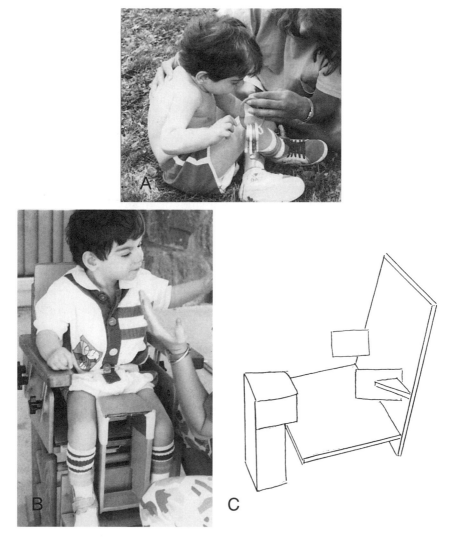

Figure 10.20 Correction of this child's sitting posture requires appropriate seat depth, high back support, seat belt at 45°, an abductor running from thighs to ankles, and lateral trunk support. In the sitting device, the child's arms are free for play (A–C).

tion. Lateral supports should contact the child's trunk only when necessary. If lateral supports are placed slightly away from the body to encourage the child to do more postural "work," it is critical to determine if this demand compromises functional use of his or her arms. A child may not be able to control his or her trunk and arms simultaneously. The higher the lateral supports, the more control they provide. The two supports should be opposite each other, unless tone in the trunk is asymmetrical; in that case, the supports should be low on the convex side and high on the concave side to correct the scoliosis. Care should be taken that the supports are not so high that they press into the axilla, nor so far apart that they hold the humeri in an abducted position. Improperly placed lateral supports interfere with shoulder mobility and hand use.

Laptrays or table surfaces can be designed to contribute to the child's correct shoulder and trunk positioning. It is important that they be provided only after optimal positioning has been attained through design of the seating or standing unit. With an improperly fitted basic unit, a child may use a laptray to "hang" by his or her arms or to rest his or her head and upper trunk, rather than enhance arm position and function.

A laptray should provide enough surface area to support the full length of the child's arms during all movements. Hands or fingers do not hang off the edge of the tray. If the tray "wraps around" the child's trunk, the cut-out should be large enough so that it does not dig into the child's chest or interfere with his or her breathing or slight weightshifts. It should be snug enough so that his or her arms do not slip between the trunk and the tray and become wedged. In general, it is preferable to provide a transparent tray for two reasons: (1) a child can see the rest of his or her body and (2) in a wheelchair, a child or care provider can see the floor through the tray to maneuver more easily through space.

A harness made of a chest plate with four straps can prevent the child from falling forward. Often, when a harness is used, the child's sitting unit is tipped slightly backward so that the child rests against the back and does not hang into the harness. The top two straps attach to the back support directly over the shoulders. Slots may be cut into the back for proper strap placement. This ensures a snug fit and, simultaneously, discourages shoulder elevation. It also discourages lateral upper trunk flexion by keeping the shoulders at the same level. The lower straps should attach to the back or through slots on either side of the trunk, below the level of the rib cage, so they are less likely to interfere with thoracic expansion during respiration. The chest plate should be at midchest so that there is no danger of it digging into a child's neck (Figure 10.21).

If the harness causes the shoulders to become retracted, small wedges attached to the back support at the level of the scapulae can be used to nudge the shoulders forward (protraction wedge). Care should be taken that the sizes or positions of the wedges do not create rounding of the upper trunk. If retraction is mild and the scapulae are mobile, then the protraction wedge may be used without a harness.

The child's use of a laptray can enhance arm and hand function by diminishing pathology in his or her shoulders. Although it cannot directly affect humeral rotation by flexing the shoulders, the pattern of internal rotation, extension, and protraction is modified. In addition, the humeri can be adducted horizontally, bringing the arms toward the midline, by using humeral wings. These also help to correct the position of humeri that are extended as part of a retraction/external rotation pattern. The "wings" are surfaces attached perpendicular to the laptray. They push the humeri

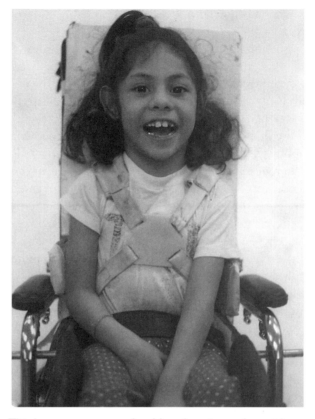

Figure 10.21   This harness prevents shoulder elevation and provides trunk support

forward, preventing humeral extension or horizontal abduction. They should provide contact along the length of the humeri and be high enough so that the child cannot lift his or her arms over them and get trapped behind them. By holding the child's arms in the desired position and running a pencil mark along the humeri on the tray, proper placement of the "wings" can be marked.

The child's use of a laptray can contribute to trunk control by supporting his or her arms, thereby relieving the trunk of the weight of the arms. In this situation, the tray supports the arms, not the trunk. In addition, passive shoulder flexion that places the humeri in an almost horizontal position helps to elongate the thoracic spine as long as the child is not hanging by his or her arms on the tray. Position of a laptray or table surface can range from midtrunk to just below the axillae, depending on the child. It may be difficult for children who demonstrate inadequate shoulder flexion or tightness in shoulder extension to keep their elbows and forearms on the tray surface because the arms are inclined to slide back from the tray edge. Two possible solutions include the use of a "wrap-around" tray or the use of humeral wings. Using a harness in conjunction with "wings" helps to stabilize the chest and position the arms effectively.

Two issues prompt concern when using a laptray on a seating or standing unit that tips back. First, if the laptray is perpendicular to the back of the unit, it will be angled toward the child in an easel-like fashion when the unit is tilted back. The tilt of the laptray can be controlled with adjustable hardware to keep it horizontal when the unit is tipped back. Second, by tipping the child slightly backward, gravity tends to push the humeri backward. It may be necessary to consider humeral wings that may not be otherwise needed when the child sits in a full, upright position.

The therapist may choose to tilt the laptray like an easel if it helps correct trunk or head position. By resting his or her forearms on an easel surface, the child may use greater degrees of shoulder flexion. This may elongate the upper trunk, enhancing the upright position. Also, tilting the laptray places visual stimuli closer to eye level. This may encourage the child to keep his or her head in a more upright position, rather than to look downward and initiate a flexion pattern in neck and trunk when reading or drawing (Figure 10.22).

Because of the complexity of the head, shoulder, and arm interaction, the therapist must be flexible and try several approaches to meet the child's needs. Correction in the child's shoulders may provide more freedom of head movement or, conversely, may create a need for external head support. For example, by correcting a pattern of shoulder retraction and external rotation and straightening of the upper back, the child may no longer need compensatory neck extension to align his or her head with his or her body. Another child, with the same corrections, however, may require a head support.

The first approach to improve inadequate head control or dysfunctional positioning of the head caused by tone problems is to correct total body position. Given enough external body support and reduction of physical stress, the child may be able to exercise control over his or her head on his or her own. Alignment of the child's body and modification of tone can reduce associated reactions and the need for compensatory movements in the neck. It should be remembered, however, that many pathological reflexes are elicited by head movement. In such cases, correction of head position can enhance body position. For example, slight flexion of a hyperextended neck may reduce extensor tone throughout the body and maintaining the head in midline may eliminate body asymmetry caused by the influence of an asymmetrical tonic neck reflex.

Head position also is related to the source of visual or auditory stimulation. Most children hyperextend their necks when seated in a chair to look at and speak with an adult who stands before them. The position of the child in the environment or the stimulus in relation to the child must be considered when attempting to correct head position.

The simplest support for the head may be a high seat back. This provides a resting place but no lateral or anterior controls. In conjunction with a slight tip-back of

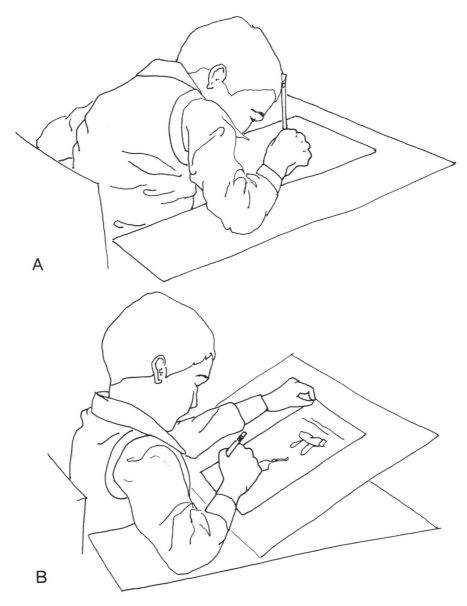

Figure 10.22 (A) Flexion pattern, including overflow into hands, is created when this child looks down at his work. (B), Angling the work surface changes the position of the head and modifies associated tone.

the unit, gravity assists in preventing passive, floppy forward flexion yet still encourages active neck flexion against slight resistance. The latter example may enhance active control of the head in some children. Another child may use an undesirable pattern of total flexion to right his or her head when tipped back. Three drawbacks to the high back for head support are (1) the hard flat back may not provide enough surface support for the rounded back of the head; (2) the point of contact of the seat back with the head may provide a tactile cue that stimulates neck extension against the surface; and (3) if the child's occipital area is big, the head will be forced forward and out of alignment with the back, causing neck flexion with a downward position or compensatory extension at the base of the cranium.

Another simple control consists of lateral head supports with a high back. Care should be taken that these supports not interfere with the visual field or cover the ears. In addition, if the lateral supports touch the cheeks, a rooting reflex may result.

Neck rings and neck collars contribute to head control with no interference to sensory receptors on the head and face. A neck ring attaches to the seat back and cradles the base of the cranium. It should be placed at a height that provides slight traction on the neck, elongating the neck and providing constant contact with the base of the skull. The neck ring reproduces the shape of the therapist's hand were the therapist to place his or her thumb and forefinger around the back of the child's neck with the occiput resting on the web space and the base of the temporal bones on thumb and fingertips. A neck collar made of medium density foam, cut in width to fit between the shoulders and the base of the skull snugly, supports and elongates the neck and can be used independent of the seating unit. To allow for slight neck flexion or jaw movements, the front of the neck collar should be connected in a yoke-like fashion.

Some supportive headrests are sculpted so that they conform to the head and neck. If a child requires the support of a sculpted headrest or, in some cases, the less supportive head ring, it is likely that the child will be unable to prevent his or her head from falling forward when in an upright position. A slight backward tilt of the seating unit assists in keeping the head in contact with the support. When a child is tipped back more than 5° or 10° for the sake of trunk control, however, it is necessary to right the head as much as possible by angling the head support or pushing it forward to flex the neck and align the head in space. The therapist must experiment with the child to find the optimal relationship among head, trunk, and angle in space.

In extreme cases, a child may have a complete lack of head control. Three options can be explored, all of which have possible drawbacks.

1. A full neck collar immobilizes the head and may interfere with jaw movements or swallowing.
2. A severe recline of the seating unit (up to 40° tipped back) with a head support limits the child's visual field or possibly compromises swallowing.
3. Stabilization of the head in a slightly reclined position can be achieved by strapping the forehead to the seat back or by wearing a helmetlike device with a chin strap attached to the back of the seat. A forehead strap alone may result in passive compensatory neck extension because the head slides down out of the strap. The helmet may be hazardous to the integrity of the cervical spine if the child's body

slides down when the head is immobilized, or pressure from the chin strap may create problems with swallowing.

In general, demands on active head control in the severely involved child should be minimized when the child is seated so that efforts can be directed toward intake of information, interaction with the environment, and fine motor or oral-motor skills. The therapist should keep in mind that developing active components for head control may be addressed by using various positions and equipment such as standers, scooter boards, and prone wedges.

Supported Standing Position

- Erect spine, liberated arms
- Neutral or slightly posterior pelvic tilt
- Hips extended with neutral rotation
- Knees stable but not locked in hyperextension
- Ankles in 90° flexion, neutral eversion/inversion
- Improved circulation and bone growth from upright weightbearing
- Increased alertness from upright position and extensor activity
- Decreased effects of flexor hypertonicity in neck and trunk when weightbearing on extended hips and knees

The supported standing position should not be used for potential ambulators exclusively (Figure 10.23). This position provides increased opportunities of function for those children who are least likely to walk by enhancing circulation, growth, and alertness; it also provides opportunities for head and arm control for children who have moderate to severe disabilities and is an alternative to long-term sitting (Manley & Gurtowski, 1985; Motloch & Brearley, 1983; Noronha, Bundy, & Groll, 1989).

The therapist first must decide which surface of the child's body is to be supported in standing. Providing support to the ventral surface by using a "prone" stander at an 80° to 85° angle to the floor provides a close-to-normal standing position and requires slightly more extensor activity. If upright at 90°, the prone stander tends to throw the child's body backward in space, and he or she may flex over the top edge of the stander to compensate. A supine stander provides dorsal support for children who show very high or very low tone. For example, when slightly reclined in a supine stander, the very floppy child who has minimal head control is provided with total support. The child who has too much extensor tone and who throws his or her head, shoulders, and upper trunk back in a prone stander is encouraged to use flexion to right himself or herself intermittently in a slightly reclined supine stander.

Through a series of trials and observations, the therapist can determine the optimal angle of a standing board to the floor. Postural demands and postural responses change as the stander is tipped farther forward or backward. In a prone stander,

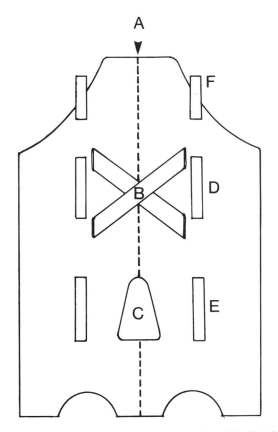

Figure 10.23 Possible components of a prone stander. (A), Height is determined by child's need for ventral support, anywhere between the waist and sternoclavicular joint. When the support is cut high (as in this example), sides must be cut out to allow for shoulder mobility. (B), Hip straps come through slots right alongside the hips. They cross from the posterior crest of one side to the hip joint of the other side, placing pressure over the sacrum. (C), Abductor wedge keeps the legs aligned symmetrically and determines the amount of hip abduction. It runs above and below the knees but does not come in contact with the perineum. (D), Hip guides may be added for additional lateral stability, especially in the presence of a functional scoliosis. (E), Lateral leg guides prevent the external rotation/knee flexion pattern that often causes children with low tone to collapse in standing. (F), Lateral trunk supports may be necessary and should be placed as low as possible.

demands on headrighting are less in an upright position than in a horizontal position. The child who cannot maintain a righted head in a prone lying position may be successful in a prone stander at 75°. In this case, with head control and tolerance in the prone position as the primary goal, the prone stander actually may be lowered as the child masters head control in increasingly higher horizontal positions.

The height of the stander determines how much support is provided to the trunk (and head in a supine position) and how much postural work must be done by the child. The therapist's goal is to make some postural demands without causing fatigue or undesirable associated reactions that result from physical stress.

As with sitting, the hips and legs should be positioned first. In the prone stander, crossed straps should stabilize the pelvis in the same way as in the prone position. If lateral shifting of the pelvis occurs, which would create a compensatory curve in the trunk, lateral pelvic blocks similar to lateral trunk supports should be placed on either side of the pelvis. With hips in neutral, the knees are directly below the hips. Occasionally, some hip abduction is desired. In either case, depending on the degree of abduction desired, a rectangular- or trapezoid-shaped block should be placed between the knees. This spacer or abductor should extend above and below the knees to distribute pressure. Its primary purpose is to keep the legs aligned and symmetrical. If the child abducts and rotates his or her hips externally, knee flexion no longer is blocked by the surface of the stander because the knees will be facing laterally. Lateral supports at the level of the knees bring the hips into a more neutral abduction/adduction position and prevent collapse at the knees.

Padding in front of the knees on the prone stander relieves pressure and prevents knee flexion. Too much padding causes the knees to hyperextend. If the knees hyperextend regardless of padding, the joint can be flexed by realigning the feet so that the ankle is slightly back of the knee. If the child wears foot orthoses, then the upper straps must be loosened because this position requires some ankle dorsiflexion.

Holes must be cut in the bottom of the standing board to accommodate the toes. Care must be taken to align these cut-outs with the hips and legs. Blocks placed laterally or medially to the child's feet can maintain the foot position if necessary. A nonskid surface could be just as effective (Figure 10.24).

The integrity of the ankle and foot must be evaluated in standing. Although this skill is beyond this chapter, ankle/foot orthoses must be provided for standing if pathology exists in that area.

The need for and placement of lateral trunk supports can be determined once the lower body position is corrected and stable. The chest support or upper edge of the prone stander may end anywhere between the bottom of the sternum to just below the clavicle, depending on need. If the chest support is cut high, it should be curved down away from the midline (something like the end of an ironing board) to free the shoulder girdle for movement.

As in the sitting position, height and angle of the laptray contribute to correcting posture. A low laptray may encourage weightbearing on extended arms. A child who has inadequate extension, however, may flex over the top of the chest support in an attempt to rest on the laptray. In such cases, a laptray at nipple level helps elongate the upper trunk and provide support for the arms as the child masters head control. The need for humeral wings should be assessed if the child retracts and extends his or her shoulders.

In the supine stander, a hip strap is unnecessary because the child extends

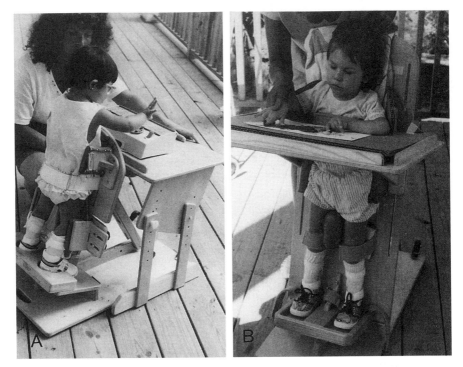

Figure 10.24   Two examples of standers: (A), prone stander; (B), supine stander.

against the back support when chest and knee straps are applied. Care should be taken that the chest strap not dig into the axillary area. Hip blocks may be desirable to prevent lateral movement and any resultant asymmetries. As with the prone stander, abductor/spacer blocks or lateral adductors should be considered to align hips and legs. Padding should be placed behind the knees if there is any indication of hyperextension at that joint. Ankle straps that come from behind the heel over the instep at a 45° angle or medial or lateral foot blocks may be needed to maintain foot placement.

A supine stander that has a laptray supports the arms, provides a working surface, and encourages the child to use some active neck and upper trunk flexion to right his or her head and come forward to the working surface. Because the supine stander is tilted backward to some extent, humeral wings may be necessary to assist the child in keeping his or her shoulders and arms forward against gravity. If head supports are needed, this is determined in the same way as for the partially reclined sitting position.

Functional Skills

The previous section discussed common positions in which central stability is provided artificially to decrease pathological movement, encourage components of postural responses, and liberate the head and arms. Intervention in this section addresses the function/dysfunction continua that relate to hand control, mobility, feeding, and toileting, all of which involve more than postural responses. These functions also require cognition, perception, attention, motor planning, and fine motor skills. Postural control is a foundation for the development of these functions. The absence of postural control impedes the development of skills in these areas. The sections that follow describe postural components or equipment related to these functions.

Ability to Place, Maintain, and Control Hand Position

Although it is desirable to have shoulder and arm mobility in all planes, this is not always a realistic goal. If expectations must be limited, then the most functional ranges of shoulder and arm movement are those that contribute to midline activity so that the child can bring objects toward his or her eyes, ears, and mouth for learning and survival. In this case, desirable ranges of volitional movement include neutral toward slight protraction; neutral toward internal rotation; 0° to 90° shoulder flexion, abduction, and horizontal adduction; and midranges of elbow flexion/extension and forearm rotation. The development of control in these ranges can be addressed in two ways: (1) by establishing skill in shoulder and elbow mobility and stability in developmental positions (enhancing the development of components of movement) and (2) by providing as much support as necessary to the body and arms so that the child can perform a few isolated movements. (This improves distal function by reducing the need for postural reactions through external support.)

With a child who has moderate to severe disabilities, the therapist may choose to devise a specific pattern of movement related to one function. Examples of specific patterns of movement may be a hand-to-mouth pattern for feeding or a simple elbow movement to activate a switch. The first step is to provide an optimum base of support to modify tone and reduce demands on the rest of the body and yet enhance attention to task. Sidelying, sitting, prone standing, and supine standing should be considered. The second step is to determine how many arm movements the child can control and which ones need to be supported artificially by a laptray or other equipment components. For example, humeral wings eliminate the child's need to protract actively or to adduct horizontally when bringing his or her hand to his or her mouth. If the therapist raises the laptray to axilla level, the child's movements are then limited to the horizontal plane, and demands for movements against gravity are eliminated.

In extreme cases, if a child has no control over arm movements (i.e., such as a child who has severe athetoid movements), one arm can be positioned so that movement is channeled in one direction. For example, blocks may be placed laterally and medially along the child's arm, creating a channel on the laptray. With such an arrangement, the hand can move only in the vertical plane, regardless of extraneous shoulder, elbow, or forearm movements. In this way, the child may successfully depress a switch plate. Following a training period, supports should be withdrawn.

Ability to Move Through Space

Devices can be provided that facilitate mobility for the child who has severe disabilities and who cannot move through space. Those children who have less severe involvements and who cannot move fast enough or efficiently enough to attain an end goal or who cannot keep up with peers also may benefit from such devices.

If pathological tone is increased through passive movement because of the intensity of the stimulation but affectual responses are positive, it is up to the therapist to provide a position in which unwanted overflow of tone can be controlled. For example, a child who hyperextends when swinging may be nestled in a flexed position within an inflatable tube placed on a platform swing.

Scooter boards may be effective in enhancing self-initiated movement in a child who has moderate to severe disabilities. They can also provide weightbearing, weightshifting, and rapid movement through space for the child who has milder disabilities. The scooter board consists of an appropriately fitted prone wedge placed on highly responsive ball-bearing casters (Figure 10.25). Several modifications to the prone wedge can enhance its effectiveness. These include a chest wedge to provide the correct shoulder-to-floor distance and a front wedge cut away to support only the chest and liberate the shoulder girdle (which is "ironing-board"-shaped). The back edge of the wedge should end before the ankles so that the child's feet can hang freely over the end of the board. The child who has severe disabilities may need an extension of the front edge of the wedge for intermittent head support. Directed, forward movement is not the goal in this case. Rather, the child begins to initiate movement through space whenever his or her hands begin to bear weight through his or her arms. For the child who cannot roll or crawl, this may be his or her only opportunity to experience active movement through space.

Children who are nonambulatory or who walk slowly with crutches may be less taxed when using a tricycle. A tricycle also allows them to engage with peers in gross motor activity. Tricycles can be purchased with back supports, hip straps, abductors along the handlebar uprights, and footplates with straps (Figure 10.26). The therapist needs to determine that the tricycle measurements and supports provided coincide with the child's sitting skills. Arm and hand positions also should be assessed. The handlebars can be raised to encourage an upright trunk. Adapted vertical handgrips that place the forearm in a neutral rotation also encourage an erect trunk, provided there is forearm mobility.

A powered wheelchair provides rapid mobility for the nonambulator who finds a manual wheelchair painstakingly slow to propel and requires excessive effort to move. Because switches offer great sophistication, powered chairs can be propelled by severely involved persons provided that they have an awareness of space and good judgment with regard to their safety and the safety of others. Just as an 18-month-old child can direct his or her body through space with reasonable safety, so can a child of the same maturational age learn to direct a powered chair. By provid-

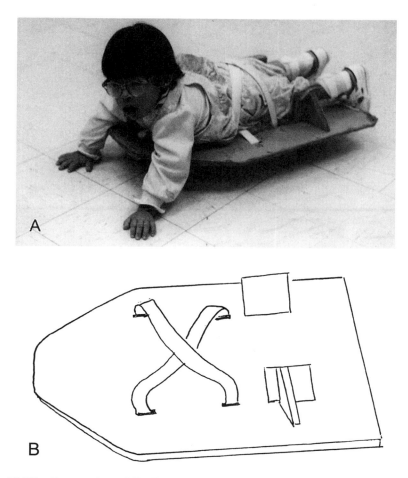

Figure 10.25   Scooter board (A, B) provides hip straps and abductors to prevent this low tone child from externally rotating her hips and dragging her legs on the floor.

ing for positioning needs in a wheelchair, the therapist combines the optimal sitting position with the most functional position of laptray and arm guides.

Ability to Feed

Positioning in a feeding program is designed to reduce the influence of low or high muscle tone on oral-motor activity to prevent situations that may trigger primitive reflexes and to provide central stability to enhance controlled distal mobility (Larnet & Ekberg, 1995). This promotes skills such as sucking, biting, chewing, and swallowing.

Tone can be modified through the choice of position and supports. A child who has very high or very low tone may need total support, such as that provided by reclined sitting or supine standing with a harness to provide shoulder control and

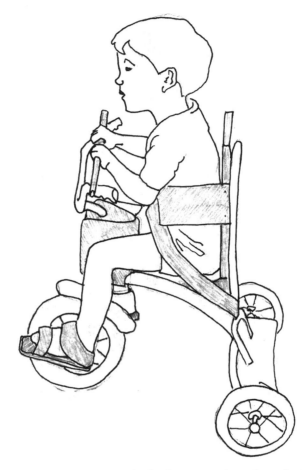

Figure 10.26 Adaptive tricycle provides back support, lateral trunk support, hip straps, abductors, foot straps, and horizontal bar to hold onto. Grasp on the original handle bar had encouraged shoulder elevation, internal rotation, elbow flexion, and ulnar deviation.

thoracic support. A child who has slightly low tone may respond well to increased postural demands (e.g., a seat with low back support or a prone stander). In other cases, the best positioning device may be the therapist's body. The child who is positioned properly in an adult's lap benefits from physical warmth, touch, and social interaction, all of which may be the most effective therapy during his or her feeding.

Head support may be needed to provide a stable base for jaw movements. A neutral or slightly flexed position of the neck contributes to controlled swallowing, reduces extensor hypertonicity, and prevents a child who has disabilities from throwing his or her head back and "bird-feeding," which is uncontrolled swallowing that uses gravity rather than musculature to get the food down. If the child has poor lip closure or lip pressure, however, keeping food in his or her mouth may be facilitated by a slight tipping back of his or her head. It is important that the neck not be extended. The appropriate position of the head can be accomplished by reclining the trunk partially and bringing the head forward to an almost-righted position.

The head support should not contact the face to avoid a rooting reflex. Activation of the rooting reflex turns the child's head away from the source of food and also may initiate asymmetries because the turning of the head can produce asymmetrical tonic neck reflex activity.

Special attention should be paid to shoulder position during feeding. High tone in elevation, retraction, protraction, or humeral rotation can compromise swallowing and the coordination of swallowing with respiration.

Ability to Void When Seated on a Toilet or Potty

The primary goal of equipment in this area is to provide support and modify tone so that the child can relax. Postural challenges should not be the issue here, instead comfort is essential. Special attention should be paid to provide adequate hip flexion and abduction in supported sitting (Figure 10.27).

Potty training for young children who have severe disabilities frequently requires a lot of time. Diversional activities are sometimes helpful to motivate and engage the child. If a younger child's potty training program includes diversional activities, then a laptray can serve the dual purpose of arm support and a play surface.

Ability to Activate the Switch for a Technology Aid

The goal of positioning is to facilitate effortless and reliable switch control. Once an optimal sitting position has been established, a therapist may find that the child benefits from additional supports (e.g., head support, harness) while learning the refinements of this task. If the hand has the potential for switch activation, it may help to temporarily provide additional supports/restraints to limit degrees of freedom of arm movements (e.g., immobilizing the arm while the child develops control of a wrist or finger movement). Another way to reduce motor demands when a severely involved child begins switch activation training may be to approach the task from a sidelying position.

The therapist and child must find the best position in space for the switch, where access to it is most efficient. If the child will be using his hand, a graphic way to identify this "sweet spot" may be to cover the laptray with paper and attach a marker to the child's hand. The most heavily colored portion of the paper usually represents the most accessible place for the switch. With less involved children, clinical observation can determine this spot. This spot may be at midline for some children and to the side for others. Once access skills emerge, it is good to gradually move the switch off to the side, leaving midline space for the placement of other activities. If the child does not have the potential to use his or her hand, the therapist and child must explore together the options for a reliable movement in any other body part.

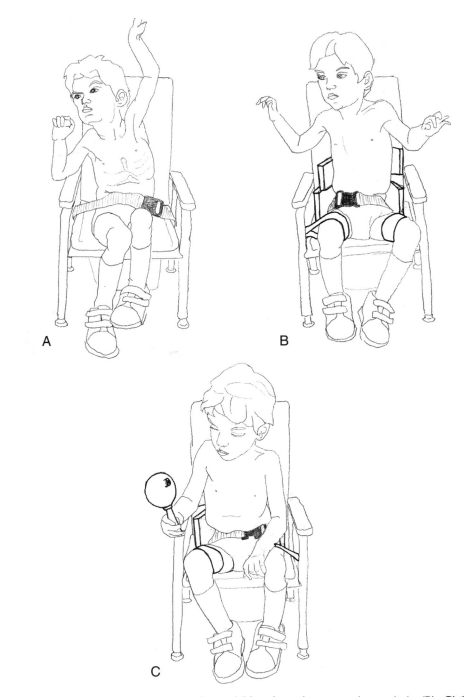

Figure 10.27 (A), Child in commercially available adapted potty with seat belt. (B), Child sitting with additional control facilitated by lateral trunk supports, hip guides, and abductor straps (dark lines). Relaxation is enhanced by the use of an activity.

A multitude of characteristics of switches are available commercially (Weiss, 1990). If the child can control more than a single movement, he or she has easier access to switches such as joysticks and keyboards. If not, the therapist must find a match between the child's motor ability and the type of switch, in terms of force and speed needed, the distance traversed to activate/deactivate, and the cognitive/perceptual components to plan coded sequences of single movements (such as may be necessary to select one word from a vocabulary of hundreds on a communication device).

If the child has an adequate agonist musculature to activate a switch but inadequate antagonist to release it (or a similar scenario), the switch can be placed in a gravity eliminated position to facilitate the weaker movement. There is an array of hardware available to position switches in this way.

Summary of Application to Practice

The last part of this chapter has addressed the more technical aspects of the biomechanical frame of reference (i.e., the practical problems of translating a therapeutic intention into a piece of equipment). This process requires some mechanical skills and an ability to manipulate three-dimensional space mentally. Although it is only one component of treatment implementation, the actual prescription or design of equipment often makes the greater demands on the novice therapist. Frequent hazards involved in this process include that concentration becomes too focused on the product (i.e., adaptive device) and the multitude of other factors that enhance posture and function are overlooked.

The diagram (Figure 10.28) illustrates an approach to postural control that is more complete than a simple device to support the child. It should be viewed as a series of "ex-centric," rather than concentric circles with the supportive device in the center. The circles widen to demonstrate a more holistic approach to biomechanical intervention. As the circles grow from the center, the factors produce effects on posture and function that are less direct and specific but that are greater in scope.

The first, smallest circle represents the most direct approach: the positioning device that physically supports the child—the "hardware" that taxes the therapist's mechanical and spatial skills. The next circle includes the physiological reactions that modulate posture (e.g., reactions to tactile cues provided by the equipment or reactions to changes in head or body position in space). The next circle represents effort—the amount of work the child must do to stay upright and interact with his or her environment. Too much effort may cause fatigue or frustration; too little effort may limit the potential for growth and change.

The circle that represents environmental factors includes those things that influence levels of arousal, attention, and tone and indirectly enhance or disrupt postural reactions. Temperature can be changed to enhance posture by altering the heat in the room, adding or removing layers of clothing, or providing close physical contact between the child and another person. The position of visual cues may affect how

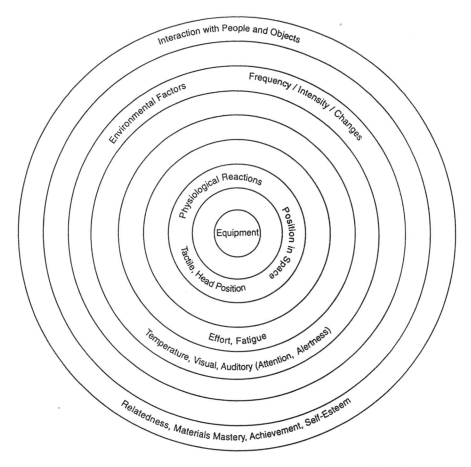

Figure 10.28 Diagram presenting an approach to postural control that is more complete than a device that merely supports the child.

the child holds his or her head, with resultant changes in tone and posture. The element of motion with visual stimulation can enhance attention or increase fatigue, depending on the child's head control and ocular motor skills. For example, practical implications include where the teacher stands or sits in relation to the child and whether the instructor moves about as he and she speaks. Another aspect of this circle is auditory stimulation. Background noise and changes in volume or tempo of voice or music enhance alertness, elicit dysfunctional startle responses, or cause a child to "shut-down," depending on the person. These factors and many others in the physical environment have a subtle yet cumulative impact on posture and function and should be incorporated into the therapist's treatment plan.

The outermost circle encompasses opportunities for interaction with people and objects. Although this appears to be the least direct channel to modify posture and function, changes often include observable phenomena. For example, significant improvement in posture may be noted when a child is drawn into a song made up about himself or herself and his or her friends or when the child is given the opportunity to apply finger paint to his or her therapist's face. Interaction with people, animals, and materials and the associated senses of mastery and self-esteem represent goals and therapeutic tools.

The occupational therapist can act as a consultant to the team to help modify the child's internal and external environment throughout the day. As part of the biomechanical frame of reference, the therapist must learn to identify and use the many forces that are greater than the force of gravity.

SUMMARY

The biomechanical frame of reference is used when a person cannot maintain posture through automatic muscle activity because of neuromuscular or musculoskeletal dysfunction. It uses external supports or equipment, either temporarily or permanently, to substitute for the lack of postural control. The frame of reference is often used as a primary approach with a child exhibiting severe physical disabilities and with other frames of reference.

The first goal of the biomechanical frame of reference is to enhance the development of postural reactions through the reduction of gravity's demands and aligning the body properly. The second goal is to improve functional performance through the use of external supports, reducing the need for and demands in postural reactions. An understanding of this frame of reference is dependent on a thorough understanding of the typical sequence of development.

Function/dyfunction continua include measures of central stability incorporating range of motion, head control, and trunk control and functional skills that incorporates control of head and arm movements, mobility, feeding, and toileting.

Application to practice involves the translation of therapeutic intentions into equipment that enhances posture and function. Through the use of "hardware" posture, central stability can be enhanced so that the child is able to engage in functional skills.

Acknowledgments

The author wishes to thank the students, parents, and staff of the United Cerebral Palsy School in Purchase, New York, for their cooperation and assistance in providing photographs for this chapter.

References

Barnes, K. J. (1991). Modification of the physical environment. In C. Christiansen & C. Baum (Eds.). *Occupational therapy: Overcoming human performance deficits.* (pp. 701–745). Thorofare, NJ: Slack.

Bergen, A., & Colangelo, C. (1985). *Positioning the client with central nervous system deficits.* Valhalla, NY: Valhalla Rehabilitation Publications.

Blair, E., Ballantyne, J., Horseman, S., & Chauvel, P. (1995). A study of a dynamic proximal stability splint in the management of children with cerebral palsy. *Developmental Medicine and Child Neurology, 37,* 544–554.

Bly, L. (1983). *The components of normal movement during the first year of life and abnormal motor development.* Birmingham, AL: Neuro-Developmental Treatment Association.

Bly, L. (1994). *Motor skill acquisition in the first year.* Tucson, AZ: Therapy Skill Builders.

Brogren, E., Hadders-Algra, M., & Forsoberg, H. (1996). Postural control in children with spastic diplegia: Muscle activity during perturbations in sitting. *Developmental Medicine and Child Neurology, 38,* 379–388.

Butler, C., Okamoto, G., & McKay, T. (1984). Motorized wheelchair driving by disabled children. *Archives of Physical Medicine and Rehabilitation, 65,* (2), 95; 197.

Colbert, A. P., Doyle, K. M., & Webb, W. E. (1986). DESEMO seats for young children with cerebral palsy. *Archives of Physical Medicine Rehabilitation, 67,* 484–486.

Fiorentino, M. (1981). *A basis for sensorimotor development–normal and abnormal.* Springfield, IL: Charles. C. Thomas.

Green, E. M., Mulcahy, C. M., & Pountney, T. E. (1995). An investigation into the development of early postural control. *Developmental Medicine and Child Neurology, 37,* 437–448.

Larnet, G., & Ekberg, O. (1995). Positioning improves the oral and pharyngeal swallowing function in children with cerebral palsy. *Acta Paediatric, 84,* 689–692.

Manley, M. T., & Gurtowski, E. (1985). The vertical wheeler: A device for ambulation in cerebral palsy. *Archives of Physical Medicine Rehabilitation, 66,* 717–720.

Motloch, W. M., & Brearley, M. N. (1983). Technical note—A patient propelled variable-inclination prone stander. *Prosthetic Orthotics International, 7,* 176–177.

Myhr, U., Von-Wendt, L., Norrlin, S., & Randell, U. (1995). Five year follow-up of functional sitting position in children with cerebral palsy. *Developmental Medicine and Child Neurology, 37,* 587–596.

Noronha, J., Bundy, A., & Groll, J. (1989). The effect of positioning on the hand function of boys with cerebral palsy. *American Journal of Occupational Therapy, 43,* 504–512.

Nwaobi, O. M. (1987). Seating orientations and upper extremity function in children with cerebral palsy. *Physical Therapy, 67,* 1209–1212.

Reid, D. J. (1996). The effects of the saddle seat on seated postural control and upper extremity movement in children with cerebral palsy. *Developmental Medicine and Child Neurology, 38,* 805–815.

Richardson A.S., P. K. (1996). Use of standardized tests in pediatric practice. In J. Case-Smith, A. S. Allen, & P. N. Pratt (Eds.) *Occupational therapy for children* (pp. 200–224). St. Louis, MO: Mosby.

Scherzer, A., & Tscharnuter, I. (1982). *Early diagnosis and therapy in cerebral palsy.* New York: Marcel Dekker.

Scherzer, A., & Tscharnuter, I. (1990). *Early diagnosis and therapy in cerebral palsy.* (2nd Ed.). New York: Marcel Dekker.

Stockmeyer, S. (1967). An interpretation of the approach of Rood to the treatment of neuromuscular dysfunction. *American Journal of Physical Medicine, 46,* 900–956.

Weiss, P. L. (1990). Mechanical characteristics of micro-switches adapted for the physical disabled. *Journal of Biomedical Engineering, 12,* 398–402.

Psychosocial Frame of Reference

LAURETTE J. OLSON

This frame of reference may be useful in working with a range of children who receive occupational therapy services. In addition to the children with specific psychiatric diagnoses, many children with learning disabilities, sensory processing or modulation deficits, or physical disabilities have experienced compromises in their relationships with family members, with peers, and in their ability to fully participate in play. Other frames of reference address the specific physical or cognitive sequelae of these dysfunctions. At times, this is sufficient; with improved sensory processing or learning strategies to compensate for deficits, children begin to participate in everyday activities without difficulty. In other cases, this does not occur. Children's difficulties in participating in everyday activities continue in spite of remediation. Family and peer relationships may be strained or weak. For example, professionals may note that particular children seem to have poor self-esteem and are withdrawn, resistive, or immature. In addition to being supportive and empathetic, it may be helpful for the occupational therapist to assess and intervene with these children using a psychosocial frame of reference. Although this frame of reference may be used in isolation in a psychosocial setting, it can be used in conjunction with many of the other frames of reference in this book. This frame of reference focuses on assessing and helping children develop play interests, skills, and interpersonal relationships that are supportive of their mental health.

THEORETICAL BASE

The theoretical base for the psychosocial frame of reference is derived from the developmental theories related to temperament, attachment, peer interactive skills, play, ability to cope, and environmental interaction. The area of psychosocial dysfunction is complex, and this chapter describes only one frame of reference directed toward understanding and providing psychosocial intervention for children.

Innate Temperament

Temperament is the inborn, inherited style with which a person approaches and responds to his or her environment. Specific behavior patterns are discernible even in the first days of life. Components of temperament include activity level, regularity of biological functions, approach/withdrawal tendencies for new situations, adaptability to change, sensory thresholds, quality of moods, intensity of mood expression, distractibility, and persistence and attention span (Chess & Thomas, 1984).

Some infants are easy to please and adapt readily to their environments. They have regular eating and sleeping patterns and are generally attentive and cheerful with their care providers. Other infants may be similar in their reaction to consistency but may withdraw and become anxious when faced with change; their adaptation is slow. Still other infants are labeled difficult; they are difficult to please, have frequent and strong displays of negative moods, have irregular eating and sleeping patterns, and are less likely to respond to care providers in a warm, cuddly fashion. Some infants may demonstrate hyperactivity, hypersensitivity, distractibility, emotional lability, or insatiability. These temperamentally difficult infants may experience their physical and social world as very stressful; similarly their caregivers may view interactions with them as equally stressful. Although the expression of one's temperament may be modified by one's social and physical environment, one's underlying temperament is generally stable. Children optimally learn to modulate their innate temperamental tendencies, which are less adaptive in their environment, so that these children are well received by other people and these children can effectively participate in everyday activities. This results in a more positive interaction with other people.

In considering the effect of children's temperaments in their psychosocial functioning, it is important to consider the compatibility of their temperaments with their parents' temperaments. In some families, the temperaments of parents and their children may be similar, mesh easily, or parents understand and empathize with offspring with different or difficult temperaments. This describes a good match; it is supportive of the development of a positive, reciprocal relationship between parents and their children. Care providers will more likely respond in a manner that is calming and organizing to children when there is a good match between the parents and their children (Chess & Thomas, 1984). When the temperaments of parents and their children are not compatible, the relationship may not be positive, and interaction may become tense, negative, and unpleasant. Negative interaction cycles tend to become repetitive, resulting in a lack of development of appropriate adaptive behaviors for the child. The child may not be soothed by parent-child interaction, and difficult behavior may become entrenched. Parent and child may avoid interaction with each other to avoid conflict.

Although every person is born with a certain temperament, its expression can be modified by the environment. Persons with more difficult temperaments are calmer, more organized, and more positive in environments that are structured to reduce physical and emotional stress. It may be difficult for parents to work on modifying how their child behaves or how their home environment is structured until they understand their own and their child's temperament.

Attachment

The quality of the early parent-child relationship is critical to a child's development and has been correlated with a child's competencies in everyday life including play skills, coping skills, problem-solving skills, peer relationships, and school performance (Figure 11.1). As a child grows, there is a unique interaction between the parent-child relationship and these competencies. For example, a child's coping skills affect how well the child gets along with his or her parents; if the child has good play skills, he or she will likely engage his or her parents. There are many factors that parents and a child bring to their relationship that affect how that relationship develops (Figure 11.2). Parents' personal experience of being parented themselves influences

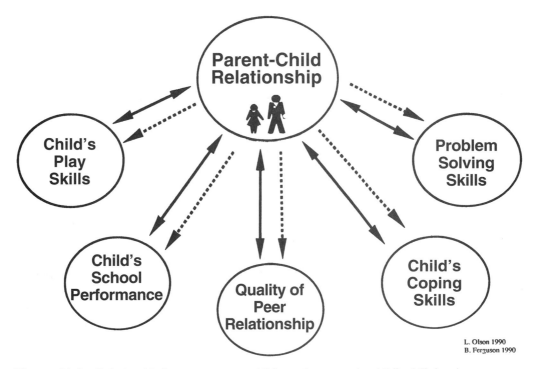

L. Olson 1990
B. Ferguson 1990

Figure 11.1   Relationship between parent-child attachment and a child's skill development.

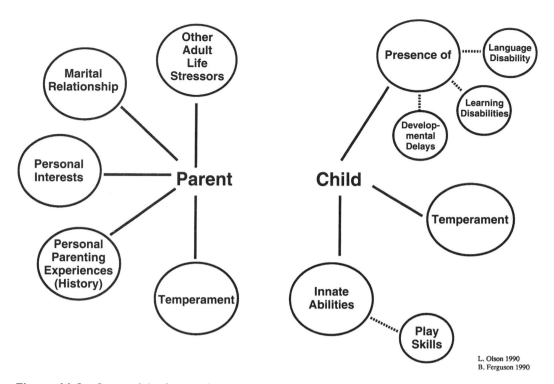

Figure 11.2 Some of the factors that a parent and a child individually bring to a parent-child relationship. These factors affect "goodness of fit."

how they parent. The presence of developmental delays or sensory processing issues can be obstacles in a parent-child relationship.

The foundation of a parent-child relationship is the attachment that develops between a parent and his or her child from birth. Care providers are responsible for providing psychological support and maintaining an environment in which the child's biological needs for nourishment and safety are met (Figure 11.3). Children optimally come to expect that if they need help, their caregivers will be readily available. This special relationship between adult and child has been called attachment relationship (Bowlby, 1969). It is an enduring, emotional, discriminating bond that develops over time (Ainsworth, 1967). Ideally, its behavioral organization is flexible so that it promotes the child's development toward becoming more autonomous and competent. As the child grows, he or she seeks out care providers less frequently, in different ways, and for different reasons. Parents should continue to adapt their caregiving approach; a 2-year-old child may need physical guidance as he or she attempts to climb high in a playground; a 6-year-old may only need a supportive glance from a caregiver sitting a distance away as he or she attempts a new and challenging feat.

In examining attachment, it is important to understand its components. The rela-

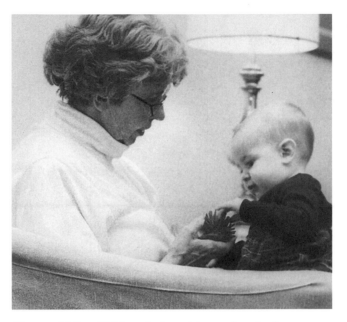

Figure 11.3   Child exploring with grandmother's support.

tionship is composed of smooth, reciprocal interactions between the child's attachment behavior and care providers' responses to that behavior. Attachment behaviors are those behaviors that a child exhibits to attract parents or care providers. They are the signals that let the care providers know that the child wants stimulation, wants to play, or is experiencing some degree of distress. These behaviors may be verbal or nonverbal; a child may cry, whine, playfully tug on a caregiver, yawn, or behave aggressively. To respond, caregivers have to first understand the child's behavior toward them and then provide the type of care that fosters the child's psychological and physical organization. This may be to provide food, physical comfort, a quiet conversation, playful interaction, or a change of environment (Figure 11.4).

The attachment relationship must be consistently nurturing so that the child knows what to expect. It is important that the child anticipate comfort, protection, and help as a matter of course. Studies have shown that when children have a secure attachment relationship with caregivers, they more likely exhibit enthusiasm, resilience, willingness to engage in challenging tasks, and competence among their peers than children who have an insecure attachment relationship with caregivers (Arend, Gore, & Sroufe, 1979; Greenberg, Speltz & DeKlyen, 1993; Lieberman, 1977; Waters, Wittman, & Sroufe, 1979). The quality of early attachment relationships exerts powerful effects on a child's later ability to establish and maintain relationships with peers and adults.

Children who have secure relationships with caregivers can also develop insecure relationships under different circumstances. For example, stress from a divorce or

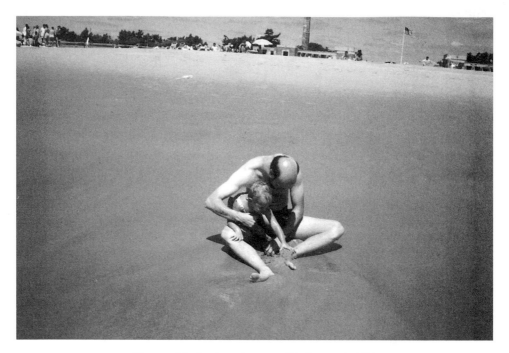

Figure 11.4 Attachment of father and child.

parental illness may change the parent-child relationship. Without careful attention to parent-child relationships, children may become less certain that their caregivers will be able to provide sufficiently for their needs. This may have a negative effect on children's ability to cope and engage in play and in peer interactions. Likewise, children who have had insecure relationships with their parents can be helped to develop more secure relationships with their parents, which then may have a positive effect on their school performance, friendships, and ability to fully participate in age-appropriate play.

Securely attached children perceive their parents and care providers as responsive and readily available. Children in these environments are reasonably confident that they can receive comfort, assistance, or encouragement when needed. Securely attached children can engage in play, seek out care providers for comfort, and then can reengage in play. When a secure attachment is developed in infancy, it is believed that the child demonstrates enthusiastic, persistent, and cooperative behavior during play. Secure children engage in problem-solving activities, and, when they become frustrated, they seek appropriate assistance from adults (Figure 11.5).

Insecurely attached children are not certain of the extent to which they can rely on care providers. This insecurity may prevent these children from becoming involved in activities because they are never sure that a secure home-base will be available to them. They may engage in play but do not necessarily seek comfort when stressed. The anx-

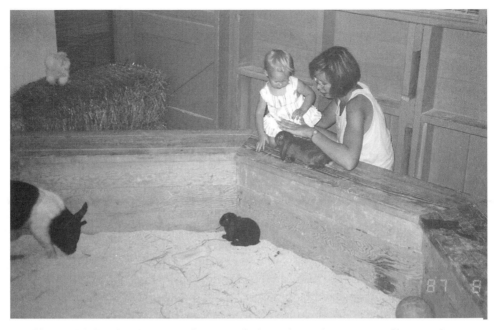

Figure 11.5   Child unsure of an animal, depends on the support of her mother.

iety caused by their uncertainty and by the inevitable challenges arising in play, remains unsoothed and, therefore, compromises their ability to fully relax and engage in play. These children may not seek comfort because they fear rejection. Similarly, they may be easily frustrated by challenges that they feel that they cannot master alone and, consequently, give up. Resistant and acting-out behaviors (Matas, Arend, & Sroufe, 1978) and socially withdrawn behaviors in children (Lieberman, 1977) have been correlated with their exhibiting an insecure attachment to their caregivers.

An insecure attachment may develop from a dysfunction in the child, in the parent, or because of a combination of vulnerabilities that the parent and child bring to the relationship. Some children with developmental disabilities may offer their parents inconsistent or unclear cues about their physical and social needs. Therefore, these parents may be unable to adequately meet those needs. These children may not be easily soothed or respond as fully as their siblings did to parent initiations at play. Parents may withdraw from interaction out of frustration. They may initiate less play with their children because they have been unsuccessful at engaging or they may develop more intrusive strategies to force their children to interact with them. These children may not be confident that their needs will be met or that the help that they want will be available when they are looking for it. Their play and social skills may suffer as they may have less stimulation from their parents to develop the play and social skills they need or the stimulation that they receive may be too intense for them and lead to their further withdrawal.

Parents may have their own vulnerabilities that make them less available as caregivers. One of the most common conditions is depression (Maxmen & Ward, 1995). New mothers are especially vulnerable to postpartum depression. Parents of children born with difficult temperaments or developmental disabilities are also more likely to experience depression. Depressed parents speak less often and with less intensity, gaze less frequently, and are slower to respond to their children's attempts to engage them. Infants as young as 3 months of age reciprocate their depressed mother's negative and less effortful interactive behavior and also begin to evoke negative responses from other adults (Downey & Coyne, 1990).

Peer Interactive Skills

Although adult-child relationships are different from child-child relationships, parent-child interaction serves as a catalyst for the development of peer interactive skills. The ability to make eye contact and to initiate and respond to playful overtures is reinforced by the resulting pleasure and comfort of parent-child relationships. The child is attracted to other people and anticipates the same attentiveness and pleasure in play that he or she has experienced with adult care providers. A child soon learns, however, that other children are different from adult playmates who often follow his or her lead. Other children are as demanding as he or she is and want their own desires accommodated; other children will not do things the way the child wants, unlike many adults. Conversely, other children are more like him or her in size, skill level, vigor, and interest, which makes them ultimately engaging.

If children are going to play together, they must figure out whose wishes will direct the group. Among equals, no one point of view is automatically better than another. Each person is free to pursue his or her own point of view through various avenues. The result may be separate, solitary activity unless some form of negotiation occurs. Ideally, children first learn to take turns and then gradually learn the sophisticated skills of presenting ideas, listening to each other, and working out compromises. During the preschool years, children learn to take turns in some activities such as going down a slide; in other situations, they often remain content with parallel activities. Five- and 6-year-old children explore the ideas of taking turns and some compromising through activities such as simple board games or playing house. Older children work hard to compromise and cooperate with greater consistency and extent in the interest of participating in more complex and interesting games and activities (Figure 11.6).

During childhood, the depth and complexity of friendships develop. At the age of 6 years, particular activities interest the child and he or she will seek companionship accordingly. A friend is someone to play with and with whom he or she can share objects in a concrete, reciprocal fashion. Gradually, who the other child is becomes more important. Children learn that some peers are more compatible than

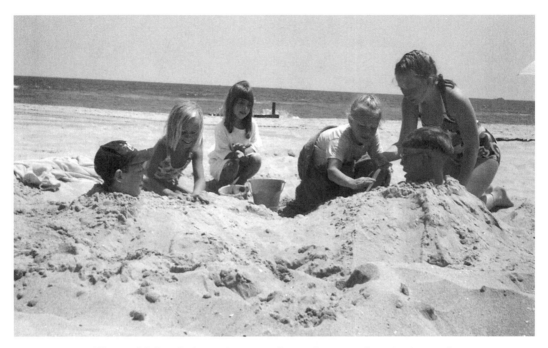

Figure 11.6   Girls working together to bury two boys in the sand.

others as a result of their particular interests, skill levels, and temperaments. By the age of 9 years, friendship has a new and deeper meaning. Friends help each other and share secrets. By the age of 11 years, children are concerned with the welfare of their friends and seek secure relationships based on mutual trust. Shared interests and abilities form the foundation of long-term friendships (Figure 11.7).

Group interaction provides an effective way to promote growth in children's psychosocial and play skills. In a supportive environment, their desire for peer acceptance and ultimately friendship will often lead to more rapid modification of play and social behaviors. When other children object to their not sharing or following the rules, children more easily acquiesce to the group norms than when an adult sets a limit. Children also learn what other children like and don't like and compare it to their own preferences. They will often modify what they do and what they say so that they can fit in with their peers.

Through peer group interaction, children come to realize that, just like themselves, other children are good at some activities and have difficulties with others. This is unlike children's general experiences with adults who help them and whose level of skill seems beyond children's reach. With peers, there are opportunities to offer help and accept help. In the process, children develop empathy for others, caregiving skills, and a sense of themselves as a productive member of a group.

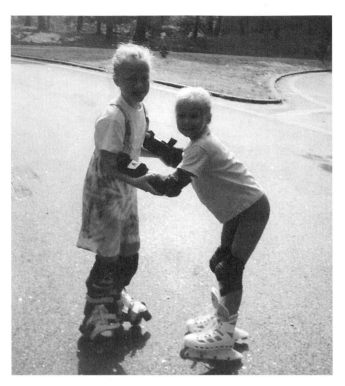

Figure 11.7 Two friends sharing an interest.

Play

Play is activity for its own sake; it is not a means to an end. It exists for the intrinsic pleasure of the moment and includes the exploration and recombination of sounds, movements, objects, and concepts (as in stories), all for the joy that the process brings. A healthy child is invested and motivated for play. Without conscious effort, play results in the development of physical, cognitive, psychological, and basic social skills. It helps a child learn to manage the everyday stresses of life and to interact appropriately with family and peers. Children may use physical play or games to release tensions and aggressive feelings; constructive or manipulative play to bind attention with their own creations; or imaginary play to test out and explore the behaviors that they observe (Figure 11.8).

Play behaviors begin in early infancy and are encouraged by the parent-child relationship. Parents or care providers and children engage each other because of their natural attraction. The mutually pleasurable experience that ideally occurs increases the probability that the interaction will occur often. In a healthy interaction, the care provider mirrors children's play behavior but also gradually helps children to elaborate on their play themes or ideas. This keeps the play challenging and interesting. Reciprocally, the child elaborates on the care provider's additions to the play. This

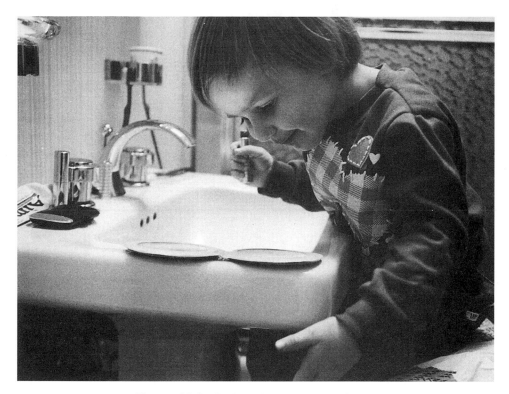

Figure 11.8 Little girl playing with makeup.

two-way communication leads to a mutual molding of behavior and maintains the interest of both players.

Parent-child play is also supportive of the child's development of a secure attachment and basic learning, interaction, problem solving, and coping skills. Securely attached children perceive themselves as competent and then are more open to opportunities where they can continuously build skills.

Children with warm, interdependent relations with their parents are more likely to comply with parental requests. Parents who are responsive to their children in play induce positive moods in the children and hence experience greater compliance to their requests than parents who are not responsive to their children in play (Lay, Waters, & Park, 1989). It is believed that the attachment process may provide the motivation for prosocial behavior; children will be motivated to change their behavior to ensure a continued supportive relationship with their parents. The first step in working toward children complying with parental demands is establishing a positive rapport in play (Barkley, 1987; Bloomquist, 1996). Children who experience high levels of supportive parenting are buffered from the negative impact of family adversity such as poverty or chronic parent illness (Petitt, Bates, & Dodge, 1997).

Peer interaction skills evolve from those interaction skills that children develop through their parent-child relationship. The parent-child relationship is the model upon which a child bases all relationships that follow. Children who have secure and supportive parent-child relationships tend to develop more positive peer relationships. In addition, peer interaction skills develop in tandem with and are interdependent with the development of play skills. A child who has good play skills will likely have an easy time engaging with other children. Children with good social skills will have the opportunity to expand and elaborate on their play skills through their interaction with other children.

The interests and skills of other children stimulate and challenge a child to expand his or her repertoires even more. Consider the child in the playground who is hesitant to climb or to do a flip on the monkey bars. As this child associates with other children who are competent in the activities, he or she can observe other children attempting these same activities. Because of the motivation to be liked and accepted by his or her peer group, the child most likely will attempt to join in the activity.

Through successful peer interactions, children develop friendships that further support their psychosocial development. Friendships enhance a child's self understanding and acceptance of himself or herself through learning about his or her similarities and differences and what the child's friends value in him or her. He or she also learns to empathize with others, which will enable him or her to work successfully with others.

All children have strengths and limitations that enhance or inhibit their abilities to engage with others. Children who have strong language skills can learn more quickly to communicate their needs and interact better verbally with other children and adults. Children who have specific motor strengths or are particularly creative may easily attract adults or other children to play with them. Children with innate vulnerabilities may be at a disadvantage socially and may have difficulty developing activity skills. They may be on the sidelines or openly excluded because they lack particular physical or language-base skills. Enhancing these children's areas of strengths and assisting them in developing basic or compensatory skills for participation in group activities with peers is critical for their psychosocial development.

Play is distinct from recreation. Although individuals play throughout life, play is a prerequisite to developing skills to participate in recreational activities such as organized sports or clubs. In play, each player is flexible in his or her approach to the materials used in play; he or she has the power to engage with the materials like others do or to approach them differently. In this way, the materials, the use of one's own body, and any human interaction in play is explored and developed. New ways of moving or playing together are discovered. Children explore the different ways that materials can be used and come to find their favored way. They experiment with different ways of moving their bodies around objects and around each other. Rules are continuously changed and renegotiated to keep the activity pleasurable and satisfying for all players. The exploration of the bounds of activity through play is preparation for accepting the predetermined group rules and the need to develop specific skills for participation in organized recreational activities.

Types of Play

Over time, many distinct types of play have been observed and consistently identified by developmental theorists, teachers, and therapists as being important for children's development. These include sensorimotor, imaginary, constructional, and game play. Although each type of play is specific, overlap occurs as children frequently combine forms of play. A 9-year-old child may build a boat, and then use it in imaginary play. There is no right or wrong in play (as there is in recreational activities). During play, children discover the consequences of their actions and the types of reactions that may be provoked; some are more desirable than others. Children then build on what they have previously learned, using new experiences to elaborate and enhance their skills.

During the first 2 years of life, infants engage in *sensorimotor play*. They become aware of their bodies and acquire an understanding of their sensorimotor abilities. Children spend endless hours moving their bodies and limbs, experiencing different sensations. First, they gain the ability to move their trunk and limbs and then the entire body through space. This process makes them aware of how body parts feel, taste, look, and move, and they spontaneously integrate this knowledge to coordinate locomotion and intentional interaction with objects and people. The feel, reaction, and response of objects and other people are incorporated into the everexpanding knowledge base of the physical world, resulting in the development of motor, perceptual, and cognitive skills (Figure 11.9). Although sensorimotor play is predominant in the first 2 years of life and other forms of play become more dominant at later stages of development, sensorimotor play is pleasurable; sensorimotor play is sought out throughout childhood and adulthood (Figure 11.10).

Through *imaginary play* and with increasing physical skill, children expand their play in ways that lead to a better understanding of the socialized world around them. Children learn about people and their characteristics and functions. Children use objects representationally to imitate the actions of the adults around them. Imaginary play grows in complexity and is used to gain a better understanding of societal roles. Social interactions are reenacted and real experiences are modified to create a pretend world that can be controlled. Children make believe that they are other people or animals. They reenact complex or confusing events. It is common for children to play out a baby's birth, a doctor's visit, or medical operations that they have experienced or heard about. They may expand on these occurrences or change the outcomes. Through this process, important events, people, and the rules in their world are better understood. Anxiety and tension are reduced, and negative experiences can be resolved. Gradually, children's internal control over their behavior grows as a result of imaginary play. Taking on the role of mommy and dealing with a pretend

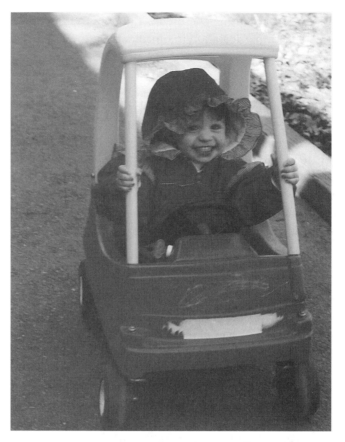

Figure 11.9   Little girl exploring movement.

baby helps a child identify with his or her real mother and helps him or her gain a better understanding of the antecedents of punishment and the process of reconciliation. Manipulating people and objects in fantasy is a prelude to dealing with a reality that cannot be so easily controlled.

Through *constructional play*, children naturally enhance the development of their fine motor and cognitive skills and their confidence and ability to handle challenges. As children play with scrap materials and recombine them in various ways, they discover new uses for things. This creative process occurs spontaneously through play, not with a preconceived plan. The child is relaxed and allows himself or herself to examine all possibilities. He or she often expresses surprise and pleasure with what he or she has created (e.g., what he or she first thought would be a building has turned into a car and then a space mobile). Problem-solving skills are developed in addition to a growing sense of mastery and self-efficacy (Figure 11.11).

Through *game play*, children develop internal control and an understanding of rules. This occurs through the process of deciding what rules are important to main-

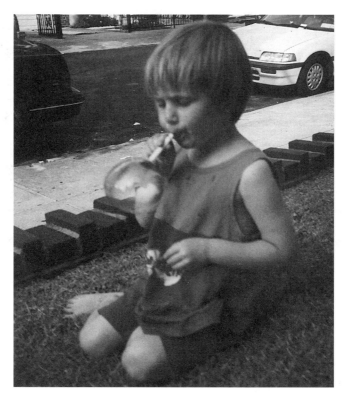

Figure 11.10   Sensorimotor play of an older child.

tain their interest, decrease frustration, and mediate the competing wishes of all play-ers. The need for all players to agree mutually to contain personal impulses for the greater enjoyment of the group becomes apparent in game play. Young children of-ten change the rules and haphazardly enforce them as they attempt to master the physical and cognitive skills necessary to play the games while maintaining their self-esteem. Games also have impulse satisfaction built into them. Children get to mo-mentarily attack another but must pull back after their point has been made or play is over. Children get to triumph over another, to metaphorically crush another with-out any real life consequences. This can be especially satisfying when a child tri-umphs over an idealized opponent who is much stronger in real life (Figure 11.12).

   As they continue to learn, children begin to value challenge and coordinated in-teraction of larger group activities. Children learn that games can be more engaging and invigorating when many must put their skills together to beat an opponent that is another group of children. To play baseball, a team needs strong hitters and chil-dren who can play different positions. Similarly, children learn that in other activi-ties (e.g., construction), if a group of children work together, they can split up tasks so that they finish bigger constructions more rapidly than if they had worked alone.

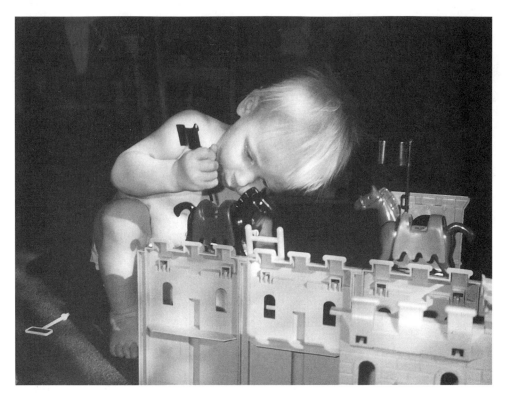

Figure 11.11 Constructional play.

In the process, they also have the pleasure of company of peers. To accomplish this, rules of reciprocal and cooperative social interaction (e.g., compromise) become important to apply to maintain the activity. Rules are heavily enforced. Rules add meaning, organization, and challenge; they provide a way for all participants to play with some harmony and, ideally, to subordinate personal wishes and impulses in the interest of group achievement. Children who break the agreed-upon rules or whose behavior doesn't support the group goal are strongly censored by their peers. This has a powerful impact on socialization of all group members because there is a naturally strong desire to be accepted by peers.

Bundy (1997) suggests that *playfulness* may be more important than actual motor or cognitive play skills. Playfulness requires a sense of intrinsic motivation, internal control, and suspension of reality in an activity. This is the essence of play; the joy and organizing power of play to one's sense of self lies within these dimensions. Although motivations change, as people grow from childhood to adulthood, a degree of playfulness optimally remains in many human activities.

Play sets the stage for work (Erikson, 1959). Through play, children develop mature motor, task, and social interaction skills. Children become increasingly goal-

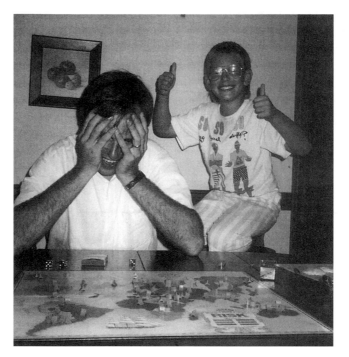

Figure 11.12. Boy's triumph over his father.

directed and interested in being productive members of their families and communities. They also gain a sense of playfulness in all activity that supports their investment in doing. Children in middle childhood have longer attention spans and now have the perseverance and interest to practice or work on repetitive activities for considerable periods of time. They will participate even in distasteful parts of an activity to be independent or in anticipation of the pleasure that they will experience later in an activity (Figure 11.13). A young gymnast will repeatedly practice the same routine with his or her coach; a youngster interested in making money will shovel many driveways over many hours on a snowy day. Besides the intrinsic rewards inherent in successful participation in an activity, the extrinsic rewards of potential fame, admiration, money, or responsibility are increasingly enticing for older children. They are no longer playing at work but truly working and further developing their work skills. This becomes the foundation for the ability to work as adolescents and adults.

To be able to have the capacity to participate in early work-related activities in childhood, children need to have a basic level of competence, an ability to cope with stresses in the environment, be reality focused, and have an investment in life. Competence emerges out of the opportunity provided by play activities that build skills toward workmanship. *Workmanship* includes attention to the quality and quantity of one's work. The ability to cope with the environment is learned through managing

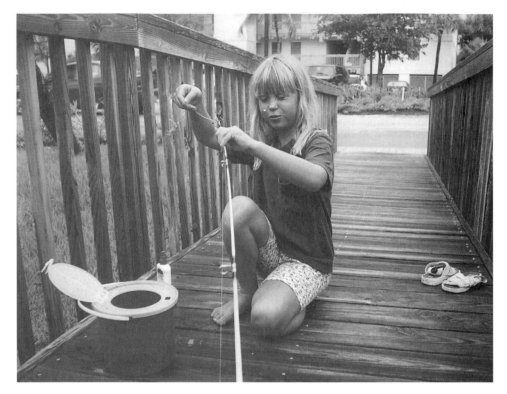

Figure 11.13 Child managing to bait a fish hook in anticipation of fishing.

anxiety and stress in the challenges that activities and social interaction provoke. Working through and mastering that anxiety and stress promotes the child's development of productive, active, and flexible behavioral strategies. When a child has the psychological strength to integrate and express contradictory realities, emotions, and demands, he or she is able to remain reality focused in tasks as opposed to reverting to fantasy. The child begins to feel that he or she has some control over himself or herself in his or her environment. He or she develops culturally acceptable means to channel aggressive or libidinal impulses. The child can take out his or her frustration in vigorous activity; the child can experience the praise and admiration that he or she longs for through exemplary task performance. An investment in life grows out of feelings of pleasure and competence that the child experiences as he or she successfully participates in activities. This pleasure in doing gives the child the optimism and perseverance to continuously approach new activities with the belief that his or her efforts will reap success and satisfaction (Cotton, 1984).

Children begin to exhibit *work behaviors* in activities in which they may exhibit intense interest or talent. Children who are gifted musically will work for hours until they can play an instrument or a particular piece of music without error. A young dancer or gymnast will adhere to a rigorous practice schedule to master complex routines for a show or competition. These children embrace the concept that "practice makes perfect" and accept the structure and instruction from their coaches or teachers that is necessary to achieve their ideal.

Children also begin to exhibit work behaviors in everyday activities. Caring for pets further develops their giving care. They must put aside their own desires for periods of time to take care of the basic needs of their pet. As children train pets and take care of them, they become sensitive to the animals' cues and learn to respond empathetically. They experience the role of giving care.

In school and at home, children take on responsibilities for maintaining their physical environment and learn to adhere to schedules for activity performance and completion.

Ability to Cope

Ability to cope is the manner in which children deal with new and difficult situations. Children develop their basic coping skills through their experience with care providers who promote their ability to cope with the world around them. Children send verbal and nonverbal signals to their care providers when they are experiencing physical or psychological stress. The care providers interpret those signals and attempt to manipulate the environment to reduce the child's stress and to promote the child's ability to adapt to the situation. Children develop strong coping skills when parents are able to facilitate coping methods that are compatible with children's personal temperament and that promote active engagement with their physical and social world.

As children develop, they take increasing responsibility for regulating their own behavior in response to stress by gradually becoming more aware of their changing emotional state and then initiating an appropriate action or interaction that reduces internal emotional pressure. When children are generally successful in resolving the stresses that new or challenging situations bring, children are said to be resilient. *Resilience* is the ability to return to a state of emotional equilibrium in a short time after stress is experienced; in this way, activity engagement can begin or be resumed. This means that the child is emotionally calm and able to focus on play or on a required activity. At times, when uncertain or insecure, to regain equilibrium, a child may retreat into safety, take time out, or delay a response until the unfamiliar is more carefully examined. In the aftermath of stressful or overwhelming occurrences, this process may involve self-comforting, playing out traumatic experiences, and using fantasy to transform reality temporarily (Anthony, 1987).

A child's resilience is challenged in ordinary ways on a daily basis. For example, if a resilient child is rejected by his or her playmates, the child needs to recognize his or her rejection, decide what led to it, and then respond in a way that produces acceptance or does not worsen the injury to his or her self-esteem. A child may retreat to the safety of his or her home to talk to a parent, but the child will re-enter peer play by figuring out how to make amends, seeking more compatible playmates, or finding other interesting activities.

If a child has difficulty performing a construction task, he or she may change the building approach so that the chances of success become greater. The child may switch to another activity if overwhelmed, or he or she may seek help from an older child or adult. In any case, the child will find a way to confront the difficult situation in a positive way that relieves frustration and injury to his or her self-esteem. The child may withdraw, but only for a brief time, to compose himself or herself. The child who has developed the ability to cope is invested in his or her environment and in the many types of play and activity available. The motivation to play and to be involved is, therefore, stronger than any impulse to give in to frustration.

Environmental Interaction

Children's living environments must be examined for their capacity to provide safety, support, space, and facilities for functional skill development. A *safe environment* has mechanisms to reduce the impact of any inherent or sudden risks. This may mean greater availability of family supports if a parent is chronically ill; safe community play space if a family lives in a cramped apartment; or additional educational supports for a child who exhibits learning deficits. Negative events that occur during human interaction should be neutralized by support and other positive opportunities that promote the children's feelings of security, self-efficacy, and self-esteem. The design of the environment and the requisite supplies available will change, depending on the culture. The primary environments for all children are home, school, and community.

Home

A good home environment has sufficient supplies to feed, clothe, and provide warmth and shelter for all family members. There is adequate security from danger by physical design or the vigilance of the care providers. In addition, there are resources for play and for the transmission of cultural values, rituals, and life roles. What is available for play and how elaborate these materials are depends on socioeconomic and cultural variables. For example, play things may be gender specific and may closely resemble adult tools; they may be pots and pans or expensive crafted toys. The most important element in a good home environment is the availability of a consistent, caring adult, who provides structure and sets guidelines for the child so that he or she is socialized to function within his or her community. The adult is sensitive to the child's innate abilities and vulnerabilities. This helps the child minimize his or her weaknesses and capitalize on his or her strengths. If a child is having difficulty, this adult adjusts his or her approach to the child to foster the child's physical or psychosocial development or seeks assistance outside of the family.

School

It is important that the child be physically safe and have his or her basic biological needs met in the school setting. Space, supplies, and equipment are available to assist him or her to learn. On the most basic level, books, paper, and writing utensils must be available. The wealth of the school district determines what additional resources become mandatory. Of primary importance to the school environment is the availability of a caring teacher who provides the necessary structure and support so that a child can invest his or her attention on learning. Through educational activities, the teacher expands and adds to children's previously acquired living skills and offers new opportunities to develop innate abilities and to compensate for vulnerabilities. The teacher also structures group prework and leisure activities to promote the development of the social skills necessary for community living and working. Other professionals, including occupational therapists, are often called upon to assist teachers when children present with psychosocial, learning, or physical vulnerabilities.

Community

In his or her community, a child should be able to explore his or her physical environment safely. Within a well-structured community, peers and adult role models should be readily available. A community contains space, resources, and the freedom to engage in various play and community activities.

Summary

Each child is born with an innate temperament that may help or hinder him or her in establishing a secure attachment relationship with his or her care providers. Throughout childhood, it is important that a child's care providers understand the child's temperament and personal style and then interact with the child in a way that facilitates the child's personal development. In this way, a secure attachment relationship and pleasurable parent-child interaction is facilitated. The quality of this primary relationship critically affects the development of coping, play, and peer interaction skills. As a child grows, each skill area influences the others. When a child increases his or her skill in one area (e.g., learning to cope more effectively with stress or expanding his or her ability to play), it is likely that the child's increased competence will lead to more positive family and peer relationships. This, in turn, fosters an increased desire to master more developmental tasks. The ability to play is thought to be directly related to the ability to work.

Children grow and develop within the contexts of home, school, and the community. Although environments vary greatly, depending on culture and socioeconomic class, their adequacy to meet the basic needs of the child and family always should be examined.

FUNCTION/DYSFUNCTION CONTINUA

Function/dysfunction continua provide therapists with descriptions of observable behaviors that are clinically relevant and identify function and dysfunction in children.

Indicators of Function and Dysfunction for Temperament Adaptation

Temperament is a person's spontaneous, innate style and approach to environments, events, and people. As a child experiences and acclimates to the environments in which he or she will be raised, he or she learns what to expect. His or her daily life becomes routinized to some degree, and temperament may not be so evident. During infancy, the child's temperament is apparent because a child is constantly being exposed to new stimuli and is adjusting to the routines of his or her environments. When a child's temperament is functional, the child can adapt to family, school, and community demands effectively and within a short amount of time.

In the psychosocial frame of reference, the child may have difficulty regulating his or her activity level and attention span to participate in the activities that he or she is required to participate in when a child's temperament is dysfunctional. Such a child may have difficulty dealing with new situations or adapting to changes in routines. These difficulties will likely interfere with the child's ability to fit in and be accepted by other persons within his or her environment. A child who exhibits a dysfunctional temperament may not be open to learning in the ways that are expected of a child in his or her environment, may not respond appropriately to nurturing and guidance, or may not be able to participate in peer play groups. When a child has a difficult temperament, the child has trouble adapting to the demands of his or her environment. This may contribute to pervasive, negative effects on attachment relationships, coping, play, and peer interactive skills (Chart 11.1).

Indicators of Function and Dysfunction for Attachment

Parent-child attachment is the special relationship between an adult and a developing child that is critical for the child's growth and development. The adult is drawn to the child who attracts him or her as a caregiver by emitting attachment behaviors that suggest a need for care and protection. As the child's caregiver, the adult protects the child from danger and offers physical sustenance, emotional security, and instruction in basic life skills necessary for survival. In the process of interacting and caring for the child, the adult and child initiate and respond playfully and affectionately with each other. This strengthens the adult's desire to take care of the child and the child's desire to seek out that adult. As the adult continuously cares for the child and experiences being able to effectively assuage the child's fears and meet the child's physical and emotional needs, the attachment grows more secure. The adult is con-

Chart 11.1   Indicators of Function and Dysfunction for Temperament Adaptation.

Temperament Adaptation	Inadequate Temperament Adaptation
FUNCTION: Ability to respond to the environment appropriately	DYSFUNCTION: Inability to respond to the environment appropriately
INDICATORS OF FUNCTION	**INDICATORS OF DYSFUNCTION**
Easily adheres to a regular routine for meeting biological needs	Biological schedule is erratic or inconsistent with environmental demands
Activity level is appropriate for situational expectations	Activity level is inappropriate for situation
Orients to relevant sensory input and is able to ignore environmental distractions	Responds to everyday sensory input with fear or irritation or cannot inhibit awareness of irrelevant sensory input
Mood is appropriate to situation	Mood is generally negative
Emotional response is appropriate to situation	Emotional expression is intense and poorly regulated
Attends to an activity for an appropriate length of time, given age and situation	Attention span is inappropriate given age and situation; it can be either too short or too long
Adapts appropriately to new situations	Adaptation to new situations is erratic; it may be characterized by disorganization or withdrawal

fident in his or her ability to meet the child's needs and the child is confident that the parent will be available and competent in meeting any need.

This first attachment relationship is the model upon which all future attachment relationships are based. Throughout one's life, one develops attachment relationships with other caregivers, including grandparents, teachers, peers, spouses, or partners.

A child who is securely attached is also generally compliant to structure, rules, and limits provided by caring adults because he or she is motivated to remain in the good standing with his or her caregivers. The child is aligned with his or her adult caregivers, is confident that they will help him or her if the child is in need, and that they will offer him or her praise and love for his or her accomplishments. A secure attachment can be powerful in developing prosocial behaviors in children (Greenberg, Speltz & DeKlyen, 1993).

The child who exhibits dysfunctional attachment behavior does not have caregivers who are able to provide adequate care or he or she is not able to sufficiently attract care providers to get basic needs met. This is referred to as insecure attachment. This dysfunction may be the result of having experienced inconsistent, neglectful, or abusive parenting, or it also may be related to a child's innate deficits such as a difficult temperament or physiological dysfunction that interferes with the child's ability to emit clear signals to his or her caregivers. The child with dysfunctional attachment behaviors will have a difficult time interacting with caregivers. The child may be resistive to caregiver demands, have difficulty seeking help when needed, and may respond aggressively or regressively to support or help from any caregiver. The child does not expect, or is uncertain about, the likelihood of nurturance or good will from adults.

When parents (one or both) exhibit dysfunctional or inconsistent care giving behaviors, a child may demonstrate functional attachment behaviors if he or she has had consistent contact with sensitive care providers outside his or her immediate family. If a child does not have the opportunity to develop a secure attachment relationship with any consistent adult, the child will likely have difficulty establishing secure attachment relationships with peers as friends and later with adult life partners (Chart 11.2).

Indicators of Function and Dysfunction for Peer Interaction

Functional peer interaction is exhibited when a child is accepted in an age-appropriate and developmentally appropriate group. A child who can approach peers in a positive way to initiate play and who responds in kind to most overtures by peers demonstrates functional peer interaction. In the interest of becoming involved in group play, the child takes turns and increasingly develops the skills of compromise, cooperation, and negotiation. The child is responsive to the verbal and nonverbal cues his or her peers give to indicate their emotional states and their reactions to him or her. The child can change his or her approach to succeed in a social situation if the cues the child receives from others suggest a need for change. Willingness to help peers in play and to accept help are also skills that the child exhibits. These behaviors facilitate closer bonds with peers and support the child's development of friendships. Through friendships, a child receives emotional support and companionship that facilitates the child's emotional well-being and competence in daily activities.

The inability to respond to peers appropriately leads to being ignored or rejected by peers. The child may be socially isolated as a result of poor peer interaction skills.

Chart 11.2 Indicators of Function and Dysfunction for Temperament Attachment.

Attachment	Insecure Attachment
FUNCTION: Ability to form adequate attachments with care providers	DYSFUNCTION: Inability to form adequate attachments with care providers
INDICATORS OF FUNCTION	**INDICATORS OF DYSFUNCTION**
Clearly signals care providers about concerns and needs	Provides inconsistent or unclear signals about needs and concerns
Engages in mutual pleasurable activity with care providers	Does not or rarely initiates or responds to playful interchanges; does not engage in mutual pleasurable activities with care providers
Initiates and responds to playful interchanges with care providers	Avoids or rejects care provider's attempts to assist him in challenging or distressing situations
Seeks care providers for support, reassurance, and assistance in challenging situations and activities	Overly and indiscriminately dependent or does not seek help and support as needed
Generally responsive to support, structure, and limits set by authority figures	Generally resistive to support, structure, and limits from authority figures
Accepts help and support as needed but seeks appropriate autonomy	

He or she may not initiate play in a positive way. This child may attempt to bully peers or may be intrusive to get his or her needs met. Another child who exhibits poor peer interaction may be overly dependent and passive and therefore is rejected by peers because he or she is immature. The child ignores or is insensitive to social cues from others and, therefore, does not alter unsuccessful methods of peer engagement. Help from peers may not be accepted because it is perceived as threatening to the child's self-esteem. The child may not offer to help peers or may be overly intrusive or domineering when trying to help. The end result is a lack or paucity of friendships (Chart 11.3).

Indicators of Function and Dysfunction for Play

Functional play is demonstrated when a child approaches all play activities with a willingness to experiment and explore. He or she spontaneously seeks out individual and group experiences. The child engages with vigor and continuously elaborates on an activity to maintain its interest and vitality. Through this process, he or she develops basic skills for all performance areas. Although the child may enjoy and learn spontaneously from all activities, he or she is drawn naturally to some activities over others because of personal interests and capabilities. Through sensorimotor play, the child continuously learns about, integrates, and enjoys the sensory and motor abilities and responses of his or her body. Imaginary play allows the child to work through confusing or conflicting events, to allay anxiety, and to understand better the structure and rules of social living. Through constructional play, the child develops perceptual, motor, and cognitive skills. Finally, through game play, the child develops internal control and turns aggressive impulses into socially acceptable strategies for achieving a dominant position over others, getting needs met, and for collaborating with others to achieve a goal. This is critical for successful functioning within work groups.

Chart 11.3   Indicators of Function and Dysfunction for Peer Interaction.

Peer Interaction	**Lack of Friendship and Collaboration with Peers**
FUNCTION: Ability to interact successfully with peers	DYSFUNCTION: Inability to interact successfully with peers
INDICATORS OF FUNCTION	**INDICATORS OF DYSFUNCTION**
Approaches peers positively to initiate play	Avoids peers or approaches peers aggressively or intrusively
Takes turns with peers	Resistant to turn taking, even with adult intervention
Responds to verbal and nonverbal social cues	Exhibits little awareness of or response to verbal and nonverbal social cues
Negotiates with peers	Unable to negotiate with peers
Compromises with peers in the interest of group play	Refuses to compromise with peers
Is willing to help and accept help from peers	Unable to offer help or accept it
	Uses aggression typically to reach his or her personal goals or withdraws from situation

A child who exhibits deficits in play skills does not participate actively in play activities. When the child does participate, it is not with full investment and he or she does not build sufficiently on prior play experiences. Rigidity toward activities may limit the child's potential to fully explore and learn. As a result, the child's underlying perceptual, motor, cognitive, emotional, and social skills do not develop adequately. He or she may appear depressed, disorganized, and less competent than his or her peers (Chart 11.4).

Indicators of Function and Dysfunction for the Ability to Cope

The child who has developed the ability to cope has a broad range of interests and resources that gratify him or her. These things provide the child with a basis for success and skill; he or she feels confident. When challenged or overwhelmed, the child engages in productive problem-solving, using various methods flexibly depending upon environmental responses. The child is able to do this because he or she has underlying skills that will allow the child to solve his or her problem and he or she has confidence in abilities. In this way, the child maintains positive involvement with his or her environment. Ability to cope is closely related to the child's innate temperament and how the child has learned to adapt it to the demands of his or her environments. The child's underlying sensory processing function and the child's security in his or her attachment relationships influences his or her ability to cope. The child who is secure in his or her attachment relationships usually is more adaptable and, thus, able to cope more effectively because the child is confident that he or she will receive help and support if he or she needs it in the process of meeting a challenge.

A child is dysfunctional when he or she does not expect to get pleasure from an activity. The child may avoid activities and tend not to be invested in them. Few activities provide gratification; therefore, the child has not developed a repertoire of skills and lacks a feeling of success. When challenged, the child often gives up in frustration and avoids involvement. He or she may not engage in spontaneous problem-

---

Chart 11.4 Indicators of Function and Dysfunction for Play Skills.

Play Skills	**Inadequate Play Skills**
FUNCTION: Ability to engage successfully in individual and group play	DYSFUNCTION: Inability to engage successfully in individual and group play
INDICATORS OF FUNCTION	**INDICATORS OF DYSFUNCTION**
Approaches play with vigor and interest	Approach to play is tentative or avoidant
Fully explores and experiments in new play situations	Does not explore and experiment in new play situations
Expands on prior play experiences	Has narrow range of play interest
Is flexible during play with peers	Has rigid approach to play
Play is repetitive, fragmented, or child ceases involvement rapidly	Does not successfully initiate play with other children
Follows the sequence and structure of group play activities	Unable to follow the sequence and structure of group play activity
Accepts rules in group play	Does not accept or follow rules of group play

solving activities and may become bored and emotionally labile. The child does not seek or seem to expect help or support. If a child is sensitive to loud noises or potential physical contact in the process of overcoming a challenge, the sensory input may overwhelm the child beyond his or her coping capacities, in addition to the task challenge. In this case, it would be important to address sensory processing or modulation issues through the use of the sensory integration frame of reference (Chart 11.5).

Indicators of Function and Dysfunction for Environmental Interaction

The theoretical base for the psychosocial frame of reference addresses the importance of the environment in the provision of safety, support, and facilities for functional skill development. The child's three primary environments are the home, school, and community. It is impossible to present all function/dysfunction continua relative to environmental interaction that encompass the varied situations and experiences to which children currently are exposed; therefore, function/dysfunction continua are presented in a general manner in this section. Therapists should carefully consider children's environments and determine what indicates function or dysfunction in these situations.

At the functional end of the continuum, a home environment provides safety, security, support, and developmental stimulation to the child. The physical living space of the home is safe from intruders, has no safety hazards, and is relatively clean. It includes materials for participating in developmentally appropriate activities. Most important, the caregivers are interested and focused on keeping a child safe and meeting his or her developmental needs. These caregivers are consistently available and provide the child appropriate limits and structure. Problems in this area are evident when there is an unsafe physical environment or when adult caregivers do not offer a secure and supportive home environment with appropriate developmental stimulation. Caregivers may not be consistently available to offer the child support and affection, may not provide the child with appropriate limits and structure, or they may make harsh and inappropriate demands on the child (Chart 11.6).

Chart 11.5   Indicators of Function and Dysfunction for the Ability to Cope.

Ability to Cope	Inability to Cope
FUNCTION: Ability to adapt to various situations	DYSFUNCTION: Inability to adapt to various situations
INDICATORS OF FUNCTION	**INDICATORS OF DYSFUNCTION**
Engages in new experiences	Avoids new experiences
Spontaneously attempts new experiences	Needs much encouragement to attempt new tasks
Is excited by new tasks	Expresses fear, reluctance, or withdrawal when faced with new tasks
When challenged in play, seeks solutions to master the activity or finds a satisfactory substitute activity	When challenged in play, will withdraw or revert to more infantile behaviors
Returns to a state of equilibrium after stress	Takes an extended period of time to recover from stress

---

Chart 11.6   Indicators of Function and Dysfunction for Home Environment.

Adequate Home Environment	**Inadequate Home Environment**
FUNCTION: A physical environment that and adult caregivers who provide safety, security, support, and developmental stimulation	DYSFUNCTION: A lack of a physical environment that and adult caregivers who provide safety, security, support, and developmental stimulation
INDICATORS OF FUNCTION	**INDICATORS OF DYSFUNCTION**
A living space that is safe from intruders, has no safety hazards, and is relatively clean	A living space that is not safe from intruders, has safety hazards, and is not clean
A living space that includes materials for participating in developmentally appropriate activities	A living space that does not have materials necessary for participating in developmentally appropriate activities
A caregiver who is interested and focused on keeping a child safe and meeting his or her developmental needs	No caregivers who are interested and capable of keeping the child safe or meeting his or her developmental needs or caregivers who put a child in physical danger
A caregiver who is consistently available to offer a child support and affection as the child requests support and affection	No caregiver who is consistently available to offer a child support and affection
A caregiver who is consistently available and capable of offering a child appropriate limits and structure	No caregiver who is consistently available or capable of offering a child appropriate limits and structure or a caregiver who makes harsh and inappropriate demands on a child

School environments include the teachers who support the child's development of academic, social, and living skills. A functional school environment is safe and has adequate space and materials for learning. Teachers facilitate and support positive interactions among children and adjust their teaching styles to the learning needs of each child. Problems in the school environment arise when space and materials are inadequate for learning or when a teacher is unable to facilitate positive interactions among children and has an inflexible teaching style (Chart 11.7).

Community environments are functional when they support children's play and interaction with others in their neighborhood activities. At the functional end, community resources are safe for sensorimotor play and recreation and adult role models provide leadership. At the dysfunctional end of the continuum, the environments are unsafe and adult role models are not involved or do not provide leadership (Chart 11.8).

GUIDE TO EVALUATION

The major concern of the occupational therapist who uses the psychosocial frame of reference for assessment is how the child functions in his or her daily life. The purposes of an occupational therapy evaluation of the child are to: 1) determine the child's skills, abilities, strengths, and challenges in everyday life and 2) determine whether the child's environment is adequate to encourage use of the child's skills in developmentally appropriate activities. In this frame of reference, the psychosocial implications of the activities are of primary concern to the therapist.

Chart 11.7 Indicators of Function and Dysfunction for School Environment.

Adequate School Environment	Inadequate School Environment
FUNCTION: An environment that and teachers who support a child's development of academic, social, and living skills	DYSFUNCTION: An environment that and teachers who do not support a child's development of academic, social, and living skills
INDICATORS OF FUNCTION	**INDICATORS OF DYSFUNCTION**
A classroom that has the materials necessary for academic learning	A classroom that does not have the materials necessary for academic learning
Space for children to productively interact with each other in play and in learning activities	A lack of space for children to interact with each other in play and in learning activities
Teachers who facilitate and support positive interactions among children	Teachers who do not facilitate or support positive interactions among children
Teachers who adjust their teaching styles to the learning needs of children	Teachers who do not adjust their teaching styles to the learning needs of children

Chart 11.8 Indicators of Function and Dysfunction for Community Environment.

Adequate Community Environment	Inadequate Community Environment
FUNCTION: An environment that and adult caregivers who support children's play and appropriate involvement in community activities	DYSFUNCTION: An environment that and adult caregivers who do not support children's play and appropriate involvement in community activities
INDICATORS OF FUNCTION	**INDICATORS OF DYSFUNCTION**
Community resources for safe sensorimotor play and recreation	No community resources for safe sensorimotor play and recreation
Adult role models who provide leadership for children's community activities	No adult role models to provide leadership for children's community activities

Consistent with the theoretical base, the six major sections of this evaluation include innate temperament, attachment, peer interaction, play, ability to cope, and environmental interaction. The order of the proposed assessment is designed to minimize any anxiety of the child and his or her family and to help the therapist gain as much information as possible. (This proposed assessment does not follow the specific order of the six major sections of the psychosocial frame of reference). All assessment in the psychosocial frame of reference should be sensitive to the child's chronological and developmental age. Some of the suggestions provided are most suitable for school-aged children.

The occupational therapy evaluation begins with a review of the historical material available on the child and family. Background material may include school and medical reports, psychological evaluations, and summaries of past treatments or interviews with caregivers. These data assist the occupational therapist in determining relevant areas for assessment and the best way to proceed with a formal evaluation. The data also give the therapist a general idea of the child's temperament, attachment relationships, ability to cope, level of play and peer interaction skills, and environments, as perceived by the parents and other professionals. Specific areas relevant to occupational therapy may need a more detailed assessment.

When the child is able to, it is important to get the child's perceptions of his or her relationships with his or her care providers, his or her play skills, peer relationships, ability to cope, and comfort in and satisfaction with his or her environments. This is crucial to understand what areas concern the child most, especially for the school-aged child. The areas that a child identifies should have priority in the assessment and intervention. A criticism of psychiatric and psychosocial treatment of children is that services frequently focus on the concerns of adults in a child's life. These concerns are often different from a child's concerns. Adults are frequently more concerned with disruptive behavior or poor academic performance. Children may be more concerned with not having friends and not feeling competent in activities. To engage a child in intervention, it is critical to address the child's concerns.

It is often easier and more productive to gather information about the child's major concerns when the child is engaged in a simple, nonstressful, enjoyable play activity. The child most likely will relax and be able to talk more easily with the therapist as he or she plays. The therapist should be organized in his or her approach and be direct and honest with the child about his or her desire to understand better how the child plays and gets along at home, in school, and in the neighborhood. It is equally important that the therapist be sensitive to the child's cues relative to his or her willingness and ability to tolerate an interview. At times, conversation is interspersed with periods of reciprocal play between the therapist and the child. Children share some information through nonverbal behavior and play. The amount and type of information that a therapist collects in a play interview depend upon the environment in which the therapist works and what he or she potentially can help a child with.

In a play interview, the therapist may collect information about the following topics:

- Play activities that the child enjoys when he or she is alone, with peers, and with his or her family: This gives a therapist a window into a child's strengths; absence of a range of activities is also telling.

- Activities that bore or frustrate the child or activities that the child perceives as too hard for him or her including play and academic tasks: This may provide useful information in considering further assessment of a child's coping, motor, and/or cognitive skills.

- Activities that the child wants to be better able to participate in including play and academic tasks: This information may help the therapist direct intervention initially to motivate the child.

- The child's perceptions of his or her experiences with teachers and classmates: This may help a therapist understand the child's school-based attachment relationships and peer interaction skills. This information may be helpful if intervention is recommended.

- What an average day in the child's home and community is like (this may include an activity configuration dictated to the therapist or written or drawn by the child): This way
  a therapist learns about the richness of a child's daily life or the poverty of activity that
  may be critical to address.
- The child's relationship with different family members (who the child feels that he or she
  gets along with best): With this information, a therapist learns something about a child's
  caregiving environment and who may be important to a child to include as a part of therapy if therapy is recommended.
- The child's understanding of friendship (who the child's friends are, what they are like,
  how they treat him or her, and how the child treats them) is especially important if a
  therapist plans on working with a child in a group setting.

When play deficits are suggested by the child's history or the child's self-report,
screening competency in play should be the next step in the occupational therapy
psychosocial assessment. Often deficits in basic play skills make participation in play
with peers or family members difficult or even impossible. The child may be emotionally labile, act out, or refuse to participate because the challenges presented by
typical play activities are beyond his or her capabilities. Other children may exclude
or ostracize the child because he or she cannot play as skillfully as others in his or
her age group.

Conversely, a child may have good underlying play skills but exhibit poor coping
or social skills. The child may share perceptions that other children dislike him or
her or treat him or her poorly or that he or she is "no good" at activities that are important to the child. This may be what a therapist observes, but it is important to understand the child's views. A person's perceptions can drive behaviors as much as his
or her actual skills. Although it is difficult for the therapist at times, it is important to
make distinctions among deficits in basic play skills, coping skills, and social skills.

To complete this aspect of the assessment, the therapist should observe the child
in a play activity appropriate for his or her age and environment. This includes sensorimotor, imaginary, constructional, and gross and fine motor game play. No formal assessment tools are available to explore play at this level, so the therapist must
choose appropriate activities based on his or her understanding of child development
and the activities common in the child's environment. The *Test of Playfulness* (ToP)
(Bundy, 1997) is presently being developed; it will help therapists use their observations of children's play to rate children's intrinsic motivation, internal control, and
ability to suspend reality in their play. This will be a important tool for evaluating
children's psychosocial functioning.

Sensory, motor, or neurologic deficits may be causative factors in play deficit.
Standardized tools are available to assess these areas, such as the *Bruininks-Oseretsky
Test of Motor Proficiency* (Bruininks, 1978) and the *Sensory Integration and Praxis Tests*
(Ayres, 1989). Because they are time-consuming to administer, they are used most
often in psychosocial practice once play deficits are identified or if there is a strong

suspicion of contributing underlying deficits. Data gained from these assessments may be useful to determine whether another frame of reference is necessary for intervention.

The therapist should also observe social skills in a structured group activity and in free play. With age-appropriate expectations in mind, the following should be noted:

- Initiations and responses with peers
- Turn-taking, compromising, and negotiating in activities
- Aggression toward and from peers
- Incidences of helping and being helped by peers

A therapist may also decide to use the *Social Skills Rating System* (Gresham & Elliot, 1989). This is a questionnaire about a child's social skills that is designed for children at the elementary and junior high level. It is given to the child, the child's teacher, and parents.

The opportunity to observe parent-child interaction in the context of an activity is also helpful in providing insight into how parents have adapted to a particular child or how difficult interactions may be for the parents and the child. The quality and process of interaction should be noted along the following lines:

- Engagement in mutual or parallel activity
- Parents' and child's verbal and nonverbal expression of enjoyment, frustration, or anger
- The child's communication of needs and desires during the activity, and the parents' subsequent response
- Structure set by the parent and the child's response to it
- Resolution of frustrations and problems during interaction

When feasible, a play history interview should be conducted with the primary care provider. This allows for a deeper understanding of the child's development to his or her current interests and level of functioning. Specific questions should relate to the types of play and specific activities that the child has enjoyed, avoided, or resisted over his lifetime. This interview may also include the child's reactions to his or her care providers, siblings, and peers and how the child's temperament and coping styles are expressed at home. The data can help put the parent-child interaction into perspective. Takata (1974) developed a *Play History* instrument that assesses how children have progressed through six play epochs that she identifies occurring developmentally through childhood. They are the sensorimotor; symbolic and simple constructive; dramatic and complex constructive; and pre-game, game, and recreational epochs. Takata's *Play History* is a useful tool to have in one's repertoire.

The *Coping Inventory* (Zeitlin, 1985) helps to analyze how adaptively the child copes in caring for himself or herself and how the child responds to environmental demands. It is a rating scale that a therapist may use after observing a child in a few activities. Ability to cope with oneself and to cope with the environment are rated in the dimensions of active to passive; productive to nonproductive; and flexible to rigid.

- Does the child actively confront challenges?
- Are the child's strategies generally successful?
- Does the child use a range of strategies suggesting an ability to choose the most appropriate strategy for a specific situation?

The therapist reflects on how the child manages everyday challenges and stressors in the activities that he or she observes him or her doing and the effects that the environment may have had on his or her responses. Many children, even those who have overall deficits in their ability to cope, are likely to have some assets in one or more areas that can be used to foster adaptation in daily activities. A therapist is likely to discover this through a systematic analysis of a child's coping skills in activity.

After gathering all or some of these data, the therapist must integrate and interpret them into an overall picture of the child's functional assets and deficits. It is important to identify the central areas that should be addressed in the intervention process. From a functional perspective, it can be anticipated that if intervention is directed toward the key problem areas, then problematic behavior will decrease overall and the child will experience greater success in his or her daily activities.

As it has been described here, a full psychosocial occupational therapy evaluation is difficult to complete unless the therapist has the opportunity to observe a child in a variety of activities over a period of time and the therapist has the time to do a comprehensive individual evaluation. This may be possible in some educational settings or in therapeutic milieus such as day hospitals or residential settings. A complete evaluation is the ideal; however, in many settings, it is not possible, and the therapist must use his or her judgment to decide which sections of the suggested assessment are necessary and viable in the particular setting.

POSTULATES REGARDING CHANGE

It is believed that a child is born with innate temperament (Chess & Thomas, 1984). Although temperament is inborn, this does not preclude change through environmental influence. When a child displays a difficult temperament, the environment and the approach of his or her care providers are critically important for the child's adaptation. Without proper support, the child is vulnerable to psychosocial dysfunction.

1. If the therapist assists a child's care providers in establishing a routine for those activities that are difficult or disorganizing for the child, then the child will become calmer, more cooperative, and organized around that daily activity.

2. If the therapist assists care providers in understanding the discomfort of a child with a difficult temperament and how it can be managed in the child's and the family's best interest, then the care providers and child will have more positive interactions.

3. If the therapist helps the child develop cognitive strategies to confront activities that produce overwhelming anxiety, then the child will more likely be able to approach and participate in these activities.

To increase the likelihood of a parent providing the necessary physical and emotional support, it is important for the parent/child interaction to be viewed as primarily positive or rewarding. The child requires a sense of security to grow into a healthy, functioning adult. He or she needs to expect comfort and assistance when stressed or overwhelmed. When this is not the case in his or her home, then the therapist should attempt to provide an opportunity for a child and his or her care provider or an alternate care provider to experience positive mutual interaction. Positive events that do not occur in some families create as much stress and are as damaging to a child's mental health as are negative interactions that do occur (Mash, 1984). Six postulates regarding change are concerned with building a positive relationship between children and parents or care providers.

4. If a therapist provides a structured and supportive environment in which parent and child can enjoy mutual play, positive engagement between parent and child will be promoted.

5. If a therapist demonstrates ways that care providers can facilitate a child's positive engagement and functioning and provides an activity in which this can be practiced, then a parent or care provider will be more likely to promote the same behaviors in the child in the future.

6. If a therapist assists care providers in experiencing comfort and competence in activities with their child, then they more likely will relax and see positive behavior and characteristics in their child.

7. If the therapist can assist the child in clearly stating or showing his or her parents or care providers what he or she needs in relation to an activity, then it is more likely that the parents or care providers will respond to those needs.

8. If the therapist helps a parent identify what made an interaction between parent and child positive and successful in a therapy session and assists the parent in creating such an environment, then a parent will more likely attempt to recreate similar positive interactions with their child.

9. If a therapist helps a parent modulate over- or underinvolvement with their child through modeling, gentle cuing, and consultation before or after activity, then parents will likely experience greater positive feedback from their child.

With peer interaction, the meaning of the situation is decided through the natural negotiation that occurs between children. The development of effective interaction skills is a step-by-step process. First, children need to be able to approach peers positively to initiate an interaction. They then have to be able to respond reciprocally, be supportive, and help each other, when appropriate. Finally, children need to be able to have realistic expectations for the particular situation. Four postulates regarding change are concerned with peer interactions:

10. In a safe and accepting environment, if a child sees the opportunity to do an enjoyable and intrinsically rewarding activity, then the child will more likely attempt to cooperate with peers in a group activity.
11. If a child learns to help another successfully and to accept help, then the child will be more likely to seek out others for mutual activity.
12. If a child learns the basic social skills needed to play with other children, the child's positive peer interaction will likely increase and his or her interests and activity skills may also expand in kind.
13. If a therapist assists a child working with other children to identify the rules necessary for group play, then the child is more likely to accept rules and limits. Furthermore, the child will be more likely to censor himself or herself and others within such a group.

Play involves exploration, experimentation, and imitation for the sake of pleasure and serves as the basis for specific aspects of learning and for the development of many skills. When engaged in play, children develop physical, cognitive, psychological, and social skills without conscious effort. The following four postulates regarding change apply to play:

14. In a safe environment, if a therapist provides the child with a play activity that is intrinsically motivating, the child will then invest time and energy in that activity.
15. If a therapist provides a child with a sensorimotor activity that is pleasurable to the senses, the child will then initiate and engage in that play activity.
16. If a therapist guides a child's play, the child will be more open to elaborating on that play and more likely to maintain interest in that activity. Consequently, the child will be more likely to seek out similar play activities independently.
17. If a therapist introduces an activity that has properties similar to those of an activity that the child enjoys, then the child will most likely approach the new activity.

Having the ability to cope means that a child can most often deal with new and difficult situations. Five postulates regarding change are concerned with the child's developing the ability to cope.

18. If a therapist assists a child in approaching a new activity in a way that decreases fear, then the child will be more likely to participate in that activity.

19. If a therapist gradually introduces opportunities to explore risk-taking in activities, then the child will more likely tolerate the activity.
20. If a therapist introduces strategies to cope with a challenge within an activity, then a child will more likely attempt to use one of the strategies to meet the challenge.
21. If a therapist provides firm limits and a safe and quiet place for the child to regain control during an activity, then a child will likely learn to use these external mechanisms to regain emotional control.
22. If the therapist assists the child in noting the signs of his or her increasing frustration and anxiety during challenges in activities, the child will begin to note his or her own signals and attempt to use the techniques taught to reduce his or her physical experience of frustration and anxiety.

To promote positive change in a child's mental health, the child's environments (i.e., home, school, and community) must provide safety and support and space and facilities for functional skill development. Five postulates regarding change are concerned with the child's interactions within his or her environment.

23. If a therapist assists a care provider in increasing the safety of the home or school environment for play, then the child will have more opportunity for secure exploration and will be more likely to engage in productive play.
24. If a therapist assists the care provider in creating and organizing an appropriate play space, then the child will be more likely to be engaged positively and to be more focused in activities at home and in school.
25. If a therapist assists the care provider in identifying and implementing ways to monitor and supervise the child's community-based play successfully, then the care provider will be more successful in managing the child's behavior.
26. If a therapist helps the care provider involve the child in positive community-based activities, then the child will be more likely to develop positive role models.
27. If a therapist helps the care provider to increase the opportunities for learning and involvement in appropriate activities with supportive consistent adults, then the impact of negative elements in the child's environment will be reduced significantly.

APPLICATION TO PRACTICE

Temperament, attachment, peer interaction, play, the ability to cope, and environmental interactions all have been identified specifically in the theoretical base, yet the application to practice for these areas most often overlaps. Intervention in the areas of temperament, attachment, and environmental interaction, particularly with regard to the home and community, focuses on the relationship between the child and parent or care providers. This is particularly true with infants and younger children.

Helping a parent better understand and adapt to his or her child's temperament is intertwined with parent-child attachment, how they interact with their child, and how the environment is set up. If a parent learns to adapt his or her approach to the child in a way that helps the child interact more positively with the parent, the attachment relationship will be strengthened. A parent who positively changes his or her approach to the child is likely to become sensitive to environmental factors and is more likely to alter them as needed. A therapist can help a parent alter his or her home environment and set up activities that facilitate positive play experiences between the parent and child. These positive experiences will lead to the parent feeling more positive about the child and open to discussing ways to repeat that experience. Often these experiences happen through play activities, which are important methods of facilitating positive change in an attachment relationship.

Intervention in the area of peer interaction is often intertwined with interventions to facilitate play or beginning work behaviors and the ability to cope. Children need to be able to work and play within groups because family and community life requires this. Many opportunities to learn and to be productive in daily life demand an ability to get along with others as one participates in activities. Good interpersonal relationships are critical to mental health.

Although addressing children's social interactions is important, it is also important that therapists assist children in developing their individual play and activity capacities. Typical children explore and develop many skills in the privacy and security of their own bedrooms or homes. Opportunities to play alone afford children with the capacity to explore their own thoughts and interests without being concerned about the wishes or feelings of other people. When children or adults have the capacity to be alone and to fully engage in individual activities that are consonant and reflective of who they are, they are likely to find those activities to be stress reducing, invigorating, organizing, and supportive of a positive emotional state. This, of course, can make them more attractive in social interaction. Specific occupational therapy intervention within this frame of reference can be provided individually, with a family, in a peer or multifamily group setting, and in school settings. In all cases, strong collaboration with other professionals working with these children and families is critical for successful intervention.

Parent-Child Interaction

In early childhood, when dysfunction is evident in temperament, attachment, and environmental interaction, the role of the therapist is to facilitate the relationship between the child and his or her parents or care providers. The therapist acts as a role model and advisor to parents and care providers alike. As an advisor, the therapist can enhance a parent's understanding of his or her child's temperament and make suggestions regarding the structure of daily routines that may help children respond more positively to family life. The therapist can help parents identify family priorities and develop clear behavioral goals for the child and strategies to achieve the goals. This can be particularly useful for a parent who must deal with a child who displays a difficult temperament. It helps the parent to provide a secure atmosphere with appropriate and consistent expectations that provide organization for such a child.

Role Modeling

In specific interactions, the therapist may serve as a role model by demonstrating effective ways of dealing with difficult behaviors or drawing the child into a positive interaction. The therapist may also coach a parent through an interaction or observe and then consult with the parent after the interaction. The therapist minimizes the degree to which he or she actively directs a situation to avoid becoming the sole authority figure. It is important that the therapist highlight parents' strengths in interaction after a parent-child session or during the session, if such a comment fits into the process. In this way, the therapist gives the parent authority, which promotes the child's confidence in the parent. The child sees his or her parent as competent and someone to rely on. With some families who have experienced a great deal of negative interaction, it is important to remember that people are less likely to notice positive occurrences or behaviors when they have been immersed in negative interaction (Mash, 1984). The therapist can help family members begin to notice and enjoy positive moments even if they are brief. The goal is to serve as a consultant to the parent—to enhance their everyday functioning with their children, to increase the pleasure and the satisfaction that they experience in parent-child interaction, and to assist them in exploring and sharing activities with their children that will bring parent and child into more frequent and consistent positive interaction.

Fostering positive parenting is critical. The therapist sets up a reciprocal interaction in which the child learns that he or she can share concretely his or her interest in activity and depend on care providers for help and praise. The therapist can demonstrate an active respect for the child's feelings and growing autonomy. Through whatever activity is chosen, the therapist can help the parent choose and provide gentle but firm behavioral limits and positive reinforcement for appropriate behavior. The therapist should have activity and behavioral plans that will likely accentuate the positive aspects of particular children, as opposed to their negative behavior that their parents may overly focus upon. Some parents have reported that they participated in parent-child activities with their child and the therapist because of their comfort level with the therapist. They stated that they only began to understand the value of parent-child activity and to enjoy it after they had experienced it over the course of time. To allow a therapist to intervene in a difficult parent-child relationship, parents need to feel supportive and accepted by the therapist.

Occupational therapy can play a vital role in implementing change in the parent-child relationship by facilitating productive and pleasurable interaction through play and activity. This can be accomplished by working with individual families or leading a group of multiple parent-child dyads or triads. The former is most likely to occur when a family identifies a specific problem that they wish to focus on solely; a group is not available or desirable to the parents; or difficulties in interaction are severe and are not likely to be resolved without the intensive teaching of skills. Using a group format is helpful in a school setting, hospital, or residential treatment center. In these environments, many families share similar concerns or difficulties and can provide a strong support network for each other.

Parent-Child Activity Groups

Particular methods for the parent-child activity group have been described by Olson, Heaney, and Soppas-Hoffman (1989). The concepts of attachment, coping, and play form the basis for the rationale, structure, and methods used in successful parent-child therapy. Two distinct play periods are used. In the first, parents assist children in constructional play. This activity is used because the materials presented are structured, familiar items such as boxes, paper, and tape. The activity can be enjoyed at different skill levels, and the range of complexity and variety is great. In initial attempts at mutual activity, parents and children may struggle to come up with ideas or figure out ways to build what the child imagines. By observing other families work through this process and by problem solving with the therapist, these sessions promote greater and more productive interactions. Ability to cope with the challenges presented in the activity is increased, resulting in the experience of pleasure and pride that is gained in mutual accomplishment.

In the free play period that follows, parents and children have the opportunity to choose their own activities. Many tabletop and gross motor activities are available. The task is to choose an activity that is enjoyable and growth promoting for the child and one that the parent can tolerate and enjoy. Listening to one another and making decisions based on the child's interest, along with the parent's understanding of what presently is best for the family, are some of the skills that are the focus of this part of the group. The therapist can observe first hand how a child participates in his or her favorite activities with his or her parents. Because these activities are likely to occur in the home or community, the goal at this level is to enhance pleasure and organization in the activity. Adaptations relative to the rules, boundaries, or materials used may be introduced. Throughout the course of this group intervention, a family's investment in mutual play grows, resulting in a stronger parent-child relationship and more complex play. The child becomes more attentive and receptive to his or her parent's initiatives and requests. Care providers come to understand their children better and exhibit greater confidence, skill, and pleasure in guiding the child's development.

Activity-based Intervention When Ill

Occupational therapists, in collaboration with other professionals, can help parents maintain a secure attachment relationship with their children in spite of a parent's serious physical or emotional illness. When parents are ill and cannot take care of and interact with their children in their typical way, children may exhibit angry, anxious, avoidant, ambivalent, or solicitous behavior. Although other adults will most likely fill in and provide daily care for the children, it is critical that each child's relationship with his or her ill parent be supported and regular opportunities to communicate and/or interact be facilitated. In this way, each child is assured that his or her parent is still available to him or her and that the child can still have a meaningful and positive relationship in spite of illness. It also gives children the opportunity to better understand their parent's condition by being able to observe the parent and be with him or her.

For the ill parent, the opportunity to engage with his or her children can have an equally positive emotional effect. Playful activity can soften a serious, unfamiliar, and adultlike environment (e.g., a hospital) into one that the child and adult can feel more comfortable and relaxed in. It can give direction and a means to interact when tension or emotion may be high. Besides being organizing and calming, it brings pleasure. This is especially true when an illness requires a long hospitalization or a long recuperation period. Activities should be organized and adapted to children's emotional and developmental needs and to parents' level of physical stamina and emotional state (Figure 11.14).

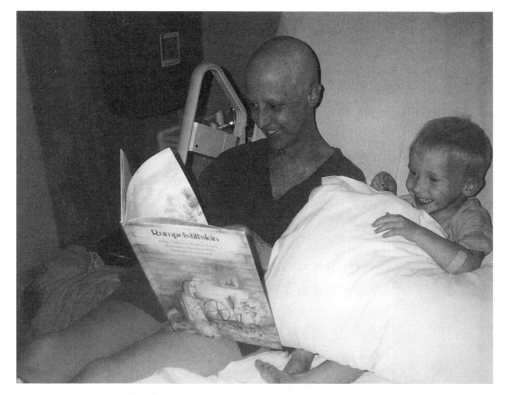

Figure 11.14 Mother and child engaging in activity in a hospital.

When a parent exhibits depression, a therapist may need to use cognitive and behavioral intervention strategies to facilitate a parent's positive mood state in parent-child interaction. People who are depressed are likely to be increasingly self-absorbed and focused. When people are more self-focused, they are more likely to be aware of their own shortcomings. Their affective reactions are more intense, anxiety awareness increases, and they are more likely to experience frustration in response to challenges in activities. A person who is depressed spends less effort, is less persistent, and expects to fail. Generally, a person who is depressed will not focus on external events, and other people will avoid them (Lewinsohn, Hoberman, Teri, & Hautzinger, 1985).

In an activity, a person who is depressed has to focus on an external event and other people around them. The occupational therapist may attempt to engage a parent with depression in an activity with his or her child. These activities should be positively reinforcing and pleasurable. Attending to an activity requires that a parent be less focused and absorbed in himself or herself. As attention is drawn away from the self and towards pleasurable interaction, it is hoped that the parent will exhibit a more positive mood state. When the parent interacts with his or her child positively, the interaction should be positive for both. It is also important to help a parent who is experiencing depression to increase his or her awareness of situations and environmental conditions that make him or her feel most relaxed and positive, including observing the pleasure that his or her child derives from focusing on parent-child activity.

Activity Groups and Peer Interactions

Children who experience dysfunction in peer interaction, play, or the ability to cope frequently profit from activity groups. Group activities facilitate physical proximity among children and provide a means and a topic for interaction. With a group leader's support and guidance, children can learn the social skills to interact with each other in a way that increases the likelihood of mutual activity or play. They can also learn how to help and seek help successfully. Over time, positive peer interaction may develop into friendship.

Activity groups operate under the premise that children are intrinsically interested in play and peer acceptance. Unless children are severely withdrawn or antisocial, they will be drawn into many activities if peers are involved. Their desires to be included in a peer group leads them to focus on the goals of others. In activity groups, the leader makes use of this natural desire to help children modify their behavior. The therapist provides a benign and supportive group environment in which children feel safe enough to explore how to positively interact with peers.

Grading the Activity

Children referred for group treatment often have experienced multiple failures and rejections from others, despite their intrinsic interest to play with others. This may be the result of deficient play, social, or coping skills. Therefore, grading the activity (so that level of play, social interaction, or level of challenge for all group members is appropriate) is important. For example, a child who needs to learn to interact more effectively with peers and who has only played simple games of luck would likely be overwhelmed if he or she first is introduced to games requiring strategy in a group. He or she would likely need a significant amount of adult support and instruction to play such a game, and this would limit the child's opportunities to work on peer interaction. The child may profit from individual instruction or coaching before he or she participates in new games with his or her peers. Sometimes, a game or activity can be adapted in part to include a member who may have weaker skills in particular activities but who may profit from observing the behavior of children who have stronger skills.

Parallel Groups. A group may function at a parallel level, a project level, or as a cooperative group (Mosey, 1986). At a parallel level, children work side by side, observe one another, but interact minimally. Children typically play at this level during the early preschool years and when they are introduced to activities that are challenging for them. For example, kindergartners are not ready to truly collaborate on a mural because they are just learning to represent their ideas on paper. When children are not ready to share supplies, cooperate, or negotiate with each other, they are most appropriate for a parallel group. They can become accustomed to working near other children, and the therapist may facilitate their observing the work or play of others and may facilitate conversation about the activity.

Project Level Groups. At a project level, children share materials and some ideas, but they continue work on and keep their own projects. Positive activity experiences and feedback from other children are important reinforcers that foster children's learning to share, cooperate, and negotiate with others in activity. The therapist may initially need to use extrinsic reinforcers such as stickers or points for good behavior that may be turned in for a small prize for some groups of children, but the intrinsic pleasure of social acceptance and friendship should be the main emphasis.

Cooperative Level Groups. At a cooperative group level, children are ready to work together on one finished project such as putting on a play, constructing a house, or designing a complex obstacle course. At this level, the children's intrinsic pleasure comes mainly from social acceptance and friendships.

Choosing Activities

Activity groups may be developed around a variety of play activities or tasks. The choice of activity depends upon the goals of the group and the interests and developmental level of the children. Imaginary play may be used to allow children to explore their feelings or wishes or to play out adult behaviors so that they may understand those behaviors. Children represent their feelings through art, while also developing fine motor skills. Constructional activities provide opportunities to build task skills; they can also be organized to facilitate collaboration among children.

clay. He made bathrooms for other members. Soon, the boys connected some of their houses into condominiums. It was about 5 months before they were able to play out any stories with the houses in the group. They appeared to need the organization and self-confidence that they derived from learning to construct first.

Club Model for Elementary School-aged Children

Florey & Greene (1997) advocate using a club model for activity groups for elementary school-aged children. They use the elements of typical after school clubs that children cherish. For example, they use club tee-shirts; all members make and put on their special tee shirt over their clothes at the start of their group meeting. Club rules are drawn up with all members contributing rules; this makes it more likely that members will follow the rules and enforce the adherence to the rules of other members. The children also come up with special handshakes and signals that mark the uniqueness of their group. Each group opens with a review of club minutes, and members are asked if they have anything new to bring up. The issues of club members are then discussed before the activity that is planned for the session is introduced.

Critical elements for group cohesion, which Florey and Greene (1997) have maximized in new group designs, are the use of rituals and depersonalized controls in their group design. This is critical to do even if a leader chooses not to use the club model that Florey and Greene discuss. Rituals are important in the lives of all people; they provide organization and structure. They make people aware of their close bonds and what they share. Rituals are calming and allow people to anticipate what will occur next. Depersonalized controls are rules about behavior that a group decides are necessary if a game or activity is going to be pleasurable or successful. They are not directed toward any person but toward the implementation of an activity. An authority figure is not passing judgment or holding the power. When a rule is broken, limits are set with the rule breaker because he or she interfered with the game or activity.

School-aged Groups

School-aged children are group- and game-focused; they have come to understand the importance of rules for the games or activities to be fun. Even children who are oppositional are more likely to abide by rules for these purposes.

Activities should be sought out that children will enthusiastically engage in. This is true even if the group goal is to develop good handwriting skills. Interspersed among, or immediately after, handwriting tasks, the therapist should include fine motor activities that are engaging for the group members. If the group is completely focused on developing psychosocial skills, the therapist may get his or her best ideas for group activities through brainstorming with the children who will be in the group. The therapist may bring a simple activity or game to the first meeting that the children will likely be enthusiastic about. During the activity, members can discuss potential ideas for upcoming groups. The therapist should work towards cultivating interest contagion for the group activities (i.e., to spread enthusiasm for particular

activities from one or a few children to the whole group) (Redl & Wineman, 1952). This will, of course, increase the positive atmosphere in the group; it will also facilitate greater group cohesion.

Dealing with Activity Group Process

In developing an activity group, it is important to remember that groups also have their own particular growth process over time. In the initial stages, group members are more dependent on the leader for structure and organization than they will be at later stages of group development. As they become accustomed to the group, members may resist the leader as they attempt to assert some control over the activities of the group. Members may appear disillusioned with the group; this is a normal part of group process. Helping members work through this leads to a more mature group stage where group norms are well respected and the group functions cohesively at its optimal developmental level. Although school-aged children require more structure and guidance from group leaders than groups of adolescence or adults do, they seek and need some control and responsibility within a group.

Throughout an activity group, a leader facilitates group and individual problem solving, encourages helping behaviors among children, participates in activity, and provides concrete task assistance as needed. Although the children may focus their conversation and interaction toward the leader, the therapist redirects interaction toward other group members whenever possible. In this way, the leader fosters positive peer interaction instead of rivalry among the children for the leader's attention. The leader may need to intervene in peer interaction within a group when difficulties arise that children can't resolve on their own. One child may regress in play and need gentle help to reorganize so that he or she can return to more age appropriate group play. A larger child may intimidate or bully other children into doing things his or her way. In the latter case, the group leader can redirect the group by appealing to all members' sense of fairness and guide the group toward negotiation. Clarification or interpretation of what the leader observes happening among the children may be helpful. This facilitates the children acquiring a greater understanding of their own behavior and that of their peers. It may reduce their anxiety about an uncomfortable situation, help clarify their own feelings, and lead to their verbalizing their own concerns because it is clear that an adult is there to support and guide them. As a result of positive participation in an activity group over a period of time, children become more secure, related, self-reliant, confident, and socially skilled; behaviors that may have interfered with peer group functioning decrease significantly.

Grading the Amount of Frustration

When children have difficulty maintaining their composure in the face of challenges in activities, the therapist needs to grade the amount of frustration inherent in the activity. When an outburst or conflict occurs, a problem-oriented discussion

helps children learn to identify their own emotional signals and then learn to resolve the situation adaptively. For example, if one child becomes angry during play, he or she may need to learn to remove himself or herself from the game to regain emotional control before the child can discuss his or her differences with his or her peers. Another child may burst into tears or destroy a project when he or she makes a mistake. With the therapist and group's help, the child may explore how he or she can deal with frustration. The child learns that he or she can ask for help when he or she gets to a certain part of a project. Or, the child learns that he or she can ask for the therapist to help to fix a mistake before destroying his or her project.

Aggressive Behavior

When children's behavior is very aggressive, it is often important to incorporate social problem–solving opportunities within an activity group. There are curriculums that specifically address this area (Shure, 1992), but a therapist may also set up opportunities or use natural opportunities within a group to promote social problem solving. This includes facilitating children's ability to think about alternative solutions to a problem, generating potential consequences of different behaviors, and analyzing why another person may have acted in a certain way. Through guided group interaction and discussion, a therapist can help children become more sensitive to interpersonal issues.

To help aggressive children develop impulse control, the therapist may guide them in recognizing their developing anger and make connections between how their body feels, what they are thinking, and what they do. Once they can identify their own signs of developing anger, children can be taught relaxation or coping techniques. This may include specific physical relaxation techniques, learning to cope through stopping and talking oneself through a situation, or learning to take effective action such as removing oneself from a stressful situation. It is important when working with aggressive children to develop a positive and warm relationship with them. These children often feel that they are disliked by others. It is unlikely that a therapist will effectively influence any change in their behavior without the children feeling accepted and valued by the therapist.

Group Resistance

If a group meets over a length of time, sooner or later, a therapist will be faced with group resistance and his or her limits will be tested by group members. Although clear rules and consequences are important to consistently enforce with the help of the group members, it is also important not to fall into the trap of becoming a corrective, directive, and coercive authority figure. Children can provoke this and if the therapist is not reflective, a power struggle may ensue that may last over a period of groups. This may set a negative tone to the group's process and interfere with the therapist's ability to be an effective clinician. It is important to develop and maintain a positive and warm relationship with group members because this will help the children to see that they are accepted and valued by the therapist, which is a necessary prerequisite to promoting change.

When dealing with resistance or a challenge to one's limits, a therapist should first attempt to appeal to the group's sense of what is right and to engage members positively. Humor may also be helpful. At times, this will lead to children refocusing their energies positively; they may either re-engage in the activity or share their issues. The group may need restructuring. Rules may not be working. An activity may be too challenging. At other times, children may need to be removed from the group for a time-out. Sometimes, it is necessary for the entire group to have a time-out within the group to reorganize. If particular children are removed, the leader should consider how he or she will reconnect with the children that he or she removes from the group, help them save face if necessary, and deal with issues related to scapegoating or creating a hero. Sometimes other members will decide that the children who are removed are bad and shouldn't be in the group; other times, they may idolize the acting-out child who "told the leader off."

The length of a group and the point at which the therapist intervenes in the process of play should be considered carefully so that the group can be refocused or the play can be terminated before the children's behavior becomes regressive or aggressive. It is always better to end a group while the children feel invested in the activity and want to participate longer than to end when they can't wait to get out of the group. This is not to say that an activity should be interrupted prematurely, but that the therapist should give the ending of the group as careful consideration as the beginning of the group. For a group to be successful, children need to have a desire to return to the group and to develop a strong interest in participation in the group.

Culture, Beliefs and Values

Groups also reflect issues of the larger society of which they are embedded. It is important that therapists reflect upon their own beliefs about culture, race, gender, and religion. Children and therapists come to a group experience with a belief system and a great deal of experience in dealing with these issues. Different subcultures within our society have varying practices related to gender, daily living, and religion that influence their approach to activities and to social interaction. These can have a significant impact on how persons participate in a group. For example, gender roles are more rigid and specific in some cultures than in others. Therefore, the choice of activity and expectations for interactions may have to be adjusted as the therapist learns about group members' culture.

At times, incidents occur in groups that reflect the prejudice and racism present in American society. Children may subtly or not so subtly exclude a child who has a different religion than other members or make racial slurs about another child. It is helpful to acknowledge these incidents and to help children understand them. Some children may have experienced themselves in similar situations as being less worthy, less competent, or less likeable instead of understanding that they were the target of racism or prejudice. Children from privileged backgrounds may have perceived themselves as better than their peers from less privileged backgrounds. The therapist may also subtly adjust the dynamics among members through the activity to promote more inclusive and accepting behaviors among members.

Sometimes, children from minority backgrounds are initially guarded or easily angered by the behavioral limits of a Caucasian therapist. They may reflect onto the therapist their anger about how they have been treated by other persons in authority from the dominant culture. Although limit setting is important, it is also important that the therapist not respond to the behavior as simply resistive behavior. The therapist's relationships with group members and the group members' relationships with each other can be dramatically altered if a therapist's hunches about prejudice or racism are sensitively explored. The therapist can listen to what may be behind anger and may ask for elaboration about similar experiences. The children can then be helped to gain control over anger that may be related to racism or prejudice and to use that anger adaptively.

Symptoms of insecurity or diminished self worth related to race or culture may be addressed nonverbally through activity. The therapist can acknowledge and model interest and acceptance of multiple cultures through incorporating activities reflecting the cultures of the children involved in the group. In a supportive environment, children enjoy talking about activities that they have enjoyed with their families and in their communities; such a discussion can be a springboard for developing group activities. When children have had little experience with activities that reflect their cultural backgrounds, a therapist may share multicultural activity books with them through which they can learn about their own and different cultures by planning interesting group activities.

Termination

How a therapist deals with the termination of an activity group or the discharge of a group member from a group is as important as how the therapist initially organizes the group. Learning how to say goodbye and to appropriately mark transitions is a critical life skill. Just as most people find special events that mark most life transitions comforting and enjoyable, children enjoy planning a special activity to mark a group's ending. The therapist should guide the children in reflecting on and reveling in what they enjoyed about the group and what they accomplished or learned. Sharing feelings about saying goodbye and helping children make the transition toward other groups or community activities are important behaviors that the therapist should model.

Facilitating Individual Play and Activity

Through individual activity intervention, a therapist can gently guide a child who exhibits limited play and coping skills to explore his or her interests. As interest in activities is captured, those activities can be used as a basis to motivate the child to develop the necessary skills to participate in activities at increasingly complex levels. In a secure environment where the only observer is a helpful therapist, a child may be more open to experimenting and exposing weaknesses in the interest of developing skills. In a group setting, he or she may be confronted by more competent children and focus on comparing finished products or skills, which may lead to a quick retreat in frustration or humiliation.

Sometimes a child is very focused on activities that "popular" children participate in even though they have little capacity for the activity. A therapist cannot dissuade the child from seeking to participate in these activities, but he or she can introduce new or related activities that the child may enjoy exploring. He or she may experience a pleasure in the new activity that hadn't been previously experienced because the previous focus was on participating in activities that interested others instead of seeking activities in which he or she had interest and/or potential capabilities. The child may also have been preoccupied with negatively comparing his or her abilities to the other players as opposed to becoming fully engaged in the activity.

Once a therapist has engaged a child successfully in individual activity, he or she carefully modulates the therapist "helping role" so that the child learns to independently participate and enjoy activities. The therapist may consult with parents so that the child begins to pursue the activities learned in therapy in their home environment. If the child agrees, parents may also be invited to observe their child in individual activity. The child can then experience his or her parents as being quietly available for support or help and learn that his or her parents can be as dependable as the therapist in facilitating his or her activity participation. The child learns to be alone and absorbed in individual activity in the presence of the supportive other. This is important for developing the capacity to be alone with oneself (Winnicott, 1965). Creativity and self-knowledge are often best nurtured in an environment that permits some solitude. When interpersonal interaction is not demanded, people can more fully immerse themselves in activity and find a different but equally important type of satisfaction (Csikszentimihalyi, 1993).

Individual activity may also serve as a bridge to activity groups. The child may gain skill, self-confidence, and the capacity to cope with challenges that make him or her more open to playing or working with peers.

Some children with severe emotional disturbance do not play, use minimal language to communicate, and initiate minimal interaction with others. Their activity focuses around basic needs, self-stimulation, or exploration of the environment that is disorganized and does not lead to effective adaptation. They may destroy things, disrupt others, or put themselves in danger. When others attempt to limit their activity, they may become physically aggressive. Often, these children benefit from individual therapeutic intervention that uses sensory and motor activities. The therapist initiates and structures activities that provide intense but organized sensory-motor input to engage the child and to promote purposeful play. If sensations are pleasurable, then the child attends and seeks to continue the activity. Once the therapist has successfully and consistently involved the child in purposeful and organized play in this way, he or she may introduce another child into the sensorimotor play.

When children exhibit severe innate deficits in social interaction (e.g., children with autism or pervasive developmental disorder), a therapist may want to develop advanced skills in assisting parents in engaging their children in interaction. Greenspan and Wieder (1997) have written extensively on their methods to help children develop two-way communication in social interaction to help parents better understand their children's atypical interactional cues and respond in ways that facilitates positive interaction between themselves and their children.

SUMMARY

This chapter presents theoretical information based predominantly on developmental psychology and organizes it into a framework for occupational therapy practice in pediatric psychosocial settings. Temperament, attachment, peer interactions, play, the ability to cope, and environmental interactions are the central issues in the development of good mental health and in the functional interventions that deal with pediatric psychosocial disorders.

Throughout childhood, the development of play, peer interaction, and the ability to cope are strongly related to the adaptation of the child's temperament to his or her environment, to the security of the child's attachment relationships, and to the adequacy of his or her environments. Each of these areas is defined specifically with regard to function and dysfunction, specific methods of evaluation, and postulates regarding change. Because all these facets are interconnected in a growing child and because they facilitate or hinder overall developmental progress reciprocally, they cannot be separated out in practice.

The discussion of application to practice focuses on addressing these complex issues in an integrated way. When the therapist attempts to improve parent-child activity interaction, he or she must consider and address the parent's understanding of the child's temperament and the adequacy of their mutual environments. The therapist may use play as a method to facilitate positive peer or parent-child interaction and to foster more adaptive coping behaviors as children confront challenges in play activities. Overall, the therapist's interventions influence many aspects of children's psychosocial functioning.

References

Ainsworth, M. (1967). Object relations, dependency and attachment: A theoretical review of the infant-mother relationship. *Child Development, 40,* 969–1020.

Anthony, E. J. (1987). Risk, vulnerability and resilience: An overview. In E. J. Anthony, & B. J. Cohler, (Eds.). *The invulnerable child.* New York, NY: Guilford Press.

Arend, R., Gore, F. L., & Sroufe, L. A. (1979). Continuity of individual-adaptation from infancy to kindergarten: A predictive study of ego resilience and curiosity in pre-schoolers. *Child Development, 50,* 950–957.

Arnold, E. (Ed.). (1978). *Helping parents help their children.* New York: Brunner/Mazel, Inc.

Ayres, A. J. (1979). *Sensory integration and the child.* Los Angeles, CA: Western Psychological Services.

Ayres, A. J. (1989). *Sensory integration and praxis tests.* Los Angeles, CA: Western Psychological Services.

Barkley, R. A. (1987). *Defiant Children: A Clinician's Manual for Parent Training.* NY: Guilford Press.

Bloomquist, M. L. (1996). *Skills Training for Children with Behavior Disorders: A Parent and Therapist Guidebook.* NY: Guilford Press.

Bowlby, J. (1969). *Attachment and loss* (Vol. 1). New York: Basic Books, Inc.

Brown, J., & Dodge, K. A. (1997). Early peer relations and child psychiatry. In J. Noshpitz, S. Greenspan, S. Wieder, & J. Osofsky (Eds.) *Handbook of child and adolescent psychiatry, Volume One: Infants and Preschoolers: Development and Syndromes* (pp. 305–320). New York: John Wiley & Sons.

Bruininks, R. (1978). *Bruininks-Oseretsky test of motor proficiency.* Circle Pines, MN: American Guidance Service.

Bundy, A. C. (1997). Play and playfulness: what to look for. In L. D. Parham & L. S. Fazio (Eds.) *Play in occupational therapy for children* (pp. 52–66), St. Louis: Mosby.

Chess, S. & Thomas, A. (1984). *Origins and evolutions of behavior disorders: From infancy to early adult life.* New York, NY: Brunner and Mazel.

Cotton, N. (1984). Childhood play as an analog to adult capacity to work. *Child Psychology and Human Development, 14(31),* 135–144.

Csikszentmihalyi, M. (1993). *The evolving self.* NY: HarperCollins Publishers.

Downey, G., & Coyne, J. C. (1990). Children of depressed parents: an integrative review. *Psychological Bulletin, 108,* 50–76.

Erikson, E. (1959). Identity and the life cycle. *Psychological Issues, 1,* 1–171.

Florey, L.L. & Greene, S. (1997). Play in middle childhood: a focus on children with behavior and emotional disorders. In L. D. Parham & L. S. Fazio (Eds.) *Play in occupational therapy for children* (pp. 126–143), St. Louis: Mosby.

Greenberg, M. T., Speltz, M. L., & DeKlyen, M. (1993). The role of attachment in the early development of disruptive behavior problems. *Development and Psychopathology, 5,* 191–213.

Greenspan S., & Wieder, S. (1997). Multisystem developmental disorder. In J. Noshpitz, S. Greenspan, S., Wieder, S., & Osofsky, J. (Eds.). *Handbook of child and adolescent psychiatry, Volume One: Infants and preschoolers: development and syndromes* (pp. 561–572). New York: John Wiley & Sons, Inc.

Gresham, F. M., & Elliott, S. N. (1990). *Social Skills Rating System.* Circle Pines: MN: American Guidance Service.

Jackson, N. F., Jackson, D. A., Monroe, C. (1983). *Skill Lessons & Activities: Getting Along with Others.* Champaign, IL: Research Press.

Lewinsohn, P. M., Hoberman, H. M., Teri, L., & Hautzinger, M. (1985). An integrative theory of depression. In S. Reiss & R. R. Bootzin (Eds.) *Theoretical issues in behavior therapy.* London: Academic Press, Inc.

Mash, E. J. (1984). Families with problem children: Children in families under stress. *New Directions for Child Development, 24,* 65–82.

Matas, L., Arend, R., & Sroufe, L. A. (1978). Continuity of adaptation in the second year: The relationship of the quality of attachment later competence. *Child Development, 24,* 65–81.

Maxmen, J. S., & Ward, N. G. (1995). *Essential psychopathology and its treatment* (2nd Ed). New York: W.W. Norton & Co.

Mosey, A. C. (1986). *Psychosocial components of occupational therapy.* New York: Raven.

Olson, L., Heaney, C., & Soppas-Hoffman, B. (1989). Parent-child activity group treatment in preventive psychiatry. *Occupational Therapy in Health Care, 6(1),* 29–43.

Pettit, G. S., Bates, J. E., Dodge, K. A. (1997). Supportive parenting, ecological context, and children's adjustment: a seven-year longitudinal study. *Child Development, 68,* 908–923.

Redl, F., & Wineman, D. (1952). *Controls from within: Techniques for the treatment of the aggressive child.* New York: The Free Press.

Reed, K. (1984). *Models of practice in occupational therapy.* Baltimore: Williams & Wilkins.

Reilly, M. (1974). *Play as exploratory learning.* Beverly Hills, CA: Sage.

Sapon-Shevin, M. (1986). Teaching cooperation. In G. Cartledge & J. F. Milburn. (Eds). *Teaching Social Skills to Children* (pp. 270–302). NY: Pergamon Press.

Shure, M. (1992). *I Can Problem Solve: An Interpersonal Cognitive Problem-Solving Program.* Champaign, IL: Research Press.

Slavson, S. R., & Schiffer, M. (1975). *Group psychotherapy for children.* New York: International Universities Press.

Takata, N. (1974). Play as a prescription. In M. Reilly (Eds.). *Play as Exploratory Learning* (pp. 209–246). Beverly Hills, CA: Sage.

Waters, E., Wittman, J., & Sroufe, L. A. (1979). Attachment, positive affect and competence in the peer group: Two studies in construct validation. *Child Development, 50,* 821–829.

Winnicott, D. W. (1965). *The maturational processes and the facilitating environment: studies in the theory of emotional development.* London: Hogarth.

Zeitlin, S. (1985). *Coping inventory.* Bensonville, IL: Scholastic Testing Service.

Acquisition Frame of Reference

CHARLOTTE BRASIC ROYEEN / MAUREEN DUNCAN

OVERVIEW

The purpose of this chapter is to acquaint the reader with a basic understanding of the acquisitional frame of reference, theories upon which it is based, and the practice implications of its use. The first section of this chapter covers historical perspectives and theoretical foundations. Assumptions, concepts, definitions, postulates, and hypothesis of the frame of reference are presented. Organization of the theoretical base subserving the acquisitional frame of reference is delineated and the function/dysfunction continua, guide for evaluation, postulates regarding change, and application to practice.

INTRODUCTION

The acquisitional frame of reference focuses on the acquisition, or learning, of specific skills required for the optimal performance within the environment. Intervention is provided with this focus in mind. Activities are given solely for the purpose of acquiring specific skills. Mastering each skill or subskill required of an activity is the primary goal (Mosey, 1986).

The acquisitional frame of reference is a conglomeration of learning theory concepts prominent in the 1950's, 1960's, and 1970's. For the most part, learning theories are based on the hypotheses and experimental research of prominent psychologists. Pavlov's early work on classical conditioning of dogs (Pavlov, 1941) opened the door for subsequent research into what is called "learning theories." Among the theorists most prominent and influential to the development of the acquisitional frame of reference were B. F. Skinner's theory of operant conditioning (Skinner, 1953, 1954, 1971,1974) and Alfred Bandura's observational learning (regarded as a cognitive and social learning theory) (Bandura, 1965, 1977). Other learning theorists include Edward Lee Thorndike (1932), Clark Leornard Hull (1951, 1952), Edwin Ray Guthrie (1935), and Edward Chace Tolman (1932, 1958).

The acquisitional frame of reference uses principles and assumptions based on the above learning theories. In addition, Carl Rogers' work on the use of unconditional positive regard and the role of therapists in the treatment setting provides basic theoretical information on how the therapist approaches intervention (Rogers, 1951, 1957; Rogers & Freiberg, 1994). Additionally, the acquisitional frame of reference pertains to application of learning theory and some of Rogers' principles with children who have a skill deficit. Principles taken from operant conditioning and observational learning form the theoretical base of the acquisitional frame of reference. Additionally, in this frame of reference, the therapist uses two important legitimate tools of the profession: the teaching learning process and activity analysis.

HISTORICAL PERSPECTIVE

Occupational therapists' use of the acquisitional frame of reference flourished in the late 1960's and early 1970's (Hollis, 1974; Norman, 1976; Rugel, Mattingly, Eichinger & May, 1971; Sieg, 1974; Smith & Tempone, 1968; Trombly, 1966; Wanderer, 1974). Mosey (1986) described the acquisitional frame of reference as the linking of learning theories prominent at this time.

The acquisitional frame of reference can be used to address cognitive and motor skill deficits (Mosey, 1986). According to Mosey (1986), the acquisitional frame of reference closely resembles the developmental frame of reference in that the therapist works on skill development. While there appear to be many similarities between the developmental frame of reference and acquisitional frame of reference, there are several key concepts that distinguish them from each other.

The developmental frame of reference views the development of skills as occurring along a continuum: skill development is age dependent. Children learn new skills when they have reached the developmental level necessary to support the skill. In the developmental frame of reference there is a hierarchy of skills. Skills must be learned at a certain stage of development before other skills can be acquired. Thus learning is viewed as stage specific. This is not true of the acquisitional frame of reference. Although the developmental level of the child is acknowledged, no particular emphasis is placed upon it. Behaviors are simply broken down into small subskills and built upon each other, resulting in complex skill development (Figure 12.1). Conversely, components of the acquisitional frame of reference are found within the developmental frame of reference.

Many frames of reference incorporate principles of acquisitional theory into their knowledge base. To illustrate, the sensory integrative frame of reference incorporates child-directed principles taken from the work of Rogers (Hinojosa, Kramer, & Pratt, 1996). Further, concepts from the acquisitional frame of reference can be supplemental to other frames of reference such as psychosocial, biomechanical, and occupational.

Recently, there has been a resurgence in behavioral therapy intervention that is based upon acquisitional theory. This is particularly true of the work of Ivan Lovass

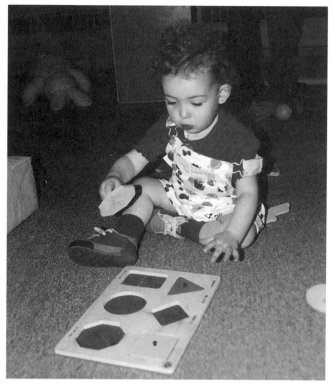

Figure 12.1 Skill development focusing on a subskill.

in the treatment of autistic children (Lovaas & Bucher, 1974), which is better known today as the applied behavioral approach.

THEORETICAL BASE OF ACQUISITIONAL FRAME OF REFERENCE

In the acquisitional frame of reference, behavior is viewed as a response to the environment. The environment either reinforces and strengthens a behavior (positive reinforcement), or fails to provide a positive reinforcement by giving no reinforcement or ignoring behaviors (negative reinforcement). In the acquisitional frame of reference, the role of the environment in eliciting adaptive responses is of primary importance.

Skill Acquisition

Skill acquisition is influenced by interaction between the environment and the child's behavior. Emphasis is placed on (1) context of the environment, (2) functional behaviors, and (3) learned skills. Each of these concepts will be explored in greater detail.

Content of the environment

The environmental content is the primary determinant of behavior in this frame of reference. The environmental content encompasses everything that is external to the individual, including human and non-human elements, and provides the reinforcement for behavior. If the environmental content does not afford or elicit certain behaviors, they will not emerge. An example of the environmental content would be the cultural or ethnic background of the family. *Environmental reinforcers* refers to the positive or negative stimuli that occur in the child's external environment (Figure 12.2).

Initially, the environment helps with the acquisition of a skill. As time progresses, it helps to reinforce the skill and allows the child to generalize that skill. Over time, the reinforcer from the environment changes. For example, when a parent is trying to develop independence in self care skills, the parent may reinforce every positive step the child takes towards independence. As the child gets older, the parent no longer needs to reinforce each independent act, but the peer group reinforces the child when he or she is clean or appropriately dressed (Figure 12.3). Through this, the child is able to generalize the importance of independence in self care and will bathe and dress appropriately without external reinforcement. Thus, a broad scope of experiences within the environment are essential for the acquisition of a broad array of skills.

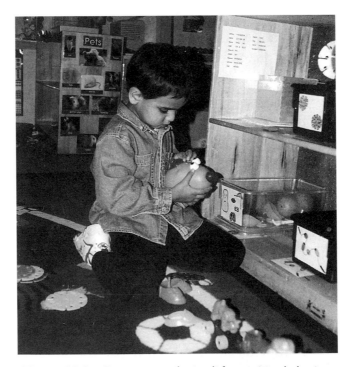

Figure 12.2 Environmental stimuli for positive behaviors.

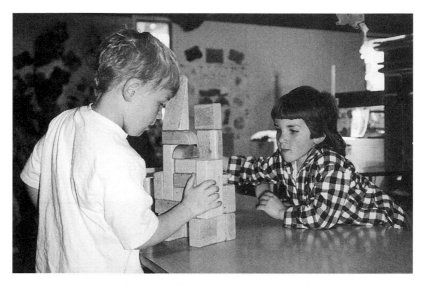

Figure 12.3   Child peers reinforcing a behavior.

Functional Behaviors

Functional behaviors refers to specific behaviors that the child needs to attain to succeed in the environment. These are the behaviors that one tries to reinforce so that the behaviors will become a more permanent part of the child's repertoire. From an occupational therapy perspective, the therapist looks at the component parts that will lead to the specific skills that the child needs to acquire. The therapist shapes or reinforces any behaviors that will contribute to the skill acquisition, which is the goal of the intervention. A set of behaviors is acquired, which will ultimately assist the child to achieve the skill. For example, when one is working with a child on self feeding, the therapist will probably begin working on grasping skills so that the child eventually acquires the ability to pick up the food and finger feed. As this intervention progresses, work on grasping skills will continue and be refined to picking up a utensil such as a spoon. Then the therapist will teach the child to use the spoon to scoop food onto it. The therapist approximates the skills that are needed to perform the final task (i.e., eating with utensils) through the use of other activities, which will lead to functional behavior. Functional behavior is dependent on context. The context is predominant in determining what is functional and what is truly necessary.

Learned Skills

Learned skills focuses on the skills that need to be acquired for performance in the specific environment. The integration of the context of the environment and functional behaviors results in learned skills. Behaviors have been shaped to the specific skills that are needed, and the environment focuses on that need. To identify those learned skills that are essential for the child, one must consider the environment and the functional behaviors that are present.

Reinforcement

Reinforcement refers to the environmental stimulus that rewards or does not reward behavior. Reinforcement takes place through the environment, which includes the social and cultural context. Skill development and it's subsequent adaptive responses to environmental stimuli is contingent, or dependent upon, positive (rewards) and negative (does not reward) reinforcement. In the acquisitional frame of reference, higher level skill development begins with the simple and progresses to the complex. Additionally, the environment is structured in such a way as to provide the learner with the greatest likelihood for success (Skinner, 1953). Reinforcement is used to encourage the development of behaviors and skills and to shape them so that they will occur more frequently.

As previously stated, *positive reinforcement* strengthens behavior by rewarding the desired behavioral response. Skill development is thus contingent upon positive reinforcement. Reinforcement can be tangible (e.g., food and money) or non-tangible (e.g., words of encouragement, praise, and hugs) (Figure 12.4). For children, reinforcement that incorporates a physical and emotional human response can be extremely powerful. While the use of positive reinforcement is the cornerstone of the development of skills and adaptive responses, the extinction of non-adaptive behaviors is dependent on the use of negative reinforcement.

Negative reinforcement is used to extinguish non-adaptive behaviors. Examples of non-adaptive behavior are the inability to make eye contact when it would be appropriate or not remaining seated when it is socially appropriate to do so. When behavior is ignored, it is negatively reinforced.

Punishment is the use of physical or verbal acts to extinguish behaviors that are perceived as not being valuable or appropriate. It is important not to categorize punishment solely as a negative reinforcement. For some children, punishment is a positive reinforcement in that it results in the acquisition of non-adaptive behaviors. To illustrate, if a child is punished for hitting another child, the child learns that they will be punished if someone sees him or her hit another child. The child may then pursue non-adaptive behavior such as hitting when no teacher or other student is around. In this example, punishment does not extinguish behavior, and it can be reinforcing it by providing attention to the individual (Skinner, 1951, 1954). For other children, punishment can serve as a negative reinforcer. When one child hits another and is then sent to "time out" as punishment, he or she may stop hitting behaviors.

Vicarious reinforcement is used to describe learning that occurs through observation. Vicarious reinforcement occurs when a child has observed the positive or negative reinforcement of behavior in other children (Bandura, 1965). Bandura proposed that learning does not only take place through direct experience; children can learn or

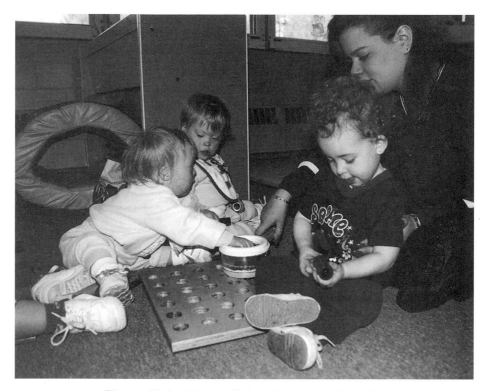

Figure 12.4 Nontangible reinforcement of a child.

acquire new behaviors simply by observing the reinforced or non-reinforced behaviors of others, hence the term *"modeling"* (Bandura, 1965, 1977). Children learn and develop skills by observing children and other models such as teachers, parents, or therapists who are performing the desired skill (Figure 12.5).

Schedules of reinforcement are the ways, time intervals, and methods of organizing reinforcement so that it will promote the acquisition (i.e., increasing or decreasing particular behaviors or skills). There are three main types of reinforcement schedules. They are continuous, partial, and intermittent. A continuous reinforcement schedule, sometimes referred to as contingency reinforcement or management schedule, is when the reward is given every time the behavior occurs. Every response is reinforced. This is thought to lead to a rapid acquisition of the behavior (Kaplan & Sadock, 1998), although this may not be the most effective reinforcement schedule for permanency of acquisition. Partial reinforcement is when reinforcement is only given some of the time that the behavior occurs, and there is no discernible pattern as to when the reinforcement will take place. Partial reinforcement is thought to be the strongest form of reinforcement in shaping behaviors (Hergenhahn, 1988). With this form of reinforcement, the subject does not know when they will be rewarded and, therefore, tends to exhibit the desired behaviors more frequently. Behaviors

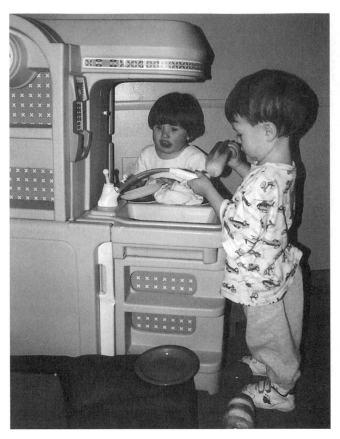

Figure 12.5   Modeling a desired skill.

shaped in this manner are also the hardest to extinguish. Intermittent reinforcement refers to reinforcement that is based on some sort of intervals. A fixed ratio would be when the reinforcement occurs at regular intervals, such as every fifth response. A variable ratio is when reinforcement occurs at varying intervals, such as every third time, then after the fifth time, and then every second time.

Shaping

Shaping means rewarding close approximations of a desired skill. For occupational therapists, this draws heavily on the understanding of activity analysis. The therapist can analyze the activity and understand its components parts. From that understanding, the therapist can shape a desired skill by building on each component part of the task. In this situation, it is important to understand the parts of the task in addition to the whole activity. Shaping of skills is accomplished in small increments with close approximations of the desired behavior rewarded (Figure 12.6). For example, if a child was learning to dress independently and put his or her pants on all

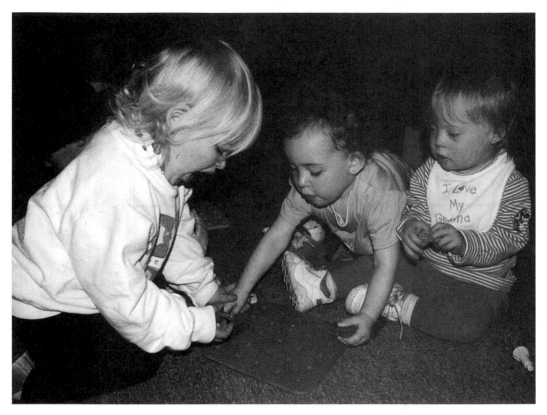

Figure 12.6 Children providing positive reinforcers.

by himself or herself, it would not matter if the pants were on backward, as long as the child did it independently. Thus, dressing is being "shaped."

Generalization

Once a behavior or skill is firmly established, the ability to maintain the skill becomes intrinsically reinforced. In other words, performing the behavior or skill correctly (performance results is the desired goal) in and by itself becomes self-reinforcing (Bandura, 1977). It is suggested that behaviors that are self-reinforcing are providing some level of meaning to the person. Some believed that it is ultimately an intrapsychic event that underlies response to reinforcement. However, intrapsychic events are not a major component of response to reinforce shaping behavior.

Functional Relationship Between the Child and the Environment

According to behaviorists, all behavior is shaped by the environment (Norman, 1976). Although not readily apparent, the environment provides positive and negative reinforcements. It is the role of the therapist to observe and identify what and how stimuli in the environment are shaping a child's behavior. In addition to the positive and negative reinforcing value the environment holds, experience and exposure to environmental stimuli provide children with the opportunity to acquire new skills.

One critical aspect of the environment is the therapist. The therapist creates the environment and sets the tone for the intervention. In this frame of reference, the works of Rogers (1951, 1957) contribute an important element, that of unconditional positive regard. This construct is used as a platform for all interventions. The therapist accepts the child for who he or she is. The atmosphere created is one of acceptance. This does not mean that all behaviors are accepted, but that child is accepted unconditionally. Children behave in ways that will gain positive reinforcement from others. Children want the love of their parents and, therefore, act accordingly. This type of environment is a powerful tool for reinforcement. According to Rogers (1995), change is more likely to occur when the therapist accepts the client at their current level of functioning.

Assumptions

This frame of reference has four major assumptions that collectively constitute the core beliefs underpinning the acquisitional frame of reference.

The first principal assumption is that intrapsychic dimensions are irrelevant to the behavior shaped by the environment. Considering the age old debate between "nature" and "nurture," this assumption states that "nurture" is all important and that all behavior is determined by the past and current environment. Consequently, there is little room for "meaning" or for intrapsychic dimensions that a person may bring to the behavior. Environment, as used here, refers to the physical, social, and cultural dimensions external to the body.

The second assumption is that the therapist accepts the child unconditionally and without judgment. This creates the environment that is conducive to learning and the development of functional skills. Children can learn by interacting and observing other children and adults. They behave in ways that will gain them positive reinforcement from others, especially people important to them such as mothers, fathers, and teachers. This assumption is a platform upon which intervention is based.

The third assumption is that competence, or the belief that one can act and have influence over the environment, results from learning skills. Thus, it is the acquisition of skills—hence the name "acquisitional frame of reference"—and not intrapsychic processes, which is of paramount importance to mastery and self-competence.

Fourth, it is believed that learning does not necessarily follow a developmental sequence. It stands to reason that according to this frame of reference, a deficit in one performance area does not predict, predicate, or necessarily correlate with a deficit or problem in another performance area. And, development of skill(s) to function in the environment does not require reconstructing, re-experiencing, or mastering previous developmental stages. Instead, specific skill(s) needed to function in a particular environment is what is paramount.

THEORETICAL POSTULATES

Theoretical postulates state the relationship between concepts in the theoretical base. Three main postulates are professed in the acquisitional frame of reference. They are

- Acquisition of skills is as a result of reinforcement, which results in learning
- Function is not stage specific
- Behaviors result from environmental interaction

Acquisition of skills refers to the idea that behavior, or observable human activity, is predominately influenced or primarily effected by the environment through negative and positive reinforcement. Positive reinforcement results in a learned behavior. Negative reinforcement results in getting rid of unwanted behaviors or maladaptive behaviors. To teach skills, therefore, behavior must be (1) reinforced directly or (2) reinforced through seeing someone else being positively or negatively reinforced. Skills, therefore, cannot be developed and refined just through repetition. Each time a child performs a newly learned skill correctly, positive reinforcement must occur. Schedules of reinforcement include (1) continuous reinforcement, (2) partial reinforcement, and (3) intermittent reinforcement, which can be a fixed ratio reinforcement or variable ratio reinforcement. General principles for management of reinforcement programs are provided in Table 12.1. In addition to these general management principals, it is important to be aware of a hierarchy of reinforcers (MacMillan, 1973). In other words, some reinforcers are stronger than others (Table 12.2).

Table 12.1   General Management Principles for Reinforcement Schedules

Generally, newly established behavior is best maintained with continuous or frequent reinforcement during its early stages. Later, it can be maintained with intermittent reinforcement, and ideally, extrinsic rewards can be dropped completely as the desired behaviors become internalized.

Punishment tends to become ineffective if not applied at most or all instances of the undesired behavior. This is one of several reasons it is generally better to concentrate on reinforcing alternative, desirable behaviors, rather than relying on punishment. Witness the dismal record of trying to enforce highway speed limits with an occasional citation, regardless of the size of the accompanying fine.

In regard to positive reinforcement, the seductive quality of variable ration, essentially random, reinforcement should be capitalized upon when practical. The knowledge that any given effort may achieve success has for years kept people in the hot sun pulling the cord of bulky lawnmowers and in stuffy casinos pulling the level of "one-armed bandits" with extraordinary frequency.

Adapted from Simons-Morton, B. G., Greene, W. H., & Gottlieb, N. H. (1995). *Introduction to health education and health promotion (2nd ed)*. Prospect Heights, IL: Waveland Press.

Table 12.2 Hierarchy of Positive Reinforcers.

Type of Reward	Example
Primary rewards	Food, M & M's, Dairy Queen treats
Toys or trifles	Plastic insects, bauble rings, stickers
Tokens and stars	Collection of items or marks to qualify for a larger reward
Seeing one's progress	Grades, charting, graphing, or otherwise visually presenting level of progress
Social approval	Verbal comments such as "Good job"; Facial expression and body language
Intrinsic reward	Feeling good about oneself for doing the target behavior

Adapted from Simons-Morton, B. G., Greene, W. H., & Gottlieb, N. H. (1995). *Introduction to health education and health promotion* (2nd ed). Prospect Heights, IL: Waveland Press.

Function is not stage specific. This statement means that the environment and events therein are more important in determining the behavior of an individual than are the developmental stages of an individual. This frame of reference assumes that individual function is more important that any identifiable stages of development. Further, the specific stages of development bear no relevance to this frame of reference. Rather, the most important determinant of behavior is the environment and what the environment elicits in terms of behavior or function. Thus, function is considered in quantitative terms (i.e., the child can do a specific task or cannot do that task). Initially, quality is secondary to the ability to perform a function, although it may become more important later. Function is the goal rather than achieving a specific developmental task. Function is not acquired in any specific order and can be acquired in any order based on the reinforcement provided to the child.

Adaptive behavior results from environmental interaction. If overall behavior is a result of environmental demand, then adaptive behavior results from interaction with an environment that has been or is designed for learning a particular skill. Adaptive behavior, as used here, refers to changes in behavior to accommodate new challenges in the environment.

FUNCTION/DYSFUNCTION CONTINUA

The acquisitional frame of reference is somewhat unique from other frames of reference in that continua of function and dysfunction are defined by the specific behavior to be acquired. That is, the child can either perform a skill needed to function in the environment or he or she cannot. Thus, there are no specific continua defined for function and dysfunction within this acquisitional frame of reference. When generating a specific function/dysfunction continua for a child, a criterion-referenced dichotomous measure is used (yes, the child can perform the specific skill; or no, the child cannot perform the skill). Or, function and dysfunction is determined by the environment within which the skill must be performed.

Furthermore, a child's developmental status provides a background only for this frame of reference; it is not of major importance. Developmental status is only considered when determining if the specific skill to be acquired is appropriate at that developmental stage. For example, a 3-year-old developmentally would not be learning to write words. That skill would not be one to work on with that child. However, a 3-year-old child should be dressing himself or herself, and that would be an appropriate skill to be acquired at that stage of life.

Once it has been determined that the skill is necessary for the child to function in his or her environment, then the specific skill is analyzed and divided into its component tasks. These tasks are further divided into component aspects. A skill specific function/dysfunction continua is developed that lists the required components to complete the skill. Any task that cannot be performed independently and is needed for the environment is considered dysfunctional. Often, tasks, which need to be acquired, must be shaped or increased in terms of frequency of occurrence.

Function/dysfunction continua can be identified for any skill that is necessary for the child to perform within the environment. It can range from simply the ability to make eye contact, to independence in activities of daily living (ADL) skills, to the ability to interact in a socially appropriate manner. Skills in the acquisitional frame of reference are always environmentally specific. It is important whether a child can do a specific skill, not how well a child can do that specific skill.

For illustrative purposes, examples of function and dysfunction within this frame of reference are provided using specific ADLs.

Indicators of Function/Dysfunction

It is difficult, if not impossible, to discuss function and dysfunction in a general manner because the behavior is so environmentally specific. Rather, behavior must be at an appropriate level for the child and always be linked to the specific content of the environment. Further, the environment is an important determinant of the behaviors to be learned. For this example, some ADLs will be used for a toddler at home. The first task would be self-feeding. Within this frame of reference, any attempt at self feeding would be acceptable as a starting point. Indicators of function would be being able to grasp the spoon (Figure 12.7), scoop food onto the spoon, and move the spoon to the mouth while losing minimal food. It would not matter if the child gets most of the food on his or her face or clothes as long as he or she attempts to

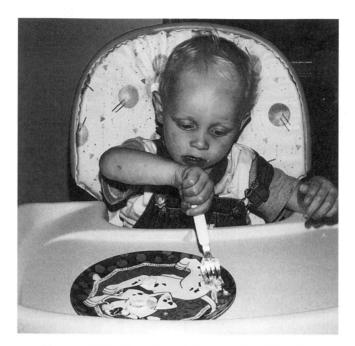

Figure 12.7 Grasping a fork to begin self-feeding.

self-feed. Further, it would not matter if self-feeding is done with much protest, as long as the child made an attempt at self-feeding. Indicators of dysfunction would be not attempting to self-feed, not being able to hold the spoon, not being able to scoop food onto the spoon, not being able to move the spoon to the mouth or dropping the majority of the food before it gets to the mouth. All attempts at self-feeding or any component parts of self-feeding would be reinforced so that behaviors could be shaped to develop good functional skills (Chart 12.1).

The next example is putting on one's pants for the same child at home. The ability to put on pants is the issue, not how well one can do this task. Indicators of function would be orienting the pants properly, being able to put one leg in, then putting the other leg in, and finally pulling up the pants. Indicators of dysfunction would be not orienting the pants properly, not being able to put one or the other leg in, or not being able to pull up the pants. Any attempt at putting on one's pants or any component parts would be reinforced so that behaviors can be shaped to develop good functional skills (Chart 12.2).

GUIDE FOR EVALUATION

This section will address how a therapist would approach the evaluation process in the acquisitional frame of reference. Essentially, the guide for evaluation in the acquisitional frame of reference begins with a general observation. The therapist needs

---

Chart 12.1   Indicators of Function and Dysfunction for Self Feeding.

Ability to Self Feed	**Inability to Self Feed**
FUNCTION: Ability to self feed	DYSFUNCTION: Inability to self feed
INDICATORS OF FUNCTION	**INDICATORS OF DYSFUNCTION**
Able to grasp and hold the spoon	Unable to grasp and hold the spoon
Able to scoop food onto the spoon	Unable to scoop food onto the spoon
Able to move spoon to mouth with minimal loss of food from the spoon	Unable to move spoon to the mouth
[Any attempts would be considered acceptable.]	

Chart 12.2   Indicators of Function and Dysfunction for a Toddler Putting on His or Her Pants

Ability to Put on Pants	**Inability to Put on Pants**
FUNCTION: Ability to put on pants	DYSFUNCTION: Inability to put on pants
INDICATORS OF FUNCTION	**INDICATORS OF DYSFUNCTION**
Able to orient pants properly	Unable to orient pants properly
Able to put one leg into pants	Unable to put one leg into pants
Able to put the other leg into pants	Unable to put the other leg into pants
Able to pull up pants	Unable to pull up pants
[Any attempts would be considered acceptable]	

---

to observe the child within the environment and be able to identify the demands of the environment to determine the required skills.

The most powerful tool the therapist possesses in implementing this frame of reference is the power of observation. Given that each performance, task, or activity is so specific to the environment at hand, most standardized tests would not be appropriate to assess a child in context using this frame of reference. The therapist combines his or her knowledge of the age-appropriate levels of tasks with an understanding of the child and the environment and it's demands. Thus, the classic expertise of therapist observation is the most powerful and appropriate guide for evaluation available for use in this frame of reference.

The therapist begins by observing, within a specific environmental setting, whether a required skill can be performed. The skills can be performed or not. This is criterion-based, in that the task, environment, and child's skill level determines what comprises the ability to perform the skill or not. Remember the evaluation determines the ability or not to perform the skill. Consideration of how well the skills are done is not part of the evaluation, although this will determine intervention to some degree. The following series of questions can assist the therapist in determining the presence of function or dysfunction.

- What are the observable skills of the individual within the environment?
- What are the physical characteristics of the environment in which the individual needs to perform?
- What are the sociocultural characteristics of the environment in which the individual needs to perform?
- What additional skills, if any, are required in the current environment?

Because the acquisitional frame of reference is accordingly *individualized,* it requires considerable skill on the part of the therapist. Each particular question should be addressed. Thus, there are no established evaluation protocols for this frame of reference, and each one developed should be specific to the child receiving intervention. The therapist must determine what skills need to be acquired by the child for the child to be successful within the environment.

Once the therapist identifies the demands of the environment and whether the child can perform these tasks, he or she needs to do a more focused observation. This will provide information about the component parts of the tasks of the environment and what is encouraging or interfering with the child's performance. This also requires classic skills of the therapist (i.e., the ability to analyze the activity and understand the component parts to determine if and how these component parts are interfering with the performance of the task and potential positive and negative reinforcers). This will help the therapist determine the more specific areas that require intervention and what reinforcer(s) will be effective within this setting.

- What are the specific component parts of the tasks?
- Which of these component parts can the child do well, and which require intervention?
- Which skills need to be shaped?
- What are identifiable positive and negative reinforcements?
- What constitutes a positive reinforcer and what constitutes a negative reinforcer for the child in question?
- Within this environment, which would be the most powerful positive reinforcers?

Assessment is, therefore, observation of performance of the skill in context. Assessment further involves the identification of the tasks required by the environment, the component parts of the tasks and the positive and negative reinforcers present in the environment which influence skill development.

POSTULATES REGARDING CHANGE

Postulates regarding change delineate the therapeutic environment that needs to be created and suggests the methods used by the therapist to facilitate change. For the acquisitional frame of reference, eight postulates have been identified. When the results of evaluation indicate dysfunction, intervention focuses on the acquisition of component parts of skills or specific skills. These learned skills are necessary to be successful within the environment.

The first 2 postulates are general postulates for this frame of reference.

1. If the therapist provides positive reinforcement specific to the child and the environment, then the child will be more likely to acquire component parts of skills or specified skills.
2. If the therapist provides negative reinforcement specific to the child and the environment, then non-adaptive behaviors will be more likely to be extinguished.

Once a deficit has been identified, the next 6 postulates relate more specifically to intervention.

3. If the therapist provides reinforcement that is specific to the child and the environment, then the child will be more likely to acquire component parts of skills or specified skills.
4. If the therapist uses a variety of schedules of reinforcement specific to the child and the environment, then the child will be more likely to acquire component parts of skills or specified skills.
5. If the therapist provides reinforcement for any attempt at a behavior, then that behavior is more likely to be acquired.
6. If the therapist reinforces component parts of a skill, then behavior will be shaped so that the skill can be acquired.
7. If a child acquires specific skills and those skills are reinforced, then the skill has the potential of being self-reinforcing and generalizable to other settings.
8. If reinforcement is consistent across settings, then skills are more likely to be acquired.

APPLICATION TO PRACTICE

The acquisitional frame of reference is frequently used in occupational therapy. It is so much a part of occupational therapy practice that therapists frequently are not aware that they are using it. Yet, a behavior or skill that is viewed as beneficial to the child is rewarded with positive reinforcement, and one that is viewed as negative meets with negative reinforcement and attempts to extinguish that behavior. The acquisitional frame of reference can comfortably stand alone as a frame of reference, or it can be used in conjunction with other frames of reference that are consistent with learning theories.

To use the acquisitional frame of reference, the occupational therapist needs to identify the specific skill or behavior that he or she wants to develop. That skill or behavior should be one that is compatible with and necessary for optimal, or at least improved, functioning within the environment. If it is a complex skill, then the therapist must first analyze it and break it down into component parts. To develop this skill or behavior, it may be necessary to first work on component parts. Once that skill, behavior, or necessary component part has been identified, the therapist needs to identify a reinforcer that is valuable to the child and the environment. It may be praise, a token, or a sticker, but it has to be something that the child wants and is compatible with the environment (Figure 12.8). Then the therapist would provide this reinforcement whenever the child makes an attempt at the desired behavior. The quality of the attempt is not important; it is solely the attempt that is important. This exemplifies the first postulate regarding change (i.e., if the therapist provides positive reinforcement specific to the child and the environment, then the child will be more likely to acquire component parts of skills or specified skills).

The same approach is used with negative or nonadaptive behaviors. The therapist would need to identify the behavior that is maladaptive. The therapist would identify a negative reinforcer that is specific and has relevance to the child and is compatible with the environment. It can be anything that the child doesn't want to occur, like being put in "time out," being sent to one's room, or having dessert withheld. This negative reinforcer is used when the behavior appears, and with repeated use, the negative

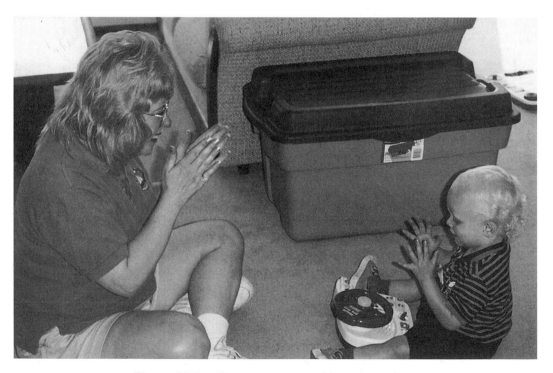

Figure 12.8 Clapping as a reward for a desired act.

reinforcer is likely to extinguished that behavior. It is critical that the positive or negative reinforcer be specific and meaningful to the child and the environment for them to be effective. The child will work harder for something that he or she values highly and will modify behavior to avoid something that he or she does not like. It is incumbent on the therapist to match the reinforcers, both positive and negative, with the child and the environment to achieve maximum success with this frame of reference.

The schedules of reinforcement presented in the theoretical base are important to the use of the frame of reference. The child will be more likely to acquire a skill or behavior if a variety of reinforcement schedules are used. The child may come to expect praise for each attempt if it is offered every time, yet the child may work harder when that reinforcement is less predictable and come at random intervals. The therapist needs to match the reinforcement schedule with the child and often needs to try different schedules to see which one works better.

The quality of performance is not initially important in this frame of reference. The child gets reinforcement for all or a majority of attempts at a task. This includes the component parts of that skill. If the child is rewarded when attempting something, then he or she is more likely to make additional attempts at the task. The focus on quality does not come until much later, if at all. At this point, it is more important to reward the child for continued work on that skill or behavior, and positive reinforcement will provide that reward. This provides the basis for the acquisition of more complex skills (Figure 12.9). As each component of a desired behavior or skill is rewarded, it gradually becomes integrated into the child's repertoire. As the skill acquisition progresses, the therapist shapes the behavior through requiring more complex skills or behaviors before a reward is given.

For example, when a child is learning to self-feed, he or she initially eats with fingers. This tends to be messy, yet the therapist will ignore the mess and provide positive reinforcement for attempts at self-feeding. When the child "graduates" to using a spoon, the therapist may give positive reinforcement for just scooping the food onto the spoon, which is a component part of eating with a spoon. This is shaping the behavior. The therapist is letting the child know that this is a valued act and is part of the skill of self-feeding (Figure 12.10). Then when the child brings the spoon with some food on it to his or her mouth, the child is rewarded again, continuing the shaping of the skill. Yet, when the child flings the spoon and the food onto the floor, the therapist would give negative reinforcement in hopes of extinguishing that behavior. The focus is on rewarding the positive attempts, ignoring the quality of performance, and using negative reinforcement to extinguish unwanted behaviors. Further, as the child is able to feed himself or herself, the behavior itself becomes rewarding, reinforcing itself. This reinforcement allows the child to begin to generalize. Self-feeding is seen as important, and the child begins to understand its importance, not just during the time of the intervention but at any time.

Once a child has been referred for an evaluation, the first step in the process is to observe the child in his or her natural environment. This may be the home setting,

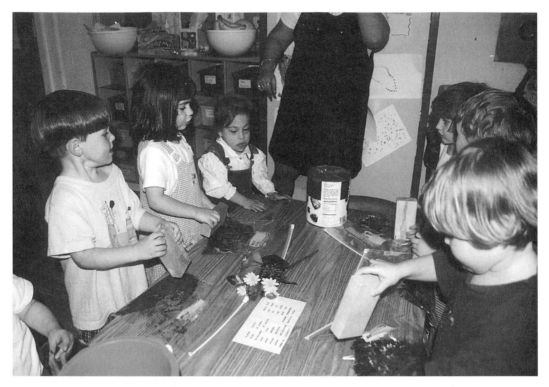

Figure 12.9   Social interaction supports skill development.

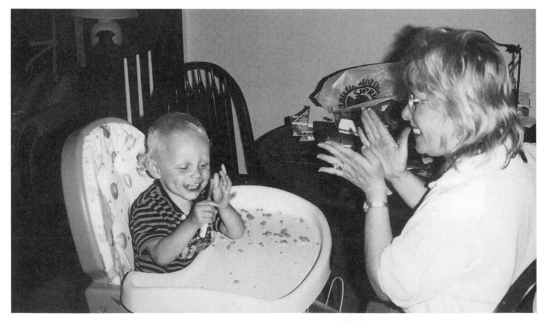

Figure 12.10   The valued skill of self-feeding.

school, or playground or at a social gathering. The therapist is observing the child's behavior and is simultaneously observing the physical and social environment and the interaction between the child and the environment (Figure 12.11). It is critical to identify what constitutes positive reinforcers and negative reinforcers (as well as potential reinforcers) within the setting. In the Midwest, Dairy Queen desserts are popular. If the child is old enough to eat ice cream, and this is a valued treat, then a Dairy Queen dessert may be a good positive reinforcer.

The following is another example, which is different and more complex. While observing Jose in the classroom, you notice the other children laughing when he disturbs the class by falling out of his chair. The children's laughter positively reinforces Jose. You also observe that Jose falls from his chair with greater frequency toward the end of the school day. As the therapist, it is a challenge to identify if Jose falls out of his chair to receive positive reinforcement, or falls out of his chair because he is unable to maintain postural stability against gravity.

Regardless of the reason for Jose's falling out of the chair, he needs to be able to maintain a sitting posture in his chair for class periods. Jose has two different issues interfering with sitting posture, both of which can be addressed with the acquisitional frame of reference. The first would be to remove the positive reinforcement Jose is receiving from the class (i.e., the laughter). This could be accomplished by working with the teacher, explaining that Jose is not being a class clown but that he

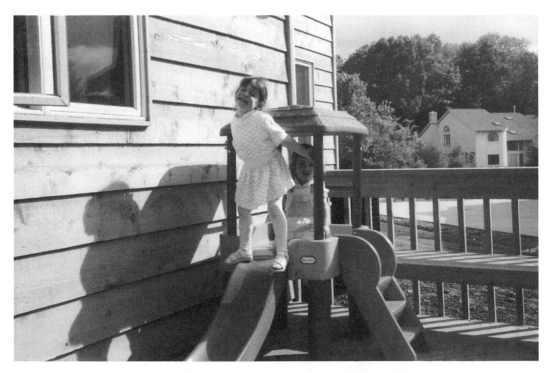

Figure 12.11 Observing children interacting in their natural environment.

has a problem remaining in his seat. The teacher can explain this to the class in a way that is not hurtful to Jose, explaining that Jose cannot help this behavior. The therapist could also work with the teacher to set up a positive reinforcement schedule for the rest of the class predicated upon not laughing when Jose falls out of his seat.

The second issue is that Jose actually does have a problem with performance components underlying sitting stability. During observation, it is noted that Jose "slumps in his chair," "props his elbows on his desk," "holds his chin in his hands," and constantly repositions himself, or "fidgets." The therapist explores the component parts of sitting stability to determine the behaviors to be shaped. A positive reinforcement schedule can then be developed that rewards Jose for the component parts of sitting stability or whenever more appropriate or desirable seating behavior is displayed. The therapist may ask the teacher to call Jose's attention to when he is sitting properly while simultaneously giving verbal approval by stating, "Good job, Jose!"

In the initial phases of intervention, Jose should be rewarded for close approximations of desired behaviors. Thus, positive reinforcement of "almost" or "sort of" sitting appropriately should be mutually decided upon by the therapist and others. Subsequently, a grading of the target behavior unfolds. Over time, higher standards of sitting or sitting for longer periods of time in the upright position should be maintained prior to receiving a reward. Monitoring of the effectiveness of the positive reward should be conducted throughout the treatment intervention to make certain that satiation does not occur. Using more than one type of reward is beneficial in preventing this from happening (Table 12.2).

It is important to note that during this intervention, all other behaviors should be ignored by all involved. This may prove challenging, and constant communication about its importance may be required for the all people involved with the child. Reinforcement may be needed for Jose and the teachers, staff, students, and parents who encompass Jose's environment. Further, the therapist may periodically have to change the reinforcers being used or modify the schedule of reinforcement for the program to be effective.

Generalization of Jose's sitting behavior can be accomplished by collaboration with all teachers and other service providers involved. That is, if all involved staff were appropriately trained or educated to (1) recognize when Jose is sitting appropriately, (2) how to reward him for such sitting, and (3) how to ignore unwanted behaviors, the likelihood of generalization across sites and settings is increased. Optimal generalization would be maximized by also working with the family. Although it not necessary for all parties involved to use the same reinforcer, everyone should be reinforcing and conversely ignoring the same behaviors.

Once the target behavior has been achieved, such as successive approximation of maintaining an upright posture in seat, switching from a continuous reinforcement schedule to some form of intermittent reinforcement or ratio schedule is appropriate. This will aid in strengthening the behavior. To continue with the previous example, the teacher will verbally praise Jose every third time, instead of every time, the target behavior is displayed. Further, when the child achieves the target behavior, the behavior will eventually become self-reinforcing and the child will be able to generalize that skill or behavior to other settings or situations.

SUMMARY

The acquisitional frame of reference focuses on the acquisition, or learning, of specific skills or subskills required to function optimally within the environment. The mastery of skills or appropriate behaviors is the primary goal of the frame of reference. The acquisitional frame of reference theoretical base is drawn from principles and assumptions based on learning theories, along with some principles from the work of Carl Rogers. Additionally, in this frame of reference, the therapist uses two important legitimate tools of the profession: the teaching learning process and activity analysis. Through the analysis of the skill or behavior to be acquired, the therapist identifies subskills or components that need to be learned. He or she then shapes skills or behaviors through the reinforcement of these components or subskills until the child achieves mastery of the behavior or skill. Mastery of the skill provides its own reinforcement, which allows the child to generalize that skill or behavior.

References

Bandura, A. (1965). Influence of a model's reinforcement contingencies on the acquisition of imitative responses. *Journal of Personality and Social Psychology, 11,* 589–595.

Bandura, A. (1977). *Social Learning Theory.* Englewood Cliffs, NJ: Prentice-Hall.

Guthrie, E. R. (1935). *The psychology of learning.* New York: Harper & Brothers.

Hergenhahn, B. R. (1988). *An introduction to theories of learning* (3rd ed). Englewood Cliffs, NJ: Prentice Hall.

Hinojosa, J., Kramer, P., & Pratt, P. N. (1996). Foundations of practice: Developmental principles, theories, and frames of reference. In J. Case-Smith, A. S. Allen, & P. N. Pratt (Eds.), *Occupational Therapy for Children* (3rd Ed.). St. Louis: Mosby.

Hollis, L. I. (1974). Skinnerian occupational therapy. *American Journal of Occupational Therapy, 28, 4,* 208–212.

Hull, C. L. (1951). *Essentials of behavior.* New Haven, CT: Yale University Press, Institute of Human Relations.

Hull, C. L. (1952). *A behavior system; an introduction to behavior theory concerning the individual organism.* New Haven, CT: Yale University Press.

Kaplan, H. I., Saddock, B. J. (1998). *Synopsis of Psychiatry* (8th ed.). Baltimore: Williams & Wilkins.

Lovaas, O. I., & Bucher, B. D. (1974). *Perspectives in Behavior Modification with Deviant Children.* Englewood Cliffs, NJ: Prentice-Hall.

MacMillan, D.L. (1973). *Behavioral modification in education.* New York: Macmillan.

Mosey, A. C. (1986). *Psychosocial Components of Occupational Therapy.* New York: Raven Press.

Norman, C. W. (1976). Behavior modification: a perspective. *American Journal of Occupational Therapy, 30, 8,* 491–494.

Pavlov, I. P. (1941). *Conditioned reflexes and psychiatry.* New York: International Press.

Rogers, C. R. (1951). *Client Centered Therapy.* Boston: Houghton Mifflin.

Rogers, C. R. (1957). The necessary and sufficient conditions of therapeutic personality change. *Journal of Consulting Psychology, 21*, 95–103.

Rogers, C. R. (1995). *On becoming a person: a therapist's view of psychotherapy.* Boston: Houghton Mifflin.

Rogers, C. R., & Freiberg, H. J. (1994). *Freedom to learn* (3rd ed.). New York: Merrill.

Rugel, R. P., Mattingly, J., Eichinger, M., & May Jr, J. (1971). The use of operant conditioning with a physically disabled child. *American Journal of Occupational Therapy, 25, 5*, 247–249.

Sieg, K. W. (1974). Applying the behavior model to the occupational therapy model. *American Journal of Occupational Therapy, 28, 7*, 421–428.

Simons-Morton, B. G., Greene, W. H., & Gottlieb, N. H. (1995). *Introduction to health education and health promotion* (2nd ed). Prospect Heights, IL: Waveland Press.

Skinner, B. F. (1953). The science of learning and the art of teaching. *Harvard Educational Review, 24*, 86–97.

Skinner, B. F. (1954). *About Behavioralism.* New York: Knopf.

Skinner, B. F. (1971). *Science and Human Behavior.* New York: Macmillan.

Skinner, B. F. (1974). *Beyond Freedom and Dignity.* New York: Knopf.

Smith, A. R., & Tempone, V. J. (1968). Psychiatric occupational therapy within a learning context. *American Journal of Occupational Therapy, 22*, 415–420.

Thorndike, E. L. (1932). *Fundamentals of learning.* New York: Teachers College, Columbia University.

Tolman, E. C. (1932). *Purposive behavior in animals and men.* New York: The Century Co.

Tolman, E. C. (1958). *Behavior and psychological man; essays in motivation and learning.* Berkeley, CA: University of California Press.

Trombly, C. A. (1966). Principles of operant conditioning related to orthotic training of quadriplegic patients. *American Journal of Occupational Therapy, 20*, 217–220.

Wanderer, Z. W. (1974). Therapy as learning: Behavior therapy. *American Journal of Occupational Therapy, 28, 4*, 207–208.

Motor Skill Acquisition Frame of Reference

MARGARET T. KAPLAN / GARY BEDELL

Knowledge about motor skill acquisition is closely tied to the fields of motor learning, motor control, motor development, and principles from learning theory. This information is often classified as contributing to the more general field known as "movement sciences." Because motor skill acquisition is a relatively new area of study and is in early stages of development, theory is constantly being modified in response to new research results and information. There is no accepted motor skill acquisition model of treatment (Gentile, 1992). However, several authors and clinicians have attempted to illustrate the application of concepts from the movement sciences to their clinical practice (Carr & Shepherd, 1987; Goodgold-Edwards & Cermak, 1989; Haugen & Mathiowetz, 1995; Poole, 1995; Sabari, 1991). These reflect individual perspectives on a developing information base and different clinical experiences and issues related to different client populations.

EVOLVING MODEL OF SKILL ACQUISITION

Gentile (1987, 1992) has developed a model of skill acquisition that is based on knowledge from the movement sciences. The movement sciences draw on research and theory from motor learning and control, human ecology, cognitive and developmental psychology, biomechanics, muscle physiology, and neurophysiology. This model is particularly applicable to occupational therapy because of the emphasis on the therapeutic use of functional tasks and the active role of the learner. This chapter will present some of the basic assumptions, concepts, and principles from this model of skill acquisition and from other sources that have been found to be useful in pediatric practice. A guide to the clinical application of these assumptions, concepts, and principles will be presented. Although information from motor control and development will be presented, this frame of reference will emphasize information based on motor learning research.

Motor Learning, Motor Control, and Motor Development

Motor learning is the study of what movement processes associated with practice or experience lead to a relatively permanent change in a person's capability for skilled action (Schmidt, 1991). Current issues in this field include the role of feedback and types of practice in learning new skills and factors that influence transfer of learning from one skill to another and among different environments. The role of the goal and the task have been investigated by researchers in motor learning and motor control. There is substantial evidence that control mechanisms used are different and learning is improved when a person is involved in a purposeful, functional activity as opposed to being involved in a repetitive, non-purposeful activity or being moved by another person (Gliner, 1985; vanderWeel, vanderMeer & Lee, 1991; Thelen et al, 1993; Carr & Shepherd, 1987). Concepts and research from both will be presented in this chapter because the studies of motor control and motor learning have blended on many issues.

Motor control is the study of how movement is controlled by the musculoskeletal and central nervous systems. The major question addressed in this field is: How do the brain and body control movements? Specific issues are usually investigated with controlled experimental research of specific aspects of postural and movement control. Current issues in this field include the exploration of models of motor control that can explain how the many possible planes of motion or degrees of freedom in the joints are controlled by the musculoskeletal and central nervous system. Some of the areas under study are synergies, motor programs, coordinative structures, and neural networks (VanSant, 1991).

Motor development is the study of how motor behavior changes over the lifespan. Current issues address age differences in motor performance with development and maturation and the influences on motor development of factors such as genetics, maturation, body dimensions, environment, motivation, and expectations. The contemporary view of motor development recognizes that changes in motor skills can be the result of any of these factors. In addition, children develop motor skills in varied ways that are influenced by personal and environmental characteristics. These characteristics interact as the child searches for solutions to motor problems. This can explain why children use various strategies to perform activities and explore the environment. This is in contrast to traditional views that describe motor development as following a rigid sequence that is based on the maturation of the central nervous system.

THEORETICAL BASE

Dynamic Systems Theory

There has been a shift away from the traditional reflex hierarchical view of motor behavior to principles based on dynamic systems theory (Mathiowetz & Haugen,

1995). The traditional view of motor behavior and development assumes that motor control difficulties are caused by problems in the central nervous system. The problems in the central nervous system cause abnormal tone, which is, in turn, the cause of motor control difficulties. The developmental sequence is seen as necessary for normal development, and the central nervous system is viewed as hierarchical with "higher" centers controlling "lower" centers. A newer way of thinking about motor behavior is the *dynamic systems theory*, which has had an important effect on the current view of how movement is organized and learned (Bernstein, 1967; Kamm, Thelen, & Jensen, 1990). This theory views movement as emerging from the interaction of many systems. The three general systems are the person, the task, and the environment. Subsystems within the person can include emotional, cognitive, perceptual, sensory, motor, and other physical systems such as cardiovascular, musculoskeletal, and neurological. Systems outside of the person that influence motor performance and skill acquisition (e.g., the characteristics and complexity of the task and the environment in which it must be performed) are also considered.

All systems interact at one point in time to accomplish a particular goal. In this view, no one system has logical priority for directing or influencing the others. This is referred to in motor learning literature as a "heterarchical view." The subsystems in charge will vary with specific task requirements and environmental demands. The resulting movement is a solution to a particular problem that emerges from this interaction. The emergent motor behavior is usually the most efficient that is available given the condition of each individual system. Each individual develops preferred movement patterns for common functional tasks through active experimentation, experience, and practice. These most efficient or preferred patterns of moving have been referred to as *"attractor states"* (Mathiowetz & Haugen, 1995). This view of how movement is organized implies that the interaction of multiple systems can be affected by change in any one of them. The subsystems within the person, task, and environment that have a potential for change are often referred to as *"control parameters"* (Mathiowetz & Haugen, 1995). Control parameters are viewed as the subsystems that constrain task performance. If these subsystems are modified or changed, a new movement pattern may emerge. Therapists consider the child's preferred and most efficient patterns of moving (attractor states) and all of the person-task-environment subsystems (control parameters) affecting the child's task performance when planning intervention. This information is foundational for understanding the most current theoretical concepts of motor learning and for providing the reader with a background for understanding this frame of reference.

Principles of Learning Theory

This frame of reference employs several principles from learning theories (Gibson, 1969; Levine, 1987; Thorndike, 1932, 1935; Travers, 1977; Vygotsky, 1978). They involve practice, experimentation, variation, instruction, and feedback.

To acquire skills, the child must have the opportunity for practice and experimentation with a variety of strategies. One of the most important factors in acquiring new motor skills is the amount of practice (Gentile, 1992). Practice is when the child has the occasion to repeatedly try to produce motor behaviors that are challenging or beyond his or her current level (Schmidt, 1991). Through practice, the child can experiment with different types of solutions for motor problems. Random practice with varied tasks appears to be more effective for long-term learning (Schmidt, 1991). Practice is most effective when the child is challenged, while still keeping the goals attainable.

To promote the development of flexible strategies, the context of practice should have variation. Through this, the child can generalize the learned strategy from one task to another and from one setting to another (Lee, Swanson & Hall, 1991; VanSant, 1991). This is critical so that the child can utilize skills acquired in the therapy session in other settings. If practice can continue in the home and other environments of the child, then learning will be improved.

The zone of proximal development (Vygotsky, 1978) is a useful concept for designing activities and tasks with achievable goals. This zone refers to the actual developmental level of the child, what the child can achieve through independent problem solving, and the level of the child's potential for achieving the tasks with adult assistance. Adult support and instruction is essential in assisting children in mastering skills that are beyond their current capabilities. This concept has been used in the area of cognitive development in the past but seems to be just as applicable in the promotion of motor skill acquisition.

Motor learning and skill acquisition is enhanced by feedback given after performance. Feedback assists the child in understanding the results of his or her movements (Levine, 1987; Thorndike, 1932, 1935; Travers, 1977). Feedback, although frequently verbal, can consist of gestures, facial expressions, auditory and tactile cues, and, when necessary, manual guidance. Whenever feedback is used, it should be succinct and appropriate to the child's cognitive, language, and sensory abilities.

One research study (Winstein & Schmidt, 1990) has shown that frequent, consistent feedback is not effective for long-term learning. Therefore, it was proposed that feedback should be given after 50% of the movement attempts. Feedback decreases as learning progresses. Feedback should be given when the child's performance has more inaccuracy than is acceptable. Further, after the child has made several attempts at a task, it is quite effective to give summary feedback of performance, rather than feedback after every try (Schmidt, 1991).

As the child moves toward mastery of a task, he or she begins to use feedback from his or her own body to get information. This helps the child to understand the outcome of movements, anticipate upcoming events, and plan alternative strategies (Brooks, 1986). As the child develops more skill, he or she is encouraged to rely more on internal feedback and self evaluation of performance rather than external feedback from others.

Concepts

This section will describe the important concepts for understanding this frame of reference. These include the child, task, skill, environment, regulatory conditions, person-task-environment match, stages of learning, practice, and feedback.

Child

Subsystems within the child include emotional, cognitive, perceptual, sensory, motor, and other physical systems such as cardiovascular, musculoskeletal, and neurological. To use the motor skill acquisition frame of reference with a child, the therapist should understand what the child's abilities are in relation to all the previously mentioned subsystems. Understanding of the complexity of the child will have an impact on the guide to evaluation as the therapist will need to understand the child in the context of his or her life, his or her abilities, and his or her limitations to use this frame of reference.

Task

A task is a sequence of activities that share a purpose and goal. Tasks have characteristics related to their complexity, degree of structure, and purpose and are influenced by the social and physical demands of the environment (Christiansen, 1991). The impact of the environment on tasks is seen in the later discussion of regulatory conditions. By nature, tasks lend themselves to analysis so that the therapist can identify their component parts. A child will choose to engage in a specific task because it has meaning and purpose for that person. *Functional tasks,* which are goal-directed and important to the child and family, are the focus of intervention in this frame of reference (Mathiowetz & Haugen, 1995). The effects of relative levels of meaning and purpose on motor learning are in the beginning stages of study. Researchers in the field of occupational therapy have investigated the effect of adding purpose to activities used in intervention programs but have not always ensured that these activities have meaning for the individual person (Riccio, Nelson, & Bush, 1990; Sietsema et al., 1993). Purpose depends on meaning, which is individual and determined by many factors (Nelson, 1988; Ferguson & Trombly, 1997). For young children, the meaning of a particular task may be inferred by their level of interest and self selection. Caregivers and older children can be asked which activities are meaningful to them. Analyses of tasks or activities are extremely helpful to the understanding of task performance. Therapists analyze tasks and activities to identify their component parts and their meaning to the individual. This analysis plays an important part in determining the child-task-environment match.

Skill

Skill is defined as consistency in achieving a motor goal with economy of effort (Gentile, 1992). *Skilled movement* involves a person finding an optimal solution to the problem of performing a goal-directed task. Skill in performing a motor task does not imply that one specific motor pattern is used. There are many possible movement patterns and strategies that could be used to accomplish a specified task. For example, it cannot be assumed that children who have demonstrated skill in feeding themselves with a spoon are all using the same neuromotor organization in their movement strategies, even if their movement looks very similar to each other.

Environment

The environment in which a child performs a task is considered a major factor relevant to task performance in this frame of reference. Occupational therapists consider the physical, social, and cultural aspects of the environment when providing evaluation and intervention. The physical environment consists of nonhuman aspects that regulate the person's access to and performance in that environment. These features include characteristics of the natural terrain, buildings, furniture, objects, devices, flora, and fauna. The physical environment is embedded with multiple sources of sensory information that have an influence on motor skill acquisition such as light, sound, color, touch, texture, and form. The critical information or the distinctive features in the environment that the child has to attend to, process, and use to perform tasks efficiently are often referred to as *"affordances"* (Gibson, 1963; Gibson, 1966).

A child's social environment includes those significant people such as family, friends, and caregivers who are available to that person and have expectations for that person. Larger social groups are also significant because they influence the person's social norms, routines, and role expectations. The social environment can be a major influence on the selection and performance of tasks, goal achievement, and the perceived roles of others with regard to the child's motor skill acquisition.

The cultural environment refers to the customs, beliefs, activity patterns, behavior standards, and expectations placed on a member of a particular group of people. It includes laws that affect access to resources and the person's opportunities for education and support (AOTA, 1994). Children, families, and other caregivers are often exposed to a variety of cultural environments. It is important to identify similarities and differences in cultural beliefs and expectations so that all individuals working with the child can support each other's roles as they relate to improving the child's motor skill acquisition.

Regulatory Conditions

Regulatory conditions are aspects of the environment that determine movement specifics such as force, timing, and distance or magnitude for successful task outcome (Gentile, 1987). Gentile (1987) classifies tasks on two dimensions based on regulatory conditions: whether the environment is stationary or in motion during the task and whether the environment varies each time the task is performed (inter-trial variability) (Figure 13.1). This system describes a continuum between open and closed tasks as defined below.

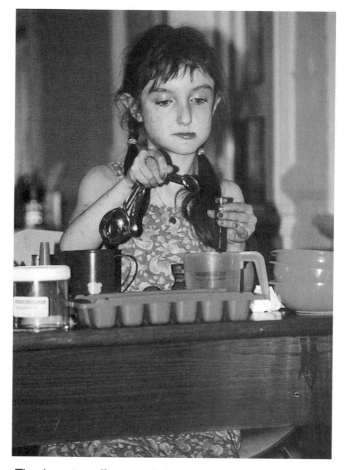

Figure 13.1 The therapist, off camera, helps the child attend to the important aspects of the task: the regulatory conditions.

Closed tasks are those in which the environment is stationary during the task performance. Some closed tasks have little variability during each performance (e.g., brushing teeth, washing hands and toileting) (Figure 13.2). Other closed tasks have more variability (e.g., self-feeding where variability is present from meal to meal with different foods, utensils, and set-up positions). Greater inter-trial variability places more demands on a child, and movement strategies must be more flexible than they need be in tasks with lesser inter-trial variability.

Open tasks are those in which the environment is in motion and include some inter-trial variability. These tasks place the most demands on a child (Figure 13.3). In addition to force and distance, movement strategies must take into account the regulatory condition of timing. Children with developmental and motor delays and disorders often have difficulty when timing becomes important to task completion.

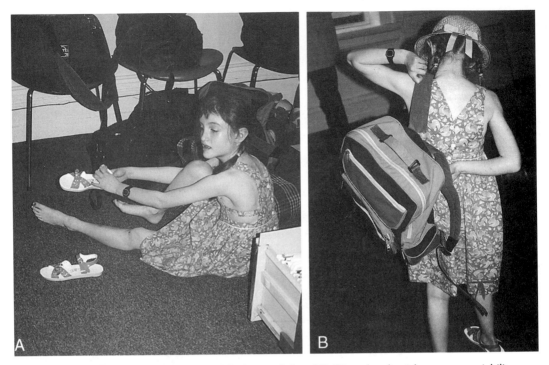

Figure 13.2 (A) Closed task with little variability. (B) Closed task with greater variability.

When a child is in early stages of learning a motor skill, Gentile's (1987) classification scheme suggests that a child should be given a closed task with lower demands before progressing to open tasks with higher demands. The type of practice needed to develop a motor skill in a closed task will entail repetitions in a less variable environment. Skill in an open task will require practice in an environment that includes variability in movement, timing, force, and magnitude.

Child-Task-Environment Match

A motor skill acquisition frame of reference is concerned with the child's ability to solve movement problems to accomplish everyday functional tasks in areas of self care, school, play, mobility, and communication. The tasks chosen to be addressed in occupational therapy must be important, meaningful, and achievable to the child based on his or her functional levels within the context of his or her family. It is important that there be a match between the capabilities of the child, the task demands, and the environmental characteristics in which the task is to be performed.

The characteristics of the task and environment can be modified to encourage the child to use different movement strategies (Kaplan, 1994). For example, a desired toy can be placed near the arm and hand that is not used as often or positioned higher in space to require increased use of shoulder extension. Hip adduction can be promoted

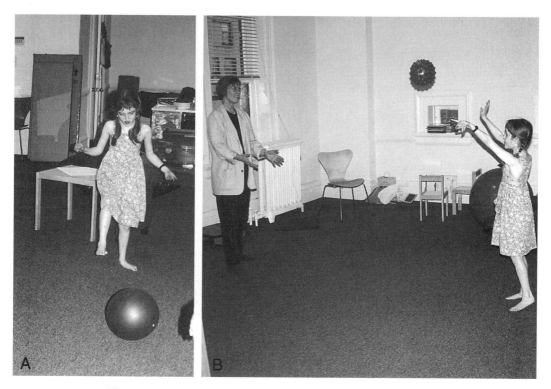

Figure 13.3   Open tasks with different demands on the child.

by having the child creep between two cushions placed close together. Toys or objects can be used that require the use of both hands or a specific type of manipulation.

Physical and sensory characteristics of the task or the environment can be important to a child's success and are often systematically manipulated during intervention. For example, a child may initially practice a task in an environment with low noise levels, subdued lighting, and little distraction from other children. The task could be adapted to include only tactile characteristics that are acceptable to the child. These sensory variables could be systematically changed as tolerated to represent the natural environment in which a child must perform the task. Other characteristics of the task can also be modified (e.g., the size, shape, texture, pliability, and amount of visual contrast and detail). Cognitive aspects of the task (e.g., number of steps, whether problem solving is required, and information processing demands) are also commonly analyzed and manipulated during intervention. The psychosocial demands of a specific task and environment may also be important to a child's ability to develop skill in that task (Figure 13.4). For example, if a child feels that their movement attempts may be successful and will meet with positive attention, they may be motivated to try harder and try more often than if there is little hope of positive feedback from others or if they are convinced that they will not be successful (Figure 13.5).

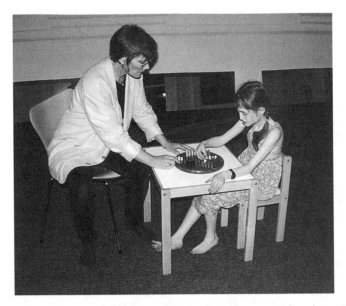

Figure 13.4 Very attentive child playing favorite board game with a therapist.

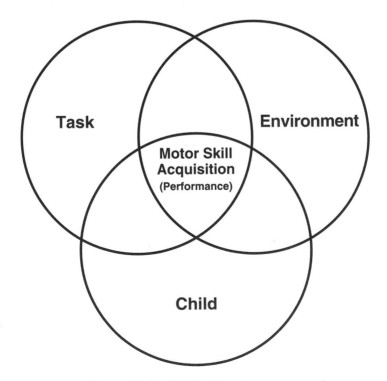

Figure 13.5 Child-task-environment match.

Stages of Learning

The acquisition of a motor skill is a process, and the requirements for practice, feedback, the role of the therapist, and the involvement of the learner are considered to vary based on the level of skill in a particular task for a particular learner. Gentile (1992) has described early and late stages of learning. During *early stages of learning*, the learner must find movement strategies to match the particular features of the task and environment to achieve the goal. To accomplish this, the child must engage in active problem solving, plan a movement, and evaluate the plan based on the outcome of the movement actually produced. This requires that the child focus on those conditions (affordances) in the environment that will determine the successful movement strategy. The learner must retain the goal and plan in memory. Then the actual movement and outcome must be compared with the information retained in memory. This process places substantial cognitive and attentional demands on the child and can present difficulty for many children with developmental delays and disorders (Figure 13.6).

At this stage, the environment needs to be structured to encourage the child to actively plan and experiment with movement strategies. One element of the environment is the adults who relate to the child. These adults can help the child to remember the goal and movement outcome and provide feedback on the outcome without focusing on the movement strategy used. Important conditions in the environment can be highlighted for the learner and he or she can be encouraged to try alternative strategies. Any movement pattern generated by the child at this early stage is acceptable. The specific movement pattern chosen by the child is considered less important than the child's active involvement and problem solving of the situation. Movement strategies that may be limiting to future or more complex movement and tasks can be modified by changing environmental conditions. For example, a child who prefers using only one hand and arm to reach for and manipulate toys or objects can be given motivating, exciting tasks or toys, for which the manipulation requires both hands.

During any movement, there are multiple joints and muscles to control, all of which can move in multiple directions. When first learning a new movement, it can be difficult to understand the most efficient way in which to control all of these possible movement options. This is sometimes called the "degrees of freedom" problem (Bernstein, 1967). In early stages of learning, the therapist should expect movements that involve co-contraction of opposing muscle groups (sometimes referred to as "fixing") and appear inefficient or awkward. These movements may be effective preliminary strategies for attempting a new motor skill when the child is experimenting with balance, coordination, and motor planning. The movement will not be smooth and flowing until the child has learned to coordinate multiple joints, muscles, and limbs and account for forces such as gravity (Gentile, 1992).

During *later stages of learning*, skill is developed in a particular task. Different tasks have different requirements based on the context and function of the action. At this

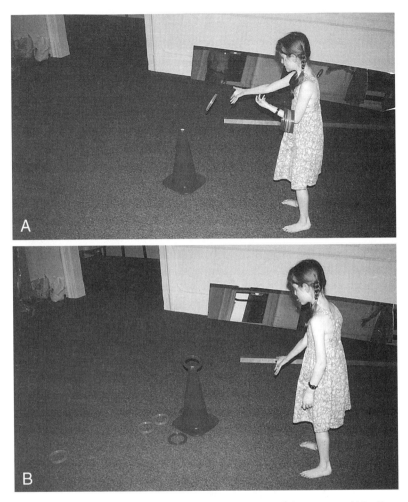

Figure 13.6 (A) The child focuses on the characteristics of the cone and it's distance from her. (B) A child has found a successful strategy after several unsuccessful attempts.

stage, a person can structure the conditions for practice and promote self-evaluation of the performance and outcome by the child. The child should be encouraged to rely less on others for informational feedback. For certain tasks, the emphasis will change from evaluating the outcome (successful or not) to more specifically monitoring and evaluating the performance and movement strategies used.

Practice

Practice and experimentation with varied strategies is essential to skill acquisition. The amount of practice is one of the most important factors in learning new motor skills (Gentile, 1992). Schmidt (1991) has defined practice as "repeated attempts to produce motor behaviors that are beyond present capabilities." The goal of practice is for the child to experiment with generating solutions to motor problems. Practice may be structured by a therapist in such a way that one task is practiced repeatedly before moving on to practice a different task. This is referred to as blocked practice. Random practice, where a person practices varied tasks in a random order, is another way to structure practice. Schmidt's (1991) review of recent research in motor learning has suggested that using random practice of varied tasks is better for long-term learning than blocked practice. Performance during the random practice session may initially appear worse than when using a blocked practice approach, but retention of learning is much improved when random practice is used. It seems that practice should be difficult and require effort to be most effective. For practice to be effective, one should strive to provide as much challenge as possible while keeping the goal achievable. Vygotsky's (1978) concept of the zone of proximal development is helpful in developing achievable goals, activities, and tasks. The zone of proximal development refers to the distance between those tasks that the child can perform completely on their own and those tasks that the child has the potential to perform with some assistance. With effective support and teaching, children can master the skills in their zone before they can master skills that are beyond it. Although this concept has been applied to cognitive development in the past, it may be useful in promoting learning of motor skills as well.

Variation in the context of practice can promote the learning of flexible strategies, which will be important for tasks in which there is more inter-trial variability. This will aid in the child's ability to more easily transfer a strategy from one context to another and may help to transfer a strategy from a therapy setting to a more natural setting in the community, school, or home (Lee, Swanson & Hall, 1991; VanSant, 1991). By analyzing the contexts in which the tasks are to be used, conditions that commonly vary can be considered when promoting skill acquisition. Practice in natural environments such as the home, classroom, and playground is optimal. If this is not possible, certain conditions may be simulated during practice.

The effectiveness of practicing a whole task versus separate parts of a task in isolation of the whole task has also been studied. Tasks that cannot easily be broken down into steps (e.g., riding a bicycle or throwing a ball) should be practiced as whole tasks. Some more complex tasks (e.g., cleaning a room) can be more easily broken down into steps and practiced as parts. However, attempting to practice balance separately from the manipulation aspect of reaching and grasping a toy or object will likely be less effective than practicing balance within the context of a functional activity such as reach and grasp of a cup for drinking or a toy for playing (Winstein, 1991).

Feedback

Feedback given after performance can affect motor learning and skill acquisition (Bly, 1996). Feedback given by others to help the child understand the outcome of his movement is often verbal but can also consist of gestures, facial expressions, auditory and tactile cues, and, when necessary, manual guidance. With increasing skill, the child will use feedback from his or her own body to get information about the outcome and to help plan alternative strategies. As time progresses, the child should be encouraged to become less dependent on feedback from others and more apt to evaluate his or her own performance. In early stages of learning, general feedback about performance, referred to as "summary" feedback, is thought to be more helpful than feedback that is more specific and detailed (Gentile, 1992).

It has been demonstrated that even in early stages of learning, constant feedback, or feedback after every attempt can impede retention of learning. Recent research studies suggest several strategies that may improve retention of skills (Winstein & Schmidt, 1990; & Winstein, 1991). Based on this research, feedback should be given after 50% of the movement attempts. As learning progresses, there should be a decrease or fading of feedback. Also, feedback given when a motor response has a greater than acceptable level of error (error range) and summary feedback after multiple attempts may be better than immediate feedback after every attempt (Schmidt, 1991). For instance, a child who is learning to feed himself or herself is not given feedback about performance after each spoonful even though some inaccuracy and spillage is observed. If the child spills the entire contents or misses the bowl, then feedback is given to help the child evaluate his or her performance and try another way to scoop and bring the spoon to his or her mouth. In this case, the therapist must decide on the error range before feedback is given. Summary feedback would be given after several spoon-to-mouth attempts and may take the form of comments like, "you are getting most of the food in your mouth" or "you are spilling much less that you did last week."

The content of the feedback used should be brief and appropriate to the child's cognitive, language and sensory abilities. For example, a child who has very limited receptive language abilities or a very young child may be given a series of hand claps, an exaggerated smile, or a pat on the back after several successful attempts. A child with limited visual abilities should be given feedback in an auditory or tactile form.

Feedback should focus on the goal of the movement or the task, not on a specific movement strategy. This is sometimes referred to as "knowledge of results" (KR) or "giving information feedback about the outcome" (IF-O) of the movement (Gentile, 1992). The feedback given would comment on the outcome, for example, "you spilled very little" or "you did it!" (Figure 13.7).

Informational feedback and suggestions can be given in different ways. The most common method is verbal, but a person can also model a different way of moving or can physically move the child using manual guidance to have them feel an alternative way of moving. Physical positioning or manual guidance is used only after other methods have been unsuccessful because it is the child who must generate the movement solution for learning to occur most efficiently (Figure 13.8). These methods can be used to encourage a child to try another movement strategy if the one they are us-

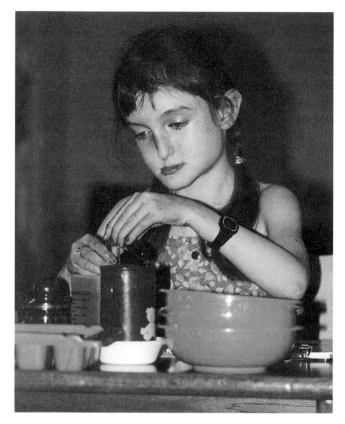

Figure 13.7 The therapist, off camera, provides verbal feedback to help the child understand that she has poured the liquid successfully.

ing is unsuccessful or inefficient. They may also be used to redirect a child to the task, remind them of the goals, or motivate the child to continue trying. Children often require help remembering the goal and attending to the characteristics in the environment, which are important to a successful outcome. The therapist may direct the child's attention to the object by using contrasting colors, by limiting extraneous sensory stimuli, or by using verbal, visual, or manual prompts to point out the salient characteristics. It may also be helpful to give feedback after a brief interval that allows the child to process his or her own feedback about the action (Gentile, 1992).

During later stages of learning, children may benefit from more specific feedback about their movement and alternate suggestions through "knowledge of performance" (KP) or "information feedback about the movement used" (IF-M) (Gentile, 1992). However, the therapist should encourage the child to become less reliant on feedback from the therapist and increase their ability to assess their own movement and performance. The content of feedback can include questions for the child to help

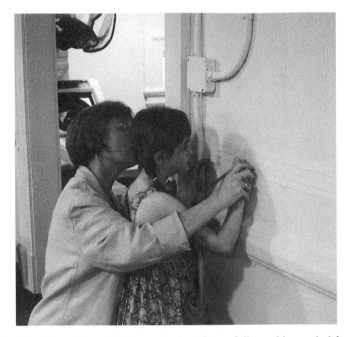

Figure 13.8 The therapist provides manual guidance followed by verbal feedback about the goal of the movement, "You stayed within the lines!"

them engage in this problem solving (e.g. "What do you think about what you did? What seemed to work well and not so well? What are some other ways you could try?).

Assumptions

There are a few basic assumptions that distinguish a motor skill acquisition frame of reference based on motor learning, control, and development principles from other frames of reference that focus on the development of motor skills. These assumptions have consequences for evaluation and intervention.

One important assumption is that functional tasks help organize behavior. The focus of evaluation and treatment is the person's ability to engage in those tasks that are meaningful. A related assumption is that successful performance of meaningful tasks emerges from the interaction of multiple personal and environmental systems. Therefore, evaluation and intervention must consider these multiple systems.

A final assumption is that the motor problems observed are the result of all the systems interacting and compensating for some damage or problem in one or more of those systems. Evaluation and intervention would seek to identify which subsystems (control parameters) can be changed or affected to enable a new or more efficient skilled motor behavior (attractor states) to emerge. This is quite different from the assumption found in other frames of reference related to motor development (i.e., motor problems observed are the direct result of neurological damage). In those frames of reference, intervention must directly influence the neurological system, which is not the case with the motor skill acquisition frame of reference.

Summary

A thorough understanding of the movement sciences is still emerging. The information presented was based on a review of available studies that are limited in the range of ages, populations, contexts, tasks, and motor skills studied. More information is needed to fully understand how children acquire more efficient motor skills. However, there is beginning support for the emphasis on functional tasks and consideration of the person, task, and environment as they interact and have an impact on emergent motor skills.

FUNCTION/DYSFUNCTION CONTINUA

The motor skill acquisition frame of reference is somewhat unique from other frames of reference in that continua of function and dysfunction are defined by the performance in the specific skill to be acquired. The child's abilities related to performing a task reflect the functional end of the continuum, while the child's inabilities or difficulties related to performing a task reflect the dysfunctional end of the continuum. That is, the child can either perform a skill needed to function in the environment, or he or she cannot. Thus, there are no specific continua defined for function and dysfunction within this acquisitional frame of reference. A criterion referenced dichotomous measure (i.e., yes, the child can perform the specific skill; or no, the child cannot perform the skill) can be used when generating a specific function/dysfunction continua for a child. Also, the task can be analyzed and the task components that the child is able to do and unable to do can be identified. Function and dysfunction is determined by the environment within which the skill must be performed. The environments in which the task will be used can be analyzed to identify the supports and constraints to performance that are present. Furthermore, a child's developmental status provides only a background for this frame of reference and is considered when determining if the skill to be acquired is reasonable to expect of the child. For example, it would be unreasonable to expect a 3-year-old child to learn to write sentences, whereas it is reasonable to expect a 3-year-old child to be learning to dress himself or herself.

Function/dysfunction continua can be identified for any task that is necessary for the child to perform within the environment. It can range from simply the ability to make eye contact, to independence in activities of daily living (ADL) skills, to the ability to interact in a socially appropriate manner. Skills in the motor skill acquisition frame of reference are always environmentally specific. Within the frame of reference, each prioritized task that is important or essential to the child is observed.

Relative to each observed task, there is one function/dysfunction continuum—the child is either able to perform the task or unable to perform the task.

Indicators of Function/Dysfunction

The indicators of function are those aspects of the task that the child is able to perform. These indicators identify the child's abilities and strengths related to task performance and are reflective of motor skill acquisition. For example, the child may be able to push his or her arms through the jacket sleeves once it has been positioned and pull up the zipper once it has been engaged by an adult.

The indicators of dysfunction are those aspects of the task that the child is unable to perform and are reflective of difficulties in motor skill acquisition. These indicators identify the child's inabilities and needs related to task performance. Using the above example, the child may be unable to pull the jacket sleeve from behind his or her back and engage the zipper. Indicators of dysfunction in this frame of reference direct one's attention to possible performance component deficits that could be remediated and characteristics of the task or environment that are too demanding and require modification (i.e., child-task-environment do not match). For example, the child may have decreased active range of motion at the shoulder girdle and have limited manual dexterity and bilateral coordination to engage the zipper. The task and environment could then be modified by encouraging an overhead versus behind-the-back approach to putting on the jacket, purchasing a jacket with velcro fasteners, or the child may benefit from performance component–based remediation of shoulder active range of motion, manual dexterity, and bilateral coordination. The demands of the task and environment need to match the developmental level and capabilities of the child.

The indicators of function and dysfunction can identify whether the child is in an early or later stage of learning. Indicators of early stages of learning include movements that are slower, use of too much or too little force, difficulty manipulating and retaining objects, dropping things easily, difficulty sequencing and timing, difficulty planning the steps of a task or movement, and frequent errors. Indicators of later stages of learning are smoother and refined movements, less use of cocontraction, better planning and sequencing of the entire task, and increased accuracy of each attempt. This evaluation information can then be used for intervention as it relates to the type of practice and feedback that can be used and task and environment modification (Chart 13.1).

GUIDE TO EVALUATION

Evaluation follows a top-down progression where occupational performance areas and contexts are assessed first and performance components are assessed secondarily because they may have an impact on the performance of functional tasks (Trombly,

Chart 13.1 Chart of Indicators of Function and Dysfunction	
Function	**Dysfunction**
INDICATORS OF FUNCTION	**INDICATORS OF DYSFUNCTION**
Child is able to perform a motor task	Child is unable to perform motor task
Child's environment supports task performance	Child's environment does not support task performance
Task requirements are within a child's capabilities with or without environmental support	Task requirements are beyond the child's capabilities with environmental support
Child-task-environment match	Child-task-environment do not match

1995). All factors that may have an impact on the child's performance must be considered in the evaluation process. It is important to note that evaluation is a dynamic process and does not necessarily follow a specific order. The following is a general guideline for evaluation. It is important for each occupational therapist to learn to observe and organize this information in a way that is efficient and effective for himself or herself. Factors related to the child, task, and environment, as well as the interaction of all three, must be evaluated as intervention can address all three areas.

The process consists of the following steps, focusing first on the child, then the task, then the environment, and finally the interaction of all three areas:

Child

1. Discussion with child, family, teacher, other care providers:

   - Identify the tasks that are most important for the child to perform effectively at home, school, and in the community. For younger children, this information may be inferred by observing the child's level of interest and self selection of tasks.

   - From these tasks, identify the tasks with which the child is reportedly having difficulty. Prioritize the tasks related to home, school, or community life on which occupational therapy intervention will focus (e.g., self-feeding, dressing, handwriting, activating computer keyboard or switch, engaging in play activities, handling money, using public transportation, maintaining one's daily living space).

   - Identify whether the motor skills to perform these tasks are within the child's capabilities or are reasonable to expect the child to perform based on the child's age and sociocultural contexts.

2. Observe the child doing each prioritized task in the environment where it is naturally performed. If this is not possible, find out about these environments and attempt to simulate them if this is feasible. Assess the task characteristics, environmental demands, and child's capabilities and stage of learning as these relate to motor skill acquisition for each specific task. In addition, standardized functional evaluations such as the *Pediatric Evaluation of Disability Inventory* (PEDI) (Haley, Coster, Ludlow, Haltiwanger, & Andrellos, 1992), *The School Function Assessment*

(Coster, Deeney, Haltiwanger, & Haley, 1998), the *Assessment of Motor and Process Skills-AMPS* (Fisher, 1992) and the *Functional Independence Measure for Children* (WeeFIM) (Hamilton, & Granger, 1991) can be used to assist with the identification, prioritization, and documentation of the child's current level of abilities.

Task

3. Analyze the requirements and characteristics of each prioritized task from a general perspective. Explore the performance components of the task, and see where the child is having difficulties with the task and which aspects of the task he or she can do well. This process of task analysis is critical in identifying whether and which aspects of the task are influencing performance. The information gained can assist with decisions about task modification, use of different tasks, or the determination of which performance components are interfering with task performance.

4. Evaluate performance components within the child that are likely to influence motor skill acquisition in this task. Only components that have a high likelihood of or are observed to be limiting task performance should be evaluated. To evaluate performance components such as muscle tone, strength, range of motion, memory, problem solving, sensory regulation, visual discrimination, coping skills, the occupational therapist can use assessments that examine these areas in more depth.

Environment

5. Analyze the demands and characteristics of the environment in which each task will be performed. Consider the physical characteristics (space, furniture, objects, work and support surface, lighting, glare, noise, distractions, overall organization), the regulatory conditions (which affect the necessary timing, force, and magnitude of movement), and the sociocultural contexts (demands, expectations, instructions, presentation of task). Environment analysis is critical in identifying whether and which aspects of the environment are influencing performance. The information gained can assist with decisions about environmental modification and exploring different environments and with a determination of which performance components are interfering with task performance.

The next few steps of the evaluation process involve looking at the interaction of the child, task, and environment.

6. Regulatory conditions are aspects of the environment that determine movement specifics that impact on the task. Tasks need to be analyzed from the perspective of Gentile's closed and open task taxonomy; number of steps; sensory-motor, cognitive, and psychosocial demands; degree of structure; and characteristics of materials: size, shape, texture, weight, pliability, and inherent visual cues and contrast.

7. Examine the following questions relative to the child's performance of tasks in relation to environment:

   • What is the child able to do? In what environments? (Indicators of function)
   • What is the child unable to do? In what environments? (Indicators of dysfunction)
   • What is interfering with motor skill acquisition that is reflected in task performance? Describe task and environmental constraints, and child performance component deficits.
   • What is supporting motor skill acquisition that is reflected in task performance? Describe task and environmental supports and child performance component capabilities.
   • What can improve the child's motor skill acquisition or task performance? Consider feedback, practice, and task or environmental modification. The information gained from asking this question and from performing the next step in this evaluation process can be directly applied to intervention (refer to postulates regarding change).

8. Explore possible modifications of the task and environment. Modify the task and/or environmental conditions, allow the child to practice the task under the new conditions, and provide feedback about motor skill performance and outcome.

9. Reassess motor skill acquisition by observing the child's task performance with the preliminary modifications, feedback, and practice provided.

10. The final step is the interpretation of evaluation and recommendations for intervention: Information about motor skill acquisition and factors that support and constrain task performance and skill acquisition is described for each prioritized task. Based on this information, goals and objectives are developed pertaining to motor skill acquisition of each task and an intervention plan is developed among the team members.

Evaluation is a dynamic process (McCaffrey-Easley, 1996). The primary focus is on the child-task-environment interaction, which is an assessment of the child while performing each prioritized task in specific environments. Observation shifts back and forth among the child's capabilities, the task characteristics, and the environmental demands. The evaluation interpretation and recommendations focus on the interaction between all three of these areas.

POSTULATES REGARDING CHANGE

Based on the emerging research in motor control, motor learning, and motor development, the following postulates regarding change guide intervention directed at motor skill acquisition. There are four general postulates:

1. If there is a match among the task requirements, environmental demands, and the child's abilities, then it is more likely that motor skill acquisition will be improved.

2. If the child understands what is to be achieved and is provided with clear information about the expected motor skill performance and outcome, then it is more likely that motor skill acquisition will be improved.

3. If the child is encouraged to independently problem solve to find his or her own optimal movement strategies to perform tasks, then it is more likely that motor skill acquisition will be improved.

4. If the child is provided with a task that is challenging (i.e, possible at the child's upper limit of capabilities or zone of proximal development) and motivating, it is more likely that motor skill acquisition will be improved.

There are 8 specific postulates:

5. In the early stages of learning, if feedback is focused on movement outcome and the critical features of the task and environment (not on movement performance), then it is more likely that motor skill acquisition will be improved.

6. In the early stages of learning, if feedback is summarized (rather than detailed) and provided when movement performance demonstrates a greater than acceptable level of error (error range), then it is more likely that motor skill acquisition will be improved.

7. In the later stages of learning, if the child is encouraged to self evaluate his or her own movement performance and outcome by focusing on inherent body and perceived environmental feedback, then it is more likely that motor skill performance will be improved.

8. If the child practices whole tasks versus parts of tasks in isolation of the whole, then it is more likely that motor skill acquisition will be improved.

9. If the child is provided with randomized practice, then it is more likely that motor skill acquisition and long-term retention will be improved. (However, the child with severe cognitive disabilities may benefit from blocked practice especially in the early stages of learning.)

10. For open tasks, if the child is provided with variability and unpredictability during practice, then it is more likely that motor skill acquisition will be improved for open tasks.

11. If the child practices and is provided feedback about motor skill performance and outcome in natural settings, then it is more likely that motor skill acquisition will be improved in those settings.

12. If the motor skill is practiced in a variety of contexts and daily routines, then it is more likely that the motor skill will be generalized, transferred to, or used in other contexts and daily routines.

APPLICATION TO PRACTICE

The motor skill acquisition frame of reference described in this chapter incorporates child-task-environmental match with the concepts of practice and feedback combined with task and environmental modification to improve motor skill acquisition. The focus of this section will be to describe in more depth how to apply the general and specific postulates regarding change to improve motor skill acquisition. Intervention is directed toward improving motor skill acquisition related to each task as specified in the goals and objectives developed from the evaluation. However, to use this frame of reference, the therapist will need to integrate his or her knowledge and skills in task/environmental analysis and modifications. This process is foundational to occupational therapy practice and has been described consistently in occupational therapy literature (Case-Smith, Pratt & Allen, 1996; Trombly, 1995).

This frame of reference can be used with children who have a wide variety of performance component problems. Information relevant to the type of problem must be considered when designing and implementing intervention. The specific methods used in this frame of reference may be different for the child with sensory regulation problems as compared with the child with hypertonicity. For example, for a child with hypertonicity, a therapist may use the motor skill acquisition frame of reference alone or in conjunction with another frame of reference like neurodevelopmental treatment; however, the therapist must always consider theories and knowledge about spasticity. The motor skill acquisition frame of reference can be used with many other approaches or by itself, but the therapist always considers available knowledge relevant to the specific problems of the child.

In this frame of reference, task performance is reflective of motor skill acquisition. Through observation of the child's task performance, the occupational therapist obtains important information about the task, environment, and child that is supporting or constraining task performance. The goal of intervention is to obtain a child-task-environment match to improve task performance. To do this, the therapist modifies the task and environment or addresses the performance component deficits or capabilities that have the potential to improve task performance.

The child needs to understand what is expected of him or her and may need to be reminded of the expected movement outcome or goal of the task to be performed. The therapist provides information feedback about critical features of the environment and the movement outcome that was performed by the child. The child can be shown how his or her movement outcome was similar and different from the expected outcome. The therapist can provide the child with a visual model of the expected outcome, such as a completed drawing or a completed dressing task with the garment positioned and oriented in the expected fashion. The child can then be encouraged to compare his or her own outcome with the visual model. For children with visual impairments, verbal and tactile information can be provided for the child to make this comparison. It is important that the outcome that is expected to be achieved is reasonable given age, ability level, and sociocultural expectations. This information can be obtained by caregivers, chart review, and criterion-referenced testing.

At times, particularly with young children or children with cognitive impairments, it may be necessary to use manual guidance to help the child understand the movement that is required for the task. In this case, the therapist would move the child through a task once or several times until the child begins to initiate the movement on his or her own. The intent of manual guidance is to use it only until the child has the idea and to withdraw it as soon as possible. The intent is not to facilitate or inhibit particular muscle groups. It is important in this approach that the child develop his or her own movement strategy and not have a strategy imposed by the therapist.

Some children with cognitive impairments may need more extensive periods of repetition or blocked practice to learn or retain new skills than others. It may be necessary to practice a task in each of the contexts in which it will be used because of the difficulty with generalization of skills and long-term retention of learning in many people with more severe cognitive impairments. Each child should be encouraged to independently problem solve to the best of his or her ability using a variety of movement strategies to achieve the goal. This will allow the child to find his or her own strategies for movement. Once the child develops personalized strategies for movement, then he or she is more likely to improve motor skill acquisition.

After the child has performed the task, it is important to wait a few seconds to allow the child to process or make use of his or her own body and perceived environmental feedback before providing additional therapist feedback. This time can vary for each child and should be monitored accordingly.

To promote motor skill acquisition in the early stages of learning, the tasks need to be challenging, motivating, and relevant to the child's life experiences. To do this effectively, the therapist needs to understand the child's skills and limitations and adapt or devise tasks that are challenging but not beyond the child's capabilities with necessary support. The therapist may use the understanding of the zone of proximal development to structure tasks that the child can do now only with some assistance but are within the child's potential range for achieving independently. Furthermore, based on the therapist's understanding of the child's environment, tasks are structured to be meaningful and relevant to the child's life.

During the early stages of learning, the therapist attempts to match the child's capabilities with the task requirements and environmental demands. This may involve the use of adaptive equipment, positioning devices, and assistive technology; modifying the task or the environment; or providing feedback to make it easier for the child to process and use critical features of the task. Once the child understands the expected movement outcome, it is important to reduce therapist feedback and encourage the child to make use of his or her inherent body and perceived environmental feedback. The therapist should provide summary or general versus detailed feedback and after the child's movement performance falls outside a given or preset error range instead of immediately after each attempt. However, some children may require more immediate or frequent feedback in the early stages of learning because of their unique learning and psychosocial preferences and needs. The therapist must weigh these factors with the information provided from research in the movement sciences when deciding on when to provide feedback.

During the later stages of learning, the child is reminded to self evaluate movement performance and outcome by focusing on his or her inherent body and perceived environmental feedback. Rather than describe to the child the difference between his or her movement outcome and the expected outcome or the specific movement strategies that were inefficient or ineffective, the therapist will ask the child questions to help him or her generate his or her own ideas and solutions about movement performance and outcome. Potential questions could be: "What do you think about what you did?," "What seemed to work well and not so well?," "What are some other ways you could try?" When the child is unable to generate his or her own ideas or solutions, the therapist can engage in this process with the child and provide more feedback about movement performance and outcome. The therapist can demonstrate to the child how he or she moved and explain why particular movement strategies may not have been effective. The therapist should suggest, demonstrate, or instruct the child in other movement strategies only if and when the child has difficulty generating alternate movement strategies on his or her own. However, therapist-generated movement strategies may not be efficient or effective in achieving the movement outcome because the therapist does not have full access to the child's inherent body and perceived environmental feedback. There is no one "normal" or "best" movement strategy to use to accomplish a particular task. The most efficient strategy for a person depends on the state of all the systems interacting in and around the person at a particular time. This is why specific physical handling strategies such as those used in the NeuroDevelopmental Treatment frame of reference are not proposed in this frame of reference.

The child should practice whole tasks. The child should not practice one isolated part of a task without the experience of doing the whole task (e.g., practicing putting the arm in the shirt sleeve without practicing putting on the whole shirt). The child may be able to do parts of the task independently and require physical assistance and more feedback from the therapist for the other parts of the task. Practicing whole tasks is important because the task, environmental conditions, and information that the child has to attend to and manage are incorporated into the practice sessions. These conditions are not addressed when practicing isolated parts of tasks, especially the timing and sequencing demands that need to be managed while performing whole tasks.

Therapists often structure treatment sessions to allow the child to practice basic skills that are important to many tasks (e.g., balance). If at all possible, balance should be practiced as part of a task, not separately, on therapy equipment such as a therapy ball or bolster. Many children have difficulty transferring skills (e.g., balance) learned on equipment (e.g., on a ball) to those tasks in which they need to use balance (e.g., dressing or reaching for and manipulating toys or eating utensils).

The therapist must structure practice conditions to include variability and unpredictability of movement, while the child practices open tasks because these are inherent characteristics of these tasks. The child can be encouraged to develop a repertoire of strategies to deal with the unpredictability of the regulatory conditions and the quickness in movements that are necessary to perform many motor skills.

A variety of tasks should be provided and practiced as soon as the child understands the specific task performance and outcome. This will allow for randomized practice, which will improve the potential for skill acquisition and long-term retention. Some children take longer to understand this and may require more blocked practice until they have demonstrated that they understand the expected task performance and outcome. Other factors (e.g., the child's information processing abilities and learning preferences) have to be considered when deciding when to transition from blocked to random practice. In addition, children with severe cognitive disabilities or children who may need more time to understand the expected movement outcome or goal may need more blocked practice. Blocked practice may need to be provided in each of the settings where the movement skill will be used because children with severe cognitive disabilities may have great difficulty in transferring the movement skills learned in one setting or for one daily routine to another.

During early and later phases of learning, the child should be encouraged to practice the movement skills in a variety of contexts, with different materials, and for different daily routines. This can provide the child with a larger repertoire and more flexible strategies in dealing with a greater number of task and environmental demands. This can improve long-term retention and generalization of the movement skills acquired. Some children with cognitive impairments may need to practice in the environment where the task is to be used with the same materials that will be used on a daily basis. In addition, some children may not benefit from simulated environments or tasks.

In the motor skill acquisition frame of reference, the goals and objectives are directed at functional task performance. The goal identifies the task performance in which effort will be directed by the child and selected caregivers. The objectives are the smaller aims that indicate whether the child is making progress toward this goal (Mager, 1975). Objectives need to be measurable and include the task performance (e.g., donning jacket; engaging and pulling up zipper), the expected level or criterion of performance (e.g., able to do three times in a week, with or without certain conditions), the necessary conditions of task performance (i.e., task modification and verbal reminder; verbal and tactile feedback; and practice) and the contexts where task performance occurs (e.g., home and classroom).

Intervention is task-oriented and context-specific because motor skill acquisition is contingent on the child's capabilities, task requirements, and environmental demands. What works for one child in one task or in one environment may not work for or in others. Therefore, it is important to carefully monitor the effectiveness of this intervention by reviewing and updating behavioral objectives and documenting observable behaviors that can indicate progress in motor skill acquisition. This is important because there is still much that is unknown about the effectiveness of the postulates regarding change that have been described in this chapter.

Other frames of reference presented in this book may be used in combination with this frame of reference. In particular, the occupational therapist may use the biomechanical, NeuroDevelopmental Treatment, sensory integration, coping, and visual information processing frames of reference. Specifically, the biomechanical frame of reference can assist with motor skill acquisition in seating, positioning, work-surface design, and set-up of task-related materials. The coping frame of reference is compatible as it relates to child-task-environmental match and focus on the psychosocial subsystems that influence motor skill acquisition. The visual information processing frame of reference also can assist with task and environmental modification. The therapist should be aware of possible conflicts arising from differences in the theoretical bases of other frames of reference, particularly assumptions; ideas about the role of the therapist, child, and family; and priorities in goals.

SUMMARY

The motor skill acquisition frame of reference described in this chapter proposes a major shift in the traditional roles and responsibilities of the therapist and the child in the intervention process. The child is seen as an active learner and as responsible for his or her own learning. The therapist is seen as a partner with the child, family, and others in the problem solving process—a facilitator of the child's acquiring new or more efficient motor skills. Instead of supplying specific strategies that are "done to" the child, this frame of reference requires the therapist to be an analyst of the child, task, and environment and to be creative in structuring a learning situation that will improve the child's ability to perform specific tasks. The emphasis on functional tasks and on active learning fits easily with traditional occupational therapy philosophy and practice.

Acknowledgments

The authors thank Paula McCreedy, MA, OT, for welcoming us in her private practice to photograph Samantha; Trish Rosen, Doctoral Candidate in the Department of Anthropology, NYU, and Dr. Faye Ginsburg for taking the photographs used in this chapter.

References

American Occupational Therapy Association. (1994). Uniform terminology for occupational therapy, third edition. *American Journal of Occupational Therapy, 48*, 1047–1054.

Bernstein, N. (1967). *Coordination and regulation of movements.* New York: Pergamon Press.

Bly, L. (September/October, 1996). What is the role of sensation in motor learning? What is the role of feedback and feedforward? *NDTA Network,* 1–7.

Brooks, V. B. (1986). *The Neural Basis of Motor Control,* New York: Oxford University Press.

Carr, J. H., & Shepherd, R. B. (1987). *A Motor Relearning Programme for Stroke* (2nd ed.), Rockville, MD: Aspen Systems.

Christiansen, C. (1991). Occupational therapy intervention for life performance. In C. Christiansen & C. Baum (Eds.), *Occupational Therapy, Overcoming Human Performance Deficits* (pp. 28–29). Thorofare, NJ: Slack, Inc.

Coster, W., Deeney, T., Haltiwanger, J., & Haley, S. (1998). *School Function Assessment.* San Antonio, TX: Psychological Corporation.

Ferguson, J. M., & Trombly, C. A. (1997). The effect of added-purpose and meaningful occupation on motor learning. *American Journal of Occupational Therapy, 51,* 508–515.

Fisher, A. G. (1992). *Assessment of motor and process skills* (Res. ed. 6.1J). Unpublished test manual, Department of Occupational Therapy, Fort Collins, CO: Colorado State University.

Gentile, A. M. (1987). Skill acquisition: Action, movement and neuromotor processes. In J. H. Carr, R. B. Shepherd, J. Gordon, A. M. Gentile, & J. M. Held (Eds.), *Movement Science: Foundations for physical therapy in rehabilitation* (pp. 93–154). Gaithersburg, MD: Aspen.

Gentile, A. M. (1992). The nature of skill acquisition: Therapeutic implications for children with movement disorders. In H. Forssberg & H. Hirschfeld (Eds.), *Movement disorders in children,* Medicine and Sports Sciences, Basel, Karger, 36, 31–40.

Gibson, E. J. (1963). Perceptual development. In H. W. (Ed.) *Child psychology.* Chicago, IL: University of Chicago Press.

Gibson, E. J. (1969). *Principles of perceptual learning and development.* New York: Appleton-Century-Crofts.

Gibson, J. J. (1966). *The senses considered as perceptual systems.* Boston, MA: Houghton Mifflin.

Gliner, J. A. (1985). Purposeful activity in motor learning theory: An event approach to motor skill acquisition. *American Journal of Occupational Therapy, 39,* 28–34.

Goodgold-Edwards, S. A., & Cermak, S. A. (1989). Integrating motor control and motor learning concepts with neuropsychological perspectives on apraxia and developmental dyspraxia. *American Journal of Occupational Therapy, 44,* 431–439.

Haugen, J. B., & Mathiowetz, V. (1995). Contemporary task-oriented approach. In C. Tremble (Ed.), *Occupational therapy for physical dysfunction* (4 ed.) (pp. 510–527). Williams & Wilkins.

Humphry, R., Jewell, K., & Rosenberger, R. C. (1995). Development of in-hand manipulation and relationship to activities. *American Journal of Occupational Therapy, 49,* 763–771.

Kamm, K., Thelen, E., & Jensen, J. I. (1990). A dynamical systems approach to motor development. *Physical Therapy, 70,* 763–775.

Kaplan, M. (1994). Motor learning: Implications for occupational therapy and neurodevelopmental treatment. *Developmental Disabilities Special Interest Section Newsletter, 17,* (3), 1–4.

Lee, T., Swanson, L., & Hall, A. (1991). What is repeated in a repetition? Effects of practice conditions on motor skill acquisition. *Physical Therapy, 71,* 150–156.

Levine, M. (1987). *Developmental variation and learning disorders.* Cambridge, MA: Educators Publishing Service.

Mager, R. F. (1975). *Preparing instructional objectives.* Belmont, CA: Pearson.

McCaffrey-Easley, A. (1996). Dynamic assessment for infants and toddlers: The relationship between assessment and the environment. *Pediatric Physical Therapy, 8,* 62–69.

Nelson, D. L. (1988). Occupation: Form and performance. *American Journal of Occupational Therapy, 42,* 633–641.

Poole, J. (1995). In C. Trombly (Ed.), *Occupational therapy for physical dysfunction* (4th ed.) (pp. 265–276). Baltimore: Williams & Wilkins.

Riccio, C. M., Nelson, D. L., & Bush, M. A. (1990). Adding purpose to repetitive exercise of elderly women through imagery. *American Journal of Occupational Therapy, 44,* 714–719.

Sabari, J. (1991). Motor learning concepts applied to activity-based intervention with adults with hemiplegia. *American Journal of Occupational Therapy, 45,* 523–530.

Schmidt, R. A. (1991). Motor learning principles for physical therapy. In M. J. Lister (Ed.), *Contemporary management of motor control problems: Proceedings of the II STEP conference* (pp. 49–63). Alexandria, VA: Foundation for Physical Therapy.

Sietsema, J. M., Nelson, D. L., Mulder, R. M., Mervau-Scheidel, D., & White, B. E. (1993). The use of a game to promote arm reach in persons with traumatic brain injury. *American Journal of Occupational Therapy, 47,* 19–24.

Thelen, E., Corbetta, D., Kamm, K., Spencer, J. P., Schneider, K., & Zernicke, R. F. (1993). The transition to reaching: Mapping intention and intrinsic dynamics. *Child Development, 64,* 1058–1098.

Thorndike, E. L. (1932). *Fundamentals of learning.* New York: Teachers College, Columbia University.

Thorndike, E. L. (1935). *The psychology of wants, interests, and attitudes.* New York: Appleton-Century-Crofts.

Travers, R. M. W. (1977). *Essentials of learning* (4th ed). New York: Macmillan.

Trombly, C. (1995). Occupation: Purposefulness and meaningfulness as therapeutic mechanisms. *American Journal of Occupational Therapy, 49,* 960–972.

van der Weel, F. R., van der Meer, A. L., & Lee, D. N. (1991). Effect of task on movement control in cerebral palsy: Implications for assessment and therapy. *Developmental Medicine and Child Neurology, 33,* 419–426.

VanSant, A. (1991). Motor control, motor learning, and motor development. In P. C. Montgomery & B. H. Connolly (Eds.), *Motor control and physical therapy: Theoretical framework and practical applications* (pp. 13–28). Hixson, TN: Chattanooga Group.

Vygotsky, L. S. (1978). *Mind in society: The development of higher psychological processes.* Cambridge, MA: Harvard University Press.

Winstein, C. J. (1991). Knowledge of results and motor learning—Implications for physical therapy. *Physical Therapy, 71,* 140–149.

Winstein, C. J. & Schmidt, R. A. (1990). Reduced frequency of knowledge of results enhances motor skill learning. *Journal of Experimental Psychology (Learning, Memory, Cognition), 16,* 677–691.

CHAPTER 14

Coping Frame of Reference

G. GORDON WILLIAMSON / MARGERY SZCZEPANSKI

Coping is a major component of the adaptive process that occupational therapists address in promoting optimal function (Fine, 1991). Coping is the integration and application of developmental skills for daily living. The more effectively a child copes, the more effectively a child learns (Garmezy & Rutter, 1983; Larson, 1984). Effective coping is positively correlated to academic achievement, self-esteem, and a sense of personal mastery (DiBuono, 1982; Kennedy, 1984; Zeitlin, 1985; Zeitlin & Williamson, 1994).

The coping frame of reference is based on a cognitive behavioral theoretical model. It emphasizes the development and use of coping resources that enable the child to deal with current and future challenges and opportunities. A key feature is its positive orientation, which focuses on healthy adaptation to demands and expectations rather than on pathology. The coping frame of reference is targeted to the improvement of the child's ability to cope with stress when engaged in all areas of occupational performance.

Frustrations and daily challenges affect the lives of all children. The information presented in this frame of reference is thus applicable to any child who may need assistance in developing more adaptive behaviors in response to his or her experiences.

In most instances, children who receive occupational therapy are likely to be referred for intervention for reasons other than ineffective coping. Although the coping frame of reference can be applied in isolation to address socio-emotional aspects of performance, typically it is used in conjunction with other frames of reference presented in this textbook. Because the outcome of any intervention is influenced by the child's coping competence, this approach should be incorporated into all intervention plans when it is determined that a child has limited adaptive abilities. Application of this frame of reference can be tailored to children and adolescents who have a wide range of special needs and who come from varied sociocultural backgrounds.

THEORETICAL BASE

This coping frame of reference organizes theoretical concepts related to stress and coping in children into a unique set of guidelines for occupational therapy practice.

Numerous experts in the field of child development have studied aspects of coping in children related to their coping resources, vulnerabilities, and behavioral responses to stressful events (Compas, 1987; Garmezy & Rutter, 1983; Murphy, 1976; Werner & Smith, 1982).

Coping is the process of making adaptations to meet personal needs and to respond to the demands of the environment. A child copes with his or her self when managing thoughts, feelings, and preferences. A child copes with the environment when managing the social and physical worlds. The goal of coping is to maintain or enhance feelings of well-being (i.e., children cope with circumstances and situations to feel good about themselves and their place in the world). A child's coping competence is determined by the match between needs or demands and the availability of resources for managing them. Effective coping reflects sufficient resources for handling the demands of daily life. Long-term outcomes of effective coping are the acquisition of a positive identity and the capacity for intimate social relationships (Shahmoon-Shanok, 1990).

Coping is an essential component of the broader concept of adaptation. The process of coping with stress is directed toward the generation of purposeful actions with effort. It does not include reflexes or automatic habitual behaviors that are so well established that they no longer require active effort. Such automatic or well-established behaviors are not addressed within the context of this frame of reference. Although this distinction is not always clear, it avoids a global definition of coping that encompasses all the child's interactions with the environment (Compas, 1987).

Basic assumptions for this frame of reference are that the coping process is transactional and coping strategies are learned. Coping transactions occur in the context of the social and physical surroundings and in sequential, cyclical interactions with them. The environment has an ongoing, ever-present influence on the coping process. Through transactions with the environment, children try out, practice, and integrate coping strategies into their behavioral repertoire. Coping strategies that have been acquired previously are modified in response to changing demands and environmental expectations. This frame of reference, therefore, can be considered acquisitional in nature because it assumes that one can learn to cope more effectively.

The coping process is generated by personal needs or environmental demands that result in stress. Stress is tension that is experienced physically, cognitively, or emotionally in response to an event perceived as challenging or threatening or harmful to a person's feelings of well-being (Lazarus & Folkman, 1984; Zeitlin & Williamson, 1994). Within this theoretical base, coping with stress is defined broadly and not restricted to the child managing adverse circumstances. Stress interpreted as a challenge often is associated with positive, energizing emotions. Stress interpreted by the child as potentially harmful or threatening tends to have a negative inference. *A developmentally appropriate level of stress, different for each child, facilitates motivation, learning, and mastery.*

Stress can evoke positive or negative feelings of tension based on the child's unique perception of the situation. The varied responses of children escorted to a therapy session demonstrate this point. One child may enter the therapy room, glance at toys enticingly displayed on a table, and then run from his or her mother's side to play with them. This child interprets the situation as a challenge. Another child, on entering the same therapy room and glancing at the same toys, remembers that it is time to leave his or her mother's side. This child perceives the situation as threatening and begins to cry. Still another child may view the situation initially with caution and spends a few minutes at his or her parent's side. With the therapist's encouragement, this child is able to approach the toys comfortably (Figure 14.1).

Although stress is a reaction, stressors are the actual internal or external events that elicit the reaction. Internal stressors include thoughts, feelings, interests, motivations, physical sensations, and the presence of a disability. External stressors are the demands of the environment, which can include negotiation of physical surroundings, management of objects, and interaction with people. External stressors can range in intensity from minor upsets in daily routines to major events, such as a change of residence or domestic discord. Because children frequently experience stress in relation to internal or external demands and expectations, these terms are used in this chapter in reference to stressors. The way children manage stress can be appreciated only by observing their coping transactions. Observation of transactions is the vehicle for understanding how a child's adaptation—the coping process—is expressed in daily life.

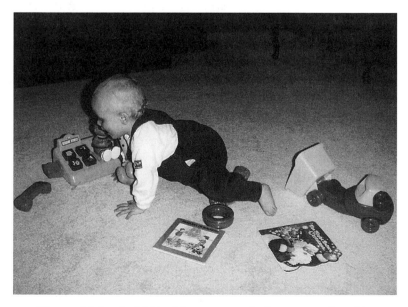

Figure 14.1   A child is able to approach the toys comfortably.

The Coping Process

Various researchers have described the coping process (Antonovsky, 1979; Haan, 1977; Lazarus & Folkman, 1984; Moos & Billings, 1982; Zeitlin, Williamson, & Rosenblatt, 1987). Drawing from their work, a coping model designed to be clinically useful has been developed. It provides a structure for observing, understanding, and analyzing the coping process in children. The model is presented from a cognitive-behavioral orientation, but it should be noted that the mental processes in children are not so clearly delineated. In the earliest years, coping is primarily emotionally driven. In the older child, the cognitive contribution becomes more influential in each step of the process.

The coping process occurs in the context of coping transactions. A coping transaction, which is a sequence of interactions between the child and the environment, consists of elements related to the child and the environment. All of these elements contribute to the outcome of the coping process. When observing coping transactions, then, it is important to appreciate the contributions of the environment, the child, and the steps of the process experienced by the child. From the child's perspective, this transactional model views coping as a four-step, interrelated process (Figure 14.2). The four steps include:

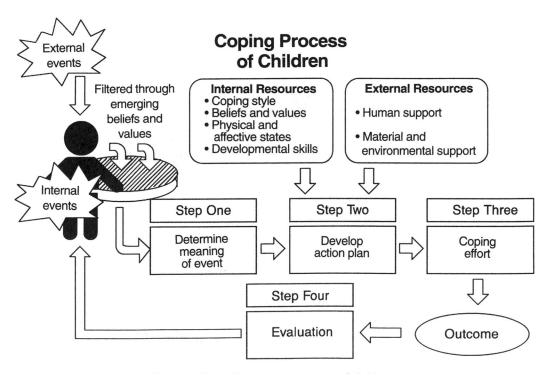

Figure 14.2 The coping process of children.

1. Determine the meaning of an event
2. Develop an action plan
3. Implement a coping effort
4. Evaluate its effectiveness

The environmental contributions to coping transactions include the creation of external demands on the child that frequently initiate the coping process, the environmental resources available to the child, and the environment's response to the child's coping effort. This environmental feedback influences how the child perceives the effectiveness of the coping effort (i.e., it contributes to the child's evaluation of how successfully the situation was managed). Analysis of coping transactions helps the therapist understand how the child copes in specific situations and functions on a daily basis.

Step 1. Determine the Meaning of an Event

The coping process is initiated by the child's experience of an internal or external event perceived as a demand or expectation that is experienced as stressful. The stress of internal demands and expectations in young children can be inferred only through their actions. Older children may be able to express internal demands verbally. Examples of these inner demands include the child's personal goals, preferences, concerns, expectations for success or failure, physical sensations, and the broad range of emotions experienced by the child.

In a child's early years, external demands and expectations are made primarily by family members and other caregivers and then later by teachers and the community. Most adults have a unique set of demands and expectations for a child's social behavior, performance, and management of daily activity that creates stress. When demands and expectations match the child's coping resources, they provide an appropriate level of stress.

Effective coping and development are hindered when the demands are too high or too low. Sample external demands and expectations particularly relevant for children include goals for developmental or academic achievement, independence in self-care, and participation in social and community activities. In addition, the physical environment imposes a unique set of external spatial and temporal demands for the child to negotiate (e.g., maneuvering in crowded surroundings, reacting to moving objects, and obtaining toys in inaccessible settings).

Cognitive and emotional processes are used by the child to appraise events as they are filtered through the child's emerging beliefs and values. The meaning of the event may be interpreted as threatening, harmful, or challenging to the child's sense of well-being. In many cases an event is perceived as stressful when a child feels the demands cannot be managed. When the event is identified by the child as a stressor, the next step is to decide a course of action.

Step 2. Develop an Action Plan

A child's decision about how to manage a stressor depends in large part on the availability of resources on which the child can draw to deal with the situation. A child's decision-making skills develop over time and become more sophisticated as abstract thinking emerges. The young child who has limited cognitive skills tends to develop an action plan based on emotions, immediate personal needs, and an evolving awareness of cause-and-effect relationships, whereas the older child may be able to think through alternatives and choices to manage the situation. The ability to predict the logical consequences of one's actions increasingly mediates the decision-making process.

Coping resources are aspects of the self and the environment that influence the child's determination of an action plan. They can be classified as internal (within the child) or external (in the environment). The major internal resources are the child's coping style, beliefs and values, physical and affective states, and developmental skills. External resources include human supports and material and environmental supports. The critical importance of these resources is discussed later in a separate section.

Step 3. Implement a Coping Effort

The third step of the coping process involves making a coping effort in response to the demand or expectation. A coping effort is what the child actually does to manage stress. In a coping effort, cognitive or behavioral coping strategies are used to handle the situation. One coping strategy may be used in isolation or several strategies may be used simultaneously. Coping efforts are usually directed toward dealing with the stressor, managing the emotions associated with the stressor, or modifying related physical tension.

Action-oriented coping efforts are specifically directed toward the stressor (demand). For instance, a child who cannot complete homework may choose to review the textbook, request parental help, or call a classmate to clarify the assignment. Coping efforts to manage emotions associated with the stressor are geared toward helping the child feel better. A child who experiences frustration may choose to withdraw from the situation that generates it, may seek comfort from others, or may use defense mechanisms to counteract or deny the feelings. Coping efforts used to manage emotions also are used frequently to modify associated physical tension. For example, a child who experiences fatigue may choose to take a break, change the activity to one that is less demanding, or persist in the activity regardless of the fatigue.

The child's coping effort produces an outcome that elicits the next important element of the coping transaction—the response of the environment to the child's coping effort. The child experiences feedback from the physical and social environments. For example, a child making efforts in learning to propel a kiddie car may receive feedback from the actual movements of the bicycle or from an adult's verbal comments (Figure 14.3).

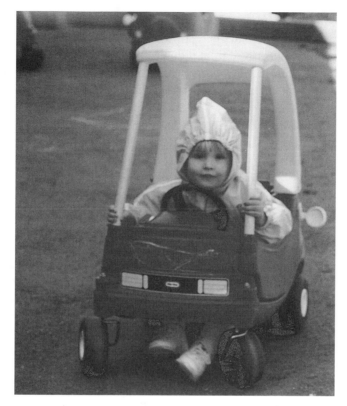

Figure 14.3   A child learning to propel a kiddie car with feedback from the movements of the car.

Step 4. Evaluate Effectiveness

The fourth step in the coping process involves the child's evaluation of the outcome of the coping effort and its resulting feedback. The evaluation includes a cognitive appreciation of the results of the coping effort in addition to the personal meaning that these results have for the child. From the child's perspective, coping efforts result in a range of positive and negative feelings about self and the environment. If the child's coping effort is effective, stress is managed by its reduction or elimination. The child feels better emotionally, a sense of well-being is enhanced or restored, and the coping cycle is completed until the next tension-generating event. Stress continues when a coping effort is not effective, and another coping cycle is generated in which similar or new strategies may be tried. A child who has a history of repeatedly unsuccessful coping may gradually develop a negative self-concept and an expectation of failure.

The child's feelings about the effectiveness of coping are internalized and then influence a sense of personal adequacy and subsequent coping efforts. Therapists must be sensitive to the child's perception of coping competence and the varying moods and emotions that result from different coping transactions. Over time, the internalization of coping effectiveness plays a critical role in determining the nature of the child's identity and the child's capacity to develop intimate relationships.

An adult's view of the goals and effectiveness of coping efforts may not be the same as the child's. Many coping efforts cannot be readily evaluated from an adult's success-or-failure paradigm; instead, the child's evaluation reflects personal thoughts and feelings that may not be apparent to an adult. Because children have idiosyncratic views of the world, they often change the goals of their activities and are fluid in shifting their expectations for outcome. For example, an adult may interpret a child's difficulty in completing a puzzle as a lack of success that will lead to frustration, whereas the child may be perfectly happy with an outcome that involves looking at the shapes and colors of the pieces. Likewise, an adult may request an action from a child that appears simple. Although complying with the request, the child may feel that the task was difficult and the situation was not managed effectively.

Coping with daily living is ongoing and continuous. A child may cope simultaneously with several stressors of varying intensity or may have to cope with a long-term stressor over time.

Coping Resources

Specific resources—internal and external—assist in the process of coping. The internal resources include coping style, beliefs and values, physical and affective states, and developmental skills. The external coping resources include human supports and material and environmental supports. Familiarity with these resources is critical to the understanding of how a child copes and to the application of this frame of reference in intervention. Adequate coping resources positively influence the child's ability to manage demands, whereas inadequate resources result in ineffective coping or a vulnerability to stress.

Internal Coping Resources

Coping Style. Coping style refers to the child's characteristic way of behaving in situations that are interpreted as threat, harm, or challenge to one's personal well-being. The coping styles of infants and toddlers can be described by the unique patterns of their sensorimotor organization, reactivity, and self-initiation (Zeitlin, Williamson, & Szczepanski, 1988). These coping characteristics are demonstrated by the integrated use of developmental skills to produce goal-directed coping efforts. In this frame of reference, coping style is viewed as a pattern of learned behaviors and not as a static personality trait.

Sensorimotor organization refers to the child's regulation of psychophysiological functions and the integration of the sensory and motor systems, including responses to auditory, visual, tactile, proprioceptive, and vestibular sensations. Representative attributes in the category of sensorimotor organization are the child's ability to self-comfort, to organize information from the different senses simultaneously for a response, to adapt to being moved by others during caregiving, to maintain an appropriate activity level, and to demonstrate visual attention.

The category of reactivity addresses the actions used by the child in response to the demands of the physical and social environments. Attributes that typify this category are the ability to respond to vocal or gestural direction, to react to the feelings and moods of others, to adjust to daily routines, to accommodate to changes in the surroundings, and to bounce back after stressful situations. In general, this type of coping behavior is elicited by external events.

Self-initiation refers to autonomously generated actions of the child that meet personal needs to interact with objects and people. Such coping behavior is intrinsically motivated. Sample attributes are the child's ability to explore objects independently using a variety of strategies, to initiate interactions with others, to apply previously learned behaviors to new situations, to demonstrate persistence during activities, and to anticipate events.

Coping styles of preschool and school-aged children can be described by the characteristic patterns used to cope with the environment and cope with self (Zeitlin, 1985). Relevant coping attributes include task-oriented behaviors such as staying with an activity until it is completed; interactive behaviors such as reacting to social cues in the environment; emotionally-based behaviors such as being able to express anger or love; and psychologically-based behaviors such as reappraising a situation that initially was perceived as threatening. Table 14.1 presents sample coping attributes relevant to preschool and older children.

Beliefs and Values. Beliefs are the ideas held as true about the self and the world. In the young child, emerging beliefs relevant to coping are related to an evolving sense of efficacy—the perceived ability to produce an effect, control events, and trust others to be responsive to needs. These beliefs usually are reflected in the child's self-esteem and can be inferred from behavior. Examples of beliefs in the older child are illustrated by such statements as "I can do it," "I am a good person," "My parents always will be there when I need them," and "I am the clumsiest kid in my school."

Values reflect a child's desires or preferences. They contribute to personal goals and serve to motivate commitments to their attainment. A value system eventually influences the child's views about what is important in life. Values in children are demonstrated in behaviors related to such issues as adult approval, academic achievement, task mastery, and preferences in play and leisure.

Beliefs and values are shaped and strongly influenced by familial and social experiences and by cultural background. They influence coping in two critical ways: First, they contribute to perceptions of events and the determination of whether an event is threatening, harmful, or challenging; and second, they serve as a motivating force for determining the initiation or avoidance of specific actions (Bandura, 1977).

Table 14.1 Sample Coping Attributes in Children Older Than 3 Years of Age

Coping with Self	Coping with the Environment
Frustration tolerance	Curiosity
Expression of personal needs and feelings	Socialization with others
Initiation of action to meet needs	Adaptation to daily routines
Ability to request help when needed	Ability to follow instructions
Balance independence with dependence	Awareness of others' feelings
Acceptance of substitutes	Acceptance of warmth and support from others
Flexibility in changing plans and behavior to achieve a goal	Resiliency following disappointment
Task persistence	Ability to become actively involved in situations
Demonstration of pleasure in successful accomplishment of activities	Awareness of and response to social expectations
	Response to new and difficult situations

Physical and Affective States. Physical state refers to general health and physiological condition, such as endurance and being well. Affective state reflects characteristic moods and emotions. Every coping transaction occurs in the context of variations in the child's physical and affective states, which can enhance coping effectiveness or create a vulnerability to stress. Chronic illness, repeated hospitalizations, a disabling condition, emotional instability, and depression, which influence physical and affective states, may result in ongoing stress for the child.

Developmental Skills. The child's levels of developmental competence and skill acquisition contribute to the range of behaviors available for coping efforts. The child's skills in the cognitive, psychosocial, communicative, and motor domains provide a basis for learning coping strategies. As the child matures, coping strategies become increasingly more complex, depending on previously acquired developmental skills. Coping with the sensation of hunger serves as an example of how developmental skills influence coping behavior: A 6-month-old infant may fuss and cry to obtain the caregiver's attention; a 1-year-old child may crawl to the mother and protest verbally; a two-year-old toddler may request "Mommy, cookie," whereas a 4-year-old child may go to the cupboard and find something to eat independently.

External Coping Resources

Human Supports. Persons in the environment who influence the child's coping efforts are considered human supports. They include parents, siblings, extended family members, peers, teachers, health professionals, and members of the community. Parents and other primary caregivers are perhaps the most significant external resources for coping in the child's early years. Parent/child interactions initially serve as the milieu in which coping efforts are initiated, practiced, and reinforced.

Through the normal course of child rearing, caregivers influence coping transactions by buffering the child's exposure to stress, making demands, modeling coping behaviors, encouraging and assisting the child in coping efforts, and giving contingent feedback. A number of factors influence the adequacy of human support, such as the quality of social interaction, nurturance, consistency, and limit setting (Figure 14.4).

Material and Environmental Supports. Material supports are items and services that money can buy. A family's material resources include the ability to provide sufficient food, clothing, shelter, and medical services and to provide appropriate toys and activities for the child. Environmental supports are the conditions of the physical surroundings such as air quality, organization of space, levels of noise and light, and opportunity for safe exploration (Figure 14.5). Environments that are chaotic, unpredictable, or overstimulating or that lack adequate stimulation may undermine the child's development and ability to cope.

Coping in Children who have Special Needs

Research indicates that preschool and school-aged children who have disabilities are less effective as a group in their coping behavior than their nondisabled peers (Kennedy, 1984; Lorch, 1981; Yeargan, 1982). In these studies, children who have disabilities were found to be more inconsistent or inflexible in their adaptive functioning. The literature also suggests that children who live in poverty tend to cope

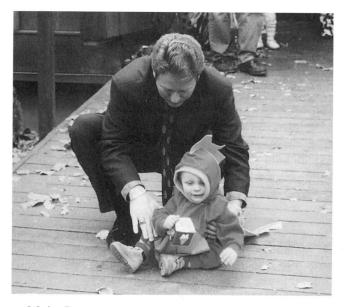

Figure 14.4 Parental support for safe exploration of environment.

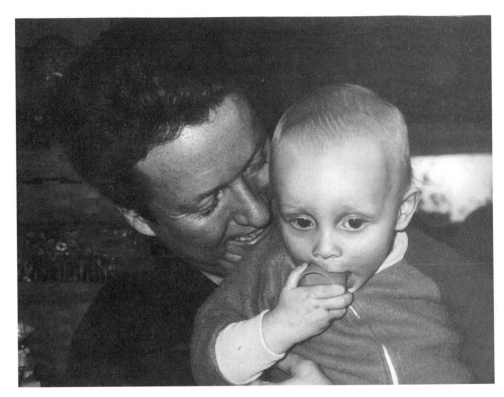

Figure 14.5   Positive father-child interaction.

less successfully than their more affluent peers (Brooks-Gunn & Furstenberg, 1987; Garbarino, 1995).

Few studies examine the coping behaviors of infants and toddlers who have special needs. The available research generally addresses a discrete component of coping, such as social interaction (Ramey, Beckman-Bell, & Gowen, 1980), environmental exploration (MacTurk, Vietze, McCarthy, McQuiston, & Yarrow, 1985), or self-generated problem solving (Brinker & Lewis, 1982). These investigations suggest that very young children who have disabilities are less competent in these coping-related domains.

Studies were conducted that were specifically designed to compare the coping styles of the two groups of children (Williamson, Zeitlin, & Szczepanski, 1989; Zeitlin & Williamson, 1990). It was found that infants and toddlers who have developmental disabilities tended to have minimally to situationally effective coping styles, whereas the nondisabled young children coped effectively more often than not. The most significant difference between the groups occurred in self-initiation. It is important to realize, however, that individual children in both groups demonstrated the entire range of coping effectiveness. This finding confirms that the presence of a disability does not necessarily imply that a child will have an ineffective coping style. Instead, it suggests that a child who has special needs may be more vulnerable to the stress of daily living.

Children who have disabilities may have fewer resources to support successful coping efforts. A neuromotor, cognitive, or communication handicap can interfere with the acquisition of developmental skills and, thereby, restrict the variety and sophistication of available coping strategies. Parents may be less accessible as a supportive external resource if they also are experiencing psychological distress or physical exhaustion from the requirements of daily caregiving (Turnbull & Turnbull, 1990). In addition, children who have disabilities often have to manage atypical stressors such as treatment regimens, hospitalization, restrictions in activity, and disruptions in daily routines (Drotar, Crawford, & Ganofsky, 1984). They tend, therefore, to face a greater number of stressors with a limited repertoire of coping resources. This vulnerability accentuates the importance for occupational therapists to assess the coping efforts of children in response to the demands and expectations placed upon them.

FUNCTION/DYSFUNCTION CONTINUA

Coping function and dysfunction can be described best as one broad, general continuum of effectiveness that reflects the child's ability to use internal and external resources to manage demands and expectations encountered on a daily basis. The continuum ranges from effective coping at the functional end to ineffective coping at the dysfunctional end. Function or dysfunction is determined by the goodness of fit between demands and expectations and the child's available coping resources. Effective coping reflects sufficient resources to meet demands of daily living and to manage stress, whereas ineffective coping reflects inadequate resources or excessive demands. The broad, general function/dysfunction continuum is discussed below. It is followed by specific function/dysfunction continua that stem from the general continuum.

Indicators of Function and Dysfunction: Effective Coping

A child is coping effectively when a child has sufficient internal and external resources to meet demands of daily life such as using a variety of available resources in a wide range of situations that require coping efforts; meeting personal needs and interacting productively with people and objects; having a healthy sense of well-being and drive toward task mastery; having cognitive skills to develop self-awareness; and having a consistent effective coping style. Problems in this area are evident when a child lacks necessary internal and external resources to manage routines, opportunities, challenges, and frustrations in daily life. He or she is unable to meet personal needs and interact productively with people and objects and has a negative sense of self. Such a child has a minimally effective coping style and may present a unique pattern of ineffective or maladaptive coping behavior (Chart 14.1).

Chart 14.1   Indicators of Function and Dysfunction for Effective Coping.

Effective Coping	**Ineffective Coping**
FUNCTION: Sufficient internal and external resources to meet demands of daily life. Demands are within the child's ability to manage.	DYSFUNCTION: Insufficient resources to meet the demands of daily life or demands inappropriately exceed child's ability to manage.
INDICATORS OF FUNCTION	**INDICATORS OF DYSFUNCTION**
Uses variety of available resources appropriately in a wide range of situations that require coping efforts	Lacks necessary internal and external resources to manage routines, opportunities, challenges, and frustrations in daily life
Meets personal needs and interacts productively with people and objects	Is unable to meet personal needs and interact productively with people and objects
Has cognitive ability to develop self-awareness	Lacks cognitive abilities to develop self-awareness
Has healthy sense of well-being and drive toward task mastery	Has negative sense of self and has expectations of failure
Displays consistently effective coping style	Displays minimally effective coping style; may present a unique pattern of ineffective or maladaptive coping behavior

---

Because coping effectiveness depends on the match between demands and coping resources, it is clinically useful to have additional function/dysfunction continua that address each of the coping resources. Intervention focuses in large part on these more specific continua that are related to coping style, beliefs and values, physical and affective states, developmental skills, human supports, material and environmental supports, and demands and expectations. These continua should be interpreted in a fluid manner. Given the complexity of daily living, the adequacy of a child's coping resources can vary, and demands can change, depending on environmental contexts.

Coping Style

Coping style refers to the way in which a child typically selects certain strategies over others to manage situations perceived as threatening, harmful, or challenging. This continuum ranges from a coping style that is consistently effective at the functional end to one that is minimally effective at the dysfunctional end. Three major levels of effectiveness are represented in this continuum: consistently effective, situationally effective, and minimally effective. Effectiveness means coping efforts are (1) appropriate for situations, (2) appropriate for the child's developmental age, and (3) used successfully to achieve desired results.

At the functional end of this continuum, the child who displays a consistently effective coping style demonstrates coping efforts that meet the above-mentioned criteria. This child has a repertoire of coping attributes that can be drawn on to produce positive outcomes. Strategies are generalized in a flexible way to unique environmental contexts. This child copes successfully with self and the environment most of the time.

The child who demonstrates a situationally effective coping style falls in the midrange of the continuum and has some coping competence. This child has coping behaviors that support the effective use of strategies in some situations but cannot generalize them to other types of situations. For example, in a therapy session the child may be able to manage when the parent is present but cannot manage independently with the clinician; or the child can manage gross motor tasks but not fine motor tasks. Thus, the ability to use coping strategies depends on environmental circumstances such as the presence or absence of human support, the type of activity, or the physical demands of the surroundings. In general, the child whose coping effectiveness is situationally determined is dependent on external resources to support coping efforts.

The child who displays a minimally effective coping style is at the dysfunctional end of the continuum and has a limited repertoire of effective coping strategies. Three characteristic patterns may be observed:

1. Coping behaviors are inconsistent and unpredictable. There is an erratic, trial-and-error quality to the child's performance.
2. Coping behaviors are rigidly repetitious in that the child continually repeats the same behavior regardless of the circumstance and fails to achieve successful results. The child cannot alter or change behavior based on the demands of the setting.
3. Coping behaviors reduce immediate stress but generate negative outcomes over time. For example, habitual use of temper tantrums may help the child to avoid or diffuse stressful events, but they have undesirable long-term consequences for learning and development.

Some examples of maladaptive coping behaviors include stereotypical body movements, persistent denial or avoidance, verbal abuse, angry reactions, nail biting, overactivity, and distractibility.

It is important to keep in mind that a child may exhibit variations in effectiveness according to particular categories of coping behaviors. For example, differences may be evident between coping with self and coping with the environment or between reactivity and self-initiation. In addition, the child may differ in the use of specific coping strategies (as depicted in the sample list of behaviors indicative of function and dysfunction related to coping style).

This continuum related to coping style is discussed in detail because of its importance to this frame of reference. The following additional continua are presented in shorter form to clarify the nature and impact of other coping resources (as well as demands and expectations). Attention to the sample behaviors indicative of function and dysfunction assists the therapist in recognizing how these resources are concretely demonstrated in the child's life (Chart 14.2).

Indicators of Function and Dysfunction for Beliefs and Values

Beliefs and values support coping to meet personal needs and demands of the environment. At the functional end of the continuum, a child trusts that personal needs

---

Chart 14.2 Indicators of Consistently Effective, Situationally Effective, and Minimally Effective Coping Style.

Consistently Effective Coping Style	**Situtionally Effective Coping Style**	**Minimally Effective Coping Style**
FUNCTION: Coping strategies are used effectively in a wide variety of situations. Coping efforts are appropriate for the child's developmental age and successfully achieve desired results.	FUNCTION: Coping strategies used effectively in one situation are not generalized to other situations. Coping efforts are variable in their appropriateness to the situation and their success.	DYSFUNCTION: Coping strategies are erratic and unpredictable, are rigidly repetitious, or reduce immediate stress but tend to generate negative outcomes over time. Coping efforts are inappropriate and usually unsuccessful.
INDICATORS OF FUNCTION	**INDICATORS OF SITUATIONAL FUNCTION**	**INDICATORS OF DYSFUNCTION**
Organizes information from the different senses for a response	Organizes certain types of sensory information but not others	Unable to tolerate sensory input
Self-regulates activity level	Variable regulates activity level	Poorly regulates activity level
Coordinates movement as required by the activity	Coordinated movement varies with type of activity	Uncoordinated movement fails to meet task demands
Adapts to daily routines and changes in schedule	Adapts to daily routines but does not tolerate change	Is unable to adjust to daily routines and changes
Engages in reciprocal social interactions	Interacts socially with some people but not with others	Is unresponsive to social interaction
Solves problems independently	Solves problems with adult support and guidance	Is unable to solve problems even with assistance
Generalizes learning to new situations	Applies acquired learning only in certain contexts	Is unable to generalize learning

---

will be met, expects success, and demonstrates high self-esteem. At the dysfunctional end, a child believes that the world is uncaring and unresponsive, anticipates failure, and demonstrates low self-esteem (Chart 14.3).

Indicators of Function and Dysfunction for Physical and Affective States

Physical and affective states support the child's coping to meet personal needs and demands of the environment and involve experiencing emotional well-being, possessing adequate physical endurance, and having the ability to regulate moods effectively. Problems in this area are evident when a child experiences overwhelming or persistent anxiety, fear, or insecurity; lacks physical endurance for age-appropriate tasks; and demonstrates erratic mood swings or depression (Chart 14.4)

Indicators of Function and Dysfunction for Developmental Skills

Developmental skills support coping to meet personal needs and demands when a child demonstrates a variety of skills appropriate to age level, when he or she ap-

---

Chart 14.3   Indicators of Function and Dysfunction for Beliefs and Values

Beliefs and Values Support Effective Coping	**Beliefs and Values Interfere with Coping**
FUNCTION: Beliefs and values support coping to meet personal needs and demands of the environment.	DYSFUNCTION: Beliefs and values interfere with coping to meet personal needs and demands of the environment.
INDICATORS OF FUNCTION	**INDICATORS OF DYSFUNCTION**
Trusts that personal needs will be met	Believes that the world is uncaring and unresponsive
Expects success	Anticipates failure
Demonstrates high self-esteem	Demonstrates low self-esteem

Chart 14.4   Indicators of Function and Dysfunction for Physical and Affective States.

Physical and Affective States Support Effective Coping	**Physical and Affective States Interfere with Coping**
FUNCTION: Physical and affective states support coping to meet personal needs and demands of the environment.	DYSFUNCTION: Physical and affective states interfere with coping to meet personal needs and demands of the environment.
INDICATORS OF FUNCTION	**INDICATORS OF DYSFUNCTION**
Experiences emotional well-being	Experiences overwhelming or persistent anxiety, fear, or insecurity
Possesses adequate physical endurance	Lacks physical endurance for age-appropriate tasks
Regulates mood effectively	Demonstrates erratic mood swings or depression

---

plies those skills spontaneously in daily functioning, and when the child acquires skills through experience and instruction. Dysfunction is evident when a child has limited skills for his or her age, when he or she cannot generalize skills in daily functioning, and when the child can only learn through highly individualized, repetitive instruction (Chart 14.5).

Human Supports

Human supports foster coping to meet the child's personal needs and demands of the environment. Indicators of function are evident when adults are nurturing and responsive to the child, when adults act as role models for appropriate behavior, and when adults give accurate, timely, and contingent feedback. Indicators of dysfunction are when adults are not available or negative toward a child, when adults model or reinforce maladaptive behaviors, and when adults give inaccurate, absent, or non-contingent feedback (Chart 14.6).

Chart 14.5 Indicators of Function and Dysfunction for Developmental Skills.

Developmental Skills Support Effective Coping	Developmental Skills Do Not Support Coping
FUNCTION: Developmental skills support coping to meet personal needs and demands.	DYSFUNCTION: Developmental Skills are absent or not used effectively in coping efforts.
INDICATORS OF FUNCTION	**INDICATORS OF DYSFUNCTION**
Demonstrates a range and variety of skills appropriate to age level	Demonstrates limited skills for age
Applies skills spontaneously in daily functioning	Is unable to generalize skills in daily functioning
Acquires skills through experience and various instructional methods	Acquires skills only through highly individualized, repetitive instruction

Material and Environmental Supports

Material and environment support fosters coping to meet personal needs and external demands when they provide adequate food, shelter, and activities to support development; when visual and auditory stimuli are appropriately regulated to foster attending behavior; and when the physical environment is organized to maximize independence. Material and environmental supports interfere with coping when the child's basic needs are not adequately met (contributing to poor health and compromised developmental competence), when the environment is overstimulating, and when the physical barriers impede independence, which causes the child to be overly dependent on others (Chart 14.7).

Demands and Expectations

Demands and expectations are appropriate when the child's social and physical environment produce appropriate stress for the child that the child can manage. Indicators of function are when the activities presented to the child at home and in school are consistent with the child's cognitive and functional abilities, when the child is provided support and guidance as needed in new and threatening situations, and when a child's personal expectations for performance are realistic. Indicators for dysfunction are evident when activities are presented to a child that are too easy or too difficult given the child's competence, when a child is expected to manage situations independently or is repeatedly placed in threatening situations without regard for coping capacity, and when a child's personal expectations are so high that they result in a persistent sense of failure or so low that they impede motivation (Chart 14.8).

Chart 14.6   Indicators of Function and Dysfunction for Human Supports.

Human Supports Foster Effective Coping	Human Supports Do Not Foster Coping
FUNCTION: Human supports foster coping to meet personal needs and demands of the environment.	DYSFUNCTION: Human supports are not available or interfere with coping.
INDICATORS OF FUNCTION	**INDICATORS OF DYSFUNCTION**
Adults are nurturing and responsive to the child.	Adults are unavailable or negative toward the child.
Adults serve as role models for appropriate behavior.	Adults model and reinforce maladaptive behavior.
Feedback regarding coping efforts is accurate, timely, and contingent.	Feedback regarding coping efforts is inaccurate, absent, or noncontingent.

Chart 14.7   Indicators of Function and Dysfunction for Materials and Environmental Supports.

Material and Environmental Supports Foster Effective Coping	Material and Environmental Supports Interfere with Coping
FUNCTION: Material and environmental supports foster coping to meet personal needs and external demands.	DYSFUNCTION: Material and environmental supports are limited or interfere with coping to meet personal needs and external demands.
INDICATORS OF FUNCTION	**INDICATORS OF DYSFUNCTION**
Adequate food, clothing, shelter, and activities to support growth and development are provided.	Basic needs are not adequately met, thereby contributing to poor health and compromised developmental competence.
Organization of physical environment maximizes independence.	Physical barriers impede independence, causing child to be overly dependent on others.
Visual and auditory stimuli are appropriately regulated to foster attending behavior.	Overstimulating environment results in short attention span and high level of distractibility.

GUIDE TO EVALUATION COPING ASSESSMENT

A comprehensive assessment identifies the child's level of coping competence and factors that influence adaptive functioning. The assessment focuses on the nature of the child's coping transactions as well as on internal and external coping resources and how the child applies these in coping efforts. In addition, daily demands and chronic stressors are identified. This section provides considerations for addressing each of these factors. A coping-related assessment can be incorporated readily in the context of an initial occupational therapy evaluation or can be conducted on an ongoing basis once the child has begun therapy. The assessment of the child's cognitive abilities is inherent in the occupational therapy evaluation. In addition, the therapist may draw on evaluation data obtained from other professionals. An in-depth assessment is indicated when the child has problems with coping.

Chart 14.8 Indicators of Function and Dysfunction for Demands and Expectations.

Demands and Expectations Are Appropriate	Demands and Expectations Are Inappropriate
FUNCTION: Demands and expectations by the social and physical environment produce developmentally appropriate stress. The child's demands and expectations are manageable.	DYSFUNCTION: Internal or external demands and expectations produce developmentally inappropriate stress (e.g., too high, too low, or inconsistent).
INDICATORS OF FUNCTION	**INDICATORS OF DYSFUNCTION**
Activities presented to child at home and in school are consistent with the child's cognitive and functional abilities.	Activities presented to child are too easy or too hard given child's competence.
Child is provided support and guidance as needed in new and threatening situations.	Child is expected to manage all situations independently or is repeatedly placed in threatening situations without regard for coping capacity.
Child's personal expectations for performance are realistic.	Child's personal expectations for achievement are so high they result in a persistent sense of failure or so low they impede motivation.

Assessment of Coping Transactions

The coping process, as previously described in the theoretical base, can be observed only in the context of coping transactions (Williamson, 1996). To assess these transactions, the practitioner needs to observe the child in various situations over time. Multiple observations in different contexts give the clinician a better sense of the ways in which elements of coping transactions facilitate or interfere with effective coping. The therapist needs to identify the demands and expectations (stressors) experienced by the child, the coping efforts that the child uses to manage demands, and the feedback that the child receives from the physical and social environments.

In assessing demands and expectations, it is necessary first to identify them and then to determine their developmental appropriateness. Demands and expectations of others can be identified through interviewing adult caregivers or through observing social interactions. Demands of the physical environment are best delineated through direct observation of the child in typical surroundings. Assessment of the child's coping efforts in response to external demands and expectations must consider (1) the repertoire of available coping strategies, (2) flexibility in their use, (3) circumstances under which they are applied, and (4) their success in managing specific stressors. In assessing the nature of the feedback in coping transactions, the therapist must appreciate how it is provided (e.g., physically, verbally); whether it gives accurate information regarding the child's performance; and whether it is offered in a timely and contingent manner.

In addition to direct observation of the child's coping transactions, information about the child's coping experiences can be gathered through parent interview. Older children and adolescents can be asked directly about their history of coping transactions. Guiding questions to the parent may include the following:

- Are any particular situations stressful for your child?
- What does your child do in these situations?
- What do you do under these circumstances?
- How does your child respond to change?
- Does your child like to explore and try new things?

The assessment of coping transactions helps the occupational therapist understand how the child manages these specific situations. To gain further information for intervention planning, it is also useful to assess the child's unique internal and external coping resources.

Assessing Coping Resources

Coping Style

To assess coping style, it is necessary to consider the overall effectiveness of the child's coping competence and to identify the most and least adaptive coping behaviors. It is important to observe the child in various situations to obtain a representative sample of the child's coping efforts and the degree of their effectiveness in managing demands and expectations. The following criteria are useful in making these clinical judgments: (1) appropriateness of the coping efforts to various situations, (2) appropriateness of the coping efforts for the child's developmental age, and (3) extent to which the efforts successfully achieve desired outcomes.

Two observation instruments are suggested to assess the child's coping style. These are the *Early Coping Inventory* (Zeitlin, Williamson, & Szczepanski, 1988) and the *Coping Inventory* (Zeitlin, 1985). The Early Coping Inventory is designed for children aged 4 to 36 months and for older children who have special needs who function within this developmental range. *The Coping Inventory* is intended for children aged 3 to 16 years.

Items in these instruments target coping behaviors that have been documented in the professional literature as being associated with adaptive functioning in children. A five-point scale is used to rate each item, ranging from ineffective to consistently effective across situations. The results of the inventories yield an overall level of coping effectiveness and identify coping style. Comparisons can be made among the different categories of the instruments. In addition, the child's most and least adaptive coping behaviors are delineated. The instruments are uniquely structured to help the clinician interpret findings and plan intervention.

Several issues need to be highlighted when assessing coping style:

1. To what extent does the child engage in self-initiated behaviors, and are these coping behaviors productive?
2. Is the child able to use coping strategies flexibly across various situations?
3. Is there a difference between how the child copes with self and how the child copes with environmental demands?
4. How does the child evaluate the effectiveness of coping efforts?

This last issue is critical because the child's evaluation of coping effectiveness strongly influences the development of self-esteem.

There are a number of instruments that assess characteristics of children that are relevant to coping (e.g., scales that address temperament, social skills, locus of control, and personality traits). In addition, a number of coping and stress instruments are available.

Beliefs and Values

Emerging or existing beliefs and values are evaluated through observation and interaction with the child. Inferences about the child's self-esteem can be made during play and purposeful, goal-directed activity. The following behaviors reflect the child's feelings about the ability to influence the environment: being willing to engage in activities, creating or accepting challenges, making efforts to complete tasks, and responding to frustration and success. This information is critical in the selection and grading of activities that foster personalized intervention. In addition, formal instruments can be useful in assessing self-esteem in school-aged children. One of these instruments is the *Piers-Harris Children's Self-Concept Inventory* (Piers & Harris, 1969), which can be administered by the advanced therapist or by other team members. Also, play and activity histories obtained from the parent or child generate information that reflects the child's preferences and interests.

With verbal older children, the clinician can explore beliefs and values directly through informal interview. Issues that can be addressed include: what the child likes to do now and wants to do in the future; what is important to the child; what ideas the child has about any present handicapping condition and about disability in general; and how the child is the same or different from other people.

A parent interview can be useful in obtaining information about the beliefs and values held by the family, which strongly influence children's beliefs and values. This interview may address such factors as approaches to managing behavior at home and the parents' perception of the child and the child's behavior, goals, and expectations for the child's future. For example, a high parental value on educational achievement may result in punishment for academic failure. Likewise, a parental value for socially acceptable behavior may result in a developmentally inappropriate concern about a toddler's inability to share, take turns, and get along with others.

Physical and Affective States

A medical history and health examination by professionals in other disciplines can contribute information about the child's physical status. Additional relevant information is obtained directly by the occupational therapist during a developmental and sensorimotor assessment (e.g., joint range of motion, muscle strength, endurance, coordination, sensory processing, functional mobility, and manipulative skills). The assessment of affective status includes observation of the appropriateness of affect and mood, range of emotional expression, and feelings of well-being. The occupational therapist provides a unique contribution to the interdisciplinary team by observing the emotional responses of the child to a variety of purposeful activities and performance demands.

Developmental Skills

To assess developmental skills as a coping resource, the therapist must be familiar with the standard practices described in this book for evaluating various developmental domains. In determining adaptive competence, the child's strengths and vulnerabilities are identified in all areas, including cognitive, psychosocial, communicative, and motor development. Because the acquisition of developmental skills does not lead automatically to effective coping, assessment focuses on what the child can do and on how well the child applies skills as integrated coping efforts within situations. Direct observation of the child in the natural contexts of activities of daily living, school, and play is critical for collecting data relevant to coping. A process-oriented, coping-related approach to developmental assessment includes identification of the circumstances in which skills are demonstrated, the degree to which the child uses skills in a self-initiated manner, the approach to and organization of structured and unstructured tasks, and the ability to solve problems. Play assessments used by occupational therapists also guide observation of the child's spontaneous use of developmental skills in a functional context.

Human Supports

Availability and quality of human supports are identified as they relate to the child's coping. During home and clinic visits, parents and other caregivers are observed in their roles as primary facilitators of development and mediators between the child and the environment. Observations of parent-child-environment interactions are made to delineate the demands and expectations created by caregivers, their role in facilitating or interfering with the child's coping efforts, and the feedback given to the child. This information contributes to the assessment of the social resources available to the child and to the assessment of the caregiver's needs in relation to parenting.

As the child enters school and participates in community activities, human supports beyond the family unit are examined increasingly. For example, observation in the classroom and playground enables the therapist to appreciate how teachers and peers influence the child's coping at school. It also is helpful to assess the potential for expanding the range of human supports available to the child. With proper guidance, previously uninvolved older siblings, grandparents, or neighbors may be recruited to assist the child.

Material and Environmental Supports

A child's needs relative to material and environmental supports vary based on age, developmental capability, and the presence of a disability. The therapist determines whether the surroundings are organized, accessible, and offer various developmentally appropriate toys. When the child has a disability, it is essential to examine the material supports that the child requires to function optimally. These supports may include mobility and positioning equipment, adaptive toys, communication aids, and architectural modifications. The *Home Observation for Measurement of the Environment* (Caldwell & Bradley, 1979) is one instrument that can be used by occupational therapists to assess the external resources of young children and their general responses to the social and physical environments.

Linking Assessment to Intervention Planning

After the assessment data pertinent to the child's coping transactions and resources have been collected, the information needs to be analyzed so that the findings can be translated into an intervention plan. The following decision-making questions can be useful when designing intervention to increase coping effectiveness:

- How and under what circumstances does the child cope effectively? Ineffectively?
- What factors facilitate effective coping and what factors interfere?
- Of the factors that interfere with effective coping, what can be changed (e.g., demands and expectations, coping resources, the environment's response to the child's coping efforts)?
- What changes will make the most difference in facilitating the child's coping competence?

POSTULATES REGARDING CHANGE

The postulates regarding change are based on the transactional nature of the coping process and how it can be influenced. These postulates address factors that influence coping and that are amenable to change, including (1) the demands of specific situations, (2) the child's coping resources for managing these demands, and (3) the environment's response to those efforts. The postulates that follow guide intervention. Although they are presented separately, these postulates usually are addressed simultaneously during therapy to promote a goodness of fit between coping resources and environmental demands.

There are three postulates regarding change in this frame of reference:

1. Effective coping is facilitated by modification of environmental demands so that they are congruent with the child's capabilities.
2. Effective coping is enhanced by expansion of internal and external coping resources.
3. Effective coping is encouraged by appropriate contingent responses to the child's coping efforts.

APPLICATION TO PRACTICE

A primary goal of intervention is to promote a goodness of fit or congruence between the child's coping resources and environmental demands and expectations. When an appropriate match occurs, learning and development are fostered, and the child experiences a sense of mastery and well-being. Intervention is designed to establish a proper fit between the child and the environment so that previously acquired coping strategies can be modified and new ones can be learned to meet current and future demands. Zeitlin and Williamson (1994) present an extensive discussion of principles and strategies of intervention for children in the early childhood years. They emphasize the steps required to develop a coping-related Individual Family Service Plan. This book also addresses the application of coping strategies with a stress model to families.

Modifying Demands

The first postulate to facilitate effective coping involves the grading of environmental demands so that they are congruent with the child's adaptive capabilities. Therapists and parents must have a thorough understanding of the child's level of functioning so that appropriate goals and expectations can be established. A slight imbalance between demands and the child's functional competence is sought, so that demands provide the challenge necessary to foster motivation and learning. The adult can grade demands and expectations for the child in numerous ways (e.g., increasing or decreasing the complexity of the demand, modifying the way in which demands are presented to the child, and providing necessary assistance or supervision for the child to be successful).

Characteristics of the physical and social environments place demands on children and influence their behavior. Therapists, therefore, must consider both environments when grading demands in intervention or adapting the home and school settings. The following examples illustrate the varied nature of demands and the ways in which they can be modified: (1) giving directions based on the child's language comprehension, (2) positioning the child physically so that toys are accessible, (3) grading sensory experiences according to the child's tolerance, (4) providing verbal guidance in anticipation of changes in activity, and (5) adapting the pace of intervention to accommodate the child's attention span and energy level.

A careful activity analysis helps the occupational therapist grade the type and sequence of intervention so that demands are appropriate. Activities therefore can be selected that are developmentally relevant and that create the proper level of challenge. The case of Jenny, a child with mental retardation, demonstrates the importance of grading demands. Jenny stubbornly refused to participate in any self-dressing activity. The therapist worked closely with the parent to devise a dressing program that was personalized to foster success and motivation. Initially, it was decided to simplify the endeavor by focusing solely on upper extremity dressing. Demands were introduced at contextually meaningful times when Jenny was motivated to accomplish the task. She enjoyed going to school and taking a bath but usually resisted going to bed. Therefore, putting on her shirt and coat before school and taking off the shirt before her bath were emphasized at home. Managing pajama tops was deferred to a later date. Likewise, donning and doffing a smock were encouraged during therapy sessions when she was to be engaged in a favorite messy activity like finger painting.

In addition, the therapist taught the parent an instructional procedure that divided the task into component parts that required Jenny to participate gradually in an increasing number of steps over time. Using a "backward-chaining" technique, the child was expected to perform only the last step, then the last two steps, then the last three steps, and so forth until the task was learned. Through these methods, demands were modified so that Jenny could acquire increased independence in dressing without eliciting resistant, maladaptive behavior.

It is important that the therapist works with parents, teachers, and other significant adults to ensure that everyone has mutually shared consistent demands and expectations for the child. This collaboration is essential to avoid confusing the child with divergent messages that can interfere with learning new coping behaviors. Likewise, it prevents the child from being overwhelmed by unrealistic demands.

Enhancing Coping Resources

The second postulate on which intervention is based involves enhancing the child's internal and external coping resources. These resources include coping style, beliefs and values, physical and affective states, developmental skills, human supports, and material and environmental supports. Many of the customary practices of occupational therapists are designed to expand these coping resources. Implementation of this postulate involves intervention to remediate or compensate for deficits in performance components (e.g., sensory processing, neuromuscular control) and to teach competencies in performance areas (e.g., play, activities of daily living). Each frame of reference described in this book contributes to helping the child acquire or develop skills that can be applied in particular situations to cope. When a child has limited coping resources, the clinician usually draws on additional frames of reference to address the child's specific needs. For example, if a sensory processing deficit interferes with effective coping, then the sensory integration frame of reference would be applied to remediate this vulnerability. The discussion that follows provides general guidelines to enhance specific coping resources.

Coping Style

The coping behaviors of many special children are erratic, inconsistent, or limited in range. Based on an assessment of the strengths and vulnerabilities of a child's coping style, intervention can be targeted to expand coping behaviors related to such attributes as self-initiation, reactivity, flexibility, activity level, and self-regulation. Coping with emotions illustrates this point. Therapy can be tailored to assist the child to control and express anger in effective ways. The therapist can (1) label the emotion as the child begins to experience the feeling, (2) model appropriate verbal expressions, (3) teach cognitive/behavioral techniques for reducing affective tension (e.g., deep breathing, counting to ten), and (4) clarify what constitutes acceptable and unacceptable behavior (e.g., "toys are for playing, not throwing").

Specific goals, objectives, and activities of intervention are founded on a knowledge of the child's most and least effective coping behaviors. As discussed previously, these behaviors may be delineated through assessment instruments, observation, or parent interviews. A list of least effective coping behaviors identifies the major factors that interfere with learning and development. This list may be reviewed to determine which of these behaviors realistically can be changed. Although most behaviors have a potential for change, some coping behaviors can be influenced more readily than others. For instance, it is basically easier to teach a child to accept help when necessary than to develop a vigorous energy level.

The coping behaviors receptive to change are formulated into goals for intervention. A goal can be directed toward changing a specific behavior (e.g., to increase the child's persistence during play with familiar toys) or it can be written in broader terms (e.g., to expand the child's flexibility). Priorities in setting goals are established by determining which changes will make the greatest difference in fostering more effective coping. To determine specific objectives for intervention, the occupational therapist must consider what behavioral competencies the child has to learn (and in what sequence) to achieve the proscribed goals.

A list of most effective coping behaviors identifies the factors that facilitate the child's performance. These coping attributes are essential to determine therapeutic strategies and activities. They are used to design intervention that builds on the child's strengths. For example, if a child's most effective coping behavior is the ability to coordinate and adapt movements to specific situations, then a therapeutic strategy to decrease passivity would emphasize motor activities. If all goes well, pleasure in successful motor performance will enhance the child's self-generated, active involvement.

It often is necessary to teach the child the specific coping strategies required to manage specific situations. The child in a wheelchair can be taught ways to negotiate the hectic environments of the school and shopping center. The child who has a learning disability can be given methods to compensate in the classroom for perceptual deficits or poor handwriting. A fearful child can learn to ride comfortably on the school bus by sitting next to a friend in a seat near the driver. The child who demonstrates limited interpersonal skills can receive instruction on how to make friends or settle arguments (i.e., coping in a social context with peers).

As previously described, children can be classified according to their coping style (i.e., as minimally effective, situationally effective, or consistently effective). The nature of intervention varies for each child. Treatment guidelines based on the adequacy of the child's coping style are presented later in this chapter.

Beliefs and Values

Coping is supported when beliefs and values contribute to a positive sense of self and facilitate the child's ability to implement effective coping efforts. A child's beliefs and values may create vulnerability to stress when they result in negative self-esteem or emotional responses that interfere with daily coping. The therapist can influence beliefs and values indirectly by providing experiences that foster a positive sense of self and competence in daily activities. For example, a child who has a physical disability may have a negative perception of self as a result of dependence on others. The child may develop a stronger sense of personal efficacy if activities are modified for more independent, self-initiated participation. For older children who are able to express their thoughts and feelings, intervention can focus on clarifying and altering their beliefs and values. It may be helpful to conduct discussions related to issues such as: "What is good about me?," "What goals do I have for myself?," and "How can I get there from here?"

When the family's beliefs and values have a negative impact on the child's coping strategies, family-based intervention may be indicated. Parents can be assisted in recognizing their own beliefs, how they are reflected in child management, and how they influence their child's behavior.

Physical and Affective States

Many standard practices in occupational therapy influence the child's physical status. Activities can be designed to develop endurance, increase strength, and improve motor control. The child's unique physical characteristics may necessitate monitoring the daily schedule to prevent fatigue, modifying the environment to maximize function, and teaching alternative methods to compensate for disabilities. Therapy to influence affective state addresses the child's moods and psychological dynamics. Intervention is graded to support an appropriate level of self-control, emotional stability, and an awake-alert state needed for effective transactions. Sample treatment strategies include careful selection of activities, behavior management techniques, and therapeutic use of self. For example, a depressed child's mood may be altered by a warm, supportive therapeutic approach and the use of a favorite activity that invites active participation. When the child's emotional needs are a primary factor interfering with effective coping, the occupational therapist may need to collaborate with a psychologist or social worker.

Developmental Skills

Because developmental skills provide a foundation for coping efforts, adaptive functioning can be facilitated by expanding the child's repertoire of available developmental competencies and by remediating performance deficits. The challenge, however, is to structure the therapeutic program so that acquisition of developmental skills is closely linked to outcomes related to coping. The child then has the opportunity to integrate and apply the skills in a functional, coping context. It is helpful to make this link by writing treatment goals that use phrases such as "in order to." For example, Pedro will improve his bilateral coordination in order to expand his play schemes, increase his self-initiated problem solving, or communicate his wants through gestures.

In some cases, intervention may focus on teaching prerequisite developmental skills that prepare a child to cope. To enhance self-initiation, a child who is physically challenged may need therapy to develop coordination of the upper extremities, instruction in operating assistive devices, or training to use eye gaze to indicate choices. It also is important that treatment objectives emphasize mastery and generalization of skills. Ample time in therapy needs to be committed to the practice of new behaviors under a variety and complexity of conditions. Therefore a level of mastery is achieved to ensure that skills are truly available under the stresses of daily living.

Human Supports

Because families serve as a major external resource to support the child's coping strategies, occupational therapists must frequently develop a collaborative relationship with parents to plan and provide relevant intervention. How parents cope with the demands of raising a special child influences overall family health and the child's life outcome (Barber, Turnbull, Behr, & Kerns, 1988; Olsen & McCubbin, 1983; Williamson, 1987; Zeitlin & Williamson, 1994). Services are thus structured to be responsive to family concerns and can take many forms. In strengthening the child's human supports, the practitioner may address issues related to caregiving, parent/child interaction, behavior management, parental role development, and informational needs regarding community resources. Through these efforts, parents expand their abilities to facilitate the child's emerging competence (Figure 14.5). The therapist also serves as an important source of human support during ongoing treatment. This support can be extended by working with the child's teacher so that the classroom setting serves as a positive, external resource that promotes adaptive functioning.

Material and Environmental Supports

Occupational therapists are specialists in adapting the physical environment to foster successful coping in the home, school, and community. For instance, the therapist may modify lighting to maximize functional vision for a child who has an ocular deficit, may provide adapted seating for a child who has motor involvement, may regulate environmental stimulation for a hyperactive child, or may recommend materials and activities that are developmentally challenging. At times, intervention may involve temporary modifications to help a child manage a transitional period of stress. For example, after surgery, the therapist may help the child who is immobilized in a cast handle self-care tasks. The practitioner also may work with the family to access needed community resources, such as daycare or after-school programs, and social services related to housing, economic assistance, and primary health care.

Providing Contingent Feedback

The third postulate is that effective coping is encouraged by providing appropriate, contingent responses to the child's coping efforts. Appropriate feedback can reinforce desired or newly acquired coping strategies, whereas inappropriate feedback can perpetuate ineffective or maladaptive coping behavior. When feedback is timely, positive, clear, and accurate in response to productive coping efforts, the child experiences a sense of mastery that contributes over time to a belief system that addresses personal worth and autonomy. Meaningful social feedback is not just verbal but can be expressed affectively through smiles, frowns, and looks of admiration or consternation. The nature of the feedback needs to be selected carefully to promote efficient learning of coping behaviors.

In considering the use of feedback, it is important to accentuate the development of self-directed, purposeful behavior. Such an approach focuses on the therapist responding contingently to the child's self-generated action. The emphasis is on a therapeutic environment that supports child-initiated activity and provides feedback that encourages the extension and elaboration of demonstrated, emerging skills. In this context, the child has the freedom to explore, solve problems, and experiment with alternative coping strategies. Attention also is required to ensure that a balanced turn taking occurs between child and therapist, with ample opportunity for the child to lead the interaction within socially appropriate limits.

Research suggests that children who have disabilities tend to assume passive, respondent roles rather than active, autonomous ones (Brinker & Lewis, 1982; Zeitlin

& Williamson, 1990). This behavioral pattern can be reinforced unintentionally by parents and professionals. When a child has a disability, parents may tend to develop a strongly dominant interactional style (Barrera & Vella, 1987; Hanzlik, 1989; Rosenberg & Robinson, 1988). Likewise, professionals may tend to implement intervention, which is highly structured and adult-directed with an emphasis on eliciting responses from the child, that then is reinforced by the therapist (Dunst, Cushing, & Vance, 1985). In both cases, the child has little opportunity to learn that intrinsically motivated behavior can be used successfully to achieve personal needs.

Direct or Indirect Intervention

In intervention planning to implement the postulates, it is useful to divide intervention strategies into two categories—direct and indirect. According to Hildebrand (1975), direct strategies influence the child's behavior through specific interaction with the adult. Traditional teaching techniques and procedures for behavior modification exemplify direct strategies. Some examples include: (1) verbal guidance to help the child solve a task, (2) the modeling of desired behaviors for the child to imitate, (3) physical prompting to assist performance of an activity, and (4) feedback through specific reinforcement schedules.

In contrast, indirect intervention strategies influence the child's behavior through management of space, materials, equipment, and other persons in the surroundings. These strategies "set the stage" for learning by modifying the environment. Sample indirect strategies include: (1) adapting the size and type of play materials, (2) eliminating distractions for the impulsive child, (3) grouping children together to foster social interaction, (4) providing a predictable sequence of activities during therapy for the child who has difficulty adjusting to change, and (5) using splints, adaptive devices, or special positioning equipment for children who have physical disabilities.

Typically, a combination of direct and indirect intervention strategies is necessary to facilitate skill acquisition and coping. Care is taken to avoid over-reliance on direct guidance in therapy because this tends to reinforce reactive, dependent coping styles. Frequently, indirect approaches through environmental modification result in the child producing the desired behavior in a self-initiated manner. Jeremy, for instance, was a toddler who had a hemiplegic type of cerebral palsy and who resisted using his affected extremity. The therapist observed, however, that he would incorporate the arm spontaneously into tasks that required the use of two hands. Bilateral activities were then introduced as an indirect intervention strategy to foster self-generated hand use (e.g., playing with a large ball, pushing a toy lawnmower, riding a rocking horse).

Intervention Based on Levels of Coping Effectiveness

The level of effectiveness of a child's coping style influences the selection of intervention strategies and the intensity of the therapeutic program. The discussion that follows provides guidelines for addressing the unique needs of children who have minimally effective, situationally effective, and consistently effective coping styles.

Minimally Effective Coping Style

A child who displays a minimally effective coping style requires intensive intervention that consists of direct teaching of developmental skills and coping behaviors. This child's coping efforts are inconsistent, or rigidly repetitious, or reduce the stress of the moment but generate negative outcomes over time (e.g., habitual withdrawal or temper tantrums). It appears that a child continues to use ineffective coping behaviors to avoid or gain control over stressful situations or because of a restricted repertoire of alternative coping strategies (Schaffer & Schaffer, 1982). The minimally effective child usually has limited developmental, behavioral, or environmental resources to draw on for coping efforts or is unable, for whatever reason, to adapt available resources to the situation. Therapy focuses on expanding the child's resources while grading environmental demands to decrease the need to use ineffective stereotypic behaviors.

Successful coping requires the integration of various developmental skills to produce functional, goal-directed coping efforts. Initially, intervention emphasizes expansion of developmental capabilities to achieve greater competence in postural control, mobility, object manipulation, cognitive processing, social interaction, and communication. In addition, treatment is designed to teach desired coping behaviors and to modify the environment to reduce opportunities for the reinforcement of maladaptive patterns. Consistency is necessary in the choice and presentation of activities, and practice is emphasized. Because the minimally effective child often is incapable of applying learned behaviors independently to new contexts, the therapist gradually introduces new activities in a variety of situations as the child's coping ability increases.

The parents and therapist need to establish priorities for intervention because it is unrealistic to address all developmental and coping-related problems at once. Likewise, it is important to determine appropriate expectations for the child's progress. A consistent and shared approach to behavior management is necessary to extinguish negative behaviors and to encourage emerging skills.

Situationally Effective Coping Style

A child who demonstrates a situationally effective coping style has some adaptive competence. Coping efforts used effectively in one situation, however, are not generalized to other situations. Intervention is geared to help this child learn to generalize the use of effective coping strategies to settings and circumstances in which the child is currently less successful. Particular emphasis is placed on indirect intervention strategies because they foster self-initiation.

To plan an intervention program, the occupational therapist must identify the nature of the situations and environments in which the child demonstrates effective coping. Sample contextual variables to consider may include (1) the presence or absence of a caregiver, (2) the degree of structure, (3) solitary or group settings, (4) the time of day when demands are presented, (5) the child's preference for certain types of sensory input, or (6) the availability of adaptive equipment for a child with a physical disability. A major therapeutic strategy is to modify the environmental characteristics of situations in which the child copes ineffectively to resemble more closely the environmental characteristics of successful coping experiences. For instance, Sean was active and flexible in routine settings but became anxious in new surroundings. His parents were taught various techniques for making novel situations more familiar and less intimidating for their son. These strategies included previewing what to expect so that he could anticipate events, having him carry a tote bag that was a comforting object, and allowing time for him to warm-up and acclimate to situations. Under these conditions, Sean was able to generalize his adaptive behaviors comfortably to new environments.

Consistently Effective Coping Style

A child who displays a consistently effective coping style uses coping efforts that are appropriate more often than not. This child is able to generalize coping strategies across a variety of situations. No child copes successfully under every circumstance, but this child has sufficient resources to modify behavior and adapt to new demands as they arise. The child who has an effective coping style may receive occupational therapy to address other therapeutic needs; therefore, coping-related intervention becomes preventive and supportive in nature. The therapist monitors the balance between environmental demands and the child's coping resources and may use indirect intervention strategies to maintain and promote productive coping efforts. Attention is also targeted toward preventing deterioration in effectiveness during stressful life events. Activities of a preventive nature can support the child and family during situations that are predictably demanding (e.g., hospitalization, modifications in the child's current program, birth of a sibling, or changes in residency).

Integrating Coping into Intervention

The principles guiding intervention when applying the coping frame of reference are intentionally broad based. Each child experiences demands in a unique manner depending upon experience and available coping resources. To improve coping, it is necessary to examine how such demands are managed in specific situations over time. Recognize that involvement in therapy is inherently stressful because it is a change process. A standard treatment protocol cannot be used because intervention needs to be personalized.

For some children, the primary therapeutic concern may be maladaptive behavior. In such cases, intervention may be based solely on a coping frame of reference. For most children, however, this frame of reference is used in conjunction with others to ensure that therapy is linked closely to adaptive functioning. For example, it helps the therapist to provide NeuroDevelopmental Treatment in a way that strengthens the child's ability to meet personal needs and to respond to the demands of the environment. The following vignettes illustrate ways that coping goals were integrated into the ongoing treatment process.

- To encourage bilateral hand use and self-initiated problem-solving strategies in an infant who has hemiplegia, toys were hung from his highchair on strings of yarn. Through trial and error the child learned to pull up on the yarn with both hands to attain the toys. In the process he expanded his ability to change strategies when necessary to achieve a goal.

- A 7-year-old child had great difficulty separating from his mother during therapy sessions. Demands were modified by grading the mother's presence over time (e.g., active involvement to an observational role to brief periods of absence). The child's coping efforts were supported by having him play with highly motivating, favorite toys during the mother's absence and using a timer to indicate when the mother would return to the room. Positive feedback and assurance were provided to reinforce the child's developing independence.

- A group of elementary-aged children who exhibited poor motor planning and interpersonal skills were engaged in making a collage to foster their sensorimotor development and cooperative play. The following therapeutic methods were used to structure the activity: (1) group determination of a common theme and title for the collage; (2) provision of diverse materials that required cutting, tearing, and other emerging manipulative skills; (3) limited supplies, which necessitated sharing; and (4) positioning of the canvas vertically on a wall, which required the children to press hard against the materials as the glue dried (i.e., proprioceptive input in antigravity holding patterns). This activity targeted both sensorimotor goals and treatment objectives related to coping with peers (e.g., responding to the feelings of others, accepting substitute ideas, sharing, taking turns, and accepting and giving praise).

A sample case is presented to illustrate how this frame of reference can be applied to enhance occupational performance and coping effectiveness simultaneously in daily life.

Joe was an 11-year-old boy of normal intelligence who had poor impulse control and specific learning disabilities related to reading and mathematics. His primary academic placement was in a self-contained special education class, but he was mainstreamed for music and physical education. Joe was referred to occupational therapy by his teacher because of behavior problems in the classroom. The teacher complained that Joe had marked mood swings—compliant behavior alternated with episodes of acting out.

The occupational therapy assessment identified some sensory integrative deficits that possibly could be contributing to his erratic behavior. However, his behavior problems appeared to be most related to a minimally effective coping style. Joe had a great fear of failure that made him averse to any academic or social situation that he interpreted as difficult. Under these conditions, he tended to react explosively. It became clear that his compliant periods occurred under circumstances in which he was left alone to play or day dream. His least effective coping behaviors were the inability to manage new or demanding situations and the associated anxiety. In contrast, his most effective coping occurred in low-demand, structured settings that were familiar and provided support and encouragement.

In consultation with the teacher, a three-pronged intervention approach was implemented in the school. First, Joe received individual occupational therapy to improve his sensory organization and sense of empowerment. Second, the teacher was helped to adapt the classroom to be less threatening. For example, (1) the class schedule was made more routine and predictable, (2) Joe's desk was placed at the end of a row next to a friend who could serve as a peer helper, (3) Joe was asked to repeat directions to ensure that he comprehended the task, and (4) reading and math lessons were graded more carefully to promote success and were conducted in shorter periods throughout the day instead of being concentrated in the morning. Adult support and guidance were provided in stressful social situations such as recess and lunch periods.

Finally, Joe participated in a small group conducted by the occupational therapist that concentrated on teaching cognitive-behavioral strategies to develop self-control and problem solving. Joe learned to identify and analyze difficult situations, to consider alternative actions and their consequences, and to plan steps for reaching desired goals. For instance, in stressful situations, he was taught to use a cognitive technique referred to as STOP (i.e., *S*top what I am doing, *T*ake a look back to see what has happened, look at my *O*ptions, and *P*lay back a different way of behaving). Over time, Joe was able to regulate his emotional reactions and resultant behavior more effectively. The small group also provided an opportunity to increase Joe's comfort level when interacting with familiar peers so that social situations would become less stressful over time.

SUMMARY

This chapter presents a frame of reference to increase the coping effectiveness of children. The transactional model of the coping process serves as a framework for the postulates regarding change, modification of environmental demands and expectations, enhancement of coping resources, and provision of contingent feedback. Direct and indirect intervention strategies are applied selectively to implement these postulates. Occupational therapy has a unique commitment to human adaptation and function that defines the very nature of effective coping. It is the intent of the authors that this frame of reference, in collaboration with others, will empower children to cope successfully with their own personal needs and environmental demands so that they can be productive in daily life.

References

Antonovsky, A. (1979). *Health, stress, and coping.* San Francisco, CA: Jossey-Bass.

Bandura, A. (1977). Self efficacy: Toward a unifying theory of behavior change. *Psychological Review, 84,* 191–215.

Barber, P. A., Turnbull, A. P., Behr, S. K., & Kerns, G. M. (1988). A family systems perspective on early childhood special education. In: S. L. Odom, M. B. Karnes (Eds.). *Early intervention for infants and children with handicaps* (pp. 179–198). Baltimore: Paul H. Brookes.

Barrera, M. E., & Vella, D. M. (1987). Disabled and nondisabled infants' interactions with their mothers. *American Journal of Occupational Therapy, 41,* 168–172.

Brinker, R. P., & Lewis, M. (1982). Discovering the competent handicapped infant: A process approach to assessment and intervention. *Topics in Early Childhood Special Education, 2*(2), 1–16.

Brooks-Gunn, J., & Furstenberg, F. F. (1987). Continuity and change in the context of poverty: Adolescent mothers and their children. In: J. J. Gallagher, & C. T. Ramey (Eds.). *The malleability of children* (pp. 171–188). Baltimore: Paul H. Brookes.

Caldwell, B. M., & Bradley, R. H. (1979). *Home observation for measurement of the environment.* Little Rock, Arkansas: Center for Child Development and Education, University of Arkansas at Little Rock.

Compas, B. E. (1987). Coping with stress during childhood and adolescence. *Psychological Bulletin, 101,* 393–403.

DiBuono, E. (1982). *A comparison of the self-concept and coping skills of learning disabled and nonhandicapped pupils in self-contained classes, resource rooms and regular classes,* Unpublished doctoral dissertation, Walden University, West Covina, CA.

Drotar, D., Crawford, P., & Ganofsky, M. A. (1984). Prevention with chronically ill children. In: M. C. Roberts, & L. Peterson (Eds.). *Prevention of problems in children* (pp. 232–265). New York: John Wiley & Sons.

Dunst, C. J., Cushing, P. J., & Vance, S. D. (1985). Response-contingent learning in profoundly handicapped infants: A social systems perspective. *Analysis and Intervention in Developmental Disabilities, 5,* 33–47.

Fine, S. B. (1991). Resilience and human adaptability: Who rises above adversity? *American Journal of Occupational Therapy, 45,* 493–503.

Garbarino, J. (1995). *Raising children in a socially toxic environment.* San Francisco: Jossey-Bass.

Garmezy, N., & Rutter, M., (Eds.). (1983). *Stress, coping, and development in children.* New York: McGraw-Hill.

Haan, N. (1977). *Coping and defending: Processes of self-environment organization.* New York: Academic Press.

Hanzlik, J. R. (1989). Interactions between mothers and their infants with developmental disabilities: Analysis and review. *Physical and Occupational Therapy in Pediatrics, 9*(4), 33–47.

Hildebrand, V. (1975). *Guiding young children.* New York: Macmillan.

Kennedy, B. (1984). *The relationship of coping behaviors and attribution of success to effort and school achievement of elementary school children.* Unpublished doctoral dissertation, State University of New York-Albany, Albany, New York.

Larson, J. G. (1984). *Relationship between coping behavior and academic achievement in kindergarten children.* Unpublished doctoral dissertation, Fairleigh Dickinson University, Teaneck, NJ.

Lazarus, R. S., & Folkman, S. (1984). *Stress, appraisal and coping.* New York: Springer Publishing.

Lorch, N. (1981). *Coping behavior in preschool children with cerebral palsy.* Unpublished doctoral dissertation, Hofstra University, Hempstead, NY.

MacTurk, R. H., Vietze, P. M., McCarthy, M. E., McQuiston, S., & Yarrow, L. J. (1985). The organization of exploratory behavior in Down syndrome and nondelayed infants. *Child Development, 56,* 573–581.

Moos, R. H., & Billings, A. G. (1982). Conceptualizing and measuring coping resources and processes. In: L. Goldberger, & S. Breznitz (Eds.). *Handbook of stress: Theoretical and clinical aspects* (pp. 212–230). New York: Free Press.

Murphy, L. B., & Moriarty, A. E. (1976). *Vulnerability, coping, and growth.* New Haven, CT: Yale University Press.

Olsen, D., & McCubbin, H. (1983). *Families: What makes them work.* Beverly Hills, CA: Sage Publications.

Piers, E., & Harris, D. (1969). *The Piers-Harris children's self-concept inventory.* Nashville, TN: Counselor Recordings and Tests.

Ramey, C. T., Beckman-Bell, P., & Gowen, J. W. (1980). Infant characteristics and infant caregiver interactions. In: J. J. Gallagher (Ed.). *Parents and families of handicapped children. New directions for exceptional children.* Vol. 4 (pp.59–83). San Francisco, CA: Jossey-Bass.

Rosenberg, S. A, & Robinson, C. C. (1988). Interactions of parents with their young handicapped children. In: S. L. Odom, M. B. Karnes (Eds.) *Early intervention for infants and children with handicaps* (159–177). Baltimore, MD: Paul H. Brookes.

Schaffer, M. P., & Schaffer, S. J. (1982). Stress related to organically-based learning disabilities. In: A. S. McNamee (Ed.) *Children and stress: Helping children cope* (pp. 8–18). Washington, DC: Association for Childhood Education International.

Shahmoon, S. R. (1990). Parenthood: A process marking identity and intimacy capacities. *Zero to Three, 11*(2), 1–9.

Turnbull, A. P., & Turnbull, H. R. (1990). *Families, professionals, and exceptionality: A special partnership* (2nd ed.). Columbus, OH: Merrill Publishing.

Werner, E. E., & Smith, R. S. (1982). *Vulnerable but invincible: A study of resilient children.* New York, NY: McGraw-Hill.

Williamson, G. G. (Ed.) (1987). *Children with spina bifida: Early intervention and preschool programming.* Baltimore, MD: Paul H. Brookes.

Williamson, G. G., Zeitlin, S., & Szczepanski, M. (1989). Coping behavior: Implications for disabled infants and toddlers. *Infant Mental Health Journal, 10,* 3–13.

Yeargan, D. R. (1982). A factor-analytic study of adaptive behavior and intellectual functioning in learning disabled children. Dissertation. Denton, TX: North Texas State University.

Zeitlin, S. (1985). *Coping inventory.* Bensenville, IL: Scholastic Testing Service.

Zeitlin, S., & Williamson, G. G. (1988). Developing family resources for adaptive coping. *Journal of the Division for Early Childhood, 12,* 137–146.

Zeitlin, S., & Williamson, G. G. (1990). Coping characteristics of disabled and nondisabled young children. *American Journal of Orthopsychiatry, 60,* 404–411.

Zeitlin, S., & Williamson, G. G. (1994). *Coping in young children: Early intervention practices to enhance adaptive behavior and resilience.* Baltimore, MD: Paul H. Brookes.

Zeitlin, S., Williamson, G. G., & Rosenblatt, W. P. (1987). The coping with stress model: A counseling approach for families with a handicapped child. *Journal of Counseling and Development, 65,* 443–446.

Zeitlin, S., Williamson, G. G., & Szczepanski, M. (1988). *Early coping inventory.* Bensenville, IL: Scholastic Testing Service.

Occupational Frame of Reference

LOREE A. PRIMEAU / JANICE M. FERGUSON

The roots of the occupational frame of reference for children can be traced back to the founding years of the profession of occupational therapy. Drawing on the philosophy of the moral treatment movement (Licht, 1948) in which patients with mental illness followed a daily regimen of exercise, work, and play, the founders of occupational therapy emphasized occupation as a point of focus and a therapeutic means (Primeau, Clark, & Pierce, 1989). From 1917, the year that the National Society for the Promotion of Occupational Therapy was formed, until the late 1940s, the profession was centered on the concept of occupation and its ability to influence human health and well-being (Kielhofner, 1997). Over the next 20 years, the profession of occupational therapy was drawn into the biomedical model of human health, in which the role of inner mechanisms of the mind and body was emphasized in determining and influencing health. The use of occupation as a point of focus and as a therapeutic means was undervalued and, in some cases, lost completely. In the 1960s, under the leadership of Mary Reilly, Ph.D., OTR, FAOTA, occupational therapy recaptured the focus on occupation with her work on occupational behavior. Today, the academic discipline of occupational science is devoted to "the study of the human as an occupational being" (Yerxa et al., 1989, p. 6).

THEORETICAL BASE

The occupational frame of reference for children organizes and synthesizes theory about occupation into a structure that can be applied to occupational therapy practice with children. Given that occupation and its use as a therapeutic means are fundamental to occupational therapy practice, it is axiomatic that every child be viewed "through an occupational lens" (Yerxa, 1995). The occupational frame of reference for children is applicable to practice with all children and can be used alone or in combination with other frames of reference.

The primary role of an occupational therapist is to enable occupation. Enabling occupation is the act of "collaborating with people to choose, organize, and perform occupations which people find useful or meaningful in a given environment" (Law, Polatajko, Baptiste, & Townsend, 1997, p. 30). Forming collaborative partnerships with people to enable them to participate in occupations of their choice and to their satisfaction is the basis of client-centered occupational therapy practice. Client-centered practice empowers people to actively participate in occupational therapy. The emphasis of client-centered practice is on collaborating with people rather than doing things for or to them. Occupational therapists who enable occupation in the context of client-centered practice "demonstrate respect for clients, involve clients in decision making, advocate with and for clients in meeting clients' needs, and otherwise recognize clients' experience and knowledge" (Law et al., 1997, p. 49). When working with children, the occupational therapist's clients include the child, parents, siblings, other family members, peers, teachers, and other adults who are responsible for the child.

Because there is a dynamic relationship between people, their environments, and their occupations (Law et al., 1996), a secondary role of occupational therapists is to enable change in people and environments (Law et al, 1997). This dynamic and interwoven relationship between the person, the environment, and his or her occupation as it occurs and develops over the lifespan results in occupational performance. *Occupational performance* is "the ability to choose, organize, and satisfactorily perform meaningful occupations that are culturally defined and age appropriate for looking after one's self, enjoying life, and contributing to the social and economic fabric of the community" (Law et al.,1997, p. 30).

Because occupational performance is dependent on interactions between people, environments, and occupation, the occupational therapist must consider the following when addressing a child's occupational performance: the relationship between a child's spirituality, performance components, and skills (person); the physical, social, cultural, and institutional environments (environment); and the occupation itself (occupation). Change in the person, environment, or occupation will result in change in occupational performance. Optimal occupational performance is achieved when the fit between the person, environment, and occupation is maximized (Law et al., 1996).

Person

The person is represented as an integrated whole consisting of a central core of spirituality and various performance components that can be observed in the person's occupational performance (Law et al., 1997). Spirituality is the child's essence of self, his or her will, motivation, and self-determination, that is expressed in his or her daily occupations, thereby creating meaning in everyday life. Spirituality is crucial to understanding the child and his or her occupational performance. Performance components are defined as basic human abilities required for successful occupational performance and have been categorized into three domains: sensorimotor, cognitive, and psychosocial (American Occupational Therapy Association [AOTA], 1994).

Not all performance components are directly observable. Often, occupational therapists must observe the child's occupational performance and then make inferences about the status of underlying performance components based on these observations (Fisher & Kielhofner, 1995a). For example, a child's cognitive abilities, such as concept formation or problem solving, are often evaluated on the basis of his or her performance in a variety of tasks. These observable actions and behaviors that are manifested in the child's occupational performance are called "skills."

Skills are dependent on the state of the child's performance components and influence his or her occupational performance. They can be classified as motor, process, and communication and interaction skills. *Motor skills* are observable actions that allow the child to move about and interact with objects in the physical environment. *Process skills* are observable in how the child organizes and adapts his or her actions in order to participate in occupations. *Communication and interaction skills* are the observable actions through which the child communicates thoughts, feelings, and intentions and coordinates his or her behavior with other people. These skills act in unison and are interdependent (Fisher & Kielhofner, 1995b).

Spirituality, performance components, and skills combine to embody the child as an interactive being engaged in a dynamic relationship with his or her environment and occupations (Law et al., 1997).

Environment

The environment has been referred to as the context of an occupation. It is defined by Law (1991) "as those contexts (situations) which occur outside individuals and elicit responses" (p. 175) from them. The environment can either enable or hinder a child's occupational performance because the environment is the context of occupation. Environments can be described or classified according to location (home, neighborhood, community, country) or attribute (physical, social, cultural, economic, legal, political). Analysis of the location and attributes of the environment is useful when determining whether it enables or hinders occupational performance (Law, 1991; Law et al., 1997).

The occupational frame of reference for children uses the term "environment" to refer to the physical, social, cultural, and institutional (i.e., economic, legal, political) attributes of the child's environment (Law et al., 1997). The term "context" is used to refer to the locations in which the child typically participates in occupations. (It should be noted that this use of the term is distinctly different from the way context is used in the 1994 AOTA document, Uniform Terminology, 3rd edition.) Within the occupational frame of reference for children, three contexts are considered: home, school, and community.

The environment enables or hinders occupational performance in terms of its ability to afford opportunities for performance and to press for particular types of performance (Kielhofner, 1995a). The environment affords opportunities for occupational performance through the potentials for action available to a child in that environment. There is freedom to choose what to do within a specific environment. For example, a playground affords a child opportunities to swing, climb, or slide on the playground equipment, build a sand castle or make mud pies in the sandbox, or play a chasing game with peers on the grassy area. The environment presses for certain types of occupational performance when it demands or requires specific behaviors. For example, the school classroom presses for particular behaviors when the teacher asks the children to work individually on their spelling assignments. They are required to remain seated at their desks and work quietly on their assigned school work, raising their hands for the teacher's assistance as needed. At the same time, environments allow for (afford) and require (press) occupational behavior, thereby influencing the child's occupational performance.

Occupation

The occupational frame of reference for children recognizes that occupation can be defined in two ways: as "that which is done" and as "active doing" (Christiansen & Baum, 1997). Occupation defined as that which is done "refers to groups of activities and tasks of everyday life, named, organized, and given value and meaning by individuals and a culture. Occupation is everything that people do to occupy themselves, including looking after themselves (self-care), enjoying life (leisure), and contributing to the social and economic fabric of their communities (productivity)" (Law et al., 1997, p. 34).

This definition classifies occupations according to three main purposes: self-care, leisure, and productivity. The purpose of self-care occupations is to look after one's self; leisure occupations are for enjoyment; and productivity occupations serve the purpose of realizing an economic or social contribution to society or providing economic sustenance (Law et al., 1997). Occupation as active doing is defined "as doing culturally meaningful work, play or daily living tasks in the stream of time and in the contexts of one's physical and social world" (Kielhofner, 1995c, p. 3) (Figure 15.1).

Occupation within the occupational frame of reference for children is based on the following assumptions.

- Children have a drive to engage in occupation.
- Occupation is complex and multi-dimensional.
- Occupation must be considered within the context of the environment.
- Occupation is experienced within the context of time.
- Occupation is a product and a process of development.

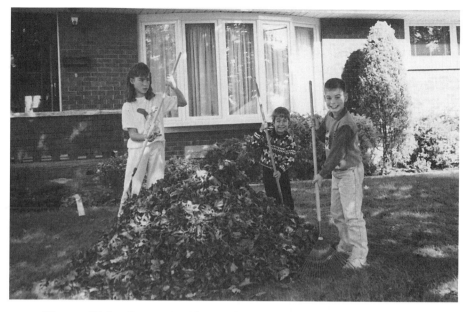

Figure 15.1   Occupation: Active doing and that which has been done.

- Occupation holds meaning for the child engaged in it.
- Occupation influences health and is a therapeutic medium.
- Occupation as a therapeutic medium can be characterized in two ways: occupation-as-means and occupation-as-ends.

Children have a drive to engage in occupation. The occupational frame of reference for children is based on the belief that children are occupational beings (Yerxa et al., 1989). They have an innate biological drive to act upon their environment, to demonstrate competence, and to experience a sense of efficacy through their actions (Clark et al., 1991; Reilly, 1962; Wilcock, 1993; Yerxa et al., 1989). This drive for competency and efficacy is expressed through engagement in occupation (Clark et al., 1991; Yerxa et al., 1989) and translates into a basic human survival need for occupation (Polatajko, 1994). Children's physical and psychological well-being rests on their ability to participate in occupations (Kielhofner, 1997; Polatajko, 1994).

Occupation is complex and multi-dimensional. Underlying the occupational frame of reference is the belief that occupation is complex and multi-dimensional. Occupation involves action within an environment and a culture that occurs across time and conveys psychological, social, symbolic, and spiritual meanings. These physical, contextual, cognitive, emotional, and spiritual dimensions interact to create occupations that are individually determined by and highly specific to the child engaged in them, and therein lies the complexity of occupation (AOTA, 1995; Polatajko, 1994; Yerxa et al., 1989).

Occupation must be considered within the context of the environment. Engagement in occupation requires children to interact with their environment, either through their actions on it or as a response to its demands or challenges (Yerxa et al., 1989). This interaction between children and their environment is reciprocal: they can affect their environment through their occupations, and their occupations can be affected by their environment. Given this relationship between children, occupation, and environment, an understanding of children's engagement in occupation is dependent on an understanding of their environment (Keilhofner, 1997) (Figure 15.2).

Occupation is experienced within the context of time. Children experience their occupations as they unfold in the course of time (Kielhofner, 1995c; Yerxa et al., 1989). Occupations constitute the ways in which a child uses time, and, therefore, they are a means of organizing time across his or her lifespan into patterns, habits, routines, lifestyles, and life stories (Christiansen & Baum, 1997; Kielhofner, 1995b; Law et al., 1997).

Occupation is a product and a process of development. Human development across the lifespan is closely related to occupation (Kielhofner, 1997). Occupation emerges as a product of development over the course of a child's lifetime (Reilly, 1969; Yerxa et al., 1989). Childhood occupations of school, play, and family chores and adulthood occupations of paid and unpaid work and leisure form a developmental continuum of occupations in which the occupations of childhood are believed to shape competence and achievement in adulthood (Primeau, Clark, & Pierce, 1989; Reilly, 1969,

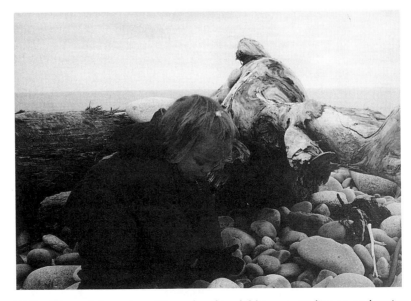

Figure 15.2 Through her play with rocks, this child is responding to and acting on the natural environment.

1974). Participation in occupation is a vehicle through which development occurs, leading to developmental outcomes or changes in a child's physical, cognitive, emotional, and social abilities (Kielhofner, 1997; Nelson, 1997). Occupation, therefore, is a product and a process of development (Kielhofner, 1997).

Occupation holds meaning for the child engaged in it. Engagement in occupation is experiential; the meaning of an occupation cannot be separated from its experience (Wood, 1995; Yerxa, 1994). Although engagement in occupation is readily observable to others, it can only be understood from the perspective of the child engaged in it (Clark et al., 1991; Nelson, 1997; Wood, 1995; Yerxa et al., 1989). Meaning is personal and cultural and arises, in part, from the child's previous experiences and associations with the occupation and the social and cultural context in which the occupation occurs. Engagement in occupation provides a source of meaning for one's life (Kielhofner, 1997; Law et al., 1997; Yerxa et al., 1989) (Figure 15.3).

Occupation influences health and is a therapeutic medium. The occupational frame of reference for children is based upon the belief that children are able to influence their health through the use of their hands as activated by their mind and will (Reilly, 1962). Engagement in occupation can lead to feelings of competence and well-being, which are believed to prevent illness and promote health (Yerxa, 1994). Within this frame of reference, it is assumed that occupation as a therapeutic medium is central to the profession of occupational therapy.

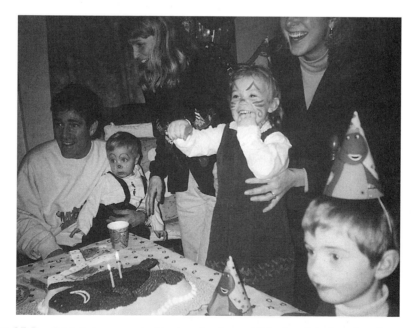

Figure 15.3   A birthday party holds meaning for a child when it is based on her personal interests and previous experiences and embedded in her cultural environment. Her engagement in this occupation will provide a source of meaning for her in the future as well.

Occupation as a therapeutic medium can be characterized in two ways: occupation-as-means and occupation-as-ends. Occupation-as-means refers to the child's engagement in occupation as the process through which change occurs (Gray, 1998; Trombly, 1995). Occupation-as-means is the therapeutic agent used to effect change in the child's occupational performance. Occupation-as-ends refers to the child's engagement in occupation as the goal or outcome of occupational therapy (Gray, 1998; Trombly, 1995). The therapeutic agency of occupation-as-ends lies in the child's successful participation in those occupations that are meaningful to him or her. In the context of health and well-being, occupation as a therapeutic medium can be envisioned as a means and an end.

Occupational Dynamics

Optimal occupational performance is achieved when the fit between the child, environment, and occupation is maximized. A child's occupational performance is enhanced by interventions that promote change in the child, the environment, and/or the occupation, thereby maximizing their fit. Within this frame of reference, change occurs through engagement in occupation (Figure 15.4). The occupational therapist, in collaboration with the child, parents, teacher, or other adults responsible for the child, designs an occupational form that has meaning for and elicits purpose in the child and/or the significant adults in the child's life and facilitates occupational performance resulting in adaptation and impact (Nelson, 1996, 1997). Change occurs through the action of the occupational dynamics of adaptation and

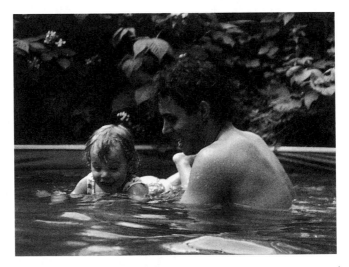

Figure 15.4   This father has facilitated his daughter's optimal occupational performance. He has maximized the fit between her, the environment, and the occupation of swimming through his choice of a safe place, playful manner, and physical support.

impact on the person and the occupational form (environment and occupation) (Figure 15.5). From this perspective, the concepts of occupational form, meaning, purpose, adaptation, impact, occupational analysis, and occupational synthesis are basic to this frame of reference, and, therefore, they are discussed in more detail.

Occupational form is the format of the occupation that is being engaged in by the person, and it refers to the specific environment in which a particular occupation occurs. It is defined as "an objective set of circumstances, independent of and external to a person . . . that elicits, guides, or structures subsequent" occupational performance (Nelson, 1988, p. 633).

Meaning arises within the person as he or she actively interprets or makes sense out of an occupational form. Meaning is created by the interaction between an occupational form (the environment and the occupation) and the person (spirituality, performance components, and skills). It is subjective, experiential, and unique to each person (Nelson, 1994, 1997). The person's developmental history influences the meaning assigned to an occupational form; different people will have different meanings for the same occupational form.

Purpose is defined as the desire for "an outcome from an anticipated occupational performance" (Nelson, 1996, p. 777). Once meaning in an occupational form has been established, then the person may experience a sense of purpose. In contrast to meaning, which arises from interaction between an occupational form and the person, purpose emerges from interaction between the person and his or her potential occupational performance. It is the goal orientation of the person engaged in an occupation. Purpose must be determined from the person's point of view, not those of others. It is a personal, affective experience that is very real to the person at that point in time (Nelson, 1994, 1997).

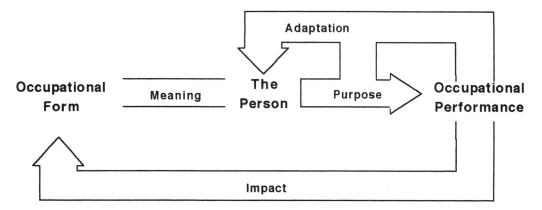

Figure 15.5 Occupational dynamics of adaptation and impact. (Reprinted with permission from Nelson, D.L. [1997]. Why the profession of occupational therapy will flourish in the 21st Century. *American Journal of Occupational Therapy, 51,* p.11–24. Copyright [1997] by the American Occupational Therapy Association, Inc.)

Meaningful, purposeful occupational performance affects the person (in spirituality, performance components, and skills) and subsequent occupational forms (in environment and occupation). *Adaptation* refers to effects of occupational performance on the person, whereas *impact* refers to effects of occupational performance on future occupational forms. Adaptation and impact are dynamic because they promote change in the person, environment, and occupation. Through the dynamic action of adaptation, participation in occupation has the potential to influence or change the person's spirituality, performance components, and skills. Through the dynamic action of impact, a person's participation in an occupation changes its subsequent occupational form. Specifically, features of the environment are affected and opportunities for engagement in different aspects of the occupation occur.

Occupational analysis is the process of identifying and examining the multidimensional aspects of an occupation. Tangible aspects, such as the materials and equipment required to perform the occupation, and intangible aspects, such as the meaning and value of the occupation, are considered (Breines, 1995). All aspects are interactional in that they impact on each other during the performance of the occupation. Occupational analysis breaks an occupation down into its component parts so that each aspect can be analyzed alone and in relation to other aspects or the occupation as a whole. A framework for occupational analysis is provided in Table 15.1.

Occupational synthesis is the process through which the occupational therapist collaborates with the child and/or adults responsible for the child to design an occupational form that is meaningful and provides purpose for his or her occupational performance. In turn, the child's occupational performance leads to adaptation in his or her spirituality, performance components, and skills and/or has an impact on his or her environment or occupation (Nelson, 1994, 1996, 1997). The term "synthesis" refers to the occupational therapist's simultaneous consideration of multiple aspects of the person, environment, and occupation in order to design an occupational form that provides the just-right challenge to the child.

Knowledge and understanding of occupational forms and elements of the person are essential for effective occupational synthesis (Nelson, 1994). When the occupational therapist considers the uniqueness of the child and his or her environment and synthesizes occupational forms that have meaning and that result in purposeful occupational performance, a therapeutic match is made (Nelson, 1997). In other words, the person-environment-occupation fit is maximized.

OCCUPATIONAL BEHAVIOR SETTINGS

An occupational behavior setting is "a composite of spaces, objects, occupational forms, and/or social groups that cohere and constitute a meaningful context" (Kielhofner, 1995a, p. 104). Occupational behavior settings afford and press for specific types of occupational performance, wielding significant influence on children's participation in occupations.

Table 15.1   Occupational Analysis

Occupational Form	
Physical Dimension	
Objects	Includes the objects present and their spatial characteristics (height, width, and depth), their positions relative to each other, their weight, temperature, texture, sounds they make, and background features such as lighting and air temperature
Human Aspects	Physical presence of people (including their size, location, etc.)
Temporal Aspects	The moment-by-moment changes in the materials over the course of the occupation (size, weight, position changes, etc.)
Sociocultural Dimension	
Symbols	Objects that society has come to a consensus regarding their meaning (e.g., a red light, national flags)
Norms	A socioculturally regulated expectation for occupational performance (e.g., norms for driving such as attending to the speed limit, using signal lights, etc.)
Sanctions	Typical social rewards or punishments associated with adhering to norms or not (e.g., speeding may result in a ticket or fine)
Roles	A set of expectations involving others (e.g., person behind the wheel of a car may be carrying out the role of a driver as well as that of a worker who is commuting to work)
Typical Use/ Variation	e.g., typical use of a pot is for cooking; of a tennis racket is to hit a tennis ball, etc.
Social Units/ Levels of Society	Symbols, norms, sanctions, roles, and typical use/variation depend in part on the social unit; include universal, cultural/subcultural, national/governmental, regional/community, institutional, organizational, family, and other groups
Language	Individual's language system provided by the sociocultural milieu
Person	
Sensory Motor	e.g., tactile, vestibular, space perception, depth perception, endurance, range of motion, strength, praxis, etc.
Cognitive	e.g., memory, problem solving, generalization of learning, concept formation, etc.
Psychosocial	e.g., interest, self-concept, social conduct, self-control, etc.
Individual Meanings	
Perceptual Meaning	Interpretations of the physical aspects of the occupational form

—continued

Table 15.1   Occupational Analysis—(Continued)

Symbolic Meaning	Interpretations of the sociocultural aspects of the occupational form
Affective	The emotional coloring given to an occupational form
Individual Purposes	
	Intrinsic and/or extrinsic, seeking sensory pleasure or avoiding sensory pain, value- or morality-oriented, conscious and/or unconscious, and the degree of purpose
Occupational Performance	
Overt Skill	Performance that is observable; reflects neuromuscular processes of action
Covert Skill	Performance that is not observable; reflects mental processes of imagery
Chains of Occupational Performance	Skills that come together in complex sequences in order to perform an occupation
Habits	Occupational performance that has been learned long ago; once acquired, little attention is required, but voluntary processes are still involved.

Adapted from Nelson, D. L. (1994). Occupational form, occupational performance, and therapeutic occupation. In C. B. Royeen (Ed.), *American Occupational Therapy Association Self Study Series, The Practice of the Future: Putting Occupation Back Into Therapy.* Rockville, MD: American Occupational Therapy Association.

Home

The home is the most pervasive context of children's lives (Csikszentmihalyi & Larson, 1984). It is where their basic needs for shelter, sustenance, social interaction, and rest are met (Kielhofner, 1995a). The bedroom, living room or family room, kitchen, dining room, bathroom, yard or garage, and basement or laundry room are occupational behavior settings in the home in which children participate in a variety of occupations. These settings were identified in a study that explored the daily life experiences of adolescents (Csikszentmihalyi & Larson, 1984). Children's range in the physical environment expands with age (Barker & Schoggen, 1973).

School

School is a shared experience of childhood that is central to children's lives (Medrich, Roizen, Rubin, & Buckley et al., 1982). Schools are the institutional context in which children are formally educated and prepared for adult life, but they are also the context for children's involvement in their peer group and culture (Csikszentmihalyi & Larson, 1984; Kielhofner, 1995a). The *School Function Assessment* (Coster et al., 1998) identifies six activity settings that exist in schools. These activity settings, referred to here as occupational behavior settings, are the classroom, transportation, transitions, mealtime/snack time, bathroom/toileting, and playground/recess. The transportation and transitions settings refer to the child's functional mobility (i.e., getting to and from school and moving around the school itself, respectively). Mealtime/snack time addresses eating in the school environment, and bathroom/toileting refers to the child's toileting and hygiene management. The occupational behavior setting of playground/recess includes free, unstructured time in the classroom, gym, or on the playground (Coster et al., 1998).

Community

The community context consists of a multi-faceted public world, which provides children with exposure to adult worlds and yet also provides opportunities for interaction with peers (Csikszentmihalyi & Larson, 1984). Children's participation in the community occurs in a wide variety of occupational behavior settings, ranging from local transportation settings (walking, riding a bike, skateboarding) and long distance transportation settings (cars, buses, trains, planes) to indoor public spaces (stores, shopping malls, movie theaters, libraries, restaurants, museums) and outdoor public spaces (streets or corners, urban parks, sports fields, beaches, protected natural areas). Other occupational behavior settings include friends' homes, churches, and community or recreational centers (Figure 15.6).

LEVELS OF OCCUPATIONAL PERFORMANCE

Occupational performance is conceptualized as a hierarchy of levels of behavior that are nested within each other (Christiansen & Baum, 1997; Nelson, 1988; Trombly, 1995). The complexity of occupational performance varies along a continuum with simpler levels of performance nested within more complex levels. There are four levels of occupational performance in the occupational frame of reference for children. They are in listed order of descending complexity: participation, complex task performance, activity performance, and component processes (Coster, 1998) (Table 15.2).

Participation

Participation is the top level of occupational performance. It addresses the child's overall pattern of participation in occupations within contexts of importance to the child and the adults responsible for the child. This level involves the child's orchestration and engagement in occupations in his or her contexts that are personally sat-

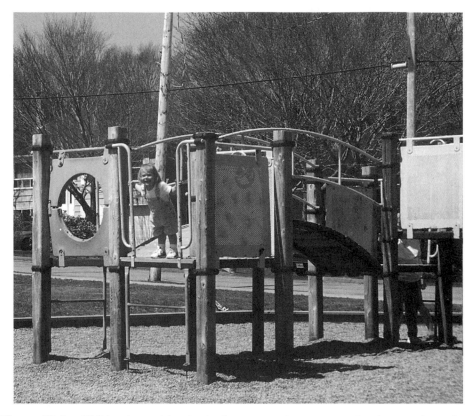

Figure 15.6 Children's participation in the community can occur in a large variety of settings. This child is playing in an outdoor public space.

isfying, growth-enhancing, responsive to opportunities and challenges of the environment, and acceptable to the adults who are responsible for the child (Coster, 1998). The child's participation in a range of occupations within the contexts of home, school, and community are of specific interest at this level. Examples of a child's participation at school include participation in occupations in the classroom, gymnasium, lunchroom, on the playground, and on the school bus. Participation in these contexts occurs in occupational behavior settings that are specific to that context.

Complex Task Performance

Complex task performance, the second level of occupational performance, focuses on the child's performance of the complex tasks that constitute the occupations in which he or she participates in these contexts. Because children's participation in occupations often occurs in contexts that have specific standards or expectations for

Table 15.2   Levels Of Occupational Performance

Participation	The child's participation in the occupations and opportunities typically expected of or available to a child of this age and culture **(contexts of home, school, and community)**
Complex Task Performance	The child's performance of important complex tasks expected of his or her same-age peers in this culture and context **(occupations of play, personal care, education, organized activities, unpaid and paid work, socialization, and functional mobility)**
Activity Performance	The child's performance of specific activities required to accomplish the major tasks expected of or desired by him or her **(motor, process, and social interaction skills)**
Component Processes	The child's basic processes or components necessary for the performance of daily tasks and activities **(performance components)**

Adapted from Coster, W. (1998). Occupation-centered assessment of children. *American Journal of Occupational Therapy, 52,* 337–344.

their behavior, this level is also concerned with the child's performance of complex tasks within each context at a level similar to that of his or her peers (Coster, 1998). Examples of complex tasks encountered by a child in a classroom include completing school work, using a computer, and working with peers in a group.

Seven occupations have been identified as relevant to children: play, personal care, education, organized activities, unpaid and paid work, socialization, and functional mobility. Each of these occupations may be broken down into complex tasks. Performance of these complex tasks is essential to children's engagement in occupations, which in turn is critical to their participation in the home, school, and community contexts (Figure 15.7).

Play

Play is the primary occupation of children (Bundy, 1993; Canadian Association of Occupational Therapists, 1996; Erikson, 1959; Parham & Primeau, 1997; Reilly, 1974; Simon & Daub, 1993). It has been classified as a productive occupation, but more often it is placed in a category of its own. Play has been variously defined as a disposition, in which the experience of play is central; as observable behavior, in which the observable characteristics are grouped into types of play; or as context, in which the play environment, particularly the cultural environment, is emphasized. Although the

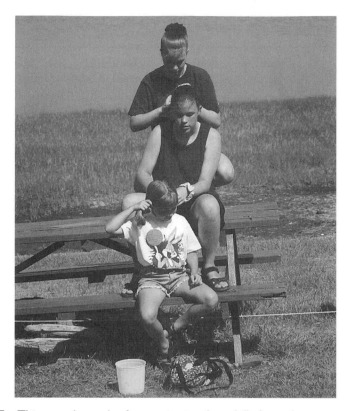

Figure 15.7 This complex task of grooming involves skills from the motor, process, and social interaction domains. (Courtesy Sandra Taylor, Wind-flowers Photography.)

experience of the player is lost when definitions of play as observable behavior are used (Parham & Primeau, 1997), these definitions are useful when determining the complex tasks that constitute play. The types of play that are considered to be complex tasks in the occupational frame of reference for children are sensorimotor play, object play, social play, motor play, imaginative play, and game play (Table 15.3).

Bundy (1997) describes children's playfulness in terms of three critical elements of play: intrinsic motivation, internal control, and suspension of reality.

- *Intrinsic Motivation.* The child is actively engaged; demonstrates overt exuberance; persists with task in the face of difficulties, obstacles, and barriers; repeats actions and activities to stay with same theme; and is interested and engaged in the process of task rather than in the product.
- *Internal Control.* The child decides what to do, how to do it, and appears self-directed; appears to feel safe; engages in challenges; modifies complexity of task; initiates and engages in play with others; shares play objects and equipment with others; and negotiates in order to have desires and needs met.

Table 15.3   Complex Tasks of Play

Sensorimotor Play	Exploring and manipulating self, people, and objects in the environment; repeating movements and actions for their sensory experiences (Morrison, Metzger, & Pratt, 1996)
Object Play	Fingering and mouthing objects; moving objects between hands; following objects visually; grasping, releasing, and dropping objects; banging, touching to skin, squeezing, and smelling objects; engaging in container play; grouping and sequencing objects; using objects in a functional manner (Pierce, 1997); engaging in construction play or manipulating objects to create or depict something (Reifel & Yeatman, 1993; Schaefer, 1993)
Social Play	Engaging in reciprocal games with adults in infancy, such as smiling and cooing at significant others; taking turns; sharing and cooperating with others (Cook & Sinker, 1993); playing in groups; taking on particular roles in play (Schaefer, 1993)
Motor Play	Crawling, running, jumping, climbing, throwing, kicking, and catching (Cook & Sinker, 1993); chasing, wrestling, and engaging in other forms of rough-and-tumble play
Imaginative Play	Conjuring up and using mental images in play (Landreth, 1993); using verbal expressions and actions to depict self as something other than self (Schaefer, 1993); initiating and responding to imagery and fantasy; sustaining use of imagery; story making and telling (Fazio, 1997)
Game Play	Understanding, accepting, and following rules (Landreth, 1993); making and breaking rules (Takata, 1974); demonstrating sense of fair play (Primeau, 1989); assuming perspectives of others (Landreth, 1993); enacting roles within games; switching roles within games (Reid, 1993)

- *Suspension of Reality.* The child pretends; clowns; engages in mischief; verbally and non-verbally jokes with and teases others; and involves objects or people in play in creative, imaginative, novel, and unconventional ways.

When these three elements are present, occupations are more likely to be experienced as play or playful.

Personal Care (Self-Care)

Occupational therapists have applied a variety of terms to this broad category of occupations, including activities of daily living, self-maintenance, and instrumental activities of daily living. A common purpose, looking after the self, is served no matter what label is used. The term "personal care" is used here to refer to those tasks that are essential to taking care of one's body, such as eating, dressing, grooming, bathing, and management of oral and toilet hygiene (Table 15.4).

Table 15.4   Complex Tasks of Personal Care

Eating	Eating and drinking a typical meal
Grooming	Brushing teeth; brushing or combing hair; caring for nose
Bathing	Washing and drying face and hands; taking a bath or shower, including water preparation
Dressing	Donning and doffing all indoor and outdoor clothes, including footwear
Toileting	Toileting tasks such as toilet management, wiping, flushing, and washing and drying hands
Bladder management	Control of bladder day and night, clean-up after accidents, and monitoring schedule
Bowel management	Control of bowel day and night, clean-up after accidents, and monitoring schedule

Adapted from Haley, S. M., Coster, W. J., Ludlow, L. H., Haltiwanger, J. T., & Andrellos, P. J. (1992). *Pediatric Evaluation of Disability Inventory* (PEDI). Version 1.0. Boston: New England Medical Center and PEDI Research Group.

Performance of personal care is linked to feelings of self-worth and successful participation in the social environment. Social and cultural norms dictate how children are expected to behave and interact with others; growing independence in personal care tasks as children mature and develop is one expectation among many. Compliance with these expectations affects how children are accepted by their peers and other people in their environment (Christiansen & Baum, 1997). Perceived social acceptance has been identified as one of the most critical contributors to overall self-worth (Harter, 1990).

Education

Education or participation in learning environments is considered to be a work or productivity occupation (AOTA, 1994; Law et al., 1997). Children's learning occurs in many settings, including preschools, day care programs, schools, their homes, and the community. Examples of educational tasks are attending to instruction; observing, imitating, and practicing skills, procedures, and techniques; managing and completing individual and group assignments; producing written work; following verbal and written instructions; and participating in group experiences (AOTA, 1994; Coster, Deeney, Haltiwanger, & Haley, 1998) (Figure 15.8) (Table 15.5).

Organized Activities

Organized activities consist of children's occupations that are adult-supervised and implemented by a formal organization or an agency. They are defined as "uses

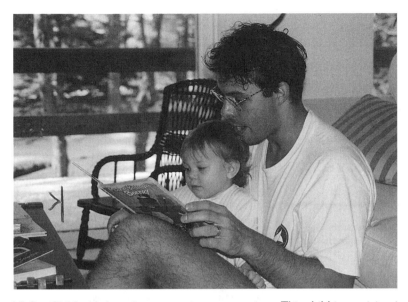

Figure 15.8 Children's learning occurs in many settings. This child is participating in the educational occupation of reading in the home.

of time that are purposive, ongoing, structured, and more or less voluntarily chosen (although parental and peer pressures may influence the process of making choices)" (Medrich, Roizen, Rubin, & Buckley, 1982, p. 158). Sports teams and leagues, clubs, extracurricular school programs/groups, and lessons are examples of organized activities. Children's participation in these types of occupations can be playful and productive; therefore, they cannot be classified as either play or productivity occupations but rather must be considered to be a blend of both.

Children's participation in organized activities can serve a variety of functions. Besides the enjoyment and fun that a child may feel while engaged in these occupations, he or she is exposed to experiences that have the potential to enhance physical and cognitive development, creativity, formation of social values, and self-discipline (Medrich et al., 1982). Organized activities typically occur in one of three formats: lessons, groups, or school programs. Lessons tend to be individual or group and are intended to convey knowledge, in the form of either skills or understanding. Groups provide opportunities for children to participate in activities as part of a social group. School programs are voluntary activities in which children can perform, receive training, socialize, and help with school operations (Table 15.6).

Unpaid and Paid Work

When one thinks about children's occupations, unpaid work and paid work do not immediately come to mind; however, most children participate in household work

Table 15.5   Complex Tasks of Education

Using Materials	Using all learning materials effectively, including such things as books, papers, notebooks, pencils, pens, erasers, chalk, scissors, glue, stapler, tape, and art materials
Set-up and Clean-up	Locating, retrieving, gathering, and putting away materials; setting up work space; tidying and cleaning work space
Written Work	Producing and sustaining written work (numbers, letters, and words) of good quality; adequate endurance for writing demands; maintaining speed in order to keep up with peers
Computer and Equipment Use	Carrying out basic functions such as turning computer on and off and accessing software; using keyboard and mouse; inserting and removing discs and tapes; completing work within time requirements
Task Behavior/Completion	Maintaining attention to task; following instructions effectively; observing, imitating, and practicing skills, procedures, and techniques; demonstrating good individual and group work habits; modifying and regulating behavior to suit the demands of the task; asking for assistance appropriately; responding well to constructive feedback

Adapted from Coster, W. J., Deeney, T. A., Haltiwanger, J. T., & Haley, S. M. (1998). *School Function Assessment* (SFA). Standardized version. Boston: Boston University.

within their families and some receive payment for their work inside and outside of the home. Children may also be involved in volunteer experiences in their communities. Unpaid and paid work tasks that children typically perform include picking up after themselves, making their beds, taking out garbage, running errands, completing yard work, caring for younger children and pets, and doing dishes (Goodnow, 1988; Medrich et al., 1982; Primeau, 1998; Rogoff, Sellers, Pirrotta, Fox, & White, 1975) (Figure 15.9).

Children's participation in unpaid and paid work has been characterized in the literature as a method of developing their prosocial or helping behaviors, introducing them to the concept of paid work in adulthood, and facilitating their independence (Goodnow, 1988). Most children complete some aspects of unpaid work in the home, typically progressing from helping others to assuming full responsibility for it. Indeed, children's participation in unpaid work in the home is often a source of tension between parents and children (Goodnow, 1988; Medrich et al., 1982). Children also complete unpaid work in the community in the form of volunteer activi-

Table 15.6   Complex Tasks of Organized Activities

Sports	Swimming, skating, tennis, martial arts, baseball, basketball, football, soccer, hockey, volleyball, and other individual and team sports
Fine Arts	Music, singing, dancing, drama, acting, drawing, painting, and arts and crafts
Religious Activities	Religious instruction and church activities
Clubs and Organizations	Boy and Girl Scouts, Brownies, Cub Scouts, Boys' and Girls' clubs, YM-YWCA
Extracurricular School Programs	Sports teams, cheerleading, chorus, band, newspaper, student council, and traffic patrol

Adapted from Medrich, E. A., Roizen, J. A., Rubin, V., & Buckley, S. (1982). *The serious business of growing up: A study of children's lives outside school.* Berkeley, CA: University of California.

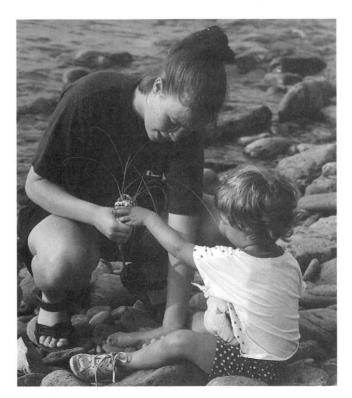

Figure 15.9   Most children participate in some form of unpaid and paid work, such as caring for younger children. (Courtesy Sandra Taylor, Wind-flowers Photography.)

ties, and they often receive payment for their work inside and outside of the home. Unpaid and paid work occupations consist of the following complex tasks:

- *Housework.* Picking up after self; shopping (Goodnow, 1988); running errands (Rogoff et al., 1975); making bed; cleaning own room and house; setting and clearing table; doing dishes; completing yard work; emptying and taking out the garbage; and preparing meals (Medrich et al., 1982).

- *Care-Giving.* Caring for siblings and other relatives; taking care of family pets (Medrich et al., 1982; Rogoff et al., 1975).

- *Community Volunteer Work.* Volunteering in community agencies and organizations, such as churches, hospitals, nursing homes, political parties, cultural institutions.

- *Part-Time Job.* Paper routes, babysitting, yard work (Medrich et al., 1982); washing windows, washing cars (Goodnow, 1988); working in fast food establishments.

Socialization

Socialization allows children to access opportunities and interact with others "in appropriate contextual and cultural ways to meet emotional and physical needs" (AOTA, 1994, p. 1051). From an occupational therapy perspective, socialization has been recognized as a self-care and leisure occupation. Socialization incorporates those tasks needed for full participation in family and community life, including functional communication, self-information (knowledge of name, address, phone number), peer interactions, problem resolution, time orientation, and self-protection (Haley et al., 1992).

Learning to get along with others is a lifelong process (Reid, 1993). Through the occupation of socialization, children learn how to meet their physical and emotional needs and how to develop and maintain relationships with others in their social environment (Figure 15.10). Socialization has two aspects: interpersonal communication and the ability to modify social behaviors according to affords and presses of the environment (Cronin, 1996). Participation in the occupation of socialization allows children to successfully navigate their social worlds (Table 15.7).

Functional Mobility

Functional mobility consists of tasks that allow one to change position or move from one place to another. Although it is recognized as a self-care occupation in the occupational therapy literature, the occupational frame of reference for children views it as more of a prerequisite for engagement in other occupations rather than an occupation in and of itself. There are two basic areas of functional mobility that are required for daily occupational performance: body transfers and body transportation (Haley et al., 1992). Body transfers include mobility in bed, using a wheelchair, and transferring from a bed, chair, wheelchair, car, tub/shower, toilet, and

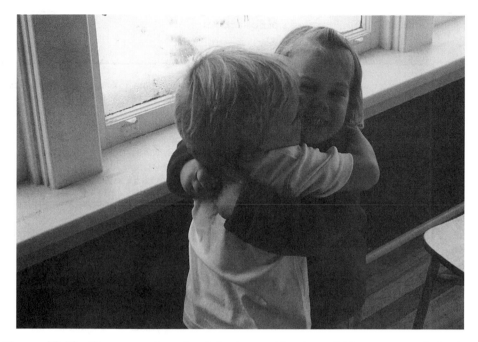

Figure 15.10   The occupation of socialization enables these children to meet their physical and emotional needs and develop a relationship with each other.

floor. Body transportation consists of locomotion indoors and outdoors, negotiation of various floor and outdoor surfaces, use of stairs, and transportation and manipulation of objects during locomotion (AOTA, 1994; Haley et al., 1992).

Functional mobility plays a significant role in children's social and cognitive development. Self-produced movement and the ability to act upon and influence the environment are primary vehicles for the child to acquire feelings of competence, mastery, and independence (Wright-Ott & Egilson, 1996). Functional mobility is a prerequisite for children's participation in occupations in the home, school, and community contexts (Table 15.8).

Activity Performance

Activity performance is the third level of occupational performance. It addresses the specific activities that are nested within the complex tasks. The focus is on the child's strengths and limitations and how they facilitate or limit his or her activity performance. Activities nested within the complex task of completing school work include manipulating papers and pencils, attending to the task at hand, organizing aspects of the work, and asking questions of the teacher as necessary. Activity per-

Table 15.7 Complex Tasks of Socialization

Functional Communication	Communicating all types of information to family, peers, and significant persons in occupational behavior settings
Following Social Conventions	Asking permission appropriately; demonstrating good manners; respecting the privacy and property of others as well as social and physical boundaries; using appropriate and inoffensive language
Compliance With Adult Directives and Rules	Cooperating with adult directives in all occupational behavior settings regarding such things as habits, routines, schedules, and required behaviors at school, church, and during mealtimes
Positive Interaction	Initiating and participating in social interactions; cooperating with others; listening well and responding appropriately; sharing; taking turns; using appropriate voice volume and tone
Behavior Regulation	Accepting and coping with change in routine; identifying problems; managing problems and/or conflicts well; recruiting assistance appropriately; maintaining control and demonstrating good frustration tolerance in all occupational behavior settings; refraining from self-stimulating behavior
Personal Care Awareness	Awareness and maintenance of personal appearance; cleaning hands and face after meals as needed throughout the day; performing nose and dental care and grooming as needed; dressing appropriately for occupations, seasons, and weather; caring for clothing as appropriate
Safety	Demonstrating caution around environmental dangers such as traffic, strangers, and unfamiliar tools and equipment; keeping inappropriate objects out of mouth; responding appropriately in emergency drills and/or real situations; reporting observed safety hazards in the environment

Adapted from Coster, W. J., Deeney, T. A., Haltiwanger, J. T., & Haley, S. M. (1998). *School Function Assessment* (SFA). Standardized version. Boston: Boston University.

formance addresses the child's current strengths and limitations in performance of these activities (Coster, 1998). The occupational frame of reference for children uses the taxonomies of motor, process, and social interaction skills from the model of human occupation to describe and define the skills required for children's activity performance (Fisher & Kielhofner, 1995b) (Figure 15.7) (Table 15.9).

Component Processes

Component processes, the fourth level of occupational performance, consists of the performance components that underlie the child's activity performance. This

Table 15.8   Complex Tasks of Functional Mobility

Maintaining and Changing Positions	Moving self to and from chair, wheelchair, standing, floor, car/other transport vehicle, tub or shower, and toilet; getting in and out as well as changing positions in child's own bed; maintaining stable seated position on floor and toilet; and maintaining functional position in seat for at least 30 minutes at a time
Travel	Moving on all types of indoor and outdoor surfaces; navigating around the various occupational behavior settings; keeping pace with peers
Manipulation with Movement	Carrying and transporting objects while traveling and changing positions in the occupational behavior settings; picking up and setting down objects; retrieving objects from storage spaces
Changing Levels	Moving up and down levels within the physical environment in occupational behavior settings
Recreational Movement	Throwing and catching a ball; running, jumping, hopping, and climbing; moving on high and low playground equipment

Adapted from Haley, S. M., Coster, W. J., Ludlow, L. H., Haltiwanger, J. T., & Andrellos, P. J. (1992). *Pediatric Evaluation of Disability Inventory* (PEDI). Version 1.0. Boston: New England Medical Center and PEDI Research Group and Coster, W. J., Deeney, T. A., Haltiwanger, J. T., & Haley, S. M. (1998). *School Function Assessment* (SFA). Standardized version. Boston: Boston University.

level addresses the contribution of the status of the child's performance components to his or her performance of activities (Coster, 1998). The component processes that underlie the activity of manipulating papers and pencils include the performance components of bilateral integration, motor control, praxis, fine coordination and dexterity, and visual-motor integration (Figure 15.11).

OCCUPATIONS OF THE CHILD

The occupational frame of reference for children identifies three contexts (i.e., home, school, and community) in which children participate in occupations to create their own unique patterns of occupational performance. Within these contexts, children engage in the occupations of play, personal care, education, organized activities, unpaid and paid work, socialization, and functional mobility. When using this frame of reference, the concern is children's participation in these occupations across all contexts.

Strategies to Maximize the Child-Environment-Occupation Fit

There are five strategies in the occupational frame of reference for children that can maximize the fit between the child, environment, and occupation. Through the

Table 15.9 The taxonomies of motor, process, and social interaction skills

Motor Domains and Skills

Posture
Relates to the stabilizing and aligning of one's body while moving in relation to objects with which one must deal

Stabilizes: Steadies one's body and maintains trunk control and balance while sitting, standing, walking, reaching, or while moving, lifting, or pulling objects
Aligns: Maintains the vertical alignments of the body over the base of support
Positions: Places one's arms and body in relation to objects in a manner that promotes efficient arm movements

Mobility
Relates to moving the entire body or a body part in space as necessary

Walks: Ambulates on level surfaces, including turning around and changing direction while walking
Reaches: Stretches or extends the arm and, when appropriate, the trunk to grasp or place objects that are out of reach
Bends: Actively flexes, rotates, or twists the body in a manner and direction appropriate to a task

Coordination
Relates to moving body parts in relationship to each other and to the environment; pertains to spatiotemporal organization of movements

Coordinates: Uses different parts of the body together to support or stabilize objects during bilateral motor tasks
Manipulates: Uses dexterous grasp and release as well as coordinated in-hand manipulation patterns
Flows: Uses smooth, fluid, continuous, uninterrupted arm and hand movements

Strength and Effort
Pertains to skills that require generation of muscle force appropriate to the action a person is undertaking

Moves: Pushes, shoves, pulls, or drags objects along a supporting surface or around a weight bearing axis
Transports: Carries objects while ambulating or moving from one place to another
Lifts: Raises or hoists objects off of supporting surface
Calibrates: Regulates or grades the force, speed, and extent of movements
Grips: Pinches or grasps in order to securely hold handles or other objects

Energy
Refers to physical exertion and sustained effort over time

Endures: Persists and completes an activity without evidence of fatigue, pausing to rest, or stopping to catch one's breath
Paces: Maintains a rate or tempo of performance across an entire task

Process Domains and Skills

Energy
Pertains to sustained and appropriately allocated mental energy

Paces: Maintains a rate or tempo of performance across an entire task
Attends: Maintains attention focused on the task

Knowledge
Refers to the ability to seek and use knowledge

Chooses: Selects appropriate tools and materials
Uses: Employs tools and materials according to their intended purposes
Handles: Supports, stabilizes, and holds tools and materials in an appropriate manner

—continued

Table 15.9   The taxonomies of motor, process, and social interaction skills

Process Domains and Skills	
	Heeds: Uses goal-directed task performance that is focused toward the completion of the intended task
	Inquires: Seeks appropriate verbal or written information by asking questions or reading directions
Temporal Organization Pertains to the beginning, logical ordering, continuation, and completion of the steps and action sequences of a task	Initiates: Starts or begins doing an action or step without hesitation
	Continues: Performs an action sequence of a step without unnecessary interruption and as an unbroken, smooth progression
	Sequences: Performs steps in an effective or logical order for efficient use of time and energy
	Terminates: Finishes or brings to completion single actions or steps without perseveration, inappropriate persistence, or premature cessation
Organizing Space and Objects Pertains to skills for organizing space and objects	Searches and Locates: Looks for and locates tools and materials through the process of logical searching
	Gathers: Collects together needed or misplaced tools and materials
	Organizes: Logically positions or spatially arranges tools and materials in an orderly fashion and in between appropriate work spaces
	Restores: Returns and puts away tools and materials, and restores immediate work spaces to original condition
	Navigates: Modifies the movement of the arm, body, or wheelchair to avoid or maneuver around existing obstacles that are encountered in the course of moving the arm, body, or wheelchair through space
Adaptation Relates to the ability to anticipate, correct for, and benefit by learning from the consequences of errors that arise in the course of action	Notices and Responds: Responds appropriately to nonverbal environmental and perceptual cues that provide feedback regarding task progression
	Accommodates: Modifies one's action or location of objects within the workpiece in anticipation of or in response to circumstances or problems that might arise in the course of action or to avoid undesirable outcomes
	Adjusts: Changes environmental conditions in anticipation of or in response to circumstances or problems that arise in the course of action or to avoid undesirable outcomes
	Benefits: Anticipates and prevents undesirable circumstances or problems from recurring or persisting
Social Interaction Domains and Skills	
Acknowledging Refers to actions that facilitate communication and interaction	Turns: Actively positions one's body to face one's social partner
	Looks: Makes visual contact with one's social partner
	Confirms: Acknowledges the reception of social messages
	Touches: Appropriately uses touch or other physical contact during social interaction
Sending Pertains to directing messages of information and for communicating	Greets: Uses appropriate words, phrases, and ceremonies to greet one's social partner
	Answers: Gives relevant replies to questions
	Questions: Requests factual information appropriate to the situation and level of familiarity among social partners

—continued

Table 15.9 The taxonomies of motor, process, and social interaction skills—(Continued)

	Complies: Agrees, accepts offerings, meets requests, and uses empathy
	Encourages: Makes supportive statements or gives positive feedback
	Extends: Sends messages that help to keep the conversation going
	Clarifies: Assures that one's social partner is following the conversation or interaction
	Sets limits: Expresses limits or refusals
	Thanks: Uses appropriate words, phrases, and ceremonies to acknowledge received favors
	Concludes: Appropriately terminates conversations or social interactions
Timing	Approaches: Uses appropriate strategies to initiate interactions
Refers to matching one's messages with those of the social partner and with the expectations of the environment	Places self: Positions oneself at an appropriate distance from one's social partner
	Assumes position: Assumes a physical posture that is appropriate to the type of interaction and level of familiarity
	Matches language: Uses language and level of address that is appropriate to the situation and social partner
	Discloses: Shares and discusses personal information, experiences, feelings, emotions, and opinions appropriately
	Expresses emotion: Displays affect in a manner that is compatible with one's social partner's affective tone and expectations of the situation

Fisher, A., & Kielhofner, G. (1995). Skill in occupational performance. In G. Kielhofner (Ed.), *A model of human occupation: Theory and application* (2nd ed., pp. 113–137). Baltimore: Williams & Wilkins.

---

process of occupational synthesis, the therapist uses these strategies to design occupational forms that will lead to adaptation and/or impact (see Figure 15.5). These strategies are establish/restore, alter, adapt, prevent, and create (Dunn, Brown, & McGuigan, 1994). They target the person, the environment, the occupation, or a combination of these to promote change, thereby maximizing the person-environment-occupation fit.

Establish/Restore

Establish and restore is aimed at promoting change within the person. The occupational therapist identifies the child's strengths and limitations and how they facilitate or limit his or her occupational performance. As a remedial approach, the focus of this strategy is on establishing or restoring age-appropriate skills that will facilitate the child's ability to engage in occupations (Dunn et al., 1994).

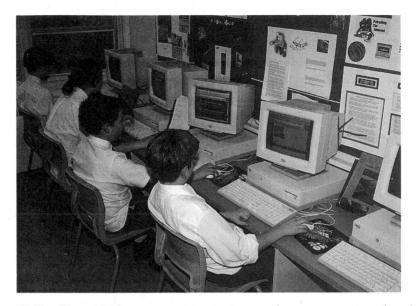

Figure 15.11   These children are participating in one of many occupations found in the school context (Participation). The educational occupation of computer use (Complex Task Performance) involves their motor and process skills, including their manipulation of the mouse and choice of appropriate computer programs (Activity Performance). Performance components that underlie these skills include fine coordination/dexterity, visual motor integration, recognition, and interest (Component Processes). (Courtesy Sandra Taylor, Wind-flowers Photography.)

Alter

Alter targets the environment as the locus for change. Environments that are compatible with the child's skills and abilities are identified by the therapist (Dunn et al., 1994). The child's current skills are accepted as they are, and the environment that maximizes those skills is selected.

Adapt

Adaptation promotes change in the environment and/or the occupation. Features of the environment or occupation are adjusted to support the child's occupational performance (Dunn et al., 1994). Using adaptive or compensatory approaches, the occupational therapist changes aspects of the environment and/or the occupation so that the child's occupational performance is enhanced.

Prevent

The person, environment, and/or occupation are targeted to prevent the development of occupational performance problems (Dunn et al., 1994). Often, the occupational therapist anticipates that a child may experience difficulties in his or her occupational performance unless intervention is provided to prevent their occurrence. The likely course of events can be circumvented by promoting change in the child, the environment, and/or the occupation.

Create

The environment and/or the occupation are created to be areas of change. The occupational therapist creates environmental and/or occupational circumstances that promote optimal occupational performance (Dunn et al., 1994). Unlike the previous strategies, this strategy does not assume that dysfunction in the child's occupational performance exists or is likely to develop. It is aimed at the creation of an environment and opportunities for engagement in occupations that will enrich the child's experience and facilitate his or her optimal occupational performance.

FUNCTION/DYSFUNCTION CONTINUA

This frame of reference is concerned with children's occupational performance in occupations across the contexts of home, school, and community. Function/dysfunction continua are conceptualized and organized around the levels of occupational performance. The four function/dysfunction continua are (1) participation, (2) complex task performance, (3) activity performance, and (4) component processes.

Indicators of Function and Dysfunction for Participation

A child's occupational performance is functional when he or she participates in occupations in his or her occupational behavior settings in the home, school, and community contexts that are personally satisfying, growth enhancing, responsive to opportunities and challenges of the environment, and acceptable to the adults who are responsible for the child. Indicators of function are when the child is satisfied with his or her participation in occupations; when the social environment (parents, teachers, and other adults responsible for the child) views the child's participation as adequate in occupations; when the child participates in occupations that are available to him or her (affords) and that are expected of him or her (presses); and, when the child participates in occupations at a level similar to children of the same age and culture.

Indicators of dysfunction in participation are when a child does not or is unable to participate in occupations in his or her occupational behavior settings that are personally satisfying, growth-enhancing, responsive to opportunities and challenges of the environment, and acceptable to the adults who are responsible for the child and when the child does not participate in occupations at a level similar to children of the same age and culture (Chart 15.1).

Chart 15.1   Indicators of Function and Dysfunction for Participation.

Ability to Participate	Inability to Participate
FUNCTION: Child participates in occupations in a variety of settings.	DYSFUNCTION: Child is unable to participate in occupations in a variety of settings.
INDICATORS OF FUNCTION	**INDICATORS OF DYSFUNCTION**
Child participates in occupations in his or her occupational behavior settings in a variety of contexts that are personally satisfying.	Child does not or is unable to participate in occupations in occupational behavior settings in a variety of contexts.
	Child participates but not to the level of personal satisfaction.
Child participates in occupations in his or her occupational behavior settings in a variety of contexts that are growth enhancing.	Child participates in occupations but they are not growth enhancing.
Child responsive to opportunities and challenges of the environment.	Child is not responsive to opportunities and challenges of the environment.
Child's participation is adequate for the social environment as deemed by the adults responsible for the child.	Child's participation is not adequate for the social environment as deemed by the adults responsible for the child.

Indicators of Function and Dysfunction for Complex Task Performance

Function/dysfunction continua at the level of complex task performance are concerned with the child's ability to perform complex tasks that are necessary for engagement in occupations. Each of the occupations of play, personal care, education, organized activities, unpaid and paid work, socialization, and functional mobility may be broken down into complex tasks.

For each of these complex tasks, indicators of function are that the child is satisfied with his or her performance of the complex tasks that are required for participation in occupations in his or her occupational behavior settings. The child's performance of complex tasks, which are required for participation in occupations in his or her occupational behavior settings, is considered adequate by the social environment (parents, teachers, and other adults responsible for the child). The child does not require assistance with his or her performance of the complex tasks that are required for participation in occupations in his or her occupational behavior settings beyond that usually provided to children of the same age and grade level. The child performs all complex tasks that are required for participation in occupations in his or her occupational behavior settings without modification of tools, materials, procedures, or time requirements beyond those usually provided for children of the same age and grade level.

Indicators of dysfunction for each of the complex tasks are that the child is not satisfied with his or her performance of the complex tasks that are required for participation in occupations in his or her occupational behavior settings. Performance of complex tasks that are required for participation in occupations in his or her occupational behavior settings is not considered adequate by the social environment (parents, teachers, and other adults responsible for the child). The child requires assistance with his or her performance of the complex tasks beyond that usually provided to children of the same age and grade level. The child requires modification of tools, materials, procedures, or time requirements beyond those usually provided for children of the same age and grade level in order to perform the complex tasks that are required for participation in occupations in his or her occupational behavior settings (Chart 15.2).

Indicators of Function and Dysfunction for Activity Performance

Function/dysfunction continua at the level of activity performance are concerned with the child's performance of specific skills that constitute the complex tasks required for participation in occupations. The three areas of activity performances are motor skills, process skills, and social interaction skills.

Indicators of function in each of the three skill areas are that the child is satisfied with his or her performance of the skills that are required for complex task performance in his or her occupational behavior settings. The social environment (parents, teachers, and other adults responsible for the child) considers the child's performance of the skills that are required for complex task performance in his or her occupational behavior settings to be adequate. The child does not require assistance with his or her performance of the skills that are required for complex task performance in his or her occupational behavior settings beyond that usually provided to children of the same age and grade level. The child performs all skills that are required for complex task performance in his or her occupational behavior settings without modification of tools, materials, procedures, or time requirements beyond those usually provided for children of the same age and grade level.

Indicators of dysfunction in each of the three skill areas are the child is not satisfied with his or her performance of the skills that are required for complex task performance in his or her occupational behavior settings. The social environment (parents, teachers, and other adults responsible for the child) does not consider the child's performance of the skills that are required for complex task performance in his or her occupational behavior settings to be adequate. The child requires assistance with his or her performance of the skills that are required for complex task performance in his or her occupational behavior settings beyond that usually provided to children of the same age and grade level. The child requires modification of tools, materials, procedures, or time requirements beyond that usually provided for children of the same age and grade level to perform the skills that are required for complex task performance in his or her occupational behavior settings (Chart 15.3).

Chart 15.2 Indicators of Function and Dysfunction for Complex Task Performance	
Ability to Perform Complex Task	**Inability to Perform Complex Task**
FUNCTION: Child performs complex tasks necessary to engage in occupations (i.e., Play, Personal Care, Education, Organized Activities, Unpaid and Paid Work, Socialization, Functional Mobility).	DYSFUNCTION: Child is unable to perform complex tasks necessary to engage in occupations (i.e., Play, Personal Care, Education, Organized Activities, Unpaid and Paid Work, Socialization, Functional Mobility).
INDICATORS OF FUNCTION	**INDICATORS OF DYSFUNCTION**
Child participates in the various complex tasks in a manner that is personally satisfying.	Child cannot or is unable to participate in the various complex tasks in a manner that is personally satisfying.
Child's performance of complex tasks is adequate for the social environment in his or her occupational behavior setting as deemed by adults responsible for the child.	Child's performance of complex tasks is not adequate for the social environment in his or her occupational behavior setting as deemed by adults responsible for the child.
	Child requires assistance for complex tasks with personal care beyond that usually provided to children of the same age level.
	Child requires modification of tools, materials, procedures, or time requirements for performance of complex tasks beyond those usually provided for children of the same age level.

Indicators of Function and Dysfunction for Component Processes

Function/dysfunction continua at the level of component processes address the performance components that underlie the child's activity and complex task performance. Impairment at this level should always be addressed in the context of its repercussions on the child's ability to perform the activities and complex tasks that are required for participation in occupations in his or her occupational behavior settings. Component processes, or performance components, are described and defined in detail in Uniform Terminology, 3rd edition (AOTA, 1994); they will not be provided here.

A child's component processes are considered functional when he or she has adequate structures and processes to support activity performance and complex task performance in his or her occupational behavior settings. The child has the component processes required for performance of the activities and complex tasks that are necessary for participation in his or her occupational behavior settings.

A child's component processes are dysfunctional when he or she has inadequate structures and processes to support activity performance and complex task performance in his or her occupational behavior settings.

Chart 15.3   Indicators of Function and Dysfunction for Activity Performance.

Ability to Perform Specific Activities	Inability to Perform Specific Activities
FUNCTION: Child has the motor, process, and social interaction skills for complex task performance.	DYSFUNCTION: Child does not have the motor, process, and social interaction required for complex task performance.
INDICATORS OF FUNCTION:	**INDICATORS OF DYSFUNCTION:**
Child is satisfied with performance of the skills required for complex tasks.	Child is not satisfied with his or her performance of the skills required for complex tasks.
Child's performance of the skills required for complex tasks is satisfactory as deemed by adults responsible for the child.	Child's performance of skills required for complex tasks is not satisfactory for the social environment as deemed by adults responsible for the child.
	Child requires assistance for the performance of skills required for complex tasks beyond that usually provided to children of the same age level.
	Child requires modification of tools, materials, procedures, or time requirements for the performance of skills required for complex tasks beyond that usually provided to children of the same age level.

GUIDE FOR EVALUATION

In this frame of reference, the evaluation process is guided by specific beliefs about how to assess children. These beliefs specify that assessment of a child's occupational performance is client-centered, is dynamic, is context-specific, and measures levels of occupational performance with a top-down approach. A top down approach addresses each level of the child's occupational performance.

Client-Centered Assessment

The occupational therapist and the client collaborate to create an evaluation process that is based on their combined expertise, experiences, and perspectives. Client-centered assessment includes the child (in accordance with his or her ability to be included) and the other people who are involved with him or her in determining what will be assessed, how it will be assessed, and what the goals or outcomes of intervention will be. In order to do this, the occupational therapist must foster clear and open communication with them, guide them to identify assessment needs and their strengths and limitations from their own perspectives, and provide them with information that will assist them to make choices about the evaluation process. Client-centered assessment is most true to the child when it is conducted in his or her natural settings using real-life occupations that are meaningful to him or her whenever possible (Townsend, 1997).

Dynamic Assessment

This assessment strategy recognizes the child's strengths in occupational performance and uses them to develop a plan for intervention, thereby promoting client-centered practice. Dynamic assessment helps the occupational therapist to identify how the child learns and approaches tasks, gain an appreciation of what types and amount of change can be expected through intervention, and determine intervention methods that are most likely to enhance the child's occupational performance. Dynamic assessment employs a test-teach-test strategy. This strategy first asks the child to attempt a task to establish what he or she can do independently. Next, the occupational therapist intervenes to teach the task by providing assistance in the form of prompts or aids or by modifying the task itself, including its complexity, presentation, or steps required to complete it. Finally, the same or a similar task is presented to determine whether the intervention has resulted in improvement in the child's task performance (Missiuna, 1987).

In addition to assessing the child's potential for change, dynamic assessment also assesses the environment for its potential for change. Separate from the exploration of task performance, the occupational therapist focuses on the conditions or features in the environment that enable the child to perform the task, including supports available in the environment (Dunn, 1993; Law, 1993). Considering the environment in the assessment provides the therapist with the opportunity to assess how the child's occupational performance may be enhanced through environmental adaptations. The Pediatric Evaluation of Disability Inventory (Haley et al., 1992) and the School Function Assessment (Coster et al., 1998) are examples of assessment tools that take into account the level of assistance and the amount and type of modifications required by the child for successful task and activity performance.

Information gathered through a dynamic assessment moves the therapist beyond assessing the child and/or his or her environment as separate entities. This understanding of the interaction between the child, environment, and occupation facilitates the occupational therapist's identification of where and how to aim interventions that will maximize the child-environment-occupation fit and enhance the child's occupational performance.

Context-Specific Assessment

Context-specific assessments provide information on the child's participation in relevant contexts (e.g., home, school, and community) and how he or she performs related complex tasks and activities in the various occupational behavior settings in each context. This information allows the occupational therapist to identify where intervention is needed to facilitate the child's participation in these contexts (Haley, Coster, & Binda-Sundberg, 1994).

Top-Down Approach to Assessment of Occupational Performance

Many occupational therapy frames of reference for children are developmentally-oriented, focusing on the child's performance components in relation to normal development. This focus on the performance components believed to be underlying occupational performance is described as a bottom-up approach. Using a bottom-up approach, occupational therapists make a mental leap from identifying an occupational performance problem to assessing and treating an inferred performance component deficit that is believed to be the basis for that problem. The connection between the occupational performance problem and the performance component deficit is often not made explicit to the child, parents, and other professionals involved with the child (Coster, 1998; Trombly, 1993).

A top-down approach primarily addresses the person's occupational performance in the contexts in which it occurs (Mathiowetz, 1993; Trombly, 1993). The focus of assessment using a top-down approach is at the top level of occupational performance, the child's participation in the home, school, and community contexts. At this level, the occupational therapist, the child, and the adults who are responsible for him or her identify what the child wants to do, needs to do, or is expected to do and the extent to which he or she is able to orchestrate and engage in these occupations within the home, school, and community contexts.

Assessment continues at the levels of complex task and activity performance to determine the child's ability to perform specific complex tasks and activities that affect his or her participation in these contexts. Finally, an assessment of component processes is done, if necessary, to determine the underlying impairments that may be affecting the child's performance of the complex tasks and activities required for his or her participation at home, school, and in the community (Coster, 1998). Assessment at each of these levels helps the occupational therapist to understand why the child's participation is limited and what can be done about it (Table 15.10).

Table 15.10 provides examples of assessments at each level of occupational performance. The ultimate goal of intervention in the occupational frame of reference for children is to enable the child to participate in occupations in the home, school, and community contexts; therefore, assessment at the levels of participation and complex task performance (occupations) are of particular interest. Table 15.10 demonstrates that many of the assessments at these lower levels of occupational performance are not occupation-based; therefore, the relationship between these levels and the child's participation in occupation is not clear.

Table 15.10   Assessments

Levels of Occupational Performance	Assessments	Occupation Based	Non-Occupation Based
Participation	Classroom Environment Scale—*Trickett & Moos, 1973*	■	
	Home Observation for Measurement of the Environment (HOME)—*Caldwell & Bradley, 1979*	■	
	Pediatric Evaluation of Disability Inventory (PEDI) —*Haley et al., 1992*	■	
	Play History—*Takata, 1969*	■	
	School Function Assessment (SFA)—*Coster et al., 1998*	■	
	Work Environment Scale—*Moos, 1981*	■	
	Qualitative Methods (participant observation, interviews, document review)	■	
Complex Tasks Performance	Assessment of Motor and Process Skills (AMPS)— *Fisher, 1995*	■	
	Canadian Occupational Performance Measure (COPM)—*Law et al., 1994*	■	
	Functional Independence Measure for Children (Wee FIM)—*Hamilton & Granger, 1991*	■	
	Interest Checklist—*Matsutsuyu, 1969*	■	
	Knox Preschool Play Scale—*Knox, 1997*	■	
	PEDI—*Haley et al., 1992*	■	
	SFA—*Coster et al., 1998*	■	
	Test of Playfulness (ToP)—*Bundy, 1997*	■	
	Qualitative Methods (Participant observation, interviews, document review)	■	
Activity Performance	AMPS—*Fisher, 1995*	■	
	Bruininks-Oseretsky Test of Motor Proficiency— *Bruininks, 1978*		■
	Gross Motor Function Measure (GMFM)— *Russell et al., 1989*		■
	Erhardt Developmental Vision Assessment— *Erhardt, 1988*		■
	Peabody Developmental Motor Scales— *Folio & Fewell, 1983*		■
	PEDI—*Haley et al., 1992*	■	
	Preschool Play Scale—*Knox, 1997*	■	
	SFA—*Coster et al., 1998*	■	
	The First STEP (Screening Test for Evaluating Preschoolers)—*Miller, 1993*		■
	Wee FIM—*Hamilton & Granger, 1991*	■	
	Qualitative Methods (Participant observation, interviews, document review)	■	
Component Processes	Bayley Scales of Infant Development—*Bayley, 1993*		■
	Beery Developmental Test of Visual Motor Integration—*Beery, 1989*		■

—continued

Table 15.10 Assessments—(Continued)

Levels of Occupational Performance	Assessments	Occupation Based	Non-Occupation Based
	Bruininks-Oseretsky Test of Motor Proficiency— *Bruininks, 1978*		■
	Motor-Free Visual Perception Test (MVPT)— *Colarusso & Hammill, 1972*		■
	Miller Assessment for Preschoolers (MAP)— *Miller, 1982*		■
	Sensory Integration and Praxis Tests (SIPT)— *Ayres, 1989*		■
	The First STEP—*Miller, 1993*		■

It is important to note that though the guide to evaluation uses a top-down model of assessment, intervention may use a bottom-up approach, depending on the unique needs of the child, his or her family, and the environment.

POSTULATES REGARDING CHANGE

There are fourteen postulates regarding change that guide intervention in the occupational frame of reference for children. The first four postulates are general postulates that act as overarching principles for intervention and address how change occurs in this frame of reference. They are:

1. If the therapist engages the child in occupation as a therapeutic medium, then change will occur in the child, environment, and/or occupation.
2. If the therapist uses a client-centered approach to create opportunities for the child to engage in occupation, then the child and/or adults responsible for the child will be able to choose, orchestrate, and satisfactorily participate in occupations that are personally satisfying, meaningful, and developmentally appropriate.
3. If the therapist creates opportunities for the child to participate in personally satisfying, meaningful, and developmentally-appropriate occupations, then the child and the adults responsible for him or her will view the child's occupational performance as satisfactory.
4. If the therapist creates opportunities that promote change in the child, environment, and/or occupation that maximizes the fit between the child, environment, and occupation, then the child's occupational performance will be optimized.

The remaining ten postulates regarding change address how the occupational therapist creates opportunities that enhance occupational performance.

5. If the therapist uses occupational synthesis to design an occupational form that is meaningful to the child and elicits his or her purposeful occupational performance, then change will occur in the child (adaptation) and change will occur in subsequent occupational forms (impact).
6. If adaptation occurs, then change will occur in the child's spirituality, performance components, and/or skills.
7. If impact occurs, then change will occur in the child's environment and/or occupation.
8. If the therapist uses occupation-as-means to address the levels of occupational performance, then the child's occupation-as-ends (participation in meaningful occupations in the contexts of home, school, and community) will be enhanced.
9. If the therapist ensures that intervention at the lower levels of occupational performance (i.e., activity performance and component processes) has an explicit focus on occupation-as-ends, then the child's occupation-as-ends is best achieved.
10. If the therapist devises interventions that establish or restore developmentally appropriate skills and allow the child to engage in occupations, then the fit between the child, environment, and occupation will be maximized.
11. If the therapist identifies alternative environments (alter) that are compatible with the child's skills and abilities, then the fit between the child, environment, and occupation will be maximized.
12. If the therapist adapts the environment and/or occupations so that they are compatible with and support the child's skills and abilities, then the fit between the child, environment, and occupation will be maximized.
13. If the therapist expects a child may experience difficulties in occupational performance without intervention, then the therapist provides intervention that will promote the child-environment-occupation fit to prevent problems from occurring.
14. If the therapist designs (creates) environments or occupations that enrich, then the fit between the child's environment and occupation will be maximized.

APPLICATION TO PRACTICE

In this frame of reference, occupation-as-means is the primary therapeutic medium used by the therapist to effect change in the child, environment, and occupation, thereby maximizing their fit and promoting the child's optimal occupational performance (occupation-as-ends). Occupation-as-means refers to the child's engagement in occupation as the process through which change occurs.

Given that the meaning of an occupation cannot be separated from its experience, the success of occupation-as-means as a therapeutic medium depends upon the meaningfulness of the occupation to the person engaged in it. Use of meaningful occupation is not a tool that can be pulled from the therapist's tool kit; it must be developed from the beginning of the relationship between the therapist and client, and it continues to evolve throughout the duration of their collaborative partnership. Although the process of discovering the meaning of occupations in a client's life is ongoing and complex, it is expedited when the therapist holds the view that therapy is entering the lives of the child and his or her family rather than the view that the child and family are entering therapy (Helfrich and Kielhofner, 1994).

How does the therapist enter the life of the client? First, a strong therapeutic rapport between the client and the therapist in the context of a collaborative partnership provides optimal conditions for the therapist to truly learn about and understand the child within the context of his or her life. A positive therapeutic rapport is likely to occur when the therapist fosters a relationship in which he or she and the client concentrate on and attend to each other, communicate effectively, coordinate their verbal and non-verbal interactions with each other, and experience feelings of enjoyment and positivity (Tickle-Degner, 1995).

Once the therapist has entered the life of the child and family and discovered the meaning of occupation in their lives, he or she is in a position to develop interventions based on meaningful occupation. An occupation is meaningful when it is fun or pleasurable or relevant to the context or situation. In this frame of reference, play is an occupation-as-means for children because it is an important aspect of their development and fun. Other real life occupations are used in intervention based on their importance and meaning to the child (Pierce, 1998). The therapist's ability to select, design, and adapt occupations that are meaningful to the child and family is dependent on the extent to which he or she has entered their lives and determines the power of meaningful occupation as a therapeutic medium.

Levels of Occupational Performance

Occupation-as-means is used at any level of occupational performance to facilitate the child's successful participation in meaningful occupations. The therapist selects and adapts occupations for the child to practice in order to facilitate his or her ability to engage in these occupations. In addition, the therapist designs occupations that target skill or performance component deficits that are affecting the child's occupational performance. Specifically, occupations are adapted and practiced at the levels of participation and complex task performance so that the child is able to participate in them. In addition, occupations are designed and structured so that skills at the level of activity performance are mastered or performance components at the level of component processes are remediated. Regardless of the level of occupational performance at which occupation-as-means is used, the overall goal of intervention in this frame of reference is to enable the child to participate in the occupations of play, personal care, education, organized activities, unpaid and paid work, socialization, and functional mobility in the contexts of home, school, and community.

In this frame of reference, the therapist considers all levels of the child's occupational performance when developing a plan for intervention. For example, a mother states that her daughter is always late for the school bus in the morning (participation). The therapist determines through an evaluation that the child is having difficulty dressing herself (complex task performance) because she is unable to stabilize her trunk (activity performance) while sitting on her bed due to her limited postural control (component processes). Identification of impairment at the component processes level and limitation at the activity performance level clarifies the cause of the child's occupational performance problem and guides the therapist's intervention. At this point, the occupational therapist may choose another frame of reference to address the deficits in the component processes. The therapist also adapts aspects of the dressing task so that the child is able to practice dressing herself. The ultimate goal of intervention is to enable the child's successful completion of the occupation of personal care (complex task) in time for her to catch the school bus (participation).

Intervention to Maximize Child-Environment-Occupation Fit

Optimal occupational performance is achieved when the fit between the child, environment, and occupation is maximized. Interventions that promote change in the child, the environment, and/or the occupation, thereby maximizing their fit, enhance the child's occupational performance. Using the processes of occupational analysis and synthesis, the therapist applies the intervention strategies of establish/restore, alter, adapt, prevent, and create to design occupations that effect change in the child, environment, and/or occupation.

Establish/Restore

Arising from remedial approaches, this strategy emphasizes identifying and then addressing, through intervention, any limitations or problem areas in the child's performance. The therapist first identifies those component processes that are interfering with the child's performance, and then intervenes, through remediation, to improve or develop the skills or abilities necessary for the occupation. This may involve the use of another frame of reference or occupation-as-means.

Alter

The therapist identifies existing environments that are compatible with the child's skills and abilities rather than changing his or her current environment. For example, an adolescent boy with a traumatic brain injury who has a part-time job in a fast food restaurant reports that he has problems managing the multiple tasks involved in working at the front counter, that is, taking customers' orders, using the cash register, and collecting food items. The occupational therapist can recommend to his employer that the boy's work environment be altered to that of the food preparation area, which is away from the noise and distractions of the front counter. This existing work environment provides the best match for his cognitive abilities and skills. With this recommendation, the therapist maximizes the fit between the boy and the social and physical environment of his paid work occupation, thereby facilitating his successful job performance. The focus of this strategy is matching the environment to the individual's skills and abilities to maximize occupational performance.

Adapt

Using adaptive or compensatory approaches, the therapist changes aspects of the environment and/or the occupation so that the child's occupational performance is enhanced. In the case of a school-aged girl with cerebral palsy that affects her handwriting and ability to complete written work in class, the occupational therapist may suggest that she use a computer, keyboard, and printer instead of a pencil and paper. The girl's desk in the classroom can be modified to accommodate the computer set-up and ensure that she maintains correct posture and positioning while she works. Her physical environment is adapted, as are aspects of her school work to maximize the fit between her, her environment, and her occupation (as a student), which in turn enables her successful participation in the classroom setting.

Prevent

The therapist uses prevention when he or she expects that a child may experience difficulties in occupational performance without intervention. For example, the therapist may identify potential problems between a boy with developmental dyspraxia and his parents, particularly in the area of their expectations for his participation in unpaid work in the home, such as making his bed and cleaning his room. The therapist can provide information to the parents about developmental dyspraxia and its effects upon their son's ability to complete his household chores in a timely manner. This knowledge can help them set realistic expectations for his performance and can limit any feelings of frustrations that may occur with their unrealistic expectations. In this case, the occupational therapist can facilitate change in the child's social environment (the expectations of his parents) to maximize the fit between this environment, his skills and abilities, and his participation in unpaid work occupations, leading to an increased likelihood of his successful occupational performance.

Create

The therapist creates environmental and/or occupational circumstances that promote optimal occupational performance. This element is not based on a deficit but instead on the potential to enhance performance. For example, an occupational therapist working with families can educate the parents about play embedded in household work. The therapist's provision of this information can lead to the creation of opportunities for the parents to incorporate play with their children into their unpaid work occupations. This thereby maximizes the fit between the family members and their environments and occupations so that the occupational performance of all family members is enhanced.

Occupation-as-Ends

The overall goal of intervention in this frame of reference is occupation-as-ends (i.e., to enable the child and the adults responsible for the child to choose, organize, and perform occupations in the contexts of home, school, and community). The therapeutic agency of occupation-as-ends lies in the child's optimal occupational performance. Occupation-as-ends can be facilitated through use of the therapeutic medium of occupation-as-means.

SUMMARY

The occupational frame of reference for children organizes and synthesizes theory about occupation into a structure that can be applied to occupational therapy practice with children. The occupational frame of reference for children is applicable to practice with all children and can be used alone or in combination with other frames of reference.

Because occupational performance is dependent on interactions between people, environments, and occupation, the occupational therapist must consider the relationship between the following when addressing a child's occupational performance: a child's spirituality, performance components, and skills (person); the physical, social, cultural, and institutional environments (environment); and the occupation itself (occupation). Optimal occupational performance is achieved when the fit between the person, environment, and occupation is maximized.

Occupational performance is conceptualized as a hierarchy of levels of behavior that are nested within each other. There are four levels of occupational performance in the occupational frame of reference for children: participation, complex task performance, activity performance, and component processes. Children participate in occupations in three contexts (i.e., home, school, and community) to create their own unique patterns of occupational performance. Within these contexts, children engage in the occupations of play, personal care, education, organized activities, unpaid and paid work, socialization, and functional mobility.

Function/dysfunction continua are organized around the levels of occupational performance; participation, complex task performance, activity performance, and component processes. The evaluation process in the occupational frame of reference for children uses various methods of assessment to evaluate the child's occupational performance. It is a client-centered, dynamic process that is context-specific and measures levels of occupational performance with a top-down approach.

There are 14 postulates regarding change that guide intervention in the occupational frame of reference for children. The first four postulates address general beliefs about how change occurs in this frame of reference and act as overarching principles for intervention. The remaining ten postulates regarding change address how the occupational therapist promotes change in the child, environment, and occupation that maximizes the child-environment-occupation fit and enhances occupational performance.

The following five strategies in the occupational frame of reference for children maximize the fit between the child, environment, and occupation: establish/restore, alter, adapt, prevent, and create. Through the process of occupational analysis and synthesis, the therapist uses these strategies to design occupational forms that will lead to adaptation and/or impact.

Occupation-as-means is the therapeutic process through which the therapist facilitates change in the child, environment, and/or occupation, which will enable the child's successful occupation-as-ends. The strategies of establish/restore, alter, adapt, prevent, and create direct the therapist's actions to maximize the child-environment-occupation fit. Occupation-as-ends or the child's successful participation in occupations in the contexts of home, school, and community is the ultimate goal of intervention based on the occupational frame of reference for children.

References

American Occupational Therapy Association. (1994). Uniform terminology for occupational therapy: Third edition. *American Journal of Occupational Therapy, 48,* 1047–1054.

American Occupational Therapy Association. (1995). Position paper: Occupation. *American Journal of Occupational Therapy, 49,* 1015–1018.

Ayres, A. J. (1989). *Sensory Integration and Praxis Tests* (SIPT). Los Angeles: Western Psychological Services.

Barker, R. G., & Schoggen, P. (1973). *Qualities of community life.* San Francisco: Jossey-Bass.

Baum, M. C., & Law, M. (1997). Occupational therapy practice: Focusing on occupational performance. *American Journal of Occupational Therapy, 51,* 277–288.

Bayley, N. (1993). *Bayley Scales of Infant Development* (2nd ed.). San Antonio, TX: Psychological Corporation.

Beery, K. E. (1989). *Beery Developmental Test of Visual Motor Integration* (3rd ed.). Cleveland, OH: Modern Curriculum Press.

Breines, E. B. (1995). *Occupational therapy activities from clay to computers: theory and practice.* Philadelphia: F.A. Davis.

Bruininks, R. (1978). *Bruininks-Oseretsky Test of Motor Proficiency.* Circle Pines, MN: American Guidance Service.

Bundy, A. C. (1993). Assessment of play and leisure: Delineation of the problem. *American Journal of Occupational Therapy, 47,* 217–222.

Bundy, A. C. (1997). Play and playfulness: What to look for. In L. D. Parham & L. S. Fazio (Eds.), *Play in occupational therapy for children* (pp. 52–66). St. Louis, MO: Mosby-Year Book.

Caldwell, B. M., & Bradley, R. H. (1979). *Home Observation for Measurement of the Environment* (HOME). Little Rock, AR: University of Arkansas.

Canadian Association of Occupational Therapists. (1996). Practice paper: Occupational therapy and children's play [Insert]. *Canadian Journal of Occupational Therapy, 63,* 1–20.

Christiansen, C., & Baum, C. (1997). Understanding occupation: Definitions and concepts. In C. Christiansen & C. Baum (Eds.), *Occupational therapy: Enabling function and well-being* (2nd ed.) (pp. 2–25). Thorofare, NJ: Slack.

Christiansen, C. H., Schwartz, R. K., & Barnes, K. J. (1993). Self-care: Evaluation and management. In J. A. DeLisa (Ed.), *Rehabilitation medicine: Principles and practice* (2nd ed) (pp. 178–200). Philadelphia: J. B. Lippincott.

Clark, F. A., Parham, D., Carlson, M. E., Frank, G., Jackson, J., Pierce, D., Wolfe, R. J., & Zemke, R. (1991). Occupational science: Academic innovation in the service of occupational therapy's future. *American Journal of Occupational Therapy, 45,* 300–310.

Colarusso, R. P., & Hammill, D. D. (1983). *Motor-Free Visual Perception Test.* Novato, CA: Academic Therapy.

Cook, J. L., & Sinker, M. (1993). Play and the growth of competence. In C. E. Schaefer (Ed.), *The therapeutic powers of play* (pp. 65–80). Northvale, NJ: Jason Aronson.

Coster, W. (1998). Occupation-centered assessment of children. *American Journal of Occupational Therapy, 52,* 337–344.

Coster, W. J., Deeney, T. A., Haltiwanger, J. T., & Haley, S. M. (1998). *School Function Assessment* (SFA). Standardized version. Boston: Boston University.

Cronin, A. F. (1996). Psychosocial and emotional domains of behavior. In J. Case-Smith, A. S. Allen, & P. N. Pratt (Eds.), *Occupational therapy for children* (3rd ed) (pp. 387–429). St. Louis, MO: Mosby-Year Book.

Csikszentmihalyi, M., & Larson, R. (1984). *Being adolescent: Conflict and growth in the teenage years.* New York: Basic Books.

Dunn, W. (1993). Measurement of function: Actions for the future. *American Journal of Occupational Therapy, 47,* 357–359.

Dunn, W., Brown, C., & McGuigan, A. (1994). The ecology of human performance: A framework for considering the effect of context. *American Journal of Occupational Therapy, 48,* 595–607.

Erhardt, R. P. (1988). *Erhardt Developmental Vision Assessment.* Tucson, AZ: Therapy Skill Builders.

Erikson, E. (1959). Identity and the life cycle. *Psychological Issues, 1,* 1–171.

Fazio, L. S. (1997). Storytelling, storymaking, and fantasy play. In L. D. Parham & L. S. Fazio (Eds.), *Play in occupational therapy for children* (pp. 233–247). St. Louis, MO: Mosby-Year Book.

Fisher, A. G. (1995). *Assessment of Motor and Process Skills* (Rev. ed.). Fort Collins, CO: Three Star Press.

Fisher, A., & Kielhofner, G. (1995a). Mind-brain-body performance subsystem. In G. Kielhofner (Ed.), *A model of human occupation: Theory and application* (2nd ed.) (pp. 83–90). Baltimore: Williams & Wilkins.

Fisher, A., & Kielhofner, G. (1995b). Skill in occupational performance. In G. Kielhofner (Ed.), *A model of human occupation: Theory and application* (2nd ed.) (pp. 113–137). Baltimore: Williams & Wilkins.

Folio, M. R., & Fewell, R. R. (1983). *Peabody Developmental Motor Scales.* Chicago: Riverside.

Goodnow, J. J. (1988). Children's household work: Its nature and functions. *Psychological Bulletin, 103,* 5–26.

Gray, J. M. (1998). Putting occupation into practice: Occupation as ends, occupation as means. *American Journal of Occupational Therapy, 52,* 354–364.

Haley, S. M., Coster, W. J., & Binda-Sundberg, K. (1994). Measuring physical disablement: The contextual challenge. *Physical Therapy, 74,* 443–451.

Haley, S. M., Coster, W. J., Ludlow, L. H., Haltiwanger, J. T., & Andrellos, P. J. (1992). *Pediatric Evaluation of Disability Inventory* (PEDI). Version 1.0. Boston: New England Medical Center and PEDI Research Group.

Hamilton, B. B., & Granger, C. V. (1991). *Functional Independence Measure for Children* (WeeFIM). Buffalo, NY: Research Foundation of the State University of New York.

Harter, S. (1990). Causes, correlates, and the functional role of global self-worth: A life-span perspective. In R. J. Steinberg & J. Kolligan (Eds.), *Competence considered.* New Haven, CT: Yale University Press.

Helfrich C., & Keilhofner, G. (1994). Volitional narratives and the meaning of therapy. *American Journal of Occupational Therapy, 48,* 319–326.

Kielhofner, G. (1995a). Environmental influences on occupational behavior. In G. Kielhofner (Ed.), *A model of human occupation: Theory and application* (2nd ed.) (pp. 91–111). Baltimore: Williams & Wilkins.

Kielhofner, G. (1995b). Habituation subsystem. In G. Kielhofner (Ed.), *A model of human occupation: Theory and application* (2nd ed.) (pp. 63–81). Baltimore: Williams & Wilkins.

Kielhofner, G. (1995c). Introduction to the model of human occupation. In G. Kielhofner (Ed.), *A model of human occupation: Theory and application* (2nd ed.) (pp. 1–7). Baltimore: Williams & Wilkins.

Kielhofner, G. (1997). *Conceptual foundations of occupational therapy* (2nd ed.). Philadelphia: F. A. Davis.

Knox, S. (1997). Development and current use of the Knox Preschool Play Scale. In L. D. Parham & L. S. Fazio (Eds.), *Play in occupational therapy for children* (pp. 35–51). St. Louis, MO: Mosby-Year Book.

Landreth, G. L. (1993). Self-expressive communication. In C. E. Schaefer (Ed.), *The therapeutic powers of play* (pp. 41–63). Northvale, NJ: Jason Aronson.

Law, M. (1991). The environment: A focus for occupational therapy. *Canadian Journal of Occupational Therapy, 58,* 171–179.

Law, M. (1993). Evaluating activities of daily living: Directions for the future. *American Journal of Occupational Therapy, 47,* 233–237.

Law, M., Baptiste, S., Carswell-Opzoomer, A., McColl, M., Polatajko, H., & Pollock, N. (1994). *Canadian Occupational Performance Measure* (2nd ed.). Toronto, Ontario, Canada: Canadian Association of Occupational Therapists.

Law, M., Baptiste, S., McColl, M., Opzoomer, A., Polatajko, H., & Pollock, N. (1990). The Canadian Occupational Performance Measure: An outcome measure for occupational therapy. *Canadian Journal of Occupational Therapy, 57,* 82–87.

Law, M., Cooper, B., Strong, S., Stewart, D., Rigby, P., & Letts, L. (1996). The person-environment-occupation model: A transactive approach to occupational performance. *Canadian Journal of Occupational Therapy, 63,* 9–23.

Law, M., Polatajko, H., Baptiste, S., & Townsend, E. (1997). Core concepts in occupational therapy. In E. Townsend (Ed.), *Enabling occupation: An occupational therapy perspective* (pp. 29–56). Ottawa, Canada: Canadian Association of Occupational Therapists.

Licht, S. (1948). *Occupational Therapy Source Book.* Baltimore, MD: Williams & Wilkins.

Mathiowetz, V. (1993). Role of physical performance component evaluations in occupational therapy functional assessment. *American Journal of Occupational Therapy, 47,* 225–230.

Matsutsuyu, J. S. (1969). The interest check list. *American Journal of Occupational Therapy, 23,* 323–328.

Medrich, E. A., Roizen, J. A., Rubin, V., & Buckley, S. (1982). *The serious business of growing up: A study of children's lives outside school.* Berkeley, CA: University of California.

Miller, L. J. (1982). *Miller Assessment for Preschoolers (MAP).* San Antonio, TX: Psychological Corporation.

Miller, L. J. (1993). *The First STEP.* San Antonio, TX: Psychological Corporation.

Missiuna, C. (1987). Dynamic assessment: A model for broadening assessment in occupational therapy. *Canadian Journal of Occupational Therapy, 54,* 17–21.

Moos, R. H. (1981). *Work Environment Scale.* Palo Alto, CA: Consulting Psychologists Press.

Morrison, C. D., Metzger, P., & Pratt, P. N. (1996). Play. In J. Case-Smith, A. S. Allen, & P. N. Pratt (Eds.), *Occupational therapy for children* (3rd ed., pp. 504–523). St. Louis, MO: Mosby-Year Book.

Nelson, D. L. (1988). Occupation: Form and performance. *American Journal of Occupational Therapy, 42,* 633–641.

Nelson, D. L. (1994). Occupational form, occupational performance, and therapeutic occupation. In C. B. Royeen (Ed.), *American Occupational Therapy Association Self Study Series, The Practice of the Future: Putting Occupation Back Into Therapy* (Lesson 2). Rockville, MD: The American Occupational Therapy Association.

Nelson, D. L. (1996). Therapeutic occupation: A definition. *American Journal of Occupational Therapy, 50,* 775–782.

Nelson, D. L. (1997). Why the profession of occupational therapy will flourish in the 21st century. *American Journal of Occupational Therapy, 51,* 11–24.

Parham, L. D., & Primeau, L. A. (1997). Play and occupational therapy. In L. D. Parham & L. S. Fazio (Eds.), *Play in occupational therapy for children* (pp. 2–21). St. Louis, MO: Mosby-Year Book.

Pierce, D. (1997). The power of object play for infants and toddlers at risk for developmental delays. In L. D. Parham & L. S. Fazio (Eds.), *Play in occupational therapy for children* (pp. 86–111). St. Louis, MO: Mosby-Year Book.

Pierce, D. (1998). What is the source of occupation's treatment power? *American Journal of Occupational Therapy, 52,* 490–491.

Polatajko, H. J. (1994). Dreams, dilemmas, and decisions for occupational therapy practice in a new millennium: A Canadian perspective. *American Journal of Occupational Therapy, 48,* 590–594.

Primeau, L. A. (1989). *A description and comparison of game playing behavior of preadolescent boys 9 to 11 years of age with and without developmental dyspraxia.* Unpublished master's thesis, University of Southern California, Los Angeles.

Primeau, L. A. (1998). Orchestration of work and play within families. *American Journal of Occupational Therapy, 52,* 188–195.

Primeau, L. A., Clark, F., & Pierce, D. (1989). Occupational therapy alone has looked upon occupation: Future applications of occupational science to pediatric occupational therapy. *Occupational Therapy in Health Care, 6(4),* 19–32.

Reid, S. (1993). Game play. In C. E. Schaefer (Ed.), *The therapeutic powers of play* (pp. 323–348). Northvale, NJ: Jason Aronson.

Reifel, S., & Yeatman, J. (1993). From category to context: Reconsidering classroom play. *Early Childhood Research Quarterly, 8,* 347–367.

Reilly, M. (1962). Occupational therapy can be one of the great ideas of 20th century medicine. *American Journal of Occupational Therapy, 16,* 1–9.

Reilly, M. (1969). The educational process. *American Journal of Occupational Therapy, 23,* 299–307.

Reilly, M. (1974). An explanation of play. In M. Reilly (Ed.), *Play as exploratory learning: Studies of curiosity behavior* (pp. 117–149). Beverly Hills, CA: Sage.

Rogoff, B., Sellers, M. J., Pirrotta, S., Fox, N., & White, S. H. (1975). Age of assignment of roles and responsibilities to children: A cross-cultural survey. *Human Development, 18,* 353–369.

Russell, D. J., Rosenbaum, P. L., Cadman, D. T., Gowland, C., Hardy, S., & Jarvis, S. (1989). *Gross Motor Function Measure.* (GMFM) Hamilton, Ontario, Canada: Gross Motor Measures Group.

Schaefer, C. E. (1993). What is play and why is it therapeutic? In C. E. Schaefer (Ed.), *The therapeutic powers of play* (pp. 1–15). Northvale, NJ: Jason Aronson.

Simon, C. J., & Daub, M. M. (1993). Human development across the life span. In H. L. Hopkins & H. D. Smith (Eds.), *Willard and Spackman's occupational therapy* (8th ed., pp. 95–130). Philadelphia: J. B. Lippincott.

Takata, N. (1969). The play history. *American Journal of Occupational Therapy, 23,* 314–318.

Takata, N. (1974). Play as prescription. In M. Reilly (Ed.), *Play as exploratory learning: Studies of curiosity behavior* (pp. 209–246). Beverly Hills, CA: Sage.

Tickle-Degnen L. (1995). Therapeutic rapport. In C.A. Trombly (Ed.), *Occupational therapy for physical dysfunction* (4th ed, pp. 277–285). Baltimore, MD: Williams & Wilkins.

Townsend, E. (1997). *Client-centered occupational assessment.* Unpublished manuscript, School of Occupational Therapy, Dalhousie University, Halifax, Nova Scotia, Canada.

Trickett, E. J., & Moos, R. H. (1973). The social environment of junior high and high school classrooms. *Journal of Educational Psychology, 65,* 93–102.

Trombly, C. (1993). Anticipating the future: Assessment of occupational function. *American Journal of Occupational Therapy, 47,* 253–257.

Trombly, C. A. (1995). Occupation: Purposefulness and meaningfulness as therapeutic mechanisms. *American Journal of Occupational Therapy, 49,* 960–972.

Wilcock, A. (1993). A theory of the human need for occupation. *Occupational Science: Australia, 1,* 17–23.

Wood, W. (1995). Weaving the warp and weft of occupational therapy: An art and science for all times. *American Journal of Occupational Therapy, 49,* 44–52.

Wright-Ott, C., & Egilson, S. (1996). Mobility. In J. Case-Smith, A. S. Allen, & P. N. Pratt (Eds.), *Occupational therapy for children* (3rd ed., pp. 562–580). St. Louis, MO: Mosby-Year Book.

Yerxa, E. J. (1994). Dreams, dilemmas, and decisions for occupational therapy practice in a new millennium: An American perspective. *American Journal of Occupational Therapy, 48,* 586–589.

Yerxa, E. J. (1995, October). *Let's talk about occupation.* Paper presented at the Fall Forum, School of Occupational Therapy, Dalhousie University & Nova Scotia Society of Occupational Therapists, Halifax, Nova Scotia, Canada.

Yerxa, E. J., Clark, F., Frank, G., Jackson, J., Parham, D., Pierce, D., Stein, C., & Zemke, R. (1989). An introduction to occupational science: A foundation for occupational therapy in the 21st century. *Occupational Therapy in Health Care, 6*(4), 1–17.

APPLICATIONS OF FRAMES OF REFERENCE

CHAPTER 16

Frames of Reference in the Real World

JIM HINOJOSA / PAULA KRAMER

This chapter discusses the importance of using frames of reference in practice. The first section focuses on the importance of understanding the frame of reference so that the therapist can articulate it clearly when treating a child. The second section focuses on the art of practice with children, with emphasis on the therapeutic relationship. The third section presents the alternative applications. Finally, the last section begins to address the development of new frames of reference.

ARTICULATING THE FRAME OF REFERENCE

When students and entry-level occupational therapists are asked to explain what they are doing with a child or why they are doing a particular activity, some common responses are "I'm not sure"; "It was just intuition"; "I know why, but I just can't put it into words"; "I saw another therapist do it and it worked well"; or "I was taught this in school, and my instructor said it works well." It is uncomfortable to be put on the spot and often difficult to respond quickly to such a complex question. As professionals, however, therapists are obliged to understand what they are doing and why they are doing it. They also need to be able to explain the rationale for what they are doing and why they are doing it to observers, especially to parents and other professionals.

In a recent clinical experience, a fieldwork student was asked to explain what she would do during a treatment session. She stated that she intended to play with the child because the child would benefit from all types of stimulation. This response indicated a lack of understanding about the child's individual needs and a lack of clearly articulated goals. Furthermore, this suggests that the intervention was not well thought out or theoretically based. Any response or reaction from the child in this treatment situation, therefore, could not be explained from a theoretical perspective. Finally, third party payers do not reimbursement for play, but they will pay for clearly planned and well thought-out interventions. And, as therapists, it is important to be prepared to explain our interventions to those who will reimburse for the services rendered; although, this should not drive our practice.

In this example, the student's apparent lack of understanding or inability to articulate a rationale for intervention may have resulted from a theoretical perspective that had not been identified clearly. This student has predetermined that the child will benefit from any sensory stimulation but has not stated specific problem areas or expected responses from the child based on the intervention. Intervention cannot be viewed in such a simplistic way. It is a step-by-step approach that is geared towards identifying problem areas and providing a well thought-out intervention designed to bring about change. As already mentioned, the structure for developing this organized systematic approach to intervention is the frame of reference.

Returning to the example, the student may have had a clear idea of what her goals were with the child, but without the structure of the frame of reference, her intervention appears to have no theoretical rationale for treatment. Furthermore, based on her intervention, she would have difficulty measuring change without this theoretical structure.

In another example, a student was asked to explain why he placed a child who had cerebral palsy in a prone position on an adapted scooter board. He responded that it seemed like the appropriate position for the child. When the instructor explored this further, asking for additional clarification of what theoretical framework the student was using, the student was able to explain that this developmentally appropriate position facilitated the child's exploration of the environment and that he was using the biomechanical frame of reference to allow the child to interact with and learn from his environment. Although the first response indicated his initial intuition, the student was able to demonstrate a theoretical understanding of the intervention when pressed for details. Intuition often is really knowledge based.

When students or therapists respond that their actions are based on intuition, they are not recognizing their knowledge base. At times, students and therapists do not appreciate what they have learned during their professional education, so they see their actions as being intuitive. In actuality, their decisions are knowledge based, but it is difficult at that moment to articulate the theoretical rationale for the actions. Identification of the frame of reference, which is grounded in theory, again allows the therapist to cite clearly his or her knowledge base and rationale for treatment.

In addition, therapists sometimes undermine their interventions when they give simplistic rationales for what they do with a child. Much of occupational therapy looks like play to the casual observer. When the therapist says that he or she is playing with the child to provide stimulation, the response of the casual observer may be that anyone can play with a child and provide stimulation in that way. When the therapist acknowledges that he or she is working from a theoretical base, however, the therapist can demonstrate that play designed to provide specific stimulation really is a highly skilled and well thought-out intervention plan designed to bring about specific responses. The purpose of the frame of reference is to provide this blueprint for practice.

When therapists are asked what their frame of reference is, many respond, "I'm eclectic." In some cases, the therapist has not identified the various frames of reference on which his or her interventions are based. When this is the situation, the therapist may not have a clearly thought-out intervention plan. He or she may not be using a frame of reference or may not have a clear understanding of the theoretical rationale for the intervention. At other times, a therapist may label his or her approach as eclectic because the interventions are based on various sources without synthesizing them into a clearly articulated frame of reference. Again, therapeutic interventions should be based on clearly articulated frames of reference that include well-delineated theoretical bases. If the therapist picks and chooses concepts, postulates, and techniques from various approaches without concern for the consistency of the theories on which they are based, then specific outcomes cannot be anticipated. The theoretical base of a frame of reference is built on theoretical information that is congruent with each other and that presents a unified approach to the change process (consistency). When the therapist uses various approaches without concern for consistency, change cannot be explained theoretically. The frame of reference delineates what outcomes can be expected from each specified intervention. The statement, "I'm eclectic," tends to indicate a lack of theory-based intervention.

Just as a physician should not prescribe medication without knowing its consequences, a therapist should not use a procedure without understanding its consequences. The therapist selects a frame of reference based on the child's presenting problems and on the specified changes or outcomes that he or she would like to promote. Techniques or procedures not derived from a frame of reference usually do not lead to organized change in a way that can be explained. At times, a misunderstood procedure can have consequences similar to a misused medication, such as when a neurophysiological technique like vestibular stimulation is used without a clear rationale for an expected response. To use vestibular stimulation without an understanding of the sensory integration frame of reference may result in an inappropriate behavioral response or a more severe central nervous system reaction.

Finally, because occupational therapy is concerned with and uses routine daily activities as the focus for intervention, it may appear to lack the empirical scientific base of guidelines for practice used by other professions that are labeled therapeutic. Because occupational therapy with children is activity-oriented and often uses play, it is crucial that the therapeutic value of chosen activities be readily explainable. The frame of reference provides the scientific, theoretical basis that explains the complexity of the activities used in the intervention process. What appears to be simple, usually has complex theoretical underpinnings that may be clarified for the therapist through the frame of reference, which brings the theories to a level at which they can be applied.

THE ART OF PRACTICE WITH CHILDREN

Previous chapters in this book presented specific frames of reference that are important to current pediatric practice. Working with children effectively involves more than knowing about and an understanding of frames of reference; it also requires an understanding of how to put frames of reference into practice effectively. Other occupational therapists have discussed and highlighted the art of practice in a global way as it applies to the whole profession of occupational therapy (Crepeau, 1991; Gilfoyle, 1980; Keilhofner, 1983; Koomar & Bundy, 1991; Mosey, 1981a, 1981b; Peloquin, 1989, 1990, 1994). For example, Mosey presents the art of practice in a broad perspective—as part of the philosophical origins of the profession (1981a). The authors in this chapter intend to discuss the art of practice in much more specific ways—as it relates to children and the implementation of the frames of reference.

Complimentary to an understanding of the specific frames of reference that have been presented in previous chapters, the art of working with children needs to be addressed and integrated. Working with children presents interesting challenges that are different from working with adults. Children are not just miniature adults, and they need to be approached in a way that is meaningful to them. Just like adults, children have thoughts and feelings that must be taken into consideration, even though they may not be able to express them.

The therapeutic relationship is an interactive process between therapist and child. The goal is to assist effectively the promotion of positive change within the child. It does not necessarily involve equal participation of therapist and child. It is the therapist's responsibility to establish the tone of the relationship. The therapist guides the relationship, to some extent manipulating it to the child's benefit. Initially, it is important to engage the child, to get to know him or her, and to involve the child in the intervention process. The therapist often acts as a stimulator and cheerleader—a provoker of responses. At other times, the therapist must be more relaxed and give comfort.

To engage the child in effective intervention is the essence of artful practice for an occupational therapist. Unlike most adults, children may not necessarily see therapy as beneficial. The art of occupational therapy involves captivating the child through toys, objects, and games or through the therapist's own actions so that the child becomes involved in the therapeutic process. This art is almost intangible and, therefore, difficult to describe. It is more than a skill; it is a mix of creativity, enthusiasm, an ability to choose objects based on a firm foundation of knowledge, and the use of self in a way that engages the child so that a relationship can be developed and intervention can promote growth. The "trick" is to appreciate the fact that the child has to be dealt with as a whole person, not as component parts or as an aspect of an occupational performance area. And this must be done with each child individually because each child is a unique human being.

The therapeutic relationship is important to the intervention process in any frame of reference. It may be addressed specifically in the change process of the theoretical base in some cases, although, it is not discussed at all in many cases. In specific frames of reference in which it is addressed, a particular type of relationship may exist that helps foster development. For example, in the sensory integrative frame of reference, the therapist takes an active part in treatment and needs to engage playfully with the child. At the same time, he or she must allow the child to be self-directed in the treatment setting. In the acquisitional frame of reference, the need for unconditional positive regard of the child by the therapist is critical to the success of the intervention. In those situations in which the therapeutic relationship is not discussed, it is incumbent on the therapist to formulate a relationship that promotes growth and change and that is consistent with that frame of reference. The art of practice, as discussed here, relates broadly to all frames of reference.

Many characteristics color an effective therapeutic relationship. Perlman (1979) describes these characteristics as warmth, acceptance, caring/concern, and genuineness. Mosey (1981a) adds sympathy and empathy. It often is difficult to describe a therapeutic relationship because its uniqueness depends on its special components: the therapist and child. To say that it is an emotional experience based on feelings and interactions is to state the obvious. The therapeutic relationship involves sympathy and empathy. Sympathy occurs when people share common feelings that often involve commiseration. Empathy involves the projection of one's personality onto another in an effort to understand the feelings, emotions, and thoughts of another human being. Often, especially with entry-level therapists, sympathy is a strong initial part of the therapeutic relationship; however, it is important to move on to the point at which the therapist can be empathetic because empathy assists the therapist in being more effective in his or her interactions with the child.

Unconditional acceptance is an essential aspect of the relationship between therapist and child. The therapist accepts the child and his or her abilities "as is." This precludes a judgmental attitude about the child and his or her life style. Granted, the role of the therapist is to develop the strengths of the child and to remediate or minimize the deficits. The therapist, however, should not base his or her ability to care and interact on what the child is able to do or how the child progresses. When a child cannot do particular tasks or has experienced previous failures, he or she is less likely to try that activity again. The therapist needs to let the child know that the attempt to do something is more important than the activity itself.

The manner in which the occupational therapist uses the legitimate tools of the profession is part of the art of practice. As adapted by the occupational therapist, the nonhuman environment becomes a component in the art of practice. Some frames of reference delineate the therapeutic nonhuman environment. For example, the biomechanical frame of reference describes as part of the nonhuman environment the use of specific equipment to promote positive change in the child. The human, occupation, and motor skills acquisition frames of reference emphasize the importance of the environment in discussing the match between the child, the task, and the environment. Other frames of reference do not address the specific environment but may make implications about or give guidelines for effective types of environments. The therapist must create a safe therapeutic environment to use any frame of reference presented in this book effectively. To raise this legitimate tool to the level of art, the therapist must use his or her understanding of the frame of reference, along with creativity, to manipulate the environment so that it engages the child and promotes growth.

It takes time and experience to develop the art of practice. It is not something that can be presumed of an entry-level therapist, although, like some painters or musicians, some therapists have an innate talent for the art of practice. It is safe to say that the art of practice is not just skilled application of the frames of reference; rather, it is a combination of knowledge, self-confidence, self-understanding, self-acceptance, and awareness. It is hoped that the entry-level therapist becomes involved actively in exploring this process to become an artful practitioner.

ALTERNATIVE APPLICATIONS OF FRAMES OF REFERENCE

Effective practice involves the therapist's ability to match the client with the most appropriate frame of reference within the context of his or her life. After a client is referred to occupational therapy, the therapist does a preliminary screening. This helps to determine the appropriate frame of reference, and thereby, the evaluation tools that should be used for the particular client. Sometimes, this can be one specific frame of reference, but at other times, one frame of reference is not adequate enough to deal with the complexity of problems presented by the child or family. This section discusses the alternative ways that frames of reference can be applied, including the use of frames of reference alone, in sequence, in parallel, and in combination. In addition, the chapter discusses the development of new and unique frames of reference.

Single Frame of Reference

To be comfortable with and understand how to use frames of reference, the entry-level therapist must first work with one frame of reference at a time. An important distinction needs to be made here: the therapist does not use only one frame of reference with all clients. For instance, with any given child, an entry-level therapist must first concentrate on the one frame of reference that fits that particular child's needs. With another child, that same therapist may need to use another frame of reference that is more suitable.

Entry-level therapists often are not fluent with theories relevant to pediatric practice. In the clinic, their primary concern is how to help the child. This concern tends to focus them on what they are doing rather than on the reasons why they are doing something (i.e., whether the practice is [or is not] effective). To become truly competent, however, novice therapists must take the time to familiarize themselves with all aspects of the frame of reference. To do this, entry-level therapists almost always have to start out by using one frame of reference with each client. As presented in this book, the frame of reference provides a blueprint for practice based on theoretical material.

When a therapist begins to use a frame of reference, he or she first should become comfortable with the entire frame of reference by concentrating on the theoretical base. Once the theoretical base is clearly understood, then the other sections of the frame of reference (i.e., function/dysfunction continua, guide to evaluation, postulates regarding change, and application to practice) are easier to understand. The theoretical base, therefore, holds the key to understanding the important concepts for intervention. All important concepts are defined. Assumptions are stated in that section and the significant relationships between concepts and postulates are presented and described. The function/dysfunction continua, guide to evaluation, postulates regarding change, and application to practice all flow from the theoretical base.

By studying one frame of reference at a time, the therapist can become comfortable with the theoretical material and its transition into application. Through the understanding of this material, the therapist develops the ability to use each function/dysfunction continuum systematically as a means to identify the child's strengths and limitations. Based on the findings relative to the function/dysfunction continua, the therapist then can determine what areas (if any) require intervention. Intervention is applied sequentially, using the postulates regarding change as illustrated in the application to practice. It is important to note that postulates regarding change are selected and used in intervention when they are appropriate. Therefore, in many interventions, all the postulates regarding change from one frame of reference are not used. Based on these postulates regarding change, the therapist creates an environment to bring about a desired response from the child. This empirical approach to intervention based on theory differentiates the skilled, competent professional from the highly technical practitioner. The skilled, competent professional bases his or her intervention on a firm theoretical base that allows for a careful evaluation of the intervention process and its efficacy.

When one frame of reference is used properly, as outlined in this text, consistency in intervention is ensured. Concepts, postulates, and postulates regarding change agree, and consistency exists in that one segment flows from the other. As long as the therapist works with one frame of reference, all actions agree, and the theoretical principles and the application to intervention are congruent. This consistency could not be achieved if a therapist took only one concept or postulate from one section and then proceeded to application. For example, handling is a major concept in the NeuroDevelopmental frame of reference. By itself, handling does not comprise the entire frame of reference. If the therapist uses handling without the other therapeutic constructs from the theoretical base or the postulates regarding change, it is just a technique and not a way to apply the NeuroDevelopmental frame of reference. Another example is reinforcement, an important concept in the acquisitional frame of reference, but one that does not encompass the entire frame of reference.

It is important to note that when only one frame of reference is used, it ensures that concepts, postulates, and postulates regarding change are all consistent and that the end result will be a more cogent intervention process. If, during the course of intervention, the therapist notices that something is not working, then he or she can go back to the frame of reference (particularly to the theoretical base, postulates regarding change, and the application to practice sections), which should provide some insight for modifying the plan for intervention. An example of how successful a single frame of reference can be used is found in the case studies of Samantha, Andy, and Travis.

Once therapists become competent in using a frame of reference and are comfortable in the thorough understanding of its application, therapists may tend to use it exclusively with all children. Unfortunately, this may deter them from deciding, on an individual basis, which frame of reference is most appropriate for each client. At times, such exclusivity could create a certain "tunnel vision"—therapists may come to believe that the one frame of reference is superior to all others. In this case, therapists may identify with that frame of reference and begin to refer to themselves as "NeuroDevelopmental therapists" or "sensory integration therapists" instead of occupational therapists. When this occurs, a therapist may be overlooking the individual needs of the child and, instead, be working from a strong belief dedicated to one specific frame of reference. The dangers of this are twofold: (1) the child may not receive intervention that meets his or her needs, and (2) the therapist may not recognize the extent of his or her knowledge base in terms of other frames of reference. This may preclude any chance of meeting his or her client's needs, which is not best practice.

Multiple Frames of Reference

In the real world, many children cannot have their needs met through only one frame of reference. The problems of real children often are more complex than those of "paper patients" (i.e., the classic textbook case). It would be easier if one frame of reference could address all the problems of a particular child, but, in reality, frames of reference are limited by the scope of their theoretical bases. For example, in the sensory integrative frame of reference, activities of daily living (ADL) are not addressed comprehensively in the theoretical base. The theoretical base for sensory integration suggests that when a child has developed end-product abilities, he or she is then able to accomplish age-appropriate skills, which should allow him or her to perform ADL. Although this may happen for some children, other children require additional direct intervention to bring them up to an age-appropriate level in these specific tasks. This requires the use of an additional frame of reference, perhaps one that addresses specific skill acquisition like the acquisitional or motor skill acquisitional frames of reference. Such an additional frame of reference would have to focus on teaching the child specific skills to perform ADL successfully. In these situations, the occupational therapist must resort to more than one frame of reference.

To construct a relevant plan of intervention for a child who has multiple problems in the real world often requires more than one frame of reference (Mosey, 1986). When a frame of reference is used in the pure sense, as each chapter in this book suggests, then it may deal with some of the child's most significant problems at the time, but it frequently is not adequate for the entire course of treatment. Whenever the therapist considers the use of combined or sequenced frames of reference, it is necessary to develop a basic understanding of what each frame of reference entails, along with its unique approach to intervention.

Frames of Reference in Sequence

Frames of reference can be used in sequence—one frame of reference is used primarily and another frame of reference is used for a separate and more discrete problem. For example, a child who has cerebral palsy may be treated first with the Neuro-Developmental frame of reference. After seeing the child for several months, the therapist observes that the child also appears to be having visual perceptual problems. He or she evaluates the child appropriately based on the visual information analysis frame of reference. In this situation, the therapist decides to continue with the Neuro-Developmental frame of reference but, in addition, decides to use the visual information analysis frame of reference. Each frame of reference addresses different performance components and draws from different theories. Furthermore, each is based on different developmental perspectives and a belief that change occurs in different ways. The study of these two frames of reference leads the therapist to understand that neither is congruent with the other in its approach to the change process. They are not in conflict, however, when applied separately. Conflict is when constructs or postulates do not agree because they are contradictory from a theoretical perspective. In this situation, each frame of reference views the change process in a different way; therefore, neither one is compatible with the other should the therapist attempt to integrate them. The therapist decides, therefore, to use these frames of reference in sequence with the NeuroDevelopmental frame of reference as his or her basic approach. He or she decides to begin each session with the NeuroDevelopmental frame of reference, and switches to the visual information analysis frame of reference toward the end of the session. Each aspect of the intervention is clearly delineated, grounded in the theoretical base of each frame of reference. This clear demarcation is evident in the environment that the therapist creates for change and his or her use of legitimate tools. During the neurodevelopmental portion of the treatment session, the child and therapist may be on a mat, with the therapist using rolls, balls, and therapeutic handling in play activities. During the visual perception portion of the treatment session, the child may sit at a table and participate in drawing activities. The techniques and activities of intervention from each frame of reference are not integrated. The therapist is always aware of the frame of reference used at any given point in the session. An example of using two frames of reference in sequence can be seen in the case study of Judith, where the NeuroDevelopmental Treatment frame of reference was used in initial preparation for the use of Sensory Integration frame of reference.

The characteristics of sequential intervention require that one frame of reference be designated as primary, followed by others that address discrete problems in a set order. Each frame of reference maintains its own integrity, and the therapeutic goals are separate. The intervention and legitimate tools are distinct and are clearly tied to each unique theoretical base.

Over time, frames of reference may be used sequentially in another way. A therapist may use one frame of reference for a period of time to achieve particular goals. Once the child has achieved those goals, another frame of reference may be used to address other areas. For example, a therapist may use the sensory integration frame of reference to modulate sensory systems, achieve functional capabilities, and to achieve end products. But then the child may still need to improve his or her handwriting. The therapist may choose to switch to the motor skill acquisitional frame of reference.

Frames of Reference in Parallel

Frames of reference can be use in parallel—two frames of reference are used at the same time to address similar or related problems from different perspectives. Each frame of reference is used separately in different treatment sessions, different sections of one session, or even in separate intervention processes. Although these frames of reference may not share the same theoretical perspectives, they do not conflict. Two frames of reference often used in parallel are the NeuroDevelopmental and biomechanical frames of reference. A therapist may treat a child who has cerebral palsy by using the NeuroDevelopmental frame of reference. He or she has selected this frame of reference to enhance the child's movement abilities and to assist the child in developing as many normal patterns as possible. During the course of treatment, the therapist reasons that the child would benefit from adaptive equipment. He or she selects the biomechanical frame of reference to determine what equipment or devices may provide proper positioning for the child so that motor skills are improved.

The primary tool of the NeuroDevelopmental frame of reference is therapeutic handling, whereas the biomechanical frame of reference relies on specific devices and therapeutic equipment to position the child. This is not meant to oversimplify either frame of reference but, rather, to point out that they do not conflict with one another and that they work toward similar goals and, therefore, can be used well in parallel fashion. In this case, the NeuroDevelopmental frame of reference addresses the child's primary motor development, while the biomechanical frame of reference is used to address the child's static positioning needs. The NeuroDevelopmental frame of reference guides the therapist's regularly scheduled treatment sessions, whereas the biomechanical frame of reference provides proper seating equipment that positions the child throughout the day. Separately, each frame of reference addresses separate aspects of the child's motor performance; jointly, the two frames of reference facilitate intervention. For example, the coping frame of reference is generally used in parallel with other frames of reference.

Another example of frames of reference used in parallel is suggested in the acquisitional frame of reference chapter. In the application to practice section, the example of Jose stated that this frame of reference would be a good choice for the therapist to use with this child in the classroom. However, it is also suggested that the therapist may use the sensory integration frame of reference for the specific problems identified in individual intervention. This gives another type of example of how two frames of reference can be used in parallel.

The case study of Judith, discussed previously as frames of reference used sequentially, can also be viewed as an example of frames of reference used in parallel. Over time, when two frames of reference are consistently used together (although not combined) with one child to address different problems, each frame of reference maintains it's integrity and is used as it was intended to be used. This one intervention with it's two separate aspects in treatment uses both frames of reference in a parallel fashion over time. To view this as using frames of reference in parallel requires examining the intervention over a period of time such as 3 months.

Frames of Reference in Combination

Frames of reference can be used in combination in an integrative way. This can be done when the constructs of the theoretical base are consistent in that they agree about how change occurs. To use frames of reference in combination requires a skillful, experienced therapist who clearly understands each frame of reference. The therapist has to examine each frame of reference to determine whether its basic postulates are congruent with those of the other frames of reference. To use the postulates regarding change together, the basic concepts should be consistent in that they all state the same or similar things.

Two frames of reference that lend themselves to be used in combination are Sensory Integration and NeuroDevelopmental Treatment. Both are developmentally oriented and propose that specific skills and abilities are achieved in a normal sequence. When frames of reference are used in combination, the techniques of both frames of reference are integrated during each session. The coping frame of reference may be used in combination (as well as in parallel) with other frames of reference but is particularly compatible with the psychosocial frame of reference. The main characteristic of combined intervention is that two separate yet integrated frames of reference address the child as a whole. Both frames of reference are consistent with each other, and the therapeutic goals are integrated. The intervention is a blend that involves the combined use of various legitimate tools.

A skilled, competent therapist who combines two frames of reference over time may begin to view them as one. This is truly the use of two frames of reference in combination. To make this into one "new" frame of reference, the therapist must reconstruct the theoretical base, carefully exploring the concepts, postulates, and assumptions from each to interweave them into a unified theoretical base that is internally consistent. From that point, he or she must reformulate the entire frame of reference. This process is intense and requires post professional education and scholarship.

Formulation of Original Frames of Reference

The formulation of new and original frames of reference is an ongoing process for occupational therapy because, as discussed previously, it is a dynamic profession and the endemic problems change continuously. This section discusses the need for new frames of reference and serves as an overview for the process of developing new frames of reference. Additional information can be found in discussions of applied scientific inquiry for occupational therapy (Mosey 1989, 1992, 1996).

Knowledge increases and technology advances over time. This creates change in society and in the problems with which occupational therapists are concerned. One example is the recent technological strides made in neonatal intensive care that have resulted in the survival of more low-birth weight babies. This new population, with its unique needs, requires specialized intervention, which has been handled in several ways. Some therapists have modified or reformulated traditional frames of reference around the specific problems of low-birth weight infants. Other therapists have begun to evolve new frames of reference, based on new theoretical information, to work with this specific population. Each case requires advanced knowledge and skills.

As society changes, the profession adapts, mandating the search for new approaches and solutions to problems. This situation requires that occupational therapists develop new frames of reference. Therapists are still refining frames of reference that are most appropriate for intervention with infants born addicted to drugs, infants born with HIV infection, and children with pervasive developmental disorder. Another reason that may stimulate the development of new frames of reference is the need to change or add new legitimate tools or when the context or setting for therapy is changed.

A change in knowledge also precipitates the need for new frames of reference. This "new" knowledge may result from the refinement of theory, the development of new theories, or new research findings that modify the theoretical bases of old frames of reference. This may also occur when a therapist finds that specific postulates regarding change from a frame of reference no longer work or when he or she is unable to find a frame of reference that addresses a particular dysfunction.

The process of developing and articulating a frame of reference is complex. It requires a strong, scholarly knowledge base combined with advanced clinical reasoning skills. It follows the sequence discussed in Chapter 5, concentrating first on raw theoretical information, which is woven into a comprehensive and cohesive theoretical base. From this sound foundation, the therapist formulates the rest of the function/dysfunction continua, identifies behaviors indicative of function and dysfunction, specifies evaluation procedures and tools, writes postulates regarding change, and outlines an application for practice. Throughout this process, the therapist is concerned about the systematic ordering of concepts and constructs combined with internal consistency so that a clear design can be formed to link theory to practice.

SUMMARY

With experience, therapists become more adept at identifying client problems and figuring out ways to deal with different deficits. The novice therapist begins his or her understanding of the intervention process by using a single frame of reference for each client. After one becomes comfortable with the theories that guide pediatric practice, the therapist can experiment with different ways to use various frames of reference, including sequential, parallel, and combined uses. The sophisticated, scholarly therapist eventually may move toward formulating a new frame of reference to guide intervention in new areas of practice.

References

Crepeau, E. B. (1991). Achieving intersubjective understanding: Examples from an occupational therapy treatment session. *American Journal of Occupational Therapy, 45,* 1016–1025.

Gilfoyle, E. M. (1980). Caring: A philosophy for practice. *American Journal of Occupational Therapy, 34,* 517–521.

Keilhofner, G. (1983). The art of occupational therapy. In G. Keilhofner (Ed.), *Health through occupation: Theory and practice in occupational therapy* (pp.295–309). Philadelphia: F. A. Davis.

Koomar, J. A., & Bundy, A. C. (1991). The art and science of creating direct intervention from theory. In A. G. Fisher, E. A. Murray, & A.C. Bundy (Eds.), *Sensory integration: Theory and Practice* (pp.251–314). Philadelphia: F.A. Davis.

Mosey, A. C. (1981a). Occupational therapy: configurations of a profession. New York: Raven Press.

Mosey, A. C. (1981b). Introduction: The art of practice. In B. Abreu (Ed.). *Physical disabilities manual* (pp. 1–3). New York: Raven Press.

Mosey, A. C. (1986). *Psychosocial components of occupational therapy.* New York: Raven Press.

Mosey, A. C. (1989). The proper focus of scientific inquiry in occupational therapy: Frames of reference (Editorial). *Occupational Therapy Journal of Research, 9,* 195–201.

Mosey, A. C. (1992). *Applied scientific inquiry in health professions: An epistemological orientation.* Rockville, MD: American Occupational Therapy Association.

Mosey, A. C. (1996). Applied scientific inquiry in the health professions: An epistemological orientation (2nd ed.). Bethesda, MD: American Occupational Therapy Association.

Peloquin, S. M. (1989). Sustaining the art of practice in occupational therapy. *American Journal of Occupational Therapy, 43,* 219–226.

Peloquin, S. M. (1990). The patient-therapist relationship in occupational therapy: Understanding visions and images. *American Journal of Occupational Therapy, 44,* 13–21.

Peloquin, S. M. (1994). Occupational therapy as art and science: Should the older definition be reclaimed? *American Journal of Occupational Therapy, 48,* 1093–1096.

Perlman, H. H. (1979). *Relationship: the heart of helping people.* Chicago, IL: The University of Chicago Press.

Case Study: NeuroDevelopmental Treatment Frame of Reference

BETH KORBY ELENKO

BACKGROUND

Andy is a 2-year-old boy who is the youngest child in a family of Middle Eastern descent. He has two older sisters who are 3 and 7 years old, respectively. The oldest is in the first grade, and the younger sister attends a Head Start program two mornings a week. His parents are currently separated, and his mother is his primary caretaker.

Home Setting

They live in a first-floor apartment in New York City. They have a small kitchen, bathroom, living room, and two bedrooms, and there is minimal closet space. The kitchen has a small table and a wall of cupboards and appliances. The living room is filled with comfortable sofas and chairs, two dressers, and a television. The living room has a small carpeted area in the center, which is the primary play area for the children. His sisters share a bedroom with a trundle bed and another twin bed filled with doll houses and toys. Andy shares the other bedroom with his mom where he sleeps in a playpen next to his mom's queen-size bed. There is also a desk with a computer and two dressers. Although the apartment is crowded, it is clean, well-maintained, and filled with brightness and warmth. Each room has a small window, and the front window in his mom's bedroom is usually open to view the comings and goings in the neighborhood.

The girls frequently sit at the window to welcome regular visitors. Many of the neighbors in their building are of the same cultural background, and they have an open door policy. They walk each other's children to and from school, babysit, and provide a support system for one another. Andy's maternal grandparents live several blocks away and are actively involved in the care of the children, as are numerous aunts, uncles, and cousins who are frequent visitors in their home.

Birth History

Andy's mother reported an uneventful pregnancy with Andy being born at 28 weeks gestation in a breech position, weighing approximately two pounds. He required respiratory support, frequent blood transfusions, and had a grade III-IV intraventricular hemorrhage during his hospitalization in the neonatal intensive care unit (NICU). He was discharged after 6 weeks to his parents with no follow-up services.

At approximately 3 months, Andy's parents grew increasingly concerned about his development as they noted that his body was as stiff as a board. Andy's mother became frustrated when she diapered and dressed him. She could not bend him at his joints and sometimes felt that she would break him when she did. Andy cried frequently and was difficult to console. He was unable to hold his head up or reach for objects. He was able to suck on his bottle, but he spilled more than he took in and was quite underweight. They took him from physician to physician but were unsuccessful getting any assistance. Doctors told them that "he would grow out of it" and to "just be patient." In spite of this assurance that Andy would grow out of it, both parents remained extremely concerned.

When Andy was 8 months old, he was hospitalized for pneumonia. At that time, they met a neurologist who told them about early intervention services and referred them to social services requesting that the family be put in contact with an early intervention agency. Finally, they were referred to the New York State Early Intervention hotline, which is a referral base for parents who are concerned with their child's development. They were assigned to an early intervention original designee (EIOD) who referred them to a home-based early intervention program to evaluate Andy.

It was at this time that Andy's parents separated reportedly because of the extreme stress and tension as a result of Andy's needs. Andy's father could not deal with his only son having any problems and left the country. Thus, Andy's mother has to handle all of Andy's unique needs in addition to raising her two other children. At the first meeting with the service coordinator from the home-based early intervention program, she discussed her concerns and needs for Andy and the family. Subsequently, Andy was evaluated by a developmental psychologist and special educator in the family's home. Based on evaluators identified concerns and recommendations, Andy was further evaluated by an occupational therapist, a physical therapist, and a speech-language pathologist.

OCCUPATIONAL THERAPY ASSESSMENT

After Andy's initial screening, which consisted of the referral information and a general observation, the occupational therapists selected the NeuroDevelopmental

Treatment (NDT) frame of reference to guide her assessment of Andy's difficulties in movement and tone. She was primarily concerned with how his delayed development affected his gross motor, fine motor, and self-help skills. The NDT frame of reference was used within the context of a family-centered, interdisciplinary approach, stressing the integral role that families play in a child's development (Bailey, Buysse, Edmondson, & Smith, 1992; Guralnick, 1989; Hinojosa & Anderson, 1991; McCollum & Yates, 1994).

The occupational therapy assessment included information from a variety of sources, including parental interview, clinical observations, and standardized assessments. Andy was seen in his home with his sisters and mom present.

Overall Assessment of Functional Skills

This area of assessment encompasses Andy's gross motor abilities, upper extremity function, and activities of daily living in the context of Andy's play exploration and daily activities in his home. Andy's mother placed him on his back on a blanket on the floor in the living room where he gazed at his mother smiling. He was visually attentive to his environment looking all around the room, smiling. He made some sounds but was mainly quiet throughout the assessment.

Andy tried but had difficulty actively turning his head to look toward the midline or to his right side in any position. He initiated rolling over from prone-to-supine by using associated movement patterns. He would cry when his pelvis was flexed so he could be held in supported sitting or any other anti-gravity position. Andy was unable to assume any anti-gravity position on his own and had difficulty maintaining them when positioned. When Andy's mom held him, she did so with Andy in trunk and pelvic extension with poor head control and "fixing"of his upper body was observed. She reported that he spends most of the day positioned on his back so he can see what goes on around him and cries in any other position.

Andy was unable to weight bear or use his arms for support in any position. Increased tone was observed in his upper extremities when he initiated movement of his upper extremities to reach for toys or his mom in supine. The asymmetrical tonic neck reflex (ATNR) dominated his upper body movements, he held his right hand in a fisted position, and he was unable to bring his arms toward the midline. When Andy attempted to open both his hands, his thumb was positioned adducted into his palm. When an object was placed in his hand, he displayed a gross grasp briefly to hold it, and spontaneously dropped it. Andy exhibited minimal volitional movement of his upper extremities.

During the assessment of play behavior, it was observed that Andy did not attempt to explore his environment. When his sisters smiled and laughed, attempting to involve him in play, he did not seem to respond to them or react to their attempts to engage him. Their attempts to get him to reach for a toy were unsuccessful. They finally grabbed his arm and pulled it towards the toy. His mother reported that he watches television and listens to music.

Information on self-care was collected from an informal interview with his mother. She reported that she struggled to position him for feeding and bathing. During feeding, she holds Andy in her lap in an extended position with his pelvis and lower extremities between her legs. She reported that while he is able to suck fluids from a bottle, he has a great deal of spillage and poor lip closure around the nipple. He had just begun taking baby foods. Bathing is difficult because of his stiffness so she sponge bathes him or holds him in the shower with her. His stiffness made diapering and dressing him extremely difficult. She uses an umbrella stroller to transport him. He is put in a car seat when he rides in the car. She stated that she was concerned because he tends to fall over or push himself straight out of the seat belt in the car seat and the stroller.

Quality of Movement

Andy's quality of movement was assessed by observing him on the floor and during attempts to get him to interact with the therapist. Andy initially exhibited hypertonicity throughout his trunk, pelvis, and all four extremities and hypotonicity in his neck and shoulder girdle. Tone was increased in the upper extremity flexors and in the lower extremity extensor muscles. He resisted passive range of movement at any joint. The ATNR was evident especially on his left side in all positions, which dominated his movement patterns. No head righting, equilibrium, or protective responses were elicited in any positions. Andy preferred to be positioned in supine where his extensor tone predominated, and it was difficult to relax his muscle tone at his pelvis in sitting or weight bear on his upper body in prone. He cried when he was handled or moved in and out of any posture. He rolled using full body extension, with hyperextension of his head and neck to flop from prone to supine, exhibiting a lack of alignment in the transverse plane. He lacked scapular-humeral dissociation and pelvic-femoral dissociation. In prone, head and neck hypotonia and instability of the shoulder girdle interferes with his ability to lift his head from the floor. His legs and feet were extended and his upper body was observed in a "fixed" posture. This included scapular retraction; humeral elevation, internal rotation, adduction, and extension; elbow extension; forearm pronation; and wrist flexion and finger flexion.

Standardized Evaluations

Andy's assessment included standardized evaluation information because age levels are required for determination of services by New York State Early Intervention Program. These age levels do not fit Andy's true skill level because of his poor quality of movement. Further, they do not analyze the specific factors that contribute to his inability to achieve his motor skills. The *Hawaii Early Learning Profile* [HELP] (Furuno, O'Reilly, Hosaka, Inatsuka, Allman, & Zeisloft, 1984) and the *Peabody Fine and Gross Motor Scales* (Folio & Fewell, 1983) were utilized. Andy's performance on these test items revealed the scattering of abilities. On both assessments, Andy scored in the 2-to-4 month level, placing him at a greater than 33% delay in more than one area of function. This performance score qualified him for early intervention services.

Evaluation Summary

In this section, Andy's motor performance is viewed relative to the function/dysfunction continua as outlined in the NDT frame of reference.

Postural Tone

Postural tone was abnormal. Hypotonicity was observed in Andy's head, neck, and shoulders, and hypertonicity was seen in his trunk, pelvis, and all four extremities. Tone was particularly increased in the upper extremity flexors and in trunk, pelvis, and lower extremity extensor muscles. In prone, his head fell into the surface while his lower extremities withdrew and lifted up from the surface. Tremors were observed with his attempts to reach with his upper body. Andy resisted passive range of motion at any joint.

Stability/Mobility

Andy performed on the dysfunctional end of the stability-mobility continuum, demonstrating many compensatory behaviors. No head righting, equilibrium, or protective responses were elicited in any positions. Andy was unable to assume any anti-gravity position on his own and had difficulty maintaining them when positioned. He required support of equipment or therapeutic handling to provide the necessary stability. He frequently exhibited "fixing" posture when held in an anti-gravity position characteristic of scapular retraction; humeral elevation, internal rotation, adduction, and extension; elbow extension; forearm pronation; and wrist flexion and finger flexion. He was dominated by an ATNR, which held his right hand in a fisted position, and he was unable to bring his arms toward midline.

Postural Control

Andy performed on the dysfunctional end of the postural control continuum with mid-range control only. Andy preferred to be positioned in supine because his extensor tone predominated. He rolled using full body extension with hyperextension of his head and neck to turn from prone to supine. In prone, Andy's face fell into the surface and he was unable to lift his head from the floor, his legs and feet were lifted into the air, and his upper body was observed in a "fixed" posture.

Postural Alignment as Related to Three Planes of Space

Andy's lack of postural alignment in any or all of the body planes is considered dysfunctional. Andy had no head righting reactions in the sagittal plane (anterior-posterior direction) when in the prone position. He also did not exhibit head righting reactions in the sagittal and frontal (lateral direction) planes with small weight shifts in supported sitting. Postural alignment was poor because of the dominance of the obligatory ATNR. He rolled using full body extension with hyperextension of his head and neck to flop over to his back, exhibiting lack of alignment in the transverse plane.

Dissociation

Andy's movement patterns were performed in an associated or synergistic way, which is indicative of dysfunction. Associated movement patterns were demonstrated during rolling. Andy initiated rolling using full body extension with hyperextension of his head and neck to flop over to his back, which appeared to increase the extension in his trunk and lower extremities. Andy also used synergistic patterns of movement when being held with full body extension. When being moved in and out of any position, it was difficult for Andy to relax. His hands were fisted when associated with flexion of the arm and opened with extension of the arm. He lacked scapular-humeral dissociation and pelvic-femoral dissociation.

Variety of Movement

Andy had limited variety of movement, exhibiting stereotypical movements where both lower extremities persist with extension, adduction, and internal rotation in all positions. He also displayed stereotypical upper extremities' persistence of shoulder elevation and retraction in all positions. An ATNR dominated all his movement patterns.

Full Passive Range of Motion

Andy's abnormal tone and stereotypical movement patterns, with limitations in passive range of motion, were evidence of dysfunction. This puts him at risk for developing contractures and deformities in the future.

Individualized Family Service Plan Meeting

Once all of Andy's evaluations were completed, an Individualized Family Service Plan (IFSP) meeting was held among his mother, his maternal grandmother, the initial service coordinator, the special education teacher from the early intervention agency, and the EIOD. At the IFSP meeting, the individuals presented Andy's evaluation findings. The team discussed these findings in the context of the family's concerns and needs. Goals for Andy and his family were discussed, and a plan for implementation was developed. Andy's mom agreed on the outcomes and services recommended for him. The outcomes written into Andy's IFSP were his goals. The professional or professionals responsible for each intervention goal were identified based on whom the team determined would be most appropriate. The entire plan was written in non-medical, jargon-free language. It was determined that Andy should receive occupational therapy, physical therapy, speech therapy, and special education, each to be provided twice a week for 30 minutes. The following outcomes were designated for occupational therapy to address:

- developing head, neck, shoulder, and trunk control
- being able to weight bear on his arms
- using hands in front of him
- holding objects in his hands
- clapping, bringing hands together
- manipulating things around him
- increasing mobility
- sitting up without support
- holding his bottle
- learning to use his cup
- learning to use a spoon

INTERVENTION

Andy's intervention illustrates specific treatment concepts and techniques that relate to the discussion of the sequence of intervention in the NDT frame of reference. In early intervention, often the therapist who treats the child is different from the therapist who completed the initial evaluation. Consistent with this pattern, Andy was assigned another occupational therapist to provide the home-based services. In the referral information, she received the initial occupational therapy evaluation report. She was also given the IFSP with the outlined expected goals for occupational therapy.

At her initial meeting with the family, the occupational therapist's primary goal was to establish a relationship with the family and to do a brief evaluation of Andy herself. Based on the information in the IFSP, the occupational therapist verified the family's identified concerns for the family and Andy. She assessed Andy's sensorimotor performance components as he engaged with family members. Rapport was easily established with Andy's mother and sisters who were eager to learn to play with him and to help him develop. During this initial session, Andy was fussy when handled by the therapist and kept his eyes on his mother.

Andy mother's major concerns were Andy's daily management. She stated that she did not feel comfortable carrying or holding Andy and struggled with how best to support him. When asked to show how she held Andy, she demonstrated lifting Andy by his arms like a sack of potatoes and tossed him over her shoulders (Figure 17.1). Thus, intervention began with instruction and demonstrations on how to handle, carry, and position Andy to inhibit his abnormal muscle tone. Using the following postulate regarding change, if therapeutic handling is used by all professionals and family members who have contact with the child, then the child has the most opportunities to move with dynamic postural tone and a variety of patterns of movement. The therapist demonstrated techniques to the family. During these initial sessions, the occupational therapist provided several opportunities for his mother and sisters to practice holding and moving Andy around in situations that were common in the home. As his mother became more comfortable with handling, the therapist demonstrated how she could facilitate Andy's head control, trunk flexion, and a midline orientation (Figure 17.2).

After a month of intervention during which his mother was becoming comfortable handling Andy, the therapist decided to address the difficulty that she was having with daily activities such as dressing and diapering. Again, the occupational therapist demonstrated or modeled the use of specific techniques to make dressing easier. The therapist demonstrated how preparatory techniques such as elongating muscles and initiating range of motion of the extremities could be incorporated into his daily routines. His mother was shown certain methods to don and take off Andy's clothing by elongating muscles in certain positions. In Figure 17.3, Andy is prone on his

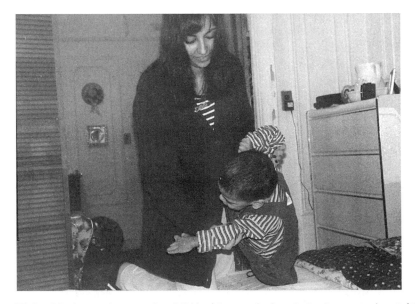

Figure 17.1   Mother picking up the child by his arms before being instructed on inhibitory carrying techniques.

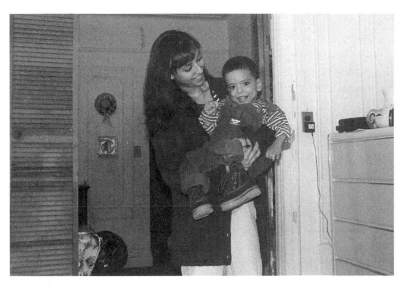

Figure 17.2 Mother carrying the child using inhibitory techniques; child has flexed hips to inhibit increased extension and promote midline orientation.

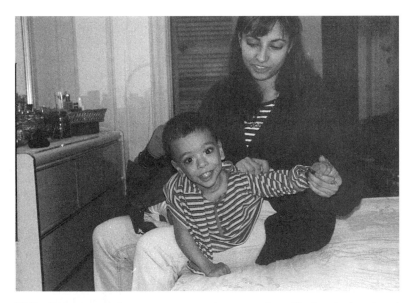

Figure 17.3 Dressing techniques were taught to mother. Mother is donning the child's shirt in prone while promoting head control and upper extremity weight bearing.

mother's lap so that he can weight bear on his upper extremities and work on holding his head up while his mother dons his shirt over his head. By bunching up the shirt sleeve, his mother could facilitate his arm in forward flexion through his sleeve rather than yank his arm through the sleeve or pull his clothing over his arm. As his mother switches to dress the other side of Andy's body, she can facilitate rolling him in a weight shift from side to side. Donning pants in prone could also be achieved in this manner by facilitating weight shifting as she pulls his pants over his legs and over his pelvis (Figure 17.4). While diapering and interacting with Andy, his mother was shown that flexion at Andy's pelvis relaxes his muscles in his spine and lower body. It was explained to her that these actions can be done during diapering so that the activity becomes easier for both of them and inhibits his tone at the same time.

With the mother more comfortable handling and playing with Andy, the occupational therapist began to focus her treatment on Andy's sensorimotor development. Treatment progressed into direct handling with preparatory activities either on the living room floor or on his mother's bed. These activities encouraged Andy's active postural control in various positions and inhibited increased tone that blocks his movement patterns. The occupational therapist used a variety of play activities with toys that were available in the home. Andy became easily excited during play activities, which added to his increased tone. Because Andy was seen in his home with limited therapeutic equipment available, the therapist frequently used her lap in addition to her hands to facilitate movement.

Andy became even more animated when his sisters interacted with him. Thus, when the sisters were home, the therapist involved them in play activities. A preparation technique for Andy was to position him in prone over the therapist's leg; in this position, the therapist encouraged head lifting and upper extremity weight bearing. In this position, he could also focus on head control and midline orientation as

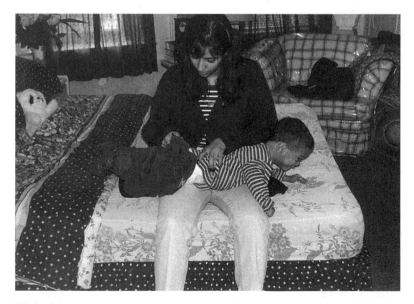

Figure 17.4 Mother demonstrating donning pants. Notice facilitation of weight shifting with mother's left hand.

he was weight bearing on his upper extremities. The therapist facilitated Andy by using proximal key points of control at his trunk or shoulder girdle to promote trunk flexion, head control, and weight bearing from prone on elbows to extended arms (Figure 17.5). Intermittent handling throughout the session allowed Andy an opportunity to activate his muscles on his own. Andy was able to maintain prone on extended arms for short periods and then collapsed at the shoulder girdle. When he did this, the therapist placed her hands on his shoulders, spread her hands while pulling up and back to elongate the pectoralis musculature laterally to facilitate his head control and weight bearing (Figure 17.6).

Andy benefitted using different key points of control because of his increased tone (e.g., providing stability at the trunk and then using handling to move the shoulder girdle so he experiences a full range of movement). This reduced his tightness and facilitated active movement. In the prone position, Andy was in a more symmetrical posture to inhibit the ATNR. In prone, he would also be oriented toward midline by using his motivation to knock things over or reach for his family members. In this way, he was encouraged to actively look up with his head and eyes and reach toward one of his sisters or blocks that they have stacked for him (Figure 17.7). He smiled and laughed when he successfully knocked the blocks over and reached again.

In prone, the therapist facilitated rolling by using key points at Andy's pelvis to roll him back toward supine. In this position, Andy was able to actively reach as a result of being in a gravity-eliminated position. Andy choose to spend most of his day

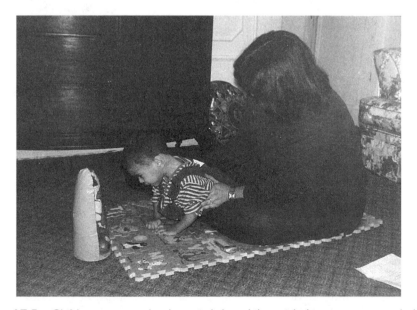

Figure 17.5 Child prone over the therapist's leg while weight bearing on extended arms. The therapist is facilitating the child at his trunk.

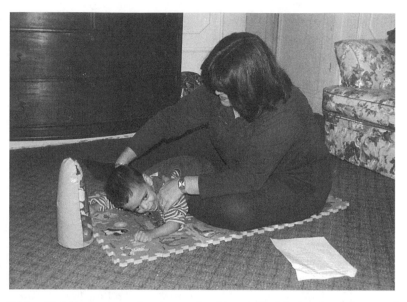

Figure 17.6 Child in prone collapsing at shoulder girdle. Notice the therapist elongating the pectoralis muscles to facilitate head lifting.

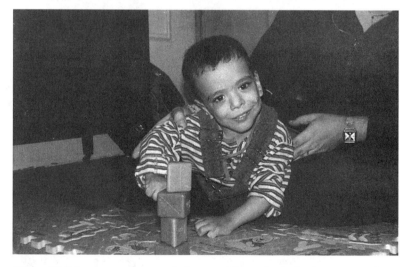

Figure 17.7 Child prone on extended arms. Therapist is facilitating reach in one extremity.

in the prone position. During therapy, the therapist spent a great deal of time facilitating Andy out of supine. From the supine position the therapist was able to facilitate rolling to sidelying, with the key point at the pelvis, and continue to prone (Figure 17.8). In sidelying, Andy was able to reach with the non-weightbearing side with facilitation at his shoulder girdle to promote a forward reach. Once he was in prone,

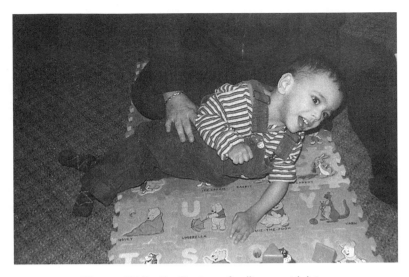

Figure 17.8   Facilitation of rolling to sidelying.

he was in a functional position. In prone, Andy was able to weight bear on his upper extremities, which relaxed his increased tone, therefore allowing him to begin to reach forward for a toy.

To transition Andy to a sitting position from prone, the occupational therapist facilitated Andy from sidelying, using key points at his pelvis and trunk, with hands placed on opposite sides of his body. When the therapist provided a downward pressure on the weightbearing side and upward pressure on the non-weightbearing trunk, Andy could be facilitated to a sitting position (Figure 17.9).

Andy could sit in a ring-sitting posture and actively control his posture for a few minutes. In this anti-gravity position, Andy attempted to hold his head up and fix his upper body to stay upright. The therapist stabilized Andy at his pelvis in a neutral position with downward pressure so that his upper body was free to move. Antigravity positions were very challenging for Andy. However, when supported, upright positions allowed Andy to reach while the therapist facilitated weight shift and trunk rotation to the opposite sides. The therapist could accomplish this by stabilizing the pelvis on one side of the body with one hand and holding the wrist on the opposite side of the body to facilitate rotational movement and weight shifting. An alternative method would be to stabilize the child in sitting between the therapist's legs and pushing gently forward with an open hand on one scapula while stabilizing the other shoulder.

The therapist facilitated Andy from ring sitting to a side-sitting position by applying downward pressure on his pelvis into the surface and then allowing him to weight bear on the therapist's leg and reach for toys. This allows Andy to weight shift and rotate his trunk in the direction of the weight bearing side. The therapist also facilitated trunk rotation to the opposite side.

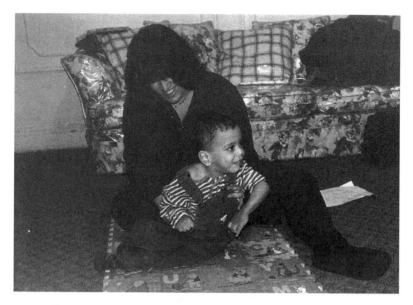

Figure 17.9   Facilitation from sidelying to sitting position.

Andy benefitted from elongating his shoulder girdle in all positions. His spasticity restricted his upper body motor control. Accordingly, elongating the shoulder girdle allows the therapist to facilitate the shoulders to move toward the weight bearing surface. Gentle traction with intermittent joint compression is applied by holding the child's arms at the wrists and hand with external rotation (Figure 17.10). This elongated tight musculature in the shoulder girdle allows for greater expansion of his chest. At other times, the therapist facilitated a weight shift from side-to-side, providing intermittent compression to the humero-scapular joint. This technique enabled Andy to work on his head righting and weight shifting, while learning that he does not need to use his upper body to fixate for postural control.

As Andy's ability to move more freely increases, the therapist graded the activities to facilitate his grasp of blocks so that he could stack them himself. The unique role of the occupational therapists is to integrate movement with functional developmentally appropriate activities. To challenge and develop Andy's cognitive skills while maximizing his motor skills, the therapist used adapted switch toys that Andy could reach to press himself to activate the switch. The switches were placed in various locations to increase elongation of his upper extremities and trunk.

As Andy begins to reach more, the therapist focuses on distal movements of wrist and fingers. With fingers extended, Andy is able to develop the ability to grasp an object when placed in his hand. Better motor control for reaching was facilitated by having him weight bear on his upper body. Andy was able to grasp an object and re-

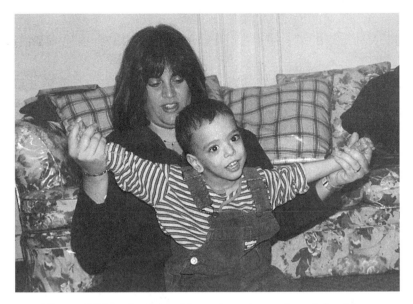

Figure 17.10 In sitting, bilateral gentle traction of shoulders.

late to it, as the therapist facilitated supination of his forearm and flexion of his fingers, by having the therapist place her hand over Andy's hand and gently moving him through these movements (Figure 17.11).

When Andy was able to hold onto an object placed in his hand for a few seconds, the occupational therapist began to focus on developing a volitional grasp. To develop a volitional grasp, the therapist closed her hand over his hand with deep pressure so that he could feel that there was an object there. He usually kept his fingers in extension when an object touched his palm. Spontaneously, Andy began to reach for an object, such as his bottle, a pencil, a block, or paper and held it between his thumb pad and inner side of his index finger adducted. However, he could only hold objects for a short period of time before he dropped them.

Andy also needed some adaptive equipment to support him during feeding, bathing, and transportation. The biomechanical frame of reference was used to augment the NDT frame of reference so that the child's needs were better met. This adaptive equipment would position Andy safely and inhibit his increased muscle tone. Further, it would free the mother's arms so that she could more easily and effectively feed, bathe, and transport him. In collaboration with his physical therapist, Andy's stroller was adapted to optimize positioning for transportation. The adapted stroller gave Andy an opportunity to experience upright posture. His high-chair was also adapted to be used during feeding.

These adaptations, which were constructed by the therapist, worked well for a few months with improving his tone and postural control because he was in an upright posture during the day, especially during feeding. Then as Andy grew and began to grow out of the adaptations that were made to his stroller, a commercial custom adapted stroller was ordered (Figure 17.12). Up until this time, Andy was bathed by holding him in the shower. The success with the custom commercial adaptive stroller provided an opportunity to explore alternative bathing methods with his mother. She acknowledged that it was becoming increasingly difficult for her to safely bathe Andy. Together, Andy's mother and the occupational therapist discussed the options available for an adapted bath chair to promote optimal positioning for ease and safety. They ordered a bath chair, which allowed Andy to sit in the bath water and enjoy the experience in a safe position, while mom, with her hands free, could focus on bathing him.

This intervention summary covered the first 3 months of Andy's intervention and highlights the use of the NDT frame of reference in a family-centered approach. While the therapist was concerned with Andy's sensorimotor development, she also was responsive to the family's needs. She was fundamentally concerned with the family's ability to handle and interact with Andy. Part of her intervention was the ongoing assessment of family members' concerns, needs, and skills to demonstrate and teach them techniques that would facilitate their handling of and interaction with Andy. For the mother, the focus was on daily living skills needed to feed, dress, bath, and transport Andy. For his siblings, the focus was on play and participation in learning activities. When using any frame of reference, it is critical that the therapist be sensitive to both the family and child's needs.

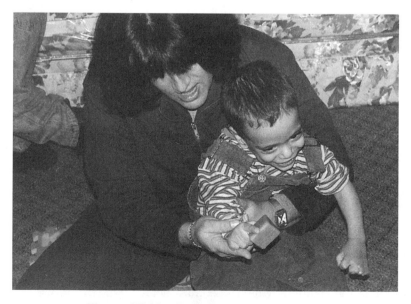

Figure 17.11   Facilitating grasping of a toy.

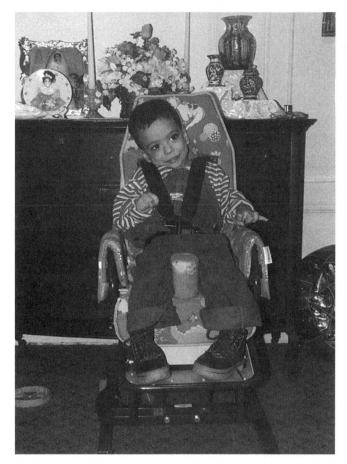

Figure 17.12   Sitting with neutral pelvis in adapted stroller.

SUMMARY

At the end of 3 months, Andy had adjusted to intervention, smiling when the therapist arrived and crying when she left. He gained control over his muscles in movement against gravity and spontaneously reached for toys, held objects volitionally, and held his head in the midline with minimal dominance of the ATNR. He started to use the prone position to engage in play activities and actively roll back and forth between prone and supine independently. In prone, he is able to transition from prone on elbows to extended arms and weight shift to reach with one extremity for a toy or person. He is able to sit on the floor briefly, with upper body support. When he attempts to reach for an object while sitting, he tends to fall to the right side or backward. In supported sitting, he is able to reach for objects at the midline, open his hand to grasp it, and hold it in his hand with a gross palmer grasp. At times, he can reach for an object out of his midline space.

He assists much more with his activities of daily living, making it easier for his mother. He reaches his arms through the sleeve of his shirt once mom initiates it over his hand. He holds his bottle with fisted hands, and now drinks from a cut-out cup without spillage. He still does not attempt to hold the cup. He enjoys finger feeding but requires hand-over-hand to get the food to his mouth once he is holding it with his thumb and index finger adducted laterally. Andy holds a spoon but needs hand-over-hand to bring the spoon to his mouth because of his increased tone, which increases even more with the anticipation of eating.

STUDY QUESTIONS

1. Why was the NDT frame of reference selected for Andy?
2. How does Andy's overall muscle tone affect his ability to reach for toys?
3. How did the occupational therapist focus on Andy's habitual patterns, and how does she attempt to improve his ability to reach for toys?
4. Why does the occupational therapist provide stability? How? Where? Could this stability be provided in other ways?
5. Why did the occupational therapist change the key points of control and provide intermittent handling with Andy?
6. What other factors make it difficult for Andy to reach for toys?
7. How does the occupational therapist facilitate active reach and grasp? What are some other ways to do this?

Acknowledgments

The author wishes to thank Al-Ameen and his mother for their willingness to be photographed to demonstrate the treatment techniques discussed in this chapter.

References

Anderson, J., & Hinojosa, J. (1984). Parents in a professional partnership. *American Journal of Occupational Therapy, 38,* 451–461.

Bailey, D., Buysse, V., Edmondson, R., & Smith, T. (1992). Creating family-centered services in early intervention: Perceptions of professionals in four states. *Exceptional Children, 58,* 298–309.

Folio, M. R., & Fewell, R. R. (1983). *Peabody developmental motor scales and activity cards.* Allen, TX: DIM Teaching Resources.

Furuno, S., O'Reilly, K. A., Hosaka, C. M., Inatsuka, T. T., Allman, T. A., & Zeisloft, B. (1984). *Hawaii Early Learning Profile (HELP).* Palo Alto, CA: Vort Corporation.

Guralnick, M. (1989). Recent developments in early intervention efficacy research: Implications for family involvement in P.L. 99–457. *Topics in Early Childhood Special Education, 9* (3), 1–17.

Hinojosa, J., & Anderson, J. (1991). Home programs for preschool children with cerebral palsy: Mother's perceptions. *American Journal of Occupational Therapy, 45,* 273–279.

McCollum, J., & Yates, T. J. (1994). Dyad as focus, triad as means: A family-centered approach to supporting parent-child interactions. *Infants and Young Children, 6* (4), 54–63.

CHAPTER 18

Case Study: Motor Skill Acquisition Frame of Reference

GARY BEDELL/MARGARET T. KAPLAN

BACKGROUND

Samantha is a 9-year-old girl with a diagnosis of dysautonomia. Dysautonomia is an autosomal recessive inherited syndrome that is characterized by a primary disturbance in autonomic nervous system function. Symptoms can include sensory regulation difficulties, motor incoordination, hyporeflexia, poor vasomotor control, labile cardiovascular reactions, diminished lacrimation, hypersalivation with aspiration and swallowing difficulties, excessive vomiting, and emotional instability (National Dysautonomia Research Foundation, 1997).

Samantha lives with her parents and her dog in an apartment building in Greenwich Village, New York City. She is in the third grade and attends a private school in her neighborhood. She currently receives occupational therapy and physical therapy two times weekly and works with a speech pathologist, who specializes in feeding and oral motor problems, once a week at a hospital. Samantha is on gastrostomy-tube feedings at night and frequently requires suctioning because of mucous build up and expectoration difficulties. However, she is beginning to tolerate greater amounts and varieties of food by mouth. She is currently eating approximately 650 calories by mouth during the day. Soft foods are easier for her to manage than hard foods. She particularly likes tuna sandwiches, cookies, and cheddar cheese.

Samantha has been receiving a full complement of services since infancy. She received outpatient rehabilitation services for sensorimotor and oral motor problems when she was an infant and toddler. She also attended an integrated classroom during her preschool years and received educational and therapeutic services to assist her with pre-academic and functional skills.

OCCUPATIONAL THERAPY EVALUATION

Information about Samantha was initially obtained by reviewing her educational file and talking to her teacher and parents. Samantha's parents explained that Samantha continues to have an occasional "medical crisis" because of poor vasomotor control and poor temperature regulation. These crises include fainting because of a rapid decrease in blood pressure, hyperthermia, spiking fevers, bronchial infections, and bacterial infections from her gastrostomy-tube. These crises occasionally require hospitalization.

Samantha's teacher and parents report that Samantha requires frequent rest breaks because of her decreased strength and endurance and her occasional attentional difficulties (Figure 18.1). In addition, they describe Samantha as a very kind and friendly child, who needs consistency in her environment and daily routines. Her parents believe that this need for predictability is based on her sensory regulation and motor control difficulties, which are common characteristics of dysautonomia. Both parents are very involved with a Familial Dysautonomia support network and have educated many of the teachers and therapists that have worked with Samantha over the years.

The evaluation followed a top-down progression—first exploring Samantha's occupational performance areas and contexts and then exploring performance components. The focus was on analyzing the child-task-environment match. There were a number of strengths and needs that were identified from the educational file review and informal discussions with the teacher and parents. Samantha's strengths include that she is ambulatory and independent in all aspects of self-care (with occasional reminders needed for quality and thoroughness). Additionally, she has very supportive and resourceful parents. She also is very social and articulate and has above-average intelligence; her reading skills are above grade-level. Samantha has good persistence and frustration tolerance for tasks that she enjoys doing such as art activities, science projects, cooking activities, and problem-solving board games.

Samantha has difficulty with most tasks that require fine controlled movements;

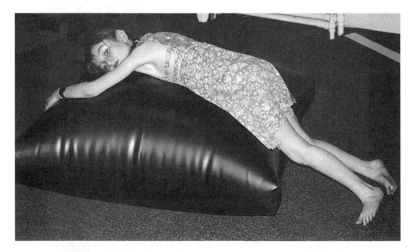

Figure 18.1   Samantha requires frequent rest breaks.

regulation of force and pressure; bilateral coordination; and increased strength, endurance, and balance. Samantha also has significant oral motor and feeding problems but is able to take small bites and sips of a few foods and liquids. She fully participates in the school lunch program and is encouraged to eat and drink as much as she can tolerate. In addition, Samantha's teacher and parents report that she occasionally makes excuses or uses social conversation to avoid certain tasks that are difficult for her, or are perceived to be so, and inconsistently asks others for assistance when needed. The tasks that Samantha reportedly is having the most difficulty with in school that will be addressed in the occupational therapy evaluation are as follows:

- Fine motor manipulation and control of materials when doing science and art projects (Figures 18.2 and 18.3)
- Carrying her food tray and opening food containers in the lunchroom while the other children are moving about
- Writing speed, endurance, and legibility for doing classroom and homework assignments
- Carrying certain classroom materials within the classroom while the other children are moving about
- Balance, running, and ball activities during physical education
- Fully participating with the other children when on the playground
- Keeping up with the other children while maintaining her balance during stair climbing
- Opening the locked heavy bathroom door with a key (Figure 18.4)

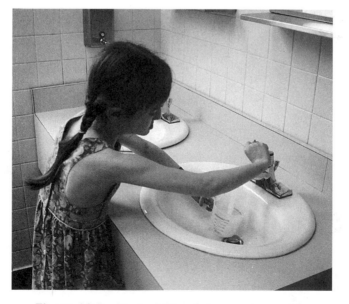

Figure 18.2 Manipulation of classroom materials.

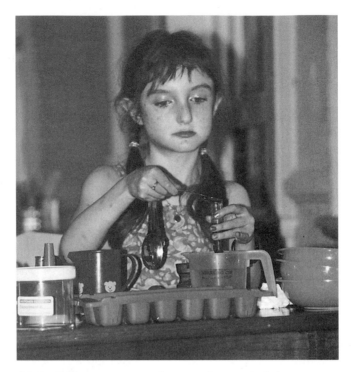

Figure 18.3 Fine motor manipulation and control of classroom materials.

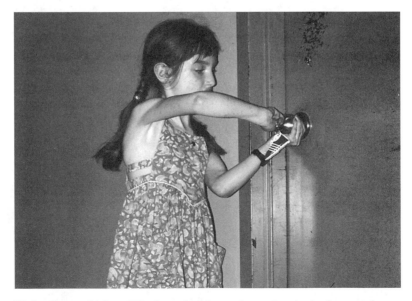

Figure 18.4 Samantha has difficulty unlocking and opening the bathroom door at school.

These tasks (with the exception of the last task, which can be considered a closed task) are all open tasks because aspects of the environment are in motion and the task requirements and environmental demands vary each time the task is attempted.

Observation of task performance

The tasks identified were observed in the contexts where, and the time when, Samantha typically performed them during the school day. While all of the above tasks were observed, two tasks will be described in-depth to demonstrate the process of evaluation when using a motor skill acquisition frame of reference: 1) Doing a science project in the classroom and 2) Carrying a lunch tray and managing food containers in the lunchroom while others are moving about. These are the same tasks that will be discussed later to demonstrate intervention.

Science Project

The science project observed required Samantha to obtain and set up all of the specified materials; obtain water from the sink and carry it back to her workstation; pour a pre-set amount of water into test tubes; and place and mix pre-set amounts of chemicals into test tubes and petri dishes using an eye dropper. These are tasks that are commonly required to participate in science labs throughout the school year. (Note: the photographs demonstrate a simulation of task performance in an occupational therapy private practice setting.)

Samantha was able to do many of the above listed parts of the science project. She was able to obtain and set up all project materials at her workstation; however, she required 5 more minutes than the other children to do this mainly because she took each item out one at a time (Figure 18.5). The other children were able to hold more objects in one hand and combine hands to hold, carry, and place objects (Figure 18.6). Samantha was able to fill up a measuring cup with water, but she filled it up too high and thus spilled some while walking back to the work station. She was able to pour water into the test tubes but did not stay within the pre-set guidelines (Figure 18.7). However, when a clear visual marker was placed on the test tube, she more closely approximated the measurement guidelines (Figure 18.8). She was able to use the eye dropper for placing and mixing the chemicals into the test tubes and petri dishes, but she did not consistently put in the correct number of drops (Figure 18.9). She also had difficulty filling up the dropper and emptying it completely.

Carrying Her Lunch Tray

In the school lunchroom, Samantha was required to stand and walk slowly in line with her classmates to initially pick up one tray from a stack; place and slide her tray on the cafeteria style counter; select and place three food items (a container of juice, a bowl of spaghetti, and a container of Jell-O) and a packet that contained plastic utensils and a napkin on her tray; take money out of her pants pocket to pay the

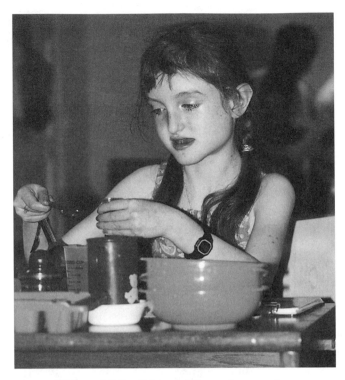

Figure 18.5 Science: filling and measuring.

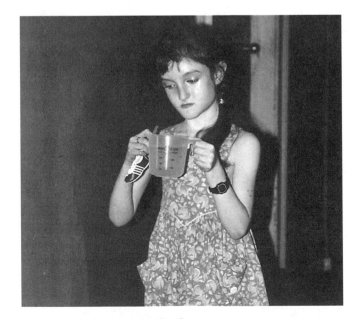

Figure 18.6 Science: carrying.

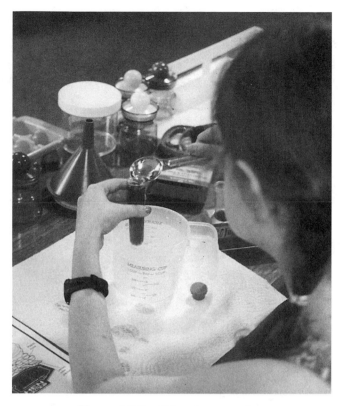

Figure 18.7 Filling the test tubes.

cashier and return her change back to her pocket; carry the tray to a table with picnic-benchlike seats where a number of her classmates were sitting. Finally, she had to open the utensil packet and food containers on her tray while seated.

Samantha was able to pick up the tray from the stack on her third attempt, after being encouraged to try different methods to do this effectively. She was able to walk along the line with the tray and obtain all food items and the utensil packet while sliding the tray along the counter. She was able to take a five-dollar bill out of her pocket, but she took more time to do this than her classmates. She dropped some of the change on her tray and the floor when retrieving it from the cashier. She picked up each of the coins and put them in her pocket one at a time.

Samantha walked tentatively and awkwardly while carrying her tray to the table. Rather than asking one of her classmates to move to allow her to pass and place her tray on the table, she waited until she was noticed. She sat at the edge of the bench and held onto the edge of the table when sitting down. By the time Samantha sat down, her classmates were almost completely done with their meal (Figure 18.10).

Samantha was unable to open the utensil package because she had difficulty generating enough force to hold and tear simultaneously. She was able to pull open the

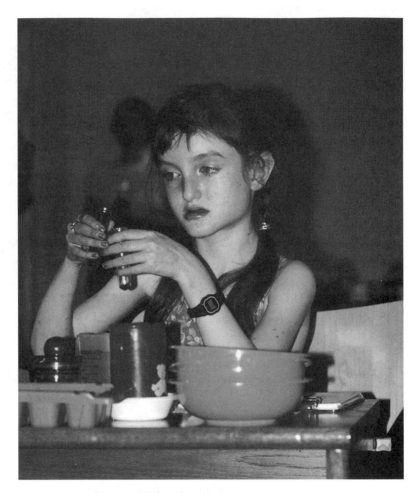

Figure 18.8 Combining correct amounts.

two sides of the juice container but was unable to complete the last step that required her to push the two sides together to form the spoutlike opening. She walked up to her teacher to ask her for help, and her teacher opened the packet and container for her.

During both of these tasks, Samantha demonstrated ability to problem solve when something was difficult for her. She tried different methods and, at times, asked adults for help, but she did not ask the other children for help. During these tasks, she exhibited asymmetrical posturing, motor overflow (e.g., excessive tongue and facial movements), and occasional drooling. She had difficulty carrying objects that were of different sizes and weights and negotiating around the other children. Decreased strength, balance, and bilateral coordination affected the quality of her performance. Her difficulty with in-hand manipulation and fine motor control and her

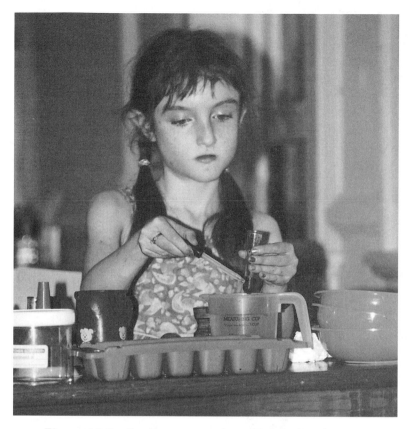

Figure 18.9 Precise measurements using the eye dropper.

immature grasp and release patterns also affected her performance. Consequently, Samantha required more time for task completion. In addition, she made a number of errors when completing tasks.

It is important to note that Samantha's performance improved when she was encouraged to use different methods to pick up the tray and when she was given a visual cue to pour the water into the test tubes more accurately. Because these methods appeared to be effective, they will also be incorporated into Samantha's intervention, which will be described in more detail later. It was evident during the evaluation that Samantha clearly understood the desired goal and many of the movements required. She had more difficulty with some of the movement components and needs to refine them to perform these tasks more accurately and efficiently. This indicates that for these tasks Samantha is not in the earliest stages of learning but is transitioning from early to later stages at the present time. Consequently, based on the specific postulates regarding change, feedback can begin to be focused on some of the movement performance rather than solely on the movement outcome. In ad-

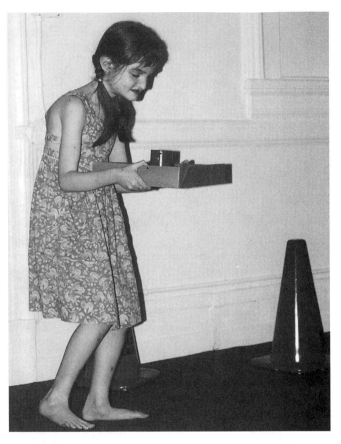

Figure 18.10 Carrying the lunch tray to a table.

dition, more detailed feedback can be given and Samantha can be encouraged to self-evaluate her own movement performance and outcome.

Goals and Objectives

Goal: Samantha will be able to accurately complete her required science projects in the classroom during the time allotted for these activities.

Objective: Samantha will be able to pour the correct amount of liquid into typically used containers without spilling given enhanced visual cues three out of four trials.

Objective: Samantha will be able to carry two objects simultaneously for setting up the workstation three out of four trials without spilling or dropping materials to improve her ability to complete the project in the allotted time.

Goal: Samantha will be able to manage her tray and food independently in the school lunchroom.

Objective: Samantha will be able to give her money to the cashier and receive change without dropping it while in the lunch line at least 3 out of 5 times per week.

Objective: Samantha will be able to open her utensil packet and juice container independently 100% of time.

Goal: Samantha will manage the luncheon routine so that she will be able to eat with other children in the cafeteria.

Objective: Samantha will be able to eat with the other children at the lunch table for at least 10 minutes (as a reflection of her improved speed and efficiency in managing her lunchroom routine).

INTERVENTION

It is important when applying the motor skill acquisition frame of reference to use the postulates regarding change to guide intervention. One general postulate states that if the child clearly understands the goal and what is to be achieved, then motor skill acquisition will be improved. By having Samantha identify the tasks that are both important and challenging for her and describe how she would like to be able to perform these tasks, it is more likely that she will be clear about the goals of intervention. It is also more likely that she will be engaged in tasks that are important, motivating, and challenging, which is another general postulate in this frame of reference.

A third general postulate states that if there is a match among the task requirements, environmental demands, and the child's capabilities, then it is more likely that motor skill acquisition will be improved. To more closely match the task requirements and environmental demands to Samantha's abilities, the team agreed on certain modifications to Samantha's school schedule and school-related tasks to allow her to fully participate in all educational and social activities with her classmates in the least restrictive environment. Samantha was allowed 10 extra minutes to finish assignments that were scheduled before having to climb stairs to go to the physical education class, art class, and lunchroom. This allowed her more time to do the assignments and prevented any possible falls or stress because of functioning in a crowded environment.

Samantha was also allowed to use a laptop computer and an audiotape recorder to take notes and do her assignments because of her difficulties with writing. However, she continued to work on her handwriting daily, with weekly monitoring from the occupational therapist related to writing speed, letter spacing, and alignment (Figure 18.11). She also was provided with a writing slant board positioned on her desk, which appeared to offer her a greater biomechanical and visual advantage when writing.

To ensure that Samantha was expected to perform tasks that were challenging but still within her capabilities, Samantha's teachers were asked to encourage her to fully participate with the other children in physical education class and when on the play-

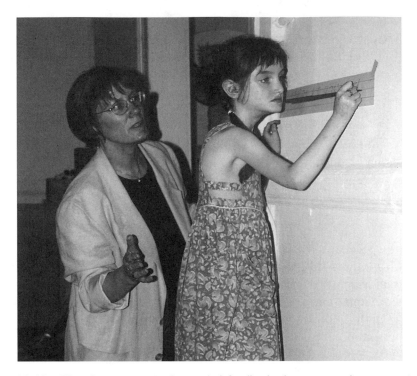

Figure 18.11 The therapist provides verbal feedback about grasp, letter spacing, and speed. Samantha is encouraged to self-evaluate her performance.

ground. If she was tired or felt uncomfortable with certain activities, she was allowed to freely move aside and return at will, without asking permission to do so. However, her teachers encouraged her to try new activities and reinforced her efforts, instead of her performance. However, for certain familiar activities, such as ball activities, she was encouraged to self evaluate her performance and generate different ways to improve her performance (Figure 18.12).

Although Samantha had trouble handling the bathroom door at school, it was also discovered that she was able to open other locked doors at home and in school. It was the weight of the school bathroom door and her decreased strength and bilateral coordination problems that limited her ability to open the bathroom door at school. It was decided that Samantha should be given the option of asking a classmate or teacher's assistant to assist her with this task because the bathroom door had to remain locked for security purposes. She was also encouraged to do as much as possible of this task when accompanied by a classmate or teacher's assistant. The occupational therapist additionally monitored her performance and provided feedback as needed on a weekly basis (Figure 18.13).

It is stated in this frame of reference that if practice and feedback in those areas occur in natural contexts and daily routines, then motor skill acquisition will be im-

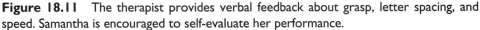

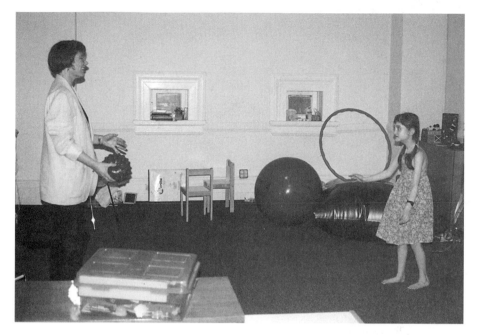

Figure 18.12 Therapist encourages Samantha to focus her attention on the ball and try a different strategy for using her arms to catch the ball.

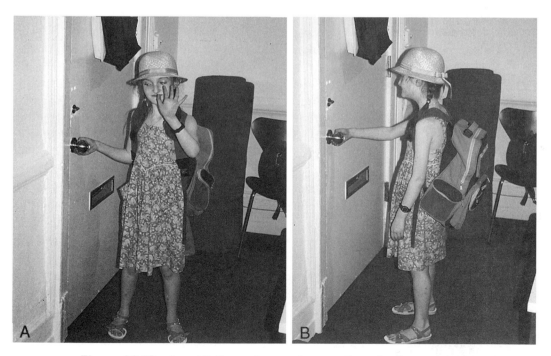

Figure 18.13 A and B, Samantha practices opening other heavy doors.

proved. Therefore, intervention will be given in the contexts in which the tasks naturally occur and at the time in which they naturally occur whenever possible. In addition, practice will include variability and unpredictability because most of the tasks selected are considered open tasks. Variability and unpredictability will be provided through the presence of other children moving about and being involved in the tasks and through the use of different task materials, positions, workstations, and contexts when practicing the selected tasks.

A randomized practice schedule will also be used because each occupational therapy session will include a variety of tasks. This may make it more likely that Samantha will be able to generalize some of the motor skills learned or refined in some of these tasks to others and that long-term retention will be improved.

Observation of task performance

The following two tasks, science project and lunchroom routine, will be described in more depth to illustrate the use of the motor skill acquisition frame of reference.

Science Project

The occupational therapist worked with Samantha in her classroom during science on a weekly basis. The therapist's role during this time was to provide feedback, suggest modifications to task materials and strategies, and encourage Samantha to practice certain motor skills to improve performance. Consistent with the postulates regarding change, she was also encouraged to practice doing the movement patterns needed to accomplish the science project and to self-evaluate her own performance. The focus was on performance; it was evident that Samantha understood all of the task requirements, but she was having difficulty with some of the movement components. The postulate regarding change, which is demonstrated here, states that in the later stages of learning, if the child is encouraged to self evaluate his or her own movement performance and outcome by focusing on inherent body and perceived environmental feedback, then it is more likely that motor skill performance will be improved.

When organizing her workstation for the science project, she was asked to first view all of the materials and then decide which objects, based on their inherent characteristics, could be managed in one hand, in each hand separately, or both hands simultaneously. Samantha was then encouraged to practice picking up two and sometimes three objects at a time (Figure 18.14).

She was told to fill up the measuring cup with water to the 1.5 cup mark and then asked to check her performance and self correct this until she was within one notch (ounce) of this marker. This strategy was also used for filling up the test tubes; however she was shown where to fill up the test tube and asked to mark this line with a red transparency pencil because of her difficulty visually discriminating the white measurement lines on the test tube.

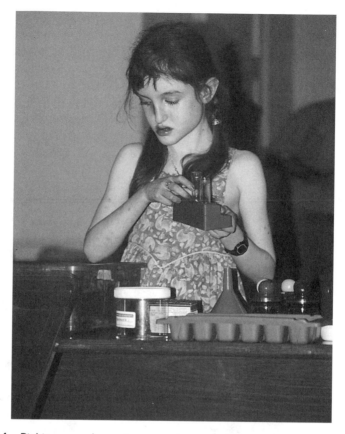

Figure 18.14   Picking up and carrying more than one object at a time to set up the activity.

Samantha was also given a limited amount of blocked practice (i.e., one task is practiced repeatedly before moving on to practice a different task) in using the eye dropper to put the correct number of droplets into the test tubes and petri dishes. She initially used a small bowl to practice this and was asked to evaluate each of her attempts. Once she acknowledged that she was having some difficulty emptying the correct number of droplets, she was given verbal feedback to squeeze the eye dropper with more or less pressure as needed and told to evaluate each attempt. When she was able to correctly place five droplets in a row, she was told to continue with the assigned experiment and to monitor her own performance (Figure 18.15). In this instance, blocked practice of a part of the whole task was used because Samantha had particular difficulty with this aspect of the project. However, this part of the project was not practiced in isolation of the whole because Samantha went on to complete the entire science project. This demonstrates the postulate regarding change that states, if the child practices whole tasks versus parts of tasks in isolation of the whole, then it is more likely that motor skill acquisition will be improved.

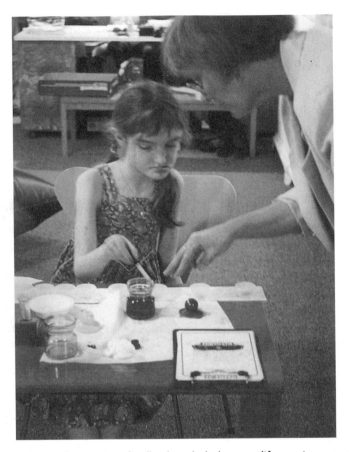

Figure 18.15 Samantha receives feedback to help her modify previous strategies during a practice session.

Completion of the experiment would result in the liquid in the test tubes both being the same color red and the contents of the three petri dishes having three different shades of blue. When Samantha was finished with the experiment, she was asked to compare her results with the teacher's results, which were presented on an adjacent workstation. She was able to make the comparisons for the test tubes but had some difficulty with the three petri dishes. Therefore, she was asked to place her petri dishes on a tray and carry and place the tray directly in front of the teacher's model to make this comparison easier. Samantha was able to see that although she closely approximated the teacher's results, she did not have three distinct shades of blue. However, with encouragement, she looked at her classmates' science projects and realized that her results were similar to theirs. Her teacher reconfirmed Samantha's assessment by providing verbal summary feedback about the general classroom performance and results at the end of the project (Figure 18.16).

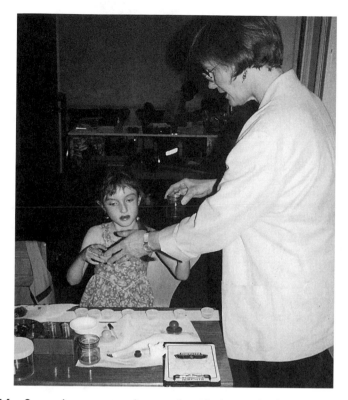

Figure 18.16 Samantha compares her result with the teacher's result to help her learn how to self-evaluate.

Samantha required additional time to complete the task because of the increased amount of practice and feedback given during this weekly occupational therapy session. However, her teacher, teacher's assistant, and some of her classmates were able to see how much Samantha was able to do on her own and the type of assistance that was necessary to improve her performance. Similar types of practice and feedback can be used with Samantha for other projects that require similar abilities. By working in the classroom, the occupational therapist was also able to assess what some of the other children were able and unable to do, provide feedback to them, and make recommendations when possible.

Samantha performed various science projects over several weeks of intervention. During this time, the conditions of practice were systematically varied by using different task materials (e.g., different size and shaped test tubes and containers, eye droppers, and liquids that had different amounts of resistance) and varied chairs and work surfaces. Less visual feedback was provided when measuring and pouring liquid. Less verbal feedback was given to regulate an adequate amount of pressure on the different eye droppers. She no longer required blocked practice to use the eye droppers accurately. Gradually fewer reminders and encouragement were given to self-evaluate her movement performance and outcome as she was able to do this on her own.

Lunchroom Routine

When receiving change from the cashier in the lunchroom, Samantha was given verbal and visual feedback to assist her with cupping her left hand and keeping it as horizontal as possible. She was encouraged to assess the characteristics of the change and retrieve what she thought she could manage and place it back into her pocket using her right (preferred) hand. She required three practice trials and a suggestion to organize what she retrieved by focusing on the coins first because these were placed on top of the bills. When it was apparent that she was having difficulty holding on to the bills, she was given verbal feedback to use her thumb more to stabilize them while continuing to cup her hand to maintain the change in her hand as well. Samantha had difficulty with this part of the lunchroom task even when additional feedback was provided, so she will continue to practice this weekly in her occupational therapy sessions. Samantha was also told that she could practice this on her own and ask the cashier to place the bills in her left hand and coins in her right hand to simplify the task for her. This demonstrates the postulate regarding change that states, if the child is encouraged to self evaluate his or her own movement performance and outcome by focusing on inherent body and perceived environmental feedback, then it is more likely that motor skill performance will be improved.

To make it easier to carry her tray back to the lunchroom table, Samantha was given verbal feedback to place all food items on the lunchtray so that the weight was evenly distributed. She was also asked to initially pick up the tray, practice at least two other ways to hold the tray, and then get a sense of which method was the most comfortable for her to carry the tray back to the table. She was reminded to say "excuse me" to the other children if they were in her way or got "too close for comfort" (Figure 18.17).

After a few unsuccessful attempts, Samantha was given verbal feedback to try a few different ways to open the packet of utensils. Additional evaluative information was obtained during this time. It was apparent that Samantha was using inadequate force and biomechanically disadvantageous positions to hold on to the packet. Additionally, she had difficulty coordinating opposing arm movements to tear it open. Her right (preferred) hand consistently generated more force than her left (non-preferred) hand. The therapist demonstrated to Samantha another way to hold the packet to assess if this would improve her performance. This position entailed holding the serrated edge of the packet using bilateral lateral pinch, stabilizing her left forearm against her trunk, and reminding her to squeeze hard with the left hand while she pulled the packet open away from her body with her right hand. She was asked to try this method and modify it on her own according to her own internal body and perceived feedback from objects in the environment. She was able to open

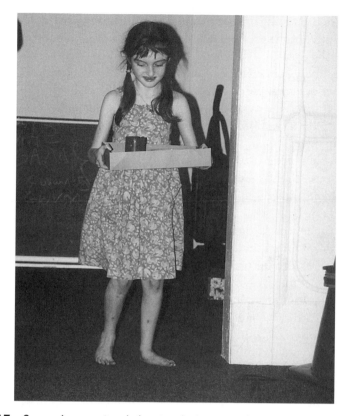

Figure 18.17 Samantha practices balancing the items on the tray and walking to her table.

the packet after eight attempts with ongoing verbal and visual feedback and manual guidance. The manual guidance was used to give her a sense of the varied gradations of pressure and force to use for opposing arm movements when tearing open the packet. This was provided by the occupational therapist placing her hands over Samantha's hands while demonstrating this bilateral "hold and move" pattern.

Similar strategies were used to assist Samantha with opening the juice container. However, Samantha still was unable to do the last step of this task and was becoming increasingly frustrated with the repeated unsuccessful attempts. Therefore, based on a discussion with the teacher and Samantha's parents, it was decided that the occupational therapist would monitor Samantha's performance of this task on a monthly basis. Samantha would also be given the option to practice this task on her own if she wanted or to ask the teacher's assistant or a classmate to help her when needed. From discussions with the teacher's assistants and observations of other children in the lunchroom, it became apparent that many other, often younger, children were also having difficulty opening this type of container. The occupational therapist and two teachers informed the principal and lunchroom manager about this and suggested ordering drink containers that these students would be able to open independently. Samantha's parents also identified a number of juice containers that Samantha was able to manage at home. A list of these and other brands were given to the lunchroom manager, who assured everyone concerned that she would begin to order one or a few of these other brands.

Over several occupational therapy sessions, Samantha was gradually given less visual and verbal feedback as she improved in her ability to maintain the change in her right hand by cupping her hand and keeping it horizontally positioned. She continued to have difficulty stabilizing the bills with her thumb, but she consistently was able to use the suggested strategy of asking the cashier to place the change in her right hand and bills in her left hand.

After two sessions, Samantha spontaneously distributed the weight of the food items on her tray without verbal feedback to do so. Consequently, she more quickly and easily carried the tray back to the lunch room table with less associated facial movements demonstrated. However, she still required occasional reminders to say "excuse me" to her classmates when they were in her way. As movement in the lunchroom is always changing, this is an open task. This demonstrates the use of the postulate regarding change stating: for open tasks, if the child is provided with variability and unpredictability during practice, then it is more likely that motor skill acquisition will be improved for open tasks.

Samantha continued to need manual guidance for two additional sessions to open the utensil packet. After these sessions, she only required visual feedback to position her hands in the biomechanically advantageous position described earlier. Verbal feedback was provided by telling Samantha to "squeeze harder" with her left hand while tearing open the utensil packet. Finally after 2 months of weekly sessions, Samantha was able to open the utensil packet after three attempts without feedback. However, she continued to require more time than her classmates to perform this task.

SUMMARY

This case study demonstrated the use of the motor skill acquisition frame of reference for Samantha. Samantha had a variety of abilities and difficulties that supported or limited task performance. It is believed that with additional practice and feedback, the time to complete the above-identified tasks should decrease as Samantha's motor skill acquisition improves and becomes more automatic or requires less conscious thinking and self-evaluation. This will allow her more time to socialize with her classmates and do the extracurricular activities that she desires. In addition, by continuing to use activities relevant to her context and curriculum, it is believed that Samantha will improve in other tasks that are important to her.

STUDY QUESTIONS

1. Why was the motor skill acquisition frame of reference selected for Samantha?

2. What other frames of reference could have been used? And why?

3. What are some other contexts where Samantha can practice similar tasks as described above?

4. Using the motor skill acquisition frame of reference, what are some other ways to address Samantha's performance of the above listed tasks?

5. Describe how you would address some of the other tasks with which Samantha had difficulty.

6. How may have the evaluation and intervention process been different if the child described in this case study had more severe cognitive impairment or more severe physical impairment?

Acknowledgments

The authors thank Samantha and her parents for allowing her inclusion in this case study; Drs. Ginsburg and Myers for providing critical information about Samantha and Dysautonomia; Paula McCreedy, MA, OT, for welcoming us in her private practice to photograph Samantha; Trish Rosen, Doctoral Candidate in the Department of Anthropology, NYU, and Dr. Faye Ginsburg for taking the photographs used in this chapter.

For further information about dysautonomia contact:
The National Dysautonomia Research Foundation
P.O. Box 21153
Eagan, MN 55121-2553
http://www.nrdf.org/

Dysautonomia Treatment and Evaluation Center
New York University Medical Center
Arnold and Marie Schwartz Health Care Center
400 East 34th St., Suite 3A
New York, NY 10016
http://www.med.nyu.edu/fd/

or

Felicia Axelrod, MD
Professor, Departments of Pediatrics and Neurology
Director of the Dysautonomia Treatment and Evaluation Center
Fax: 212-263-7041
E mail: Felicia.Axelrod@mcccm.med.nyu.edu

Case Study: Biomechanical Frame of Reference

CHERYL ANN COLANGELO

BACKGROUND

Travis is a 5-year-old boy of normal intelligence with cerebral palsy resulting in athetosis. He has documented needs in the areas of gross and fine motor development and self-care skills. He has entered kindergarten in an inclusive classroom. Occupational therapy services were requested to help Travis participate in the school program and to assure that those experiences available to his typical classmates would also be made available to him.

Home Setting

Travis lives in a middle class suburban neighborhood with two working parents and an older sister. He is cared for after school by a babysitter who is very involved in his therapeutic program. He receives home-based physical therapy twice weekly in addition to school-based services in occupational therapy.

Schooling

School medical records are abbreviated; only salient features relevant to Travis' current health management are available. Travis was born prematurely; he has a seizure disorder that has been successfully managed with medication. He has frequent, but not severe, upper respiratory infections. Other than that, he is in good health.

Travis received home-based therapy services between the ages of 9 months and 2½ years. He then attended a full day preschool program for children with special needs and received occupational therapy, physical therapy, and speech therapy thrice weekly. His parents were actively involved in his therapeutic program and received, by their report, a good deal of support and instruction in the area of home and family management. Treatment in the preschool was based on the NeuroDevelopmental Treatment (NDT) and Biomechanical frames of reference. In the spring before Travis entered kindergarten, he visited his new school with his preschool therapists to meet his kindergarten teacher. At this time, the history of Travis' treatment and adapted equipment program was shared and plans for his academic year were discussed.

The transition to kindergarten represented a change from a special needs community to that of a typical classroom where Travis would be the only child with a physical disability. The current K-5 population, as well as teachers, at this new school had never been exposed to a schoolmate in a wheelchair. Travis' parents' current concerns were that he 1) become an active, accepted member of the preschool community and 2) be provided and trained with whatever adaptations would be necessary to allow him to engage in the academic curriculum.

OCCUPATIONAL THERAPY EVALUATION

Intervention history and setting play an important role in determining what needs should be addressed, how occupational therapy services should be delivered, and which frames of reference are most appropriate. In Travis' case, where there is a transition from one setting or program to another, these factors take on increased significance.

Potential for Change in the Area of Postural Reactions

Travis has participated in direct and intensive therapy services for 4 years. He is young, has likely potential for change, and is considered to have strong cognitive skills. The therapist can expect some qualitative changes in postural skills, but this is a good time to begin the shift from an emphasis on quality of movement toward functional skills, with external supports to substitute for inadequate postural control, and more cognitive attention to executing movement. For example, rather than relying on inadequate postural responses to vestibular and proprioceptive input, Travis may learn to consciously check his body position and use his arms or external supports to realign himself before engaging in an activity. It should be remembered that for children with central nervous system dysfunction, optimal development and competence lies somewhere in the middle of the continuum of quality of movement and function with support.

Environment

The delivery of occupational therapy services is determined in part by the needs and philosophy of the providing agency. The educational system has several options for providing services to children with multiple disabilities, and priorities vary depending on the option. Many schools provide, or contract for, special classes that are restricted to children with moderate and severe disabilities. Here, sensory motor development and controlled mobility are high priorities; therapy services are intensive and time and facilities are available to address component skills. On the other end of the continuum, children with disabilities may be included in the regular classroom, where academic achievement and community participation are priorities. In this situation, the occupational therapist addresses performance skills, helping the student to maximize participation in academic activities and minimizing time out of the classroom for therapy. Each school district determines how therapy services will be delivered and how needs are addressed by their definition of scope of practice and by the time, staff, and space allotted for therapy. School-based practice often restricts the ability to address component skills in a clinical fashion but provides the therapist with a rich environment to promote change through interaction with teachers, other students, and the community. When appropriate, home-based or clinic-based therapy may be recommended to address areas such as quality of movement or home management, but these services are not the responsibility of the school district.

In Travis' case, his needs were assessed in the context of the inclusive classroom; high value was placed on classroom participation and performance skills. This was a good match for the biomechanical frame of reference. An equipment program to provide external support to *substitute* for inadequate postural mechanisms and to enhance functions (such as head control for visual attention and the ability to maintain and control hand position) would require a low level of intrusion of the therapist and fewer therapeutic demands in the classroom. In addition, Travis' history of 4 years of intensive therapy assured that the development of component motor skills had been addressed dynamically, and home-based physical therapy continued to address these.

Another aspect of the environment or context to consider is the population that comprises Travis' community of peers. Travis came from an environment in which his needs for assistance were equal to the needs of his classmates, and he was one of the most intelligent children. Adults in the program were aware of his skills and were able to place appropriate demands on him. His most significant social and verbal interactions took place with adults.

It is important to compare the perception of Travis as seen by people who are familiar with children with disabilities to those of members of his new community. His therapist must be able to see him from a point of view that has expanded beyond the clinic.

Travis is a slender, attractive boy who is alert and socially responsive. He has a moderate degree of athetosis, so that self-initiated movement is accomplished by extraneous distal movement, and control of limbs and head in mid-ranges is poor. He can sustain eye contact well when listening but poorly when speaking because of extraneous head and neck movements accompanying the effort of producing sound.

When engaged in conversation, Travis demonstrates a vocabulary that is startling in its sophistication. However, speech intelligibility is moderately impaired because of poor oral-motor control, and speech volume is low because of inadequate coordination between respiration and speech mechanisms. When with adults, he is animated and socially appropriate. Travis shows a wide range of emotions and initiates discussions regarding his physical and emotional concerns. Travis can sit independently, but he requires external support to use his hands. Hand function is very limited. He creeps independently. He is dependent in self-care and cannot propel his manual wheelchair.

This is how Travis's schoolmates, as well as many adults, perceive him: He waves his arms and shakes his body. He makes faces and baby noises. He needs to be fed and taken to the bathroom. He smiles and is happy. He doesn't fight with other children—he is nice. He likes to be helped.

Travis' schoolmates are universally solicitous of him. They anticipate his needs and incorporate him into play by placing games and toys before him and moving pieces for him. They speak to him as if he were a young sibling, rarely asking him questions that require more than a "yes" or "no" answer. They tend to avoid sharing age-appropriate anecdotes (e.g., discussion of a favorite movie) with him. Travis' teacher is concerned that he does not initiate interaction with his peers.

Travis current physical status is not likely to change dramatically, but his role and participation in his new environment can be developed.

Functional Posture and Mobility

Using the biomechanical frame of reference, the following areas are assessed in relation to school participation and performance.

Range of Motion

Travis has full active range of motion but inadequate control of mid-ranges in all extremities. He stabilizes himself by using movement at the end-ranges of joint movement. The implications of this will be discussed in the following sections.

Control of Head in the Righted Position

At rest, Travis can hold his head in a righted position when seated. He cannot sustain this when attempting to control his mouth or limbs. Thus, he cannot sustain eye contact when speaking and has difficulty looking at paperwork while he points to an answer or looking where he is going when walking with support.

Control of Trunk in an Upright Position

Travis can bench sit with his feet on the floor for up to 15 minutes, if he does not need to speak or use his hands. He seeks stability by adducting his legs. He is unable to sustain his hips in abduction with external rotation for ring sitting on the floor.

When long sitting, he has a posterior pelvic tilt with compensatory rounding of his back and neck hyperextension. His arms are not liberated for movement. Trunk control is best when he has a wide base of support, so he is most functional in a "w" sitting position, with hips in end-ranges of adduction and internal rotation (a pattern that impacts negatively on ambulation skills).

In bench sitting or floor sitting, the initiation of speaking or arm movements disrupts the symmetry of Travis's trunk because the associated large, uncontrolled movements of head and arms disrupt his balance (these peripheral movements create a shift in his center of gravity, to which he has ungraded equilibrium responses).

Control of Shoulder and Arms for Positioning Hand in Space

When sitting at rest, Travis often holds his shoulders in an elevated and retracted position to help support his head and upper trunk. When seeking more postural support, he locks his elbows into extension and props himself with fists resting on thighs; in this case, there is a pattern of adduction with internal rotation in shoulders and hips.

When reaching, given no support surface for his arms, Travis locks his elbows into extension to reduce degrees of freedom of movement because accuracy of hand placement decreases as the number of joints moving with poor control increases. His hands are directed from the shoulders, which move in wide arcs because of poor midrange control. To bring his hands closer to midline, Travis adducts and internally rotates his shoulders and flexes his elbows, stabilizing both hands against his chest.

Travis' grasp is gross and cylindrical; smaller objects are raked up and held where they fall in his hand between adducted fingers. Grasp is accompanied by flexion and ulnar deviation of the wrist. It is difficult for him to stabilize his arm for grasping; he often picks objects up as he is swiping. He cannot sustain his hand in one position in space to release an object on a target spot. Travis has minimal control for drawing and handling puzzles and classroom manipulatives, action figures, or animals for imaginative play.

Ability to Move Through Space

Travis' independent mobility is accomplished by creeping. This is done with his head down, although he can lift it intermittently to visually direct himself. He creeps with arms abducted, elbows extended, and hands fisted. Hips are widely abducted, flexed more than 90°, and unstable. He cannot coordinate movement of all four limbs, and often, rather than weight shifting laterally, he weight shifts posteriorly, bringing both hands up off the floor and forward together. This is functional only for short distances in the classroom because of time and energy expenditure. Although it is socially acceptable in the context of the kindergarten classroom, it is not an appropriate means of locomotion in other parts of the school.

Travis walks slowly if given support by an adult at the level of his rib cage or if he is allowed to grasp an adult's hands held over his head. When grasping an adult's hands above his head, he exercises little postural control; rather, he hangs by his arms while he makes stepping movements. Given trunk support, Travis uses exaggerated lateral flexion of the neck and trunk to initiate weight shift for stepping; this interferes with his ability to maintain a righted head and visual attention to where he is going. Travis walks with adducted legs, providing him with a narrow base of support. When the ball of his foot contacts the floor, he responds with a stepping reaction of immediate hip and knee flexion, so there is little time to regain stability between steps.

Travis cannot sustain a constant arm position to support himself independently with a walker or rollator (Figure 19.1). Although he can maintain grasp on the handles, he unintentionally pushes, pulls, and lifts the walker as his body weight shifts.

In the manual wheelchair, Travis cannot place and maintain his hands on the wheels long enough for effective self-propulsion.

Ability to Engage in Self-Care

Travis can finger feed hard items such as pretzels and cookies. Softer foods are crushed in his grasp. He gets his hand to his mouth by bracing his hands against his chest and bringing his head down to his hands and also by retracting and extending his shoulder with elbow flexed so that his hand is by his cheek and turning his head

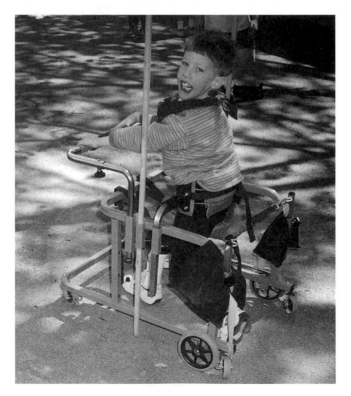

Figure 19.1 Walker.

to it (he gets stability in this end-range of shoulder movement). Travis cannot use utensils or control the flow of liquid from a cup into his mouth. He can suck liquids through a straw, but he bites on the straw for stability and creates negative pressure in his mouth by using his tongue against his palate rather than coordinating movements of lips, cheeks, tongue, and jaw. His suck pattern reinforces pathologic oral-motor movements, which interfere with effective eating and articulation.

Travis cannot sit on a toilet independently. He cannot maintain his hips at 90° flexion, so his legs adduct and he falls through the hole in the toilet seat. Sometimes he overcompensates by extending his hips, but this throws his trunk backward. He cannot stand at the urinal without assistance.

Ability to Access Switches for Technology Aids

When Travis reaches for any switch, his movements are circumductive, reaching around rather than reaching directly. Thus, prolonged time is needed for approaching and contacting the switch. He can sustain contact with a large switch plate with his hand in a fisted position (this position helps him stabilize his wrist). He approaches a keyboard with fingers extended, using his thumb to make contact. His wrist is generally flexed and ulnarly deviated. Contact with a given key is successful 25% of the time. He is unable to control a mouse.

Travis grasps a joystick with his wrist flexed and deviated. To position his hand with this wrist position, his arm is abducted with elbow flexed. Thus, he is unable to stabilize his arm against his body for added stability. Because Travis tends to seek stability distally (at the point of his hands), any shifts in trunk position create unwanted movement at the joystick.

Goals

In summary, the following are long-range goals established for the educational setting by the team of family, school staff, and therapists. These can be addressed to a significant extent, but not exclusively, by the biomechanical frame of reference. Needless to say, Travis may have other needs that are within the scope of occupational therapy but could not be addressed through this frame of reference.

1. Provide equipment to develop postural control during classroom activities.
2. Provide means for independent, appropriate movement through space.
3. Provide equipment and support that facilitate initiation of social interaction with peers.
4. Provide proper positioning and adaptations to increase participation in writing, art, and construction activities.
5. Provide positioning and adaptive equipment to increase independence in self-feeding.
6. Provide positioning and adaptive equipment to increase independence in toileting.

INTERVENTION

Often, when the biomechanical frame of reference is used, a variety of positioning devices are made available to address different goals. The appropriateness of these devices to the environment is an important consideration; what is acceptable in a hospital or special program may be intrusive or unmanageable in a public school. In Travis' case, his equipment is somewhat representative of him; it comprises a part of his introduction to the community. Cosmetics, manageability (i.e., size and weight), and the number of devices used should be considered as they effect the staff's ability to incorporate them into the daily routine. Teachers, students, and parents of those students should understand the purpose of this new equipment so that it is not alienating.

Regardless of how effective any device appears to the therapist, the ultimate use and efficacy remains with the classroom student and the teacher involved. Ongoing communication about how it may best be incorporated into the day, problems or potential problems it presents, and how the device may be modified to better suit its use in school is an essential component of the treatment program.

In the following, Travis' goals are identified in terms of his needs in school and discussed in terms of biomechanical considerations.

Postural Control in the Classroom (Central Stability; the Ability to Maintain Head and Trunk in a Righted Position)

Travis' most stable position was sitting with hips and knees at 90° flexion, using a seat belt at a 45° angle to stabilize the pelvis and maintain weight bearing on the ischial tuberosities. Without the belt, his very mobile pelvis would tilt posteriorly and he would lose the ability to regain a neutral position once his body weight was centered over the base of his spine. With his pelvis stabilized and feet strapped, the hip adduction Travis used to seek stability was no longer necessary, thus there was no need for an abductor. Travis needed his seating unit tipped back *very* slightly, just enough so that he could rest his head on the high seat back. Lateral head supports and trunk supports helped to decrease extraneous or compensatory movements in the lateral planes. The head supports allowed for some movement for visual scanning but provided enough support to assist with sustained visual attention.

Travis' wheelchair was handsome and racy looking; his classmates were honored by the role of friend and helper when selected to push Travis (accompanied by an adult aide) to "special classes" (i.e., art, music, etc.). The chair fit up to the tables in the classroom. However, the fit was not ideal. The seat back was slightly reclined, but the seat was parallel to the floor, opening the hip angle and encouraging a posterior pelvic tip. In addition, the seat belt (which was properly positioned at a 45° angle to the hips) had a large metal buckle, the top of which forced the top of the pelvis back and fixed it in a posterior tilt. As a result, Travis sat on the base of his spine rather than on his ischial tuberosities and compensated with a rounded back, decreasing his postural stability and requiring neck hyperextension for head righting.

By placing a wedge under his thighs and raising the footrests proportionately to support his feet, the slight recline was maintained and correct hip angle was recovered. The belt buckle was moved from the center to the side; this was slightly less convenient for caretakers but it eliminated the pressure that tilted the pelvis posteriorly.

Many kindergarten activities occur with the students sitting or playing on the floor. These include teacher presentations, sharing time, "reading partners" activities with older students, and large construction activities.

Travis and his teacher felt that, during sedentary floor time (i.e., calendar, weather, story time), he should be relaxed and supported with minimal postural demands being made. A commercially available floor sitter was provided, which consisted of a corner back (two upright pieces joined at a 90° angle), a deep seat with seat belt, and an abduction wedge. The corner provided lateral trunk support but encouraged rounding of the back. The seat belt was not used because it prevented independent transfers. Travis lounged comfortably in this device, sitting on the base of his spine in a semi-reclined position, bracing his perineum against the abduction wedge. Although his therapists winced at his posture, the seat was comfortable, practical for transfers, and functional for relaxed participation in listening activities. It offered more support than a beanbag chair or leaning against the wall. This was the one time during Travis' school day that Travis was free of postural demands. The bright blue floor sitter, when not used by Travis, was shared with his classmates and incorporated into their imaginative play, sometimes as a spaceship or eighteen wheeler (Figure 19.2).

During active, mobile times (i.e., construction, imaginary play) Travis could move about by creeping and transitioned independently from quadruped to "w" sitting. There was concern regarding his hip position in "w" sitting but using a floor sitter during this type of activity would restrict Travis' interactive play. The best compromise was to remove Travis' ankle-foot orthoses at this time; with the ability to plantar flex his ankles, Travis was able to sit on his heels, rather than between them, for brief periods of time.

Independent, Appropriate Mobility Through Space (Ability to Move Through Space; Ability to Access Switch for Technological Aid)

Although Travis could make his way around the classroom by creeping during floor play, this was an ineffective, unsafe, and inappropriate modality for movement around the school. Use of a scooter board, while it would have contributed to the development of component skills of head control and shoulder stability, was also inappropriate for use in hallways crowded with 5- to 10-year-old children. Supported walking and powered mobility were viable alternatives.

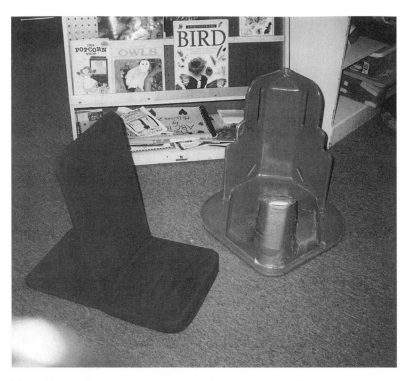

Figure 19.2 Either floor seat provides comfort and support for group listening activities but does not provide optimal positioning for speech production or hand function.

Ambulation with a walker is a long-term goal addressed by the physical therapy program at home. A modified rollator was provided for mobility at school, which made less demands on postural control and upper extremity support. It included Travis' pelvis, holding it in place even if his legs collapsed momentarily. Although there was a bar for him to hold on to, its use was not critical in supporting his body or directing the rollator, which moved in the direction that Travis' hips faced. With this external support, Travis could concentrate on sustaining visual attention to the environment and practicing controlled stepping movements. With this device (under the supervision of an aide) Travis could direct his movement through space and take opportunities to visit or peek into other rooms along the hallways. The rollator had a detachable saddle that could provide full body support when both feet were off the ground (Figure 19.3). With it, Travis could participate in recess activities, such as chasing other children and kickball, by sitting in the saddle and propelling forward with his feet.

Travis had the cognitive ability and maturity to responsibly use a powered wheelchair. His parents ordered this through a clinic, which outfitted the chair to provide the support described in the previous section. The following adaptions were provided to help Travis develop control of the joystick: A harness that limited anterior

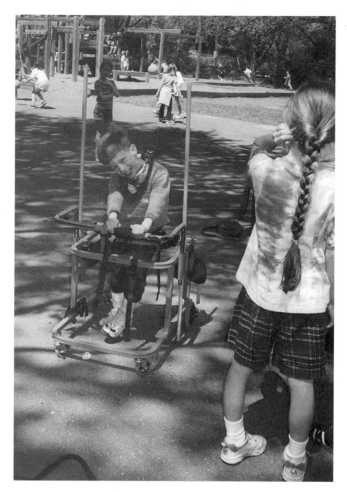

Figure 19.3   Use of the supportive saddle-seat allows the student to "run" on the playground with his friends.

and posterior movement of the upper trunk, which decreased distal movements of the arm controlling the joystick. Humeral wings were built into a lap tray to prevent large movements in the directions of shoulder retraction and abduction, keeping the arms toward the midline. The lap tray itself provided a support surface for the forearms. Travis' "sweet spot" was located where his hand rested when his shoulder was flexed forward (passively, by the humeral wing) and his elbow was extended but not locked. In order to keep Travis' forearm resting on the lap tray, the joystick (which was accessible through a hole in the lap tray) was lowered slightly. In this way, Travis did not have to extend his wrist to keep his hand on the joystick while his forearm maintained contact with the lap tray; his wrist passively fell into a neutral position when his hand rested on the joystick, and gravity helped to keep his hand in place.

The joystick mechanism was equipped with a dampening device so that it did not respond to small, extraneous movements of the arm or hand.

Social Interaction (Ability to Move Through Space; Ability to Access Technology Aids)

It was difficult for Travis' schoolmates to recognize his areas of competence because of his physical dependence and impaired articulation. In the hallways, students tended to address questions about Travis to his aides or the classmate who was pushing his wheelchair. Travis rarely responded to these overtures, being aware that students interpreted his poor articulation as inability to use language. To complicate this, Travis could often not be heard in the noisy hallways or cafeteria because of his low volume.

"Touring" in his rollator gave Travis an opportunity to take charge of his own mobility, engage in exploration, and demonstrate his competence to his peers. Although he did not initiate conversation, he approached groups of students to examine their activity and interaction. His aide redirected questions from students to Travis and "translated" by repeating Travis' words when necessary. Travis' directed mobility, and the sophistication of his verbal responses elicited new respect for him. To assist in verbal communication, Travis' speech therapist provided him with an amplifying device that he wore as a headphone. The headgear required modification so that it would stay on his head despite the excessive mobility of his head, neck, and shoulders. The rollator, with saddle, was also used to allow Travis to participate in the ice-skating outings that were part of the physical education program.

Another modality that provided Travis with the opportunity to demonstrate his competence and engage socially was the computer. Travis knew letters and their sounds as well as his classmates and understood the concepts presented in classroom software. Travis used the Intellekeys-enlarged keyboard, with arrow keys to engage the mouse. Successful access to this keyboard was facilitated by the following: the keyboard was set into a lap tray with an easel (attached to his wheelchair) so that the keyboard was flush with the easel surface (Figure 19.4). This allowed Travis to maintain his forearm on the support surface, despite lack of wrist extension. The angle of the easel encouraged an upright position of his head and neck. Humeral wings attached to the lap tray provided additional stability and limited extraneous movement of the shoulders and arms. A small ring splint extended the PIP joint of the index finger, helping Travis isolate that finger for depressing the keys. Use of this finger rather than his thumb prevented the posturing of forearm pronation with elbow flexion and shoulder internal rotation and abduction—the movement pattern that brought his arm away from his trunk and up off the support surface.

Travis was able to engage with his classmates using software for games and academic work because Intellekeys can be used with another keyboard simultaneously.

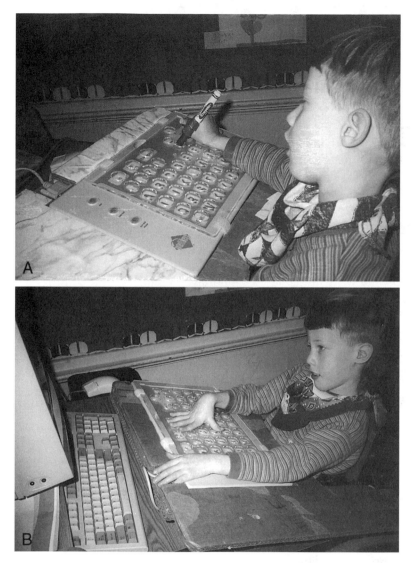

Figure 19.4 A and B, Student using recessed keyboard on easel with keyguard. Adapted marker-holder facilitates wrist extension and substitutes for lack of finger isolation.

Participation in Writing and Art and Construction Activities (Ability to Place and Sustain Hands in Desired Position)

When presented with these activities, Travis has two options for positioning. He can pull his wheelchair directly to the table with his peers, or he can use a lap tray with his wheelchair. When he pulls his wheelchair to the table, he has more proximity to his classmates and the center of activity. More external support and an increased control with a stable, fixed working surface is provided when he uses the lap tray, but the lap tray provides a barrier between Travis and his peers. Both options were used at the discretion of Travis and his teachers.

Travis could not keep his arms on the tabletop, which was a disadvantage; his arms kept sliding back when his shoulders moved into retraction with humeral extension. The lap tray wrapped around his trunk so that forearm support was available on the sides and the front of his body. Humeral wings provided further humeral stability and prevented unwanted ranges of shoulder movement. A harness was used during particularly demanding tasks but was disengaged at other times to allow Travis to play with some trunk mobility and control.

Travis engaged in two types of writing and drawing activities. One was creative expression, where color and movement were priorities and accuracy was not. This was done at the table with his classmates. Travis also wanted to learn to draw shapes and letters; this required greater control. Although Travis was not likely to be a functional writer and even though he was effective with keyboarding, the ability to form letters and write his name was important to him. To best control the formation of lines for shapes and letters, Travis used a lap tray with an easel to encourage head righting and support his arms. Also, a splint was applied to the ulnar border of his wrist to stabilize it in a neutral position so that flexion and ulnar deviation would not lever his forearm up off the support surface. Having first tried a writing splint that positioned the marker between his thumb and first two fingers, Travis chose to hold the marker independently between his index and long fingers.

With external support, Travis learned more effectively to exercise conscious control of arm and hand movements within limited range of movement. He also learned that, during bilateral activities, he could stabilize one arm against the supports rather than try to control both arms in space simultaneously.

Self-feeding

Travis' grasp on finger foods lacks smooth, coordinated control, and he lacked forearm control for accurate placement of food in his mouth. He was in danger of spearing his face with a fork and could not keep a spoon level to avoid spilling. When eating, Travis' needs for postural support were maximal because of demands placed on his hands and mouth and also because of the noise and activity level in the cafeteria. To move Travis to a quieter place for lunchtime, despite the benefits to motor control, would be counterproductive to the goals of inclusion. Component oral-motor and manipulative skills could be addressed in occupational and speech therapy pullout sessions. During lunchtime, motor demands needed to be decreased and postural supports increased. Travis used his wheelchair with head and trunk supports, a harness, and adapted lap tray.

The first approach to self-feeding incorporated a sandwich holder. This eliminated the need for the forearm and wrist control necessary to scoop or spear and bring a utensil to his mouth. Travis worked on stabilizing his arm against the humeral wing, keeping his elbow on the lap tray and using isolated elbow flexion to bring the sandwich holder toward his mouth. Maintaining forearm position in mid-position during this process so that the right end of the holder faced his mouth was dependent on Travis' conscious control. When the sandwich was within a few inches of his head, Travis braced his arm and brought his mouth to the sandwich. This avoided mishaps that may occur if his hand jerked on the way to his mouth. Managing the sandwich holder was a precursor to controlling a fork in the same manner.

The issue of cup-versus-straw drinking presented a dilemma. Travis could drink independently using a straw, but his method reinforced the oral-motor pathology that contributed to impaired articulation. The team chose a more dependent option for drinking at lunchtime because speech intelligibility was so critical to the inclusion process. Travis's aide helped him to drink from a cup, while better patterns of sucking from a straw were addressed during therapy.

Increased Independence in Toileting

A smaller ring was snapped into the toilet seat to provide greater thigh support and to prevent Travis from falling in. Horizontal bars were attached to the sides of the toilet for two purposes. First, Travis needed to hold onto them when sitting for trunk support and to pull himself forward so that his pelvis was tipped anteriorly for relaxation and proper direction of the flow of urine. Second, Travis began to learn to stand, bracing his thighs against the toilet and holding on to the bars (Figure 19.5).

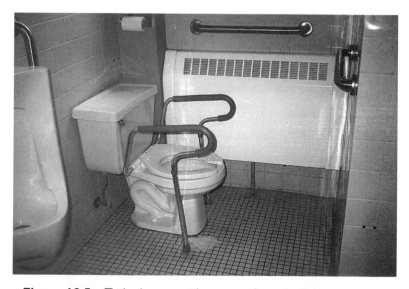

Figure 19.5 Toilet bars provide support for independent standing.

Standing provided greater potential for toileting independence because there was less need for clothing removal and the transfer from wheelchair to standing was easier than from wheelchair to sitting (especially with lowered pants). Bars were also attached to adjacent walls to assist with transfers.

SUMMARY

Priorities for Travis' first year in an inclusive school program were to help him adjust to the new environment, introduce him as an individual to the community, and help the school staff be comfortable and competent with his physical management. By the end of his kindergarten year, he was accepted as an intelligent student and social peer of his classmates. He had opportunities to interact with them, and they developed an appreciation for who he was and what he had to offer. Travis had mastered control of mobility and communication devices (i.e., power chair, keyboard, amplifier). He continued, with school staff and therapists, to work on the elements of active control necessary for self-feeding, toileting, and increased manipulative skills.

Future therapy services would need to maintain or modify his positioning program, respond to new management needs as classroom and curriculum changed, and address the dynamic motor patterns necessary for accomplishments identified by Travis as important to him.

STUDY QUESTIONS

1. Why is the biomechanical frame of reference used with Travis at this time?
2. What additional equipment may be helpful for Travis in his home environment?
3. What other frames of reference may be used in occupational therapy intervention with Travis?

Acknowledgments

The author wishes to thank the child shown in this chapter and his parents for allowing him to be photographed. This case study is not based on the child pictured.

Case Study: Combined Sensory Integration and NeuroDevelopmental Treatment Frames of Reference

CHANIE PRUZANSKY/KAY FARRINGTON

BACKGROUND

Judith was 11 months old when she was brought for evaluation because of delayed motor development and delayed fine motor skills. Primary complaints were difficulty with reaching and inability to transfer objects from one hand to the other.

Judith is the third and youngest child of an intact middle class family residing in a small two story private home in New York with a small grassy back yard with a tree and swings. Her 4½-year-old brother is in kindergarten, and her 3-year-old sister is in nursery school.

Judith was born at 38 weeks' gestation, secondary to maternal hypertension and toxemia. Her birth weight was 6 lbs, 2 oz. Judith has a history of chronic ear infections and had tubes inserted into her ears (myringotomy) at 8 months of age. Overall, she appears to be in generally good health.

Judith appeared to be a content, placid infant with an easy-going temperament. She tolerated handling well, except for extreme distress when placed in the quadruped position and on the therapy ball. Judith exhibited a wide base of support in prone and supported sitting positions. When placed in prone, she supported herself on her upper extremities with extended elbows and maintained her lower extremities in a flexed, frog leg posture. She became distressed within a short time in this position. She also became very distressed and arched her back in a supported quadruped position over the examiners knee. When placed in sitting, she was unable to extend her lower spine for erect posture.

Occupational therapy frames of reference chosen to address Judith's deficits were the Sensory Integration and NeuroDevelopmental Treatment frames of reference used in alternating sequence in each session. The NeuroDevelopmental Treatment frame of reference was used because of Judith's problems with postural tone and her lack of balance between stability and mobility. The Sensory Integration frame of reference was chosen because sensory integration is critical to treating deficits in the nervous system before other issues can be addressed.

Evaluation Based on the NeuroDevelopmental Treatment Frame of Reference

An evaluation using the NeuroDevelopmental Treatment frame of reference was used because of Judith's need for a wide base of support, her deficits in cocontraction, and her overall delayed motor development.

Postural Tone. Judith presented with generalized low postural tone with a wide base of support in prone and other positions. Patterns of fixation were present in the lower extremities, including knee hyperextension, toe clawing, and crossing of the ankles. Upper extremity positions of fixation, hand fisting, and shoulder elevation were observed especially when challenged motorically.

Righting and Equilibrium Reactions as They Relate to Postural Alignment. When in supine position with her head held off a stable surface, Judith did not tuck her chin against gravity (Figure 20.1). She did not display protective extension when tested in prone.

Stability and Mobility (Gross Motor Skills). Judith lacked stability; she avoided shifting weight and was very fearful of moving from one position to another. Her base of support appeared compromised because of her aversion to placing her feet

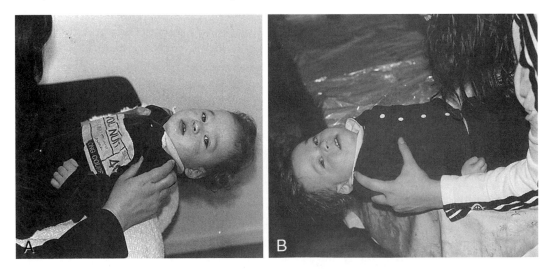

Figure 20.1 A and B, Chin tuck mature and immature response.

on a surface to bear weight. She appeared to use a static sitting posture as a result of trunk instability.

Stability and Mobility (Fine Motor Skills). Judith exhibited a high guard position in sitting, which contributed to delay of fine motor skills. She was able to place her index finger in the hole of a peg board, which indicated the beginning of finger isolation skills. She picked up small objects by using a raking pattern. She was able to hold a block in each hand and attempted to pick up a third block by holding it between the two blocks in her fists. She removed a peg from the pegboard and crumpled paper with both hands. She pulled the string of a pull toy.

Dissociation. Judith lacked dissociation in her lower extremities when she pulled up to stand. She avoided shifting her weight to one hip when kneeling or performed an inadequate shift and pivoted up on both feet almost at the same time (instead of half kneeling).

Variety of Movement. Judith's movement repertoire was very limited. Stereotypic postures in shoulder elevation and hand fisting were present at times. Furthermore, her fear and anxiety about changing positions and lack of trunk rotation limited her movement possibilities. She tended to be very static with a paucity of gross motor movement.

Range of Motion (ROM). Judith's patterns of fixation were temporary and did not impede ROM.

Evaluation Based on the Sensory Integrative Frame of Reference

An evaluation using the sensory integration frame of reference was used based on Judith's apparent sensitivity to touch and movement.

Sensory System Modulation

Tactile System. Judith did not like to be held or cuddled. She kept her hands fisted when placed in prone. It was reported that when Judith first started to crawl she supported her weight only on her finger tips and not the entire palm. She refused to hold her bottle. Judith would not bear weight on her feet. Mom reported that Judith would not stand in an "Exersaucer" possibly because of excessive sensitivity on the soles of her feet.

Auditory System. Judith was hypersensitive to loud noises such as the vacuum cleaner. Hearing problems were also suspected, especially after several months had passed and speech did not develop as expected. This resulted in a referral for a speech and hearing evaluation.

Relationship to Gravity. Judith appeared to be gravitationally insecure. She would sit on the floor with her legs widely abducted to anchor any movement and played only with those toys within arm's reach. Judith could not tolerate a sudden change in her head position or being placed on a therapy ball or the therapist's lap.

Vestibular processing appeared to be deficient and movement appeared to provoke fear (e.g., transitioning from prone to sit position elicited a fear response).

Movement Level. Judith tended to stay in one position. When facilitated from prone into a quadruped position, she arched her back, began crying, and had difficulty calming.

Oral Arousal. Judith had difficulty controlling oral secretions, at times drooling noticeably. She exhibited an open mouth posture the majority of the time.

Olfactory Arousal. Judith did not respond adversely to odors but she would sniff unfamiliar toys.

Visual System. No problems noted.

Attention Level. Judith appeared placid, and her mother initially thought she was being "such a good baby." However, she became concerned as Judith's lack of movement and fearfulness became more obvious. Judith was hyper alert to tactile and vestibular change.

Postrotary Nystagmus. Not tested because of her age.

Sensitivity to movement. Judith tolerated little rotary movement or linear acceleration. She could not tolerate swinging in prone or supine although Mom reported that Judith was comfortable on the backyard swing.

Proprioceptive Sensitivity. Judith demonstrated poor response to joint and muscle movement. She was able to sit independently but was uncomfortable being held and would react by stiffening and pulling away. She displayed head lag when pulled to sit.

Emotional Arousal. Although Judith generally appeared underaroused, she quickly became overaroused and fearful with any change in her environment.

Functional Support Capabilities

The systems previously discussed (i.e., auditory, visual, vestibular, proprioceptive, and tactile) provide the basis for development of the functional support capabilities that lead to the end-product.

Suck-Swallow-Breathe. Judith's problems in this area related primarily to sucking, oral motor control, and the integration of these areas with phonation. She exhibited poor oral motor control and drooled excessively. She also had difficulty with biting and chewing. Postural control, phonation, and vocal abilities were all delayed.

Tactile Discrimination. Judith's resistance to touching objects and her negative response to touch from others impeded her exploration of the environment. Ultimately, this may affect her ability to discriminate using touch.

Cocontraction. Judith exhibited difficulty in simultaneous contraction of flexor and extensor muscles. The area of cocontraction related to stability and mobility was further assessed in the NeuroDevelopmental Treatment assessment.

Muscle Tone. Judith had mildly low postural tone, which was also analyzed using the NeuroDevelopmental Treatment frame of reference.

Balance and Equilibrium.   Judith was excessively fearful of falling as a result of poor modulation in the vestibular system. Judith did not display protective extension forward or to either side.

Developmental Reflexes.   Prone extension and supine flexion were poor.

Lateralization.   Judith showed a preference for her right hand.

Bilateral Integration.   Judith was unable to transfer items from one hand to the other.

End-Product Abilities

End-product abilities reflect the outcome of sensory system modulation levels and the functional support capabilities. There is limited expectation of Judith achieving end-product abilities because of her age.

Praxis.   Judith was slow to reach for toys, perhaps because of lack of organization or sensitivity to movement. Her lack of movement may indicate praxis deficits. Her tactile sensitivity may also contribute to dyspraxia.

Form and Space Perception.   Judith was too young to assess this area.

Behavior.   Behaviorally, there were no overt problems; however, her fear of movement and responses to touch may be indicative of problems in this area.

Academics.   Judith was too young to assess this area.

Language and Articulation.   Judith seemed to have receptive and expressive language delays.

Emotional Tone.   Judith exhibited stress and anxiety when exposed to new activities, movement transitions, and certain toys. She demonstrated tactile defensiveness and had difficulty relating to gravity and change of head position—all of which affect her emotional tone.

Activity Level.   Judith's activity level was minimal.

Environmental Mastery.   Judith demonstrated inappropriate adaptive responses and an inability to explore her environment. Thus, she would be expected to have difficulty in mastery.

Summary of Evaluation Findings

Judith was delayed in gross and fine motor developmental milestones. She appeared to be tactile defensive, which was demonstrated when she was being held. In particular, there was defensiveness on the soles of her feet and possibly in her mouth. Sensory processing problems (in particular, sensitivity to movement) and poor motor planning skills significantly impeded her development in the areas of cognition, communication, and social emotional development.

At 11 months, Judith was delayed in all manipulative skills. She obtained an age equivalent score of 7 to 8 months on the fine motor section of the *Peabody Fine and*

Gross Motor Scales (Folio & Fewell, 1983) indicating a 3 to 4 month delay. Judith displayed the potential to improve her abilities in all areas and would benefit from early intervention services.

At the completion of the evaluation, the results were described and explained to the parents. The parents confirmed that the evaluation addressed their concerns and observations regarding their child and that they understood the evaluation results. The parents indicated that their child's responses were typical of her performance abilities.

A meeting to develop an Individualized Family Service Plan (IFSP) was held. Judith was scheduled to receive two sessions weekly, each of occupational therapy, physical therapy, speech therapy, and special education. Special education sessions were to be 1 hour, and each of the other therapies were assigned for 30 minute sessions.

A sample of occupational therapy goals and objectives related to the sensory integrative frame of reference includes:

Goal 1: To improve Judith's ability to move independently so she can explore her environment

- Judith will roll from prone to supine position.
- Judith will transition into a quadruped position and from prone to the sitting position.
- Judith will transition from sitting to standing.

Goal 2: To improve motor planning so that Judith can actively engage in age-appropriate tasks and activities

- Judith will spontaneously pick up objects and move them at will.
- Judith will wave bye-bye.
- Judith will pick up a peg and place it in a hole in a pegboard.

A sample of the occupational therapy goals and objectives related to the NeuroDevelopmental Treatment frame of reference include:

Goal 3: To improve Judith's ability to rotate her trunk and cross her midline so that she can move more freely through her environment and transition from one position to another

- Judith will play with a toy in her midline.
- Judith will be able to reach across her midline to grasp a toy she wants.
- Judith will be able to transition from sitting to quadruped.
- Judith will sit on the floor and use one hand to place a shape into a shape sorter positioned on the opposite side of her body (Figure 20.2).

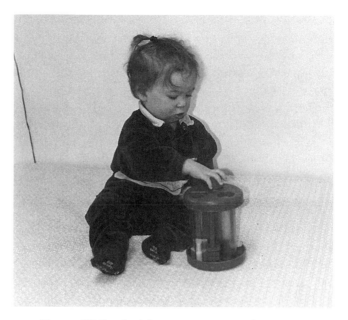

Figure 20.2 Activity to promote trunk rotation.

Goal 4: To improve fine motor skills so that Judith can manipulate toys

- Judith will be able to pick up small objects using a variety of hand grasps.
- Judith will be able to place shapes into a shape sorter.
- Judith will be able to put together large interlocking blocks (i.e., Legos).

APPLICATION OF THE NEURODEVELOPMENTAL TREATMENT FRAME OF REFERENCE

Six postulates regarding change from the NeuroDevelopmental frame of reference were used with Judith. One postulate related to postural control and base of support, one related to postural alignment, and two related to variety of movement were used. *If the therapist is able to feel the child's muscle activation and the therapist can grade her touch accordingly, then the child will receive the optimum level of input to promote active participation in movement.* For example, Judith was placed in the prone position with feet facing the therapist. The therapist's hands were on the sides of Judith's hips, controlling abduction and lifting hips up and back over knees, which encouraged Judith to extend elbows in quadruped position. As Judith was able to increase her control of movement, the therapist's handling control decreased.

To promote postural control in relationship to the base of support, the therapist must provide a sequence of intervention, beginning with preparatory activities.

These activities may include techniques that promote stability through postural alignment of the body before active movement. For example, deep pressure to the child's base of support facilitated the initiation of movement from that base of support as preparation. Judith was placed in a sitting position on a bench, and downward pressure was given to one knee. The other knee was extended with heel tapping the floor. Leg positions were then reversed followed by pressure on both knees in the 90 / 90 / 90 position. This activity strengthens sit-to-stand skills (Figure 20.3).

Proximal stability may be facilitated through weight bearing that requires cocontraction around a joint. Before Judith was standing independently, she was placed in a standing position with the therapist giving support at the hips and applying downward pressure to facilitate cocontraction around lower extremity joints. Trunk rotation and forward mobility were encouraged by weight shifting and alternately moving each hip forward.

If the therapist facilitates postural control during functional movement and the child has ample opportunity to repeat these movement patterns, then these patterns will become integrated into his or her repertoire of motor behaviors. Because Judith has low tone, the therapist facilitated her from quadruped to sitting position by handling first proximally at Judith's shoulders and gradually moving support distally to her hands. Both hands are placed on the shoulders with one hand pressing downward and the other hand pulling backward

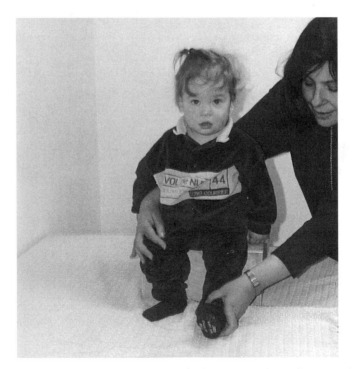

Figure 20.3 The child in sitting position with therapist applying downward pressure to one knee while tapping an opposite heel on the floor.

to facilitate rotation and the movement into sit. The hand that is pulling backward gradually moves down the arm to provide distal support using external rotation of the arm.

If the therapist facilitates postural alignment in preparation for the initiation of movement, then the child will have the potential to use appropriate muscle activation to maintain postural control during activities. Judith tended to sit with lower extremities abducted. By placing Judith's legs in neutral position (i.e., increased adduction), the therapist was able to initiate a lateral weight shift for reaching and engage her in play activities that involve reaching.

If the therapist adapts the environment to take into account the child's developmental level, needs, and interests, then the maximum amount of stimulation will be provided to encourage motor skills. Judith greatly enjoyed looking at her reflection in the mirror so the therapist placed a portable crib in front of the mirror. An eight-inch high wooden box was placed in the crib, and Judith was seated on the box. She reached forward to the rail and then pulled herself up to stand. Because Judith spent some time each day in the portable crib, the mirror and the box increased the amount of stimulation she received while in this environment.

APPLICATION OF THE SENSORY INTEGRATION FRAME OF REFERENCE

Eight general postulates regarding change were identified for Judith from the sensory integration frame of reference. They are as follows: *If the therapist provides a situation in which the child can act on his or her environment, then the child will be more likely to produce adaptive responses.* Because Judith's treatment took place at her home, the equipment selected was that which was already present in the environment and that which is easily transported:

- Outdoor swing set
- Scooter board
- Physiotherapy peanut inflatable ball
- DynaDisc
- Therapy bolster
- Sit 'n Spin
- Rough textured blanket
- Weighted vest, weighted blanket
- Baby lotion, baby powder
- Shaving cream or whipped cream
- Dried beans, rice, pasta, shredded paper, cotton balls
- Koosh balls, Koosh animals, Theraband
- Vibrating toys

- Velcro toys
- Mouth toys, whistles
- Bubbles, wet sponges, pieces of fur
- Long strings of glittery beads, colored foil
- Play-dough

These items were used in play situations with Judith.

If intervention involves several sensory systems and requires intersensory integration, then it will be more powerful and more likely to bring about an adaptive response. Activities were used that involved multiple sensory systems. For example, Judith would kneel, leaning forward on a bolster, while the therapist rolled the bolster slightly to get Judith to reach over and push with open hands on a carpet sample on the other side of the bolster. This provided tactile, proprioceptive, and vestibular input.

If the child is self-directed during therapy, then the neurologic mechanisms needed to build motor patterns (i.e., feed forward and corollary discharge) will occur. Several activities were offered, and Judith was allowed to choose and reject activities.

If the therapist provides a situation that requires an adaptive response that is developmentally appropriate, then an adaptive response is more likely to occur and more likely to promote growth. Activities used in intervention were designed to require an adaptive response. For example, Judith was held in prone across therapist's hands supported at the upper chest and across lower extremities facing a mirror. The therapist would swing the child toward the mirror and back again, encouraging spinal extension. The therapist gradually lowered her hand from the upper chest to the lower chest so that Judith was encouraged to perform a more complex adaptive response to reach for and smile at her reflection in the mirror (Figure 20.4).

If the activity presented to the child is challenging yet achievable, then it will facilitate an improved adaptive response. All activities were designed to be "doable" for Judith. Judith was encouraged gently and with gradation to attempt activities that were initially fear-provoking.

If the therapist provides the child with a sense of emotional safety, then the child will be more likely to engage in the therapy process. Because Judith was an infant, the therapist was especially careful to gauge Judith's reactions. The therapist advanced in a gradual progression so that Judith felt totally secure.

If the therapist provides the child with constant feedback during the therapy session, then the child will gain a greater understanding of what he or she is doing or what he or she has done. Praise and encouragement helped Judith understand what the therapist wanted her to accomplish. She was continually given positive feedback so that she would stay engaged in and feel positively about the activities that were devised. Multiple activities were devised to develop similar types of responses to reinforce her understanding.

If the therapist provides activities that involve controlled change and variety, then the child is more likely to make an adapted response rather than develop a learned behavior. Judith was alternately

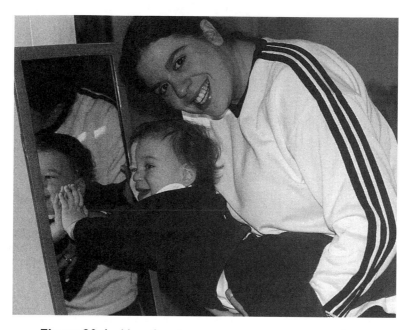

Figure 20.4   Use of a mirror to promote prone extension.

placed on the floor, a platform, a bolster, or a peanut to promote reaching. This helped her to develop balance and equilibrium reactions on different surfaces and with different levels of challenge. The use of multiple activities with similar goals increases the likelihood of an adapted response.

Modulation of vestibular input was addressed using the following postulates.

First, if modulation input is given to one system, then influence is seen in all systems because they are interdependent. In the prior example of using linear acceleration and deceleration toward the mirror, input was provided to the vestibular receptors to reduce sensory processing dysfunctions and Judith's gravitational insecurity.

Second, if the child's sensory diet is modified, then sensory system modulation is more likely to occur. Because Judith's deficits involved many sensory systems, there was a need to focus on her sensory diet. The Wilbarger Protocol was used, which includes brushing and joint compression to mitigate tactile defensiveness. A variety of movement experiences also exposed Judith to different movements at different intensities.

Third, if a child is overreactive, then the usual adaptive response will reflect survival needs and not integration; therefore, the sensory system input will have to be modified for the child to produce an adequate response. As an infant, Judith lacked adequate defenses to protect herself from too much of or the wrong kinds of sensory input. Therefore, caution was used in providing slow intensification of activities during intervention.

Fourth, if the sensory system modulation level is normalized, then functional support capabilities and end-product abilities will be facilitated. During intervention, therapy focused on sensory system modulation, which serves as the basis for the development of functional support capabilities and end-product abilities.

APPLICATION OF BOTH FRAMES OF REFERENCE

Occupational therapy intervention consisted of incorporating NeuroDevelopmental Treatment and Sensory Integration treatment techniques in a sequential manner within each session. In the beginning of each session, the NeuroDevelopmental Treatment frame of reference guided intervention, which was followed by the initiation of the sensory integration frame of reference.

A Typical Therapy Session

The therapist arrived at Judith's home and was eagerly welcomed. Judith was placed on an exercise mat on the table, and therapy began with preparatory handling to increase postural tone and increase self-initiated mobility.

NeuroDevelopmental Treatment interventions were geared toward increasing tone and facilitation of movement. Judith's shoulders and trunk were mobilized in preparation for movement with facilitation. The therapist used handling techniques involving depression of the shoulders and adduction of the scapula to mobilize Judith's shoulders and upper extremities. The therapist used handling to facilitate flexion and extension of the trunk, as well as lateral flexion and trunk rotation. This preparatory handling increased her postural tone and prepared her for more dynamic mobility.

Postural alignment was carefully monitored as preparation before sensory input. For example, her trunk was aligned over her pelvis (the base of support) when she was seated straddling the "peanut." Deep pressure into the base of support was provided to maintain her feet in contact with the floor. Trunk rotation was facilitated as she reached for shapes hidden in a rice/bean bin placed on either side of the inflatable peanut (Figure 20.5).

Based on the NeuroDevelopmental Treatment frame of reference, Judith was placed in a standing position with the therapist supporting her from behind. The therapist's hands were in front of Judith's ankles so that the therapist could lift Judith up and down gently tapping the soles of her feet alternately against the table. This provided the child with experience in weight bearing and weight shifting. While still in that position, Judith was moved in a swaying motion, shifting her weight side to side. Judith enjoyed this activity especially when the therapist sang to her (Figure 20.6).

A bolster was placed on the table, and Judith was placed in the prone position across the roll. The therapist held lower extremities as Judith extended her upper body forward. Judith began to cry so this activity was terminated.

Judith was placed in the prone position on a scooter board on the table. This activity was geared toward weight bearing on upper extremities and dissociation of

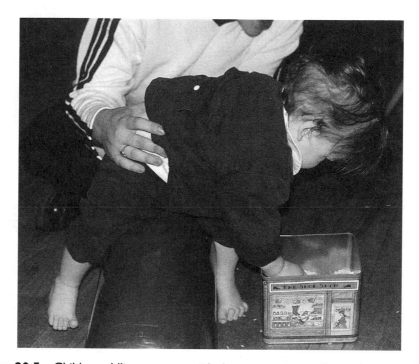

Figure 20.5   Child straddling a peanut with deep pressure into base of support. Trunk rotation facilitated as child looks for toys in rice/bean bin on the side of the peanut.

movements of the upper and lower extremities. The baby sitter sat at the end of the table. The therapist propelled Judith down the table and with arms fully extended. Judith gave the baby-sitter a "high-five." Judith became fatigued after three trials. The purpose of this activity was to encourage more controlled isolated upper extremity movements.

At this point, building upon the mobility facilitated by the NeuroDevelopment Treatment frame of reference, the therapist began to use the Sensory Integration frame of reference. Intervention began with application of a brushing program (the Wilbarger Protocol). Judith was then placed on a rough blanket on the floor in the prone position with her head facing the therapist. The therapist pulled the blanket along the floor, weaving and turning full circle (Figure 20.7). The Wilbarger Protocol and the activity described provide proprioceptive, vestibular, and tactile sensory input.

Judith was encouraged to crawl through a portable tunnel to obtain a toy. Judith discovered that the tunnel would rock with her motion and experimented with this for several minutes (Figure 20.8). This activity combined mobility with sensory input while engaged in an adaptive activity.

Judith was placed in front of a carpeted staircase with a favorite toy placed on the

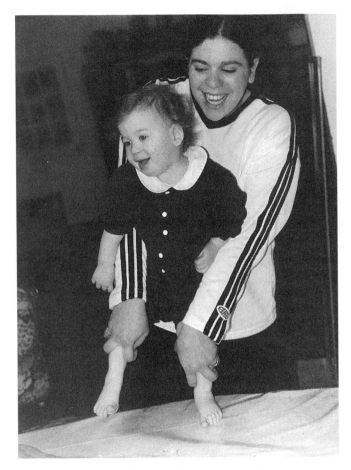

Figure 20.6 Weight shifting using swaying motion.

fourth step. The therapist started Judith up the stairs by placing first one knee and then the other on the bottom step and inhibiting abduction of the lower extremities.

Judith sat on the DynaDisc to work on her balance by reaching for toy musical instruments, such as maracas. This activity was continued on the peanut and varied with different toys.

Near the end of the session, Judith was placed in her high chair to work on oral motor skills. A box drink with a small straw was provided. The therapist squeezed the box to bring liquid to the top of straw. At first, Judith allowed the juice to run out of her mouth but later managed to swallow some of the juice (Figure 20.9).

Responses to Intervention

After 5 months of therapy, Judith has progressed significantly. Her hyperalert state has been ameliorated. Her hands are usually open; she plays with a wide vari-

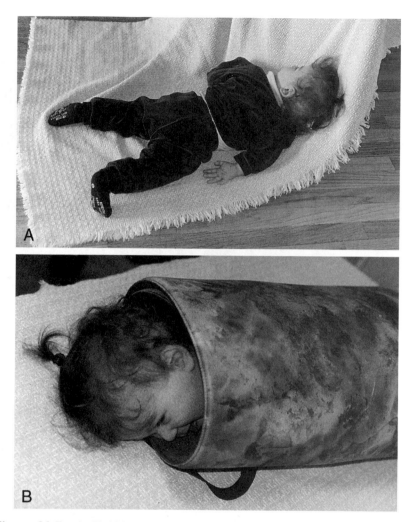

Figure 20.7   A, Child being pulled on a blanket. B, Child wrapped in a blanket.

ety of toys composed of many different textures. When the vacuum cleaner is switched on, she is able to ignore it and continues to play normally.

Judith's relationship to gravity is far more secure. She can roll from the supine to prone position and back and can transition from either the prone position or the supine position to sitting without difficulty. Improvement was noted in Judith's ability to modulate vestibular input in standing. Mom allows her to climb up and down stairs with minimal supervision. She is able to motor plan getting on the Sit 'n Spin but cannot yet coordinate herself to get onto the Sit 'n Spin. She is able to stand independently and take one to two steps. However, Judith still has difficulties with trunk rotation (Figure 20.10).

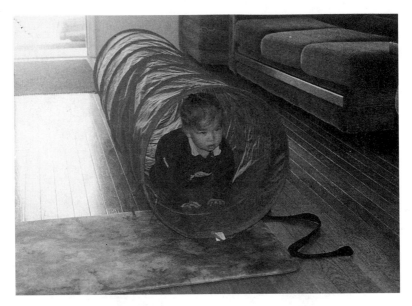

Figure 20.8 Child crawling through a portable tunnel.

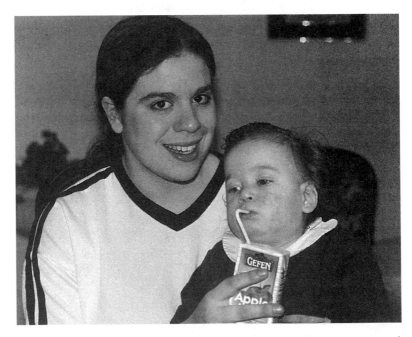

Figure 20.9 Sucking is a functional skill that may aid in overall organization and improve postural control and oral motor control.

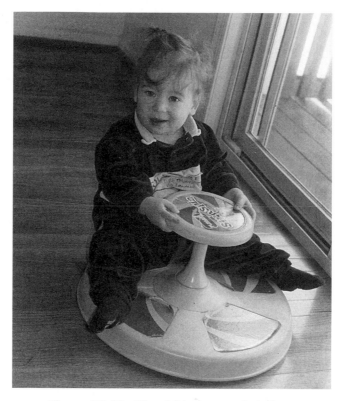

Figure 20.10 The child sitting on Sit 'n Spin.

Modulation of tactile input has allowed her to use her hands more effectively for environmental mastery. Judith can transfer objects from hand to hand since improving her grasp and release of objects. Not only does she now place a cube in a cup, but she can discriminate shapes by placing them correctly in a shape sorter. Judith can identify a desired object by pointing with her index finger and vocalizing. She scribbles on a blackboard with chalk as she is no longer sensitive to the feel of the chalk. She picks up Cheerios with a neat pincer grasp. She claps her hands and waves bye-bye.

In the area of oral motor control, Judith is still drooling significantly and is unable to blow bubbles, blow a whistle, blow out a lit candle, or drink from a straw.

IMPLICATION FOR FUTURE INTERVENTION

At 16 months of age, oral motor control and self care skills become increasingly important. Most children are able to self feed and control oral secretions, which will be a focus of intervention. Trunk rotation, crossing midline, and fine motor skills will also continue to be addressed. Examples of updated objectives are:

Goal 1: To improve self care skills for independent feeding and dressing

- Judith will hold a spoon in her hand while being spoon fed.
- Judith will begin to self feed using a spoon or fork.
- Judith will remove her shoes and socks.

Goal 2. To improve oral motor control so that she can decrease drooling and drink from a straw or adapted cup with minimal spillage

- Judith will blow a whistle.
- Judith will drink from a straw without dribbling.
- Judith will lick a lollipop.

Goal 3: To improve trunk rotation and fluidity of movement so that she can independently move from one position to another

- Judith will sit on the floor and play with a xylophone, holding the baton in her right hand while hitting the xylophone placed on her left side.
- Judith will stand by the refrigerator, remove magnets from the door, and drop them into a pot behind her (Figure 20.11).

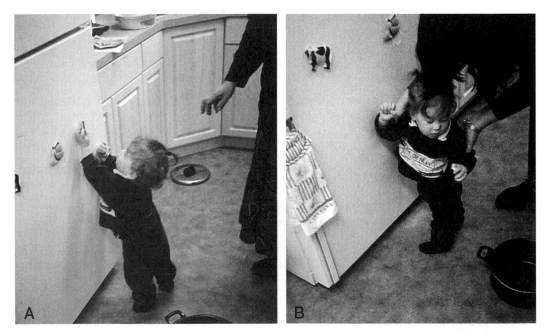

Figure 20.11 A and B, Trunk rotation.

- Judith will sit on a box, pick up bean bags from the floor beside her, and hand them to the therapist sitting on the opposite side (Figure 20.12).
- Judith will transition from quadruped to sitting and from sitting to standing.

SUMMARY

Judith was able to make maximum progress because her providers followed through consistently with the therapist's intervention recommendations. As is frequently found in interventions, Judith's parents frequently asked the therapist to make predictions as to when Judith would reach major developmental milestones. It was helpful to explain the sequence and subskills necessary prior to reaching the next milestone so her parents could understand what was going on in therapy.

Judith continues to require occupational therapy to address residual difficulties in vestibular processing that can interfere with gross motor and fine motor skills. Deficient sensory registration, modulation, and developmental dyspraxia may be interfering with speech development. Further progress in dissociation and variety of movement are necessary for fluidity of movement. Judith is an adorable little girl who has made rapid progress in 5 months. Her therapist anticipates that progress will continue at a satisfactory rate.

This case study shows the use of the NeuroDevelopmental Treatment frame of reference and the Sensory Integration frame of reference together. Each treatment session used these two frames of reference sequentially, first NeuroDevelopmental

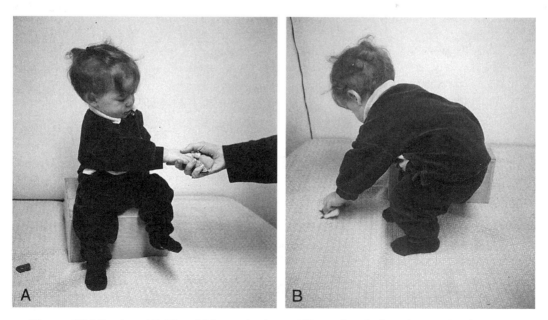

Figure 20.12   A and B, The child crossing her midline to hand a bean bag to the therapist.

Treatment, then Sensory Integration. If one looked backed at the course of intervention, it seems that the frames of reference are used in a parallel manner, each frame of reference is used consistently over a period of time, and they are not integrated in any way. It is almost as if there are two courses of intervention going on, both of which are important to the development of the child.

STUDY QUESTIONS

1. List the signs pointing to Judith's sensory defensiveness.
2. Why were Sensory Integration and NeuroDevelopmental Treatment frames of reference both used?
3. List additional goals and treatment activities that address Judith's goals.
4. Discuss how the postulates regarding change serve to address the function/dysfunction continua from which the goals are derived.
5. How could the two frames of reference be integrated to be used in a combined manner?

Acknowledgments

The authors wish to thank their supervisor Jill Anderson, M.S., OTR for her encouragement, her generosity in freely sharing her knowledge, her gentle manner and her patience in guiding them.

References

Folio, M. R., & Fewell, R. R. (1983). *Peabody developmental motor scales and activity cards.* Allen, TX: DIM Teaching Resources.

Oetter, P., Richter, E., & Frick, S. (1992). *MORE integrating the mouth with sensory and postural function.* Hugo, MN: PDP Products.

Wilbarger, P. (1991) *Occupational therapy: sensory defensiveness,* 60 minute video, PDP Products, Hugo, MN.

Wilbarger, P., & Wilbarger, J. (1991). *Sensory defensiveness in children 2–12.* Santa Barbara, CA: Avanti Education Programs.

Index

Note: Page numbers in *italics* indicate illustrations; those followed by t indicate tables; and those followed by c indicate charts.

Abuse, sensory defensiveness in, 131
Academics, 144, 155c. *See also* Learning; School
  interventions for, 201
Acceptance, unconditional, 378, 386, 523
Accommodation, visual, 256
Acquisitional frame of reference, 377–399
  application to practice of, 393–399
  assumptions underlying, 386
  behavior therapy in, 378–379
  environmental interaction in, 388, 392
  evaluation in, 390–392
  function/dysfunction continua in, 388–390, 391c
  generalization in, 385–386, 398
  historical perspective on, 378–379
  individualized nature of, 388, 392
  learning theory in, 377, 379–386
  observation in, 391, 395–397
  postulates regarding change in, 392–393
  reinforcement in, 382–384, 387, 387c, 388c, 393,
    394–395
  with sensory integration frame of reference, 529
  shaping and, 384–385
  skill acquisition in, 379–382. *See also* Motor skill acquisi-
    tion frame of reference; Skill acquisition
  theoretical base of, 377, 379–386
  theoretical postulates for, 387–388
  unconditional positive regard in, 378,
    386
Acquisitional theories, 69
Activities of daily living (ADLs). *See also* Skill(s)
  function/dysfunction continua for, 389–390
  in NeuroDevelopmental Treatment, 102
  as performance area, 11
Activity adaptation, 36–37
Activity analysis, 34–37, 393–394
Activity groups, 37
  for children, 363–371
    activity selection for, 364–366
    club model for, 367
    cooperative, 364
    culture, beliefs, and values in, 370–371
    handling aggression in, 368–369
    handling frustration in, 368–369
    handling resistance in, 369–370
    management strategies for, 368–370
    parallel, 364

    project, 364
    of school age, 367–368
    structure of, 366–368
    termination of, 371
  for parents and children, 361–363
Activity level
  evaluation of, 155c
  function/dysfunction indicators for, 152c
  sensory system modulation and, 145
Activity performance, 483t, 491–493
  component processes of, 483t, 492–493, 494t–496t,
    501
  function/dysfunction continua for, 500, 502c
Adapt, in occupational synthesis, 497, 510
Adaptation
  activity, 36–37
  coping and, 432
  occupation and, 478
Adapted chair, 298. *See also* Seating equipment
Adaptive behavior, environmental interaction and,
  388
Adult directives and rules, compliance with, 492t
Affect. *See also* Emotional tone
  coping and, 440, 446, 447c, 453, 458–459
  muscle tone and, 272
Affordances, 406
Aggression, in activity groups, 369
Alert Program, 186, 237
Alerting, 210
Alignment. *See* Postural alignment
Alter, in occupational synthesis, 497, 509–510
Ambulation aids, 578, *578*, 582, *583*
American Occupational Therapy Association (AOTA),
    Uniform Terminology of, 10
Ankle straps, for stander, 312, *312*
Anterolateral system, 126–127
Antigravity movement, 127, 148c, 153c. *See also*
    Gravity
  flexion response and, 188, *189*, *190*, *191*
  hypertonicity and, 270
  lateral neck flexion and, 266
  protraction and, 263
Arm control
  evaluation of, 284–286, 577
  facilitation of, 313
  function/dysfunction continua for, 275, 276c

Arousal
  auditory, 132
  definition of, 210
  dysfunctional, 147, 148c–149c
  emotional, 135, 148c
    evaluation of, 592
  levels of, 135, 135t
  modulation of, 128, 129t, 130, 130–131
  olfactory, 133–134, 148c
    evaluation of, 592
  oral, 133, 148c
    evaluation of, 592
  sensory system modulation and, 128, 130, 130–131
Arousal/alerting, in visual attention, 210
  facilitation of, 236–237, 237
Articulation. See Language and articulation
Assessment of Motor and Process Skills-AMPS, 420
Assistive technology, 31–33
  definition of, 31
  evaluation for, 288, 579
  for feeding, 586–587
  function/dysfunction indicators for, 277–278, 278c
  guidelines for, 289–291
  high tech, 32, 33
  low tech, 32
  for mobility, 314–315, 580–581, 582–583, 583, 584,
    585, 586
  in NeuroDevelopmental Treatment, 115, 547–548, 549
  postulates regarding change for, 289–291
  for sitting. See Seating equipment
  for toileting, 587, 587–588
  use of, facilitation of, 317–319
Asymmetrical tonic neck reflex, 259, 262
Athetosis, 270
Attachment, 325–330
  facilitation of, 359–363
  function/dysfunction continua for, 344–346, 346c
  insecure, 345
  postulates regarding change for, 355–356
Attention, visual. See Visual attention
Attention deficit disorder, vs. hyperactivity, 134
Attention level, 134, 148c, 150c, 153c
  evaluation of, 153c, 592
  function/dysfunction indicators for, 148c, 150c
Attractor states, in movement, 403
Auditory arousal, 132
Auditory defensiveness, 132
  interventions for, 184
Auditory discrimination, 135, 150c
Auditory system
  evaluation of, 591
  function/dysfunction indicators for, 148c
  in sensory integration, 128
Auditory training, 184
Ayres, A. Jean, 119–121, 124, 127

Back supports, 299, 301–302, 302
Backward chaining technique, 456
Balance and equilibrium, 136–137, 138
  CNS dysfunction and, 270–271

development of, 259–260
  evaluation of, 154c, 590
  function/dysfunction indicators for, 150c
  interventions for, 187, 187–188
  vestibular system and, 127–128, 134–135
Bandura, Alfred, 377
Base of support, 85–86, 94
Bathing, 486t, 486–487
Behavior
  reinforcement of. See Reinforcement
  sensory integration and, 144, 152c
Behavior regulation, 492t
Behavior therapy, acquisitional frame of reference and,
    378–379
Behaviorism, 378
Beliefs, coping and, 439, 445–446, 447c, 452–453, 458
Bilateral integration, 137
  evaluation of, 154
  facilitation of, 192
  function/dysfunction indicators for, 151c
Biomechanical frame of reference, 257–321
  application to practice of, 292–321, 580–588
    for central stability, 292–312, 319–321
    for functional skills, 312–321
  evaluation in, 278–288, 574–579
  function/dysfunction continua in, 273–278, 274c–278c
  goals of, 257–258, 272
  holistic approach in, 319–320, 320
  motor development and, 259–260. See also Motor devel-
    opment
  with NeuroDevelopmental Treatment frame of refer-
    ence, 528–529, 547
  occupational therapy evaluation in, 574–579
  postulates regarding change in, 289–291
  postural control and, 85–86, 93–94, 96c, 259–261,
    580–581. See also Postural control
  postural reactions to damage/dysfunction and, 268–272
  prone position and, 264–265, 265
  sidelying position and, 265–266, 266
  sitting position and, 266–268, 267
  stability development and, 260–261
  standing position and, 268
  supine position and, 262–264, 263
  theoretical base of, 257–273
Bird feeding, prevention of, 316–317
Bite-crunch activities, 196
Bladder management, 486t, 486–487. See also Toileting
Blocked practice, 413, 426
Blos' developmental theory, 70
Bobath, Berta, 83
Bobath, Karl, 83
Body transfers, 490–491, 493t
Body transportation, 491, 493t
Bolster swing, 139, 188, 199, 200
Bonding. See Attachment
Bowel management, 486t, 486–487. See also Toileting
Breathing. See Suck-swallow-breathe synchrony
Breathing abnormalities, 136
Bruininks-Oseretsky Test of Motor Proficiency, 353–354
Bubble balls, 176, 177

Case study
   of biomechanical frame of reference, 573–588
   of motor skill acquisition frame of reference, 551–571
   of NeuroDevelopmental Treatment frame of reference,
      533–550
   of NDT and sensory integration frame of reference,
      589–607
Categorization, 214–216, *216*, *217*
   facilitation of, *249*, 249–250
Central nervous system
   disorders of, motor problems and, 269–272
   hierarchical organization of, 124–125
   interconnectedness of, 125
   plasticity of, 125
Central vision, definition of, 256
Cerebral palsy, case study of, 573–588
Chair, adapted, 297–308, *298*. *See also* Seating equipment
Change
   postulates regarding. *See* Postulates regarding change
   from sensory input, 90
Changing levels, 493t
Chew-lick activities, 196
Child abuse, sensory defensiveness in, 131
Child-environment-occupation fit, maximization of,
      493–498, 509
Child-parent relationship. *See* Attachment; Parent-child
      relationship
Children. *See also* Infant; Newborn
   activity groups for, 363–371. *See also* Activity groups,
      for children
   therapeutic relationship with, 523
   unconditional acceptance of, 378, 386, 523
Chunking, for visual memory, 246
Client-centered assessment, of occupational performance,
      502–503
Clinical reasoning process, 167–168, 202
Closed tasks, 407, *408*
Club model, for activity groups, 367
Cocontraction, 136, *137*, *193*
   evaluation of, 154c, 593
   function/dysfunction indictors for, 150c
Coding and storage, of visual memories, 212
   facilitation of, 245–246
Cognitive analysis skills, 209
Cognitive integration component, 16–17
Collaborative partnerships, 470
Communication. *See also* Language and articulation
   with family, 49–50
   functional, 492t
Communication and interaction skills, 471
Community environment
   function/dysfunction indicators for, 350, 351c
   as occupational behavior setting, 481
   psychosocial aspects of, 343, 350, 351c
Compensatory movement/posture, 268–269
   patterns of, 89
Complex task performance, 482t, 482–491
   assessment of, 502–506, 505t
   function/dysfunction indicators for, 499–500, 501c
Compliance with adult conventions and rules, 492t

Component processes, 483t, 492–493, 493t–496t
   function/dysfunction indicators for, 501
Compression, in preparation and facilitation, 110, *111*
Computers, 584, *585*. *See also* Assistive technology
   in detection of relationships, 251–252
Conditioning, operant, 377
Conscious use of self, as legitimate tool, 28–29
Constant theories, 69
Constructional play, 34, 336, *338*, 347. *See also* Play
   in activity groups, for parent and child, 361–363
Constructional tasks, for detection of relationships,
      250–251, *251*
Context(s)
   cultural, 47–50
   education
      influences on, 45–50
      in systems theory, 43–45
   family, 47–50
   health
      influences on, 45–50
      in systems theory, 43–45
   occupational, 471
Context-specific assessment, of occupational performance,
      503–504
Contingency reinforcement, 383
Contractions, tonic, 261
Contrast sensitivity, definition of, 256
Control parameters, in movement, 403
Coping, 341–342
   in activity groups, 368–369
   adaptation and, 432
   affective states and, 440, 446, 447c, 453, 458–459
   beliefs and values and, 439, 445–446, 447c, 452–453, 458
   definition of, 432
   demands and expectations and, 448, 450c
   developmental skills and, 440, 446–447, 448c, 453, 459
   effectiveness of, 443–445, 446c, 461–463
      indicators of, 443–445, 444c
      intervention strategies and, 461–462
   facilitation of, 455–465
      assessment and, 454
   function/dysfunction indicators for, 348–349, 349c
   human supports for, 440–441, 447, 449c, 453–454,
      459–460
   integration of into intervention, 463–465
   material and environmental supports for, 441, 448,
      449c, 454, 460
   modification of demands and, 455–456
   physical states and, 440, 446, 447c, 453, 458–459
   postulates regarding change for, 357–358
   in special needs children, 441–443
Coping assessment, 449–454
Coping attributes, 439, 440t
Coping effort, 436
Coping frame of reference, 431–466
   application to practice of, 455–465
   evaluation in, 449–454
   function/dysfunction continua in, 443–448, 444c–450c
   postulates regarding change in, 454–455
   with psychosocial frame of reference, 529–530

Coping frame of reference—*Continued*
  theoretical base of, 431–443
Coping Inventory, 354–355, 451
Coping process, *434*, 434–438
Coping resources, 436, 438–441
  enhancement of, 456–460
  evaluation of, 451–454
  external, 440t, 440–441
  function/dysfunction indicators for, 446–448,
      447c–450c
  internal, 438–440, 440t
Coping skills, parental, 440–441, 447, 449c, 453–454,
      459–460
Coping style, 438–439
  assessment of, 451–452
  effectiveness of, 444–445, 446c, 461–463
  enhancement of, 457–458
Coping transactions, 434–438
  assessment of, 450–451
Copying skills, evaluation of, 229–230, 354–355
Corollary discharge, *140*, 142
Create, in occupational synthesis, 498, 511
Cultural context, 47–50
Cultural environment, 406
Cultural issues, in activity groups, 370–371
Culture
  definition of, 20
  in performance context, 18–20
Curative model paradigm, 51–55, 52t

Default patterns, 202
Defensiveness. *See* Sensory defensiveness
Degree of freedom problem, 411
Depression, parent-child relationship and, 330, 362
Detection of relationships, 217, *218*, *250*, 250–252,
      251
Development
  ecology of, 46–47
  frame of reference for, 7
  individual variations in, 6
  linear, 4–5
  motor, 84–89, 402. *See also* Motor development
  occupation and, 474–475
  progression of, 4
  pyramidal, 5
  rates of, 5
  sequential nature of, 4, 6, 7, 125–126
  social, 17
Developmental disabilities, coping and, 441–443. *See also*
      Coping
Developmental dyspraxia, 141
Developmental reflexes, 137, *139*, 151c. *See also*
      Reflex(es)
  evaluation of, 139, 154
  function/dysfunction indicators for, 151c
Developmental Test of Visual Motor Integration, 229
Developmental Test of Visual Perception, 229–230
Developmental theories, 3–7, 69, 70, 378, 386
Directives, compliance with, 492t
Disability rights movement, 41, 45–46

Discrimination
  emotional, 135, 150c
  racial/ethnic, in activity groups, 370–371
  sensory
    auditory, 135, 150c
    olfactory, 135, 150c
    oral, 135, 150c
    proprioceptive, 135
      evaluation of, 154c
      function/dysfunction indicators for, 150c
    tactile, 126, 136
      evaluation of, 154c, 593
      function/dysfunction indicators for, 150c
    visual, 135, 150c, 214–217, *215–217*, 246–247. *See
      also* Visual discrimination
Dissociation, 87, 97, *98*, 98c, *99*
  evaluation of, 103, 538, 591
  lack of, 89
  postulates regarding change for, 106
Distal key points, handling at, 108
Domain of concern
  interventions and, 22–23
  occupation as, 23–24
  performance areas in, 10–13
  performance components of, 13–18
  performance context for, 18–23
Dorsal column medial lemniscal system, 126–127
Dressing, 486t, 486–487
  function/dysfunction continua for, 390, 391c
Dynamic assessment, of occupational performance,
      503
Dynamic movement, 86
Dynamic systems theory, 402–403
Dynamic theories, 69
Dysautonomia, case study of, 551–571
Dysfunction, indicators of, 74–76, 76t. *See also*
      Function/dysfunction continua
Dyspraxia
  developmental, 141
  evaluation of, 154–155
  interventions for, 197–201, *198–200*

Early Coping Inventory, 451
Eating. *See* Feeding
Ecological model paradigm, 52t, 58–60
Ecology of human development, 46–47
Education. *See also* Learning; School
  function/dysfunction indicators for, 499–500, 501c
  as occupation, 486, 488t
Education contexts
  influences on, 45–50
  in systems theory, 43–45
Education for All Handicapped Children Act, 41
Educational reform, 46
Elaborative rehearsal, for visual memory, 246
Elbow mobility
  evaluation of, 284–286
  facilitation of, 313
  function/dysfunction continua for, 275, 276c
Elkind's developmental theory, 70

Emotional arousal, 135, 148c
   evaluation of, 592
Emotional control, facilitation of, 457
Emotional discrimination, 135, 150c
Emotional states, muscle tone and, 272
Emotional tone, 135. *See also* Affect
   evaluation of, 155c
   function/dysfunction indicators for, 152c
   sensory system modulation and, 145
End-product abilities, *123*, 123–124, 129t, 140–145
   academic, 144, 155c
   activity level, 145
   behavioral, 144
   emotional tone, 145
   environmental mastery, 145
   evaluation of, 154–155, 593
   form and space perception skills, 144
   interventions for, 196–202
   language and articulation, 144–145
   postulates regarding change for, 171
   praxis, *140*, 140–144
Environment
   adaptations in, for coping, 441, 448, 449c, 454,
      460
   classification of, 471
   cultural, 406
   nonhuman, legitimate tools in, 29–34
   occupation and, 474
   as occupational context, 471–472
   in occupational frame of reference, 471–472
   physical, 406
   reinforcement from, 380, 385–386
   social, 406
   for task performance, 406
      evaluation of, 420–421
   therapeutic, 523–524
Environmental content, skill acquisition and, 380
Environmental interactions, 342–343
   adaptive behavior and, 388
   evaluation of, 355
   function/dysfunction continua for, 349–350, 350c
   postulates regarding change for, 358
Environmental mastery, 145
   evaluation of, 155c
   function/dysfunction indicators for, 152c
Environmental reinforcers, 380, 385–386
Equilibrium, 136–137, *138*
   CNS dysfunction and, 270–271
   development of, 259–260
   evaluation of, 154c, 590
   function/dysfunction indicators for, 150c
   interventions for, *187*, 187–188
Erikson's developmental theory, 70
Establish/restore, in occupational synthesis, 496,
      509
Experimentation, in skill acquisition, 412–413
Eye movements
   deficits in, 222–223
   development of, 263
   evaluation of, 223–224

Family. *See also* Parent
   communication with, 49–50
   in frame of reference, 47–48
   functions of, 48–49
   interactions with, 29
   in performance context, 21
Family context, 47–50
Feedback
   in information processing model, 207, *207*
   in motor activity, 85
   in skill acquisition, 404, 413–416, 424–425
   summary, 414
Feedforward, *140*, 141–142
   in motor activity, 85
Feeding, 486t, 486–487
   evaluation of, 287, 578–579
   facilitation of, 315–317, 586–587
   function/dysfunction indicators for, 276–277, 277c,
      389–390, 491c
   reinforcement of, 395
Figure-ground test, 229, *231*
Fixation, definition of, 256
Fixing, of joints, 88, 89, 100
Flexion
   lateral neck, 266
   supine, 188, 189, *191*
Flexion response, 188, 189, *190*, *191*
   facilitation of, 189, *192—195*
Flexion swing, *194*
Floor sitter, 581, *582*
Forehead strap, 308–309
Form and space perception skills, 144
   evaluation of, 155c
   function/dysfunction indicators for, 152c
Form constancy test, 229, *232*
Frame(s) of reference, 3–4, 22–23
   acquisitional, 377–399. *See also* Acquisitional frame of
      reference
   alternative applications of, 524–531
   application to practice of, 67–68, 78–79
   articulation of, 519–521
   biomechanical, 257–321. *See also* Biomechanical frame
      of reference
   in combination, 529–530
   components of, 67–68
   context for. *See* Context(s)
   coping, 431–466. *See also* Coping frame of ref-
      erence
   in curative model paradigm, 54–55
   development of, 67–68
   developmental, 7
   in ecological care paradigm, 58–60
   evaluation guidelines for, 76–77
   family in, 47–48
   features of, 27
   function/dysfunction continua for, 74–76, 75t. *See also*
      Function/dysfunction continua
   legitimate tools, 28
   limitations of, 526–527
   as link between theory and practice, 69

motor skill acquisition, 401–427. *See also* Motor skill acquisition frame of reference
multiple, 526–527
Frame(s) of reference
NeuroDevelopmental Treatment, 83–117. *See also* Neuro-
Developmental Treatment frame of reference
occupation, 37–38
occupational, 469–512. *See also* Occupational frame of
reference
original, formulation of, 530–531
in palliative care paradigm, 56–58
parallel use of, 528–529
postulates regarding change for, 77–78. *See also* Postulates regarding change
psychosocial, 323–373. *See also* Psychosocial frame of
reference
rationales for, 519–521
in real world, 519–531
selection and application of, 60–61
selection of, 521, 526
sensory integration, 119–168. *See also* Sensory integration frame of reference
sequential use of, 527–528
single, 524–526
structure of, 67–79
theoretical base for, 68–73, 521. *See also* Theoretical
base; Theory(ies)
visual perception, 205–253. *See also* Visual information
analysis
Freezing, of joints, 88, 89
Freud's developmental theory, 70
Frick, Sheila, 184
Friendships, 330–331. *See also* Peer interaction
Frustration, in activity groups, 369
Functional behaviors, 381
Functional communication, 492t
Functional Independence Measure for Children, 420
Functional mobility
function/dysfunction indicators for, 499–500, 501c
as occupation, 490–491, 493t
Functional performance behaviors
evaluation of, 287–288
function/dysfunction indicators for, 275–278, 277c, 278c
Functional skills, evaluation of, 101–102, *102*
Functional support capabilities, 135–139
balance and equilibrium, 136–137, *138*
bilateral integration, 137
cocontraction, 136, *137*
evaluation of, 139, 153–154, 592–593
function/dysfunction indicators for, 147, 150c–151c
interventions for, 186–196
lateralization, 137
muscle tone, 136
postulates regarding change for, 171
proprioception, 136
suck-swallow-breathe synchrony, 136
tactile discrimination, 126, 136
Functional tasks, 405
Function/dysfunction continua, 74–76, 75c
for acquisitional frame of reference, 388–390, 391c

for biomechanical frame of reference, 273–278,
274c–278c
for coping frame of reference, 443–448, 444c–450c
for motor skill acquisition frame of reference, 417–418,
419c
for NeuroDevelopmental Treatment frame of reference,
90–100, 93c, 95c–98c, 100c, 101c
for occupational frame of reference, 498–501, 499c,
501c, 502c
for psychosocial frame of reference, 344–350, 345c–351c
for sensory integration frame of reference, 146–147,
148c–152c
for skills, 388–390, 446–447, 448c
for visual information analysis frame of reference, 219–233

Gallant reflex, 271
Game play, 336–338, 347, 485t. *See also* Play
Gender issues, activity groups and, 370–371
Generalization, 385–386, 398
Grasp, facilitation of, 547, *548*
Gravitational insecurity, 132
evaluation of, 591–592
Gravity
effects of, 257
equilibrium response and, 259, 260
hypertonicity and, 270
lateral neck flexion against, 266
movement against, 127, 148c, 153c
flexion response and, 188, 189, *190, 191*
postural reactions and, 259–260
protraction against, 263
righting response and, 259, 260
vestibular system and, 127
Grooming, 486t, 486–487
Group interaction, 331
Group play, 34
Group resistance, in activity groups, 369–370

Hand control
evaluation of, 284–286, 577
facilitation of, 313, 546–547
function/dysfunction indicators for, 275, 276c
for writing, 202, 203
Handling, 90, 105, 528–529
in NeuroDevelopmental Treatment, 90, 105, 108–109,
109, 110
at proximal key points, 108, *109*
therapeutic equipment for, 109, *110*
Handwriting problems, 202, 203
Harness, seating, *304*, 304–305
Head control
evaluation of, 280–281, *281*, 576
function/dysfunction indicators for, 274, 275c
in prone position, 264–265, *265*
in sidelying position, 266
in sitting position, 267
in supine posture, 262, *262*
Head position, whole-body reactions and, 271
Head support(s), 306–309
for feeding, 316–317

Health care, systems approach in, 43–45
Health care reform, 45
Health contexts
  influences on, 45–50
  in systems theory, 43–45
Hearing. *See under* Auditory
Helmet, for head support, 308–309
High guard position, 92, *95*
Hip position, in sitting, 299–302, *300, 301*
Hip straps, for stander, 311–312, *312*
History, play, 354
Home environment
  as occupational behavior setting, 480
  psychosocial aspects of, 342–343
Home Observation for Measurement of the Environment, 454
How Does Your Engine Run (Williams & Shellenberger), 185
Humeral wings, 304–306, 313, 584, *585, 586*
Hurricane game, 187, *187*
Hyperactivity
  vs. attention deficit disorder, 134
  interventions for, 181
Hypertonia, 269–270
Hypertonicity, 269–270. *See also* Muscle tone
  interventions for, case study of, 539–548, *540–549*
  joint effects of, 270
Hypotheses, 72–73
Hypotonia, 269
Hypotonicity, 269. *See also* Muscle tone

Illness, parental, parent-child relationship and, 361–362
Imaginative play, 34, 335–336, 485t. *See also* Play
Inclusiveness, in school, 41, 574–575
Independence, encouragement of, 460–461
Indicators of function/dysfunction, 74–76, 76t
Individualized Family Service Plan (IFSP), 455
  preparation of, 538–539
Individuals With Disabilities Education Act (IDEA), 46
Infant
  attachment behavior in, 325–330
  motor development in, 261–268. *See also* Motor development
  motor reflexes in, 259
Infant bonding. *See* Attachment
Information feedback about the outcome, 414, 415
Information processing model, 207, *207*–209
Intermittent reinforcement, 384
Intervention(s)
  direct vs. indirect, 461
  integration of coping into, 463–465
  theory-based, 68–73
Interview
  play, 352–353
  play history, 354
Intrinsic reinforcement, 385

Joints
  fixing of, 88, 89, 100
  range of motion of
    evaluation of, 280, 538, 576, 591
    full passive, 100, 101c

  function/dysfunction continua for, 274, 274c
  tone problems and, 270
Joystick, 583–584

Key points of control, 90
Keyboard use, facilitation of, 584, *585*
Knee straps, for stander, 312, *312*
Knowledge of results, 414, 415

Labeling, visual discrimination and, 213
Language and articulation, 144–145
  evaluation of, 155c
  function/dysfunction indicators for, 75–76, 76t, 152c
  interventions for, 201
Laptrays, 304–306, 307, 583, 584, *585, 586*
  for chair, 304–306, 307
  for stander, 311, *312*
Lateral neck flexion, 266
Lateralization, 137
  evaluation of, 154
  facilitation of, 192
  function/dysfunction indicators for, 151c
Learned skills, 381–382
Learning, 402. *See also* Acquisitional frame of reference; Skill acquisition
  function/dysfunction indicators for, 499–500, 501c
  motor, 402. *See also* Motor skill acquisition frame of reference
  observational, 377
  as occupation, 486, 488t
  stages of, 411–412, 418
  visual information analysis in, 217–219
Learning process, as legitimate tool, 37
Learning theory, 377
  motor skills acquisition and, 403–404
  reinforcement in, 383–384
  shaping in, 384–385
Legitimate tools, 27–38
  activity adaptation as, 37
  activity analysis as, 34–37
  activity groups as, 37. *See also* Activity groups
  assistive technology as, 30–33. *See also* Assistive technology
  conscious use of self as, 28–29
  in nonhuman environment, 29–34
  pets as, 30
  physical agent modalities as, 33
  purposeful activities as, 34–37
  teaching/learning process as, 37
  toys as, *31*, 39
Leisure activities. *See also* Play
  as performance area, 12–13
Lens accommodation, definition of, 256
Levels, changing of, 493t
Listening, therapeutic, 184
Log rolling, *99*
Long sitting, 267
Lovass, Ivan, 378–379

Macrosystem, 47
Mainstreaming, 41, 574–575
Maintenance rehearsal, for visual memory, 246
Managed care, 45
Management schedule, 383
Manipulation with movement, 493t
Manual guidance, 423–424
Masking, for selective attention deficit, 238, 240
Mastery. *See also* Acquisitional frame of reference; Learn-
    ing; Skill acquisition
  environmental, 145
    evaluation of, 155c
    function/dysfunction indicators for, 152c
Matching, 214, 215, 216, 222, 223
  evaluation of, 229
  facilitation of, 248–249
Maturational theories, 69
Medical model, 51–55, 52t
Memory, visual. *See* Visual memory
Mesosystem, 47
Microsystem, 47
Miller Assessment for Preschoolers, 229
Mnemonic devices, 246
Mobility
  evaluation of, 279–288, 537, 590–591
  functional
    function/dysfunction indicators for, 499–500, 501c
    as occupation, 490–491, 493t
  function/dysfunction indicators for, 275, 276c,
    499–500, 501c
  stability and, 86, 91–93, 94–96, 95c, 261
Mobility through space
  evaluation of, 286–287, 577–578
  facilitation of, 314, 314–315, 315, 581–584
Modeling, 383, 384
Moral treatment movement, 469
Mosey, Anne Cronin, 3, 67
Motor abnormalities
  CNS dysfunction and, 269–272
  musculoskeletal dysfunction and, 268–269
Motor behavior, hierarchical view of, 402–403
Motor control, 402
Motor development, 402. *See also* Biomechanical frame of
    reference
  atypical, 88–89
  base of support and, 85–86, 94
  cephalocaudal, 84–85
  components of, 86–87
  direction of, 84–85
  equilibrium reactions and, 259–260
  feedback and feedforward mechanism in, 84–85
  functional skills and, 88
  motor patterns and, 260
  normal, 84–88
  planes of, 87, 107–108
  postural alignment and, 85–86
  postural control and, 85–86, 259–261. *See also* Postural
    control
  prone position and, 264–265, 265
  protective reactions and, 260

  proximal-distal control in, 84–85
  righting reactions and, 259, 260
  sequence of, 191–192, 260–261
  sidelying position and, 265–266, 266
  sitting position and, 266–268, 267
  skilled movement and, 261–268
  stability and, 260–261
  standing position and, 268
  supine position and, 262, 262–264, 263
  weightshifting and, 264
Motor domains, in occupational frame of reference, 494t,
    500, 502c
Motor Free Test of Visual Perception, 227, 228
Motor learning, 402. *See also* Learning
  stages of, 411–412, 418
Motor patterns, 260
  development of from sensory stimulation, 259
Motor play, 485t. *See also* Play
Motor reflexes, infantile, 259. *See also* Reflex(es)
Motor restlessness, 132–133
Motor sciences, 402–417
Motor skill(s). *See also* Skill(s)
  definition of, 471
  facilitation of, 179, 195–196, 197
  in occupational frame of reference, 494t, 500, 502c
  oral, development of, 263–264
Motor skill acquisition frame of reference, 401–427. *See
    also* Skill acquisition
  application to practice of, 422–427
  associated frames of reference for, 427
  assumptions about, 416–417
  case study of, 551–571
  child in, 405
    evaluation of, 419–420
  child-task conditions in, 406–409, 410
  child-task-environment match in, 408–409, 410,
    424–425, 552, 561
    evaluation of, 420–421
  conceptual basis for, 405–416
  dynamic systems theory and, 402–403
  environment in, 406, 420–421
    evaluation of, 420–421
  evaluation in, 418–421
  evolving model of, 401–402
  feedback in, 404, 413–416, 423, 424–425
  function/dysfunction continuum in, 417–418, 419c
  interventions in, 561–570
  learning theory and, 403–404
  occupational therapy assessment in, 551–561
  postulates regarding change in, 421–422
  practice in, 404, 412–413
  regulatory conditions in, 406–408
  skill in, 405–406. *See also* Skill(s)
  task in, 405. *See also* Tasks
    evaluation of, 420
  theoretical base of, 402–417
  zone of proximal development in, 404, 413
Motor subcomponent, of sensorimotor performance com-
    ponent, 15–16
Motor tasks. *See* Tasks

Mouth input, activities for, 185–186
Mouth toys, 196, *197*
Movement(s). *See also* Biomechanical frame of reference;
    Motor development
  compensatory, 89, 268–269
  dissociation of, 87, 97, *98*, 98c, *99*
    evaluation of, 103, 538, 591
    lack of, 89
    postulates regarding change for, 106
  against gravity, 127, 148c, 153c
    flexion response and, 188, 189, *190*, *191*
  manipulation with, 493t
  phasic, 260
  quality of, 90–100, 93c–98c, 100c, 101c
    evaluation of, *102*, 103–104
      standardized, 104–105
  recreational, 493t
  sensitivity to, 134–135, 149c
    evaluation of, 592
  skilled, 261, 405–406
  variety of, 87–88, 97–98, 100c
    evaluation of, 104, 538, 591
    postulates regarding change for, 106–107
Movement Assessment of Infants (MAI), 104
Movement level, 132–133, 150c
  evaluation of, 592
  function/dysfunction indicators for, 148c
Movement speed, tone and, 270
Movement strategies, selection of, 425
Multiarthrodial muscles, tone irregularities and, 270
Muscle(s)
  multiarthrodial, tone irregularities and, 270
  phasic, 260, 261
    functions of, 272
  tonic, functions of, 272
Muscle contractions, tonic, 261
Muscle tone, 136, 150c
  abnormal, 269–270
  affect and, 272
  evaluation of, 139, 593
  fluctuating, 270
  high, 269–270
  joint effects of, 270
  low, 269
  movement speed and, 270
  in neuromuscular dysfunction, 269
  vs. postural tone, 86–87
  surface support and, 272
  temperature and, 272

National Society for the Promotion of Occupational
    Therapy, 469
Neck collars, 308
Neck proprioception, 182, 188, *192*
Neck rings, 308
Negative reinforcement, 382, 393, 394–396
Neonate. *See also* Infant
  motor development in, 261–268
NeuroDevelopmental Treatment (NDT) frame of refer-
    ence, 83–117

adaptive equipment in, 115
application to practice of, 107, 533–550
assistive technology in, 115, 547–548, *549*
base of support in, 86
with biomechanical frame of reference, 528–529,
    547
case studies of, 533–550, 589–608
certification in, 107
compression in, 110, *111*
development of, 83–84
evaluation in, 100–105, *102*, 535–538, 590–594
facilitation of autonomic movement in, 84
feedback and feedforward mechanism in, 85
function/dysfunction continua in, 90–100, 93t, 95t–98t,
    100t, 537–538
handling in, 90, 105, 108–109, *109*, *110*
hierarchical motor sequences in, 83–84
integration of activities in, 113–115
intervention in, 539–548, 595–597, 600–607
  principles of, 107–115
  sequence of, 108
  techniques in, 108–115
motor development and, 84–90. *See also* Motor develop-
    ment
play in, 113–115
positioning in, 115
postulates regarding change in, 105–107, 595
postural alignment in, 85–87
postural control in, 85–86
preparation and facilitation in, 109–113, *111–114*
reflex inhibiting postures in, 83
sensory input as change agent in, 90
with sensory integration, 529–530
  case study of, 589–607
standard skill assessment in, 535–536
theoretical base of, 84–90
weightbearing/weightshifing in, 111–113, *113*, *114*
Neurologic disorders, motor problems and, 269–272
Neuromuscular dysfunction, muscle tone in, 269
Neuromusculoskeletal subcomponent, of sensorimotor per-
    formance component, 15
Neuronal models, creation of, 142–143
Newborn. *See also* Infant
  motor development in, 261–268. *See also* Motor devel-
    opment
Nonhuman environment
  assistive technology in, 31–33
  legitimate tools in, 29–34
  overview of, 33–34
  pets in, 30
  physical agent modalities in, 33
Nonreductionism, 4
Nonverbal contact, function/dysfunction indicators for,
    75, 76t
Nystagmus, postrotary, 134, 149c

Object play, 485t. *See also* Play
Observation, in acquisitional frame of reference, 391,
    395–397
Observational learning, 377

Occupation
adaptation and, 478
characteristics of, 472–476
child-environment fit with, maximization of, 493–498, 509
definition of, 23, 472
development and, 474–475
domain of concern and, 23–24
education as, 486, 488t
environmental context for, 474
as frame of reference, 37–38. *See also* Occupational frame of reference
functional mobility as, 490–491, 493t
function/dysfunction indicators for, 499–500, 501c
health aspects of, 475
impact of, 478
meaning of, 475, 477–478, 508
as means and ends, 476, 508–511
in occupational frame of reference, 472–478
organized activities as, 486–487, 489t
personal care as, 485–486, 486t
play as, 482t, 483–485, 485t. *See also* Play
as product of development, 474–475
purposes of, 472, 477–478, 480c
socialization as, 490, 492t
temporal context for, 474
as therapeutic medium, 475–476
Occupational analysis, 478, 479t–480t
Occupational behavior settings, 478–481
Occupational dynamics, 476–478, 477
Occupational form, 477, 477, 479t
Occupational frame of reference, 37–38, 469–512
application to practice of, 507–511
assumptions underlying, 472–476
child-environment-occupation fit in, maximization of, 493–498, 509
for children, 493–498
environment in, 471–472
evaluation in, 502–506
function/dysfunction continua in, 498–501, 499c, 501c, 502c
motor domains and skills in, 494t
occupation in, 472–478
person in, 470–471
postulates regarding change in, 506–507
process domains and skills in, 494t–495t
social domains and skills in, 495t–496t
theoretical base for, 469–478
therapeutic match in, 478
Occupational performance, 480t
activity performance and, 483t, 491–492, 491–493, 494t–496t, 500, 501, 502c, 505t
assessment of, 502–506
bottom-up, 504
client-centered, 502–503
context-specific, 503–504
dynamic, 503
tools for, 505t–506t
top-down, 504–506

complex task performance and, 482t, 482–491, 499–500, 501c, 502–506, 505t
component processes in, 483t, 492–493, 494t–496t, 501, 505t–506t
facilitation of, 508–511
function/dysfunction indicators for, 498–501, 499c, 501c, 502c
levels of, 481–493, 482t
participation and, 481–482, 482t, 498, 499t, 505t
Occupational synthesis, 478, 496–498
adapt in, 497, 510
alter in, 497, 509–510
create in, 498, 511
establish/restore in, 496, 509
prevent in, 497–498, 510
Occupational therapy
art of, 522–524
client-centered, 470
clinical reasoning process in, 167–168, 202
contexts for, 45–50. *See also* Context(s)
curative model for, 51–55, 52t
default patterns in, 202
domain of concern of, 10–24. *See also* Domain of concern
ecological model for, 52t, 58–60
engaging child in, 522–524
focus of, 3, 5–6, 22–24
frames of reference for. *See* Frame(s) of reference
history of, 469
individualization of, 6–7
legitimate tools of, 27–38
palliative care model for, 52t, 56–58
pediatric service settings for, 41, 42t–43t
performance areas of, 10–24
school-based, referral base for, 184
team approach in, 61–62
terminology for, 10
therapeutic relationship in, 523
trends in, 9–10
Occupational therapy assessment
in biomechanical frame of reference, 574–579
in motor skills acquisition frame of reference, 551–561
in NeuroDevelopmental Treatment frame of reference, 534–539
Occupation-as ends, 476, 511
Occupation-as means, 476, 508–511
Ocular motor skills. *See also under* Vision; Visual
deficits in, 222–223
development of, 263
evaluation of, 223–224
Ocular pursuits, definition of, 256
Ocular vergence, definition of, 256
Olfactory arousal, 133–134, 148c
evaluation of, 592
Olfactory defensiveness, 134
Olfactory discrimination, 135, 150c
Open system, definition of, 43–44
Open tasks, 407, 409
Operant conditioning, 377

Operational theories, 69
Oral arousal, 133, 148c
    evaluation of, 592
Oral defensiveness, 132, 133
    interventions for, 183, 196, *197*
Oral discrimination, 135, 150c
Oral motor control
    development of, 263–264
    facilitation of, 179, 185–186, 186, 195–196, *196, 197*
Organized activities
    function/dysfunction indicators for, 499–500, 501c
    as occupations, 486–487, 489t
Otoliths, 127, 134
Overarousal, 147, 148c–149c
    shutdown and, *130*, 130–131
Overhead suspension system, 176
Overreactivity, sensory system, 135, 135t

Palliative care paradigm, 52t, 56–58
Paradigm(s)
    curative model, 51–55, 52t
    palliative care, 52t, 56–58
    social, 50–61. *See also* Social paradigms
Parent, coping skills of, 440–441, 447, 449c, 453–454,
        459–460
Parent-child relationship
    activity groups for, 361–363
    attachment and, 325–330. *See also* Attachment
    coping and, 440–441, 447, 449c, 453–454, 459–460
    enhancement of, 359–363
    evaluation of, 354
    parental depression and, 362
    parental illness and, 361–362
    play and, 332–333. *See also* Play
    postulates regarding change for, 355–356
    role modeling for, 360–361
    temperament and, 324–325. *See also* Temperament
Partial reinforcement, 383–384
Passive range of motion, 100, 101c
Pathological reflexes, 271. *See also* Reflex(es)
Peabody Developmental Motor Scales, 229
Pediatric Evaluation of Disability Inventory, 419
Pediatric practice, locus of, 41–45
Pediatric service settings, 41, 42t–43t
Peer interaction, 330–331
    activity groups for, 363–371
    evaluation of, 354
    facilitation of, 363–371, 373
    function/dysfunction indicators for, 346–347, 347c
    play and, 332–333. *See also* Play
    postulates regarding change for, 356–357
Peer reinforcement, 380
Pelvic blocks, 301
Pelvic position, in sitting, 299–302, 300, *301*
Perceptual processing, 15
Performance areas, 10–13, 22–23
    activities of daily living as, 11. *See also* Activities of daily
            living (ADLs)
    play or leisure activities as, 12–13. *See also* Play
    work and productive activities as, 12. *See also* Work

Performance component(s), 13–18, 22, 470–471
    cognitive, 16–17
    psychological, 17–18
    sensorimotor, 14–16
    subsets of, 14
Performance context, 18–24
    culture in, 18–20
    definition of, 18
    environmental, 18–19
    family in, 21
    temporal, 18, 21–22
Peripheral vision, definition of, 256
Person, occupational therapy view of, 470–471
Personal care, 485–486, 486t. *See also* Dressing; Feeding;
        Toileting
    function/dysfunction indicators for, 499–500, 501c
Personal care awareness, 492t
Pets, as legitimate tools, 30
Phasic movements, 260
Phasic muscles, functions of, 272
Physical agent modalities, 33
Physical environment, 406
Physical states, coping and, 440, 446, 447c, 453, 458–459
Physiological shutdown, *130*, 130–131
Piers-Harris Children's Self-Concept Inventory, 452
Planes of space
    motor development and, 87
    postural alignment in, 94–97, 97c
Play, 34, 332–341
    in activity groups, for parent and child, 361–363
    attachment and, 332–333
    benefits of, 12–13, 338–339
    as complex task performance, 482t, 483–485
    constructional, 336, *338*
    definition of, 483–484
    evaluation of, 352–353
    facilitation of, 371–373
    function/dysfunction indicators for, 347–348, 499–500,
            501c
    game, 336–338, 485t
    imaginative, 335–336, 485t
    motor, 485t
    in NeuroDevelopmental Treatment, 113–115
    object, 485t
    peer interaction and, 333–334
    as performance area, 12–13
    playfulness and, 338
    postulates regarding change for, 357
    vs. recreation, 334–335
    sensorimotor, 335, *336, 337*, 485t
    social, 485t
    therapeutic applications of, 13
    types of, 34, 335–341
    work and, 338–341
Play exploration, 12, 13
Play History, 354
Play history interview, 354
Play interview, 352–353
Play performance, 12
Play-all, 176, *177*

Playfulness, 338
  components of, 484–485
  evaluation of, 353
Position
  facilitation of, 289–291
  maintaining and changing, 493t
  prone, 264–265, *265*
  sidelying, 265–266, *266*
  sitting, 266–268, *267*
  standing, 268
    facilitation of, 309–312, *310*, *312*
  supine, *262*, 262–264, *263*, 282–283
    facilitation of, 292
  translation of, 291
Positional stability, 92–93, *94–96*
Positioning
  evaluation for, 279–288
  for feeding, 315–316, *315–317*, 586–587
  guidelines for, 290–291
  for mobility through space, 314–315, *315*, *316*
  in NeuroDevelopmental Treatment, 115
  for postural control. *See* Postural control
  for switch activation, 317–319
  for toileting, 317, *318*, *587*, 587–588
Positioning devices. *See also* Assistive technology
  guidelines for, 289–291
Positioning log, 280
Positive interaction, 492t
Positive reinforcement, 382, 393, 394, 395–398. *See also*
        Reinforcement
  hierarchy of, 388c
Postpartum depression, 330
Postrotary nystagmus, 134, 149c
Postulates, 72
Postulates regarding change, 77–78
  for acquisitional frame of reference, 392–393
  for biomechanical frame of reference, 289–291
  for coping frame of reference, 454–455
  for motor skill acquisition frame of reference, 421–422
  for NeuroDevelopmental Treatment frame of reference,
        105–107
  for occupational frame of reference, 506–507
  for psychosocial frame of reference, 355–358
  for sensory integration frame of reference, 169–171
  for visual information analysis, 233–235
Postural alignment, 85–87, *94–97*, 98c
  evaluation of, 103, 538
  facilitation of, 597
  postulates regarding change for, 106
  preparation and facilitation techniques for, 109–110
Postural control, 85–86, 93–94, 96c
  approach to, 319–320, *320*
  arm, 261, 263, 266, 275, 276c, 284–286, 313, 577
  assistive technology for. *See* Assistive technology
  components of, 261–268
  development of, 259–261
  evaluation of, 104, 279–288, 537
  facilitation of, 292–321, 580–581, 595–596
    for central stability, 292–312
    for functional skills, 312–321

hand, 275, 276c, 284–286, 313, 546–547, 577
  head, *262*, 264–267, *265*, 274, 275c, 280–281, *281*, 576
  postulates regarding change for, 105–106
  in prone position, 264–265, *265*, 283
    facilitation of, 292–295, *294*, *295*
  in sidelying position, 265–266, *266*, 283, *283*
    facilitation of, 295–297, *296*, 544–545
  in sitting position, 266–268, *267*, 282, 283–284
    facilitation of, 297–309, 545
  in supine position, *262*, 262–264, *263*, 282–283
    facilitation of, 292
  trunk, 261–268, *263*, 265–267, 274–275, 276c,
        282–284, *283*, 576, *274–275*
Postural reactions
  CNS dysfunction and, 269–272
  effort/stress and, 271
  gravity and, 259–260
  head position and, 271
  modification of, 272
  musculoskeletal dysfunction and, 268–269
Postural tone, 86–87, 91, *92*, 93t
  abnormal, 88–89, 93t
  evaluation of, 103, 537, 590
  postulates regarding change for, 105
Posture, compensatory, 268–269
Posture and Fine Motor Assessment of Infants, 104
Potty training, 317, *318*. *See also* Toileting
Practice
  blocked, 413, 426
  random, 413, 426
  in skill acquisition, 404, 412–413, 424–426
Praxis, 126, 140–145
  deficits in
    developmental, 141
    evaluation of, 154–155
    interventions for, 197–201, *198–200*
  definition of, 140
  evaluation of, 154–155, 593
  facilitation of, 197–201, *198–200*
  functions of, 140
  neuromechanisms of, *140*, 141–143
Prejudice, in activity groups, 370–371
Preparation and facilitation, in NeuroDevelopmental
        Treatment, 109–113, *111–114*
Preparatory activities, 90
Prevent, in occupational synthesis, 497–498, 510
Primitive reflexes, 270–271
Process domains and skills, 471
  in occupational frame of reference, 494t–495t, 500, 502c
Prone extension, facilitation of, 188, *189*, *190*
Prone position
  facilitation of, 544–545
  postural control in, 264–265, *265*, 283
    facilitation of, 292–295, *294*, *295*
Prone stander, 309–311, *310*, *312*
Prone wedge, 293–294, *294*, *295*
Proprioception, 127, 136
  facilitation of, 182
  neck, 182, 188, *192*
  for sensory integrative dysfunction, 182, 188, *192*, 199

Proprioceptive discrimination, 135
  evaluation of, 154c
  function/dysfunction indicators for, 150c
Proprioceptive sensitivity, 135, 149c
  evaluation of, 592
Protective reactions, 260
Proximal key points, handling at, 108, *109*
Psychological performance component, 17–18
  of domains of performance, 17–18
Psychological skills component, 17–18
  of domains of performance, 17–18
Psychosocial evaluation, 350–355
  history in, 351–352
  interview/observation in, 352–355
  purposes of, 350
Psychosocial frame of reference, 323–373
  application to practice of, 358–373
  attachment and, 325–330
  coping ability and, 341–342
  with coping frame of reference, 529–530
  environmental interaction and, 342–343
  evaluation in, 350–355. *See also* Psychosocial evaluation
  function/dysfunction continua in, 344–350, 345c–351c
  peer interactive skills and, 330–331
  play and, 332–341
  postulates regarding change in, 355–358
  resilience and, 341–342
  temperament and, 324–325
  theoretical base for, 323–343
Punishment, 382
Purposeful activities, 34–37
  analysis of, 34–37
  types of, 34

Racial issues, in activity groups, 370–371
Random practice, 413, 426
Range of motion
  evaluation of, 280, 538, 576, 591
  full passive, 100, 101c
  function/dysfunction indicators for, 274, 274c
Reaching, 261
  facilitation of, 544–545, 547
  function/dysfunction indicators for, 275, 276c
  in sidelying position, 266, *266*
  in supine position, 263, *263*
Reactivity, coping style and, 439
Recognition, in visual discrimination, 214, *215*
Recognition acuity, definition of, 256
Recreational movement, 493t. *See also* Play
Reductionism, 4–5
Reflex(es)
  developmental, 137, *139*
    evaluation of, 139, 154
    function/dysfunction indicators for, 151c
  Gallant, 271
  pathological, 271
  primitive, 270–271
  rooting, 271
    in feeding, 317
  tonic labyrinthine, 285, *285*

tonic neck, 259, 262
    asymmetrical, 271
    symmetrical, 271
Reflex inhibiting postures (RIP), 83
Registration, 211, 244
  facilitation of, 244–245
  retrieval and, 212
Regulatory conditions, for tasks, 406–408
Rehearsal, for visual memory, 246
Reilly, Mary, 469
Reinforcement, 382–384, 387, 387c, 388c, 393, 394–395
  contingency, 383
  environmental, 380, 385–386
  guidelines for, 387c
  intermittent, 384
  intrinsic, 385
  negative, 382, 393, 394–396
  partial, 383–384
  peer, 380
  positive, 382, 393, 394, 395–398
    hierarchy of, 388c
  punishment and, 382
  schedules of, 383–384, 387, 387c
  unconditional positive regard in, 378, 386
  vicarious, 382–383
Relationships, visual detection of, 217, *218*
  facilitation of, *249*, 250, 250–252
Resilience, 341–342
Resistance, in activity groups, 369–370
Restlessness, 132–133
Retrieval, of visual memories, 212, 246
Righting reactions
  CNS dysfunction and, 270–271
  development of, 259, 260
  evaluation of, 590
Ring sitting, 267, *267*
Rogers' developmental theory, 70, 378, 386
Role modeling, for parent-child interaction, 360–361
Rollator, 582, *583*, 584
Rolling
  facilitation of, 543–544
  log, *99*
  segmental, *98*
Rooting reflex, 271
  in feeding, 317
Rotation, facilitation of, 192
Rules, compliance with, 492t

Saccades, definition of, 256
Saccule, 127
Safety, 492t
  in sensory integration interventions, 175
Sandwich holder, 586–587
School
  function/dysfunction indicators for, 350, 351c
  inclusiveness in, 41, 574–575
  as occupational therapy setting, 480–481, 574–575
    referral base for, 184
  postulates regarding change for, 358

School—*Continued*
  psychosocial aspects of, 343, 350, 351c
School Function Assessment, 419–420, 481
Scooter board, 188, *189,* 199, 314, *314*
Seat belt, 300–301
  for potty chair, 317, *318*
Seating equipment. *See also* Sitting position
  back supports, 299, 301–302, *302*
  harness, *304,* 304–305
  head supports, 306–309
    for feeding, 316–317
  humeral wings, 304–306
  laptrays, 304–306, *307,* 583
  seat belt, 300–301
  specifications for, *298,* 299–309
  thigh supports, 302, *302*
  trunk supports, 302–304, *304*
Segmental rolling, *98*
Selective attention, visual, 210–211
  facilitation of, 237–239, *239–243*
  function/dysfunction indicators for, 220, 220c
Self, conscious use of, as legitimate tool, 28–29
Self-care, 485–486, 486t. *See also* Dressing; Feeding;
    Grooming; Toileting
Self-feeding. *See* Feeding
Self-initiation, coping style and, 439
Self-management skills, 18
Semicircular canals, 127, 134
Sensitivity to movement, 134–135, 149c
Sensorimotor organization, coping style and, 438–
    439
Sensorimotor performance component, 14–16
  motor subcomponent of, 15–16
  neuromusculoskeletal subcomponent of, 15
  sensory subcomponent of, 14–15
Sensorimotor play, 34, 335, *336, 337,* 347, 485t. *See also*
    Play
Sensory awareness, 14
Sensory defensiveness
  auditory, 132
    interventions for, 184
  behavior and, 144
  excitatory activities for, 180–181
  inhibitory activities for, 180
  interventions for, 180–186
    home-based, 186
    school-based, 184–186
  levels of, 180
  olfactory, 134
  oral, 132, 133
    interventions for, 183, 196, *197*
  tactile, 127, 131–132, 591, 593
  visual, 134
  Wilbarger Protocol for, 181–182
Sensory diet, 129, *130,* 176, 182, *183*
  at home, 186
  at school, 184–186
Sensory input
  as change agent, 90
  registration of, 125

Sensory Integration and Praxis Tests (SIPT), 120–121, *122,*
    353–354
Sensory integration frame of reference, 119–168
  with acquisitional frame of reference, 529
  application to practice of, 171–203, 597–607
  basic concepts of, 124–128
  behavior and, 144
  clinical reasoning process in, 167–168, 202
  definition of, 119
  end-products in, *123,* 123–124, 129t, 140–145. *See also*
      End-product abilities
  evaluation of, 147–155, 160–168
    clinical reasoning in, 167–168
    tools for, 162–166
  functional support capabilities in, 135–139
  function/dysfunction continua in, 146–147, 148c–152c
  inner drive for, 125
  interventions in, 171–203, 597–607
    adaptive response to, 178–179
    environment for, 175–178
    equipment for, 176–178, *177, 178*
    flexibility in, 174–175
    for functional support capabilities, 186–196
    general considerations in, 172–173
    guidelines for, 173–175
    safety in, 175–176
    for sensory system modulation, 180–186
    sequence of treatment in, 179–180
  with NeuroDevelopmental Treatment, 529–530
    case study of, 589–607
  postulates of, 145–146
  postulates regarding change in, 169–171, 597–600
  sensory system modulation in, 128–135. *See also* Sensory
      system modulation
  sensory systems in, types of, 126–128
  theoretical base of, 121–145, *123*
Sensory processing, 14–15
Sensory stimulation, motor pattern development from,
    259
Sensory system(s), 126–128. *See also under* Auditory; Olfac-
      tory; Tactile; Vestibular; Visual
  interrelationship of, 128
  proprioceptive, 127
  vestibular, 127–128
Sensory system modulation, 128–135, 129t
  abnormal, *130,* 130–131
  arousal and, 128, *130,* 130–131. *See also* Arousal
  evaluation of, 151–153
  function/dysfunction indicators for, 146–147
  normal variations in, 130
  postulates regarding change for, 170–171
  sensory diet and, 129, *130*
  sensory system response in, 128, 129t
  shutdown and, *130,* 130–131
Seriation, in visual memory, 245–246
Shaping, 384–385
Shoulder mobility
  evaluation of, 284–286, 577
  facilitation of, 313
  function/dysfunction indicators for, 275, 276c

Shoulder muscles, elongation of, 546
Shutdown, *130*, 130–131
Sidelyer, *296*, 296–297
Sidelying, postural control in, 265–266, *266*, 283, *283*
  facilitation of, 295–297, *296*, 544–545
Sight. *See* Vision
Sitting position
  aids for. *See* Seating equipment
  back support for, 299, 301–302, *302*
  facilitation of, 545
  generalization of, 398
  pelvic position in, 299–302, *300*, *301*
  postural control in, 266–268, *267*, *282*, 283–284
    facilitation of, 297–309, 545
  reinforcement of, 397–398
  seat belt for, 300–301
  thigh supports for, 302, *302*
  trunk supports for, 302–304, *304*
Skill(s), 405–406, 471
  analysis of, 393–394
  communication and interaction, 471
  components of, identification of, 394
  coping and, 440, 446–447, 448c, 453, 459
  definition of, 405
  function/dysfunction indicators for, 388–390, 446–447, 448c
  generalization of, 385–386, 398
  learned, 381–382
  motor, 471
    facilitation of, 179, 195–196, *197*
    frame of reference for. *See* Motor skill acquisition frame of reference
    in occupational frame of reference, 494t, 500, 502c
  process, 471
  reinforcement of, 382–384
  shaping of, 384–385
  spatial, facilitation of, 251
Skill acquisition, 379–382. *See also* Acquisitional frame of reference; Motor skill acquisition frame of reference
  definition of, 387
  environmental content and, 380
  evolving model of, 401–402
  experimentation in, 412–413
  facilitation of, 393–399, 422–427
  feedback in, 404, 413–416, 424–425
  functional behaviors and, 381
  interventions for
    direct vs. indirect, 461
    theory-based, 68–73
  learned skills and, 381–382
  manual guidance for, 423–424
  modeling and, 383, *384*
  movement strategies for, 425
  practice in, 404, 412–413, 424–426, *425*
  reinforcement in, 382–384
  reinforcement of, 382–384, 387, 387c, 388c, 393
  stages of, 411–412
Skilled movements, 261, 405–406
Skinner, B.F., 378

Social conventions, following of, 492t
Social development, 17
Social domains, in occupational frame of reference, 495t–496t, 500, 502c
Social environment, 406
Social interaction, facilitation of, 584
Social paradigms, 50–61
  curative, 51–55, 52t
  definition of, 50–51
  ecological, 52t, 58–60
  frames of reference and, 60–61
  influence of, 51
  palliative, 52t, 56–58
Social play, 485t. *See also* Play
Social skills
  group activities for, 365. *See also* Activity groups
  in occupational frame of reference, 495t–496t, 500, 502c
Social Skills Rating System, 354
Socialization
  function/dysfunction indicators for, 499–500, 501c
  as occupation, 490, 492t
Southern California Postrotary Nystagmus Test (SCPNT), 120
Southern California Sensory Integration Test (SCSIT), 120
Spasticity, 269–270. *See also* Muscle tone
Spatial planes
  motor development and, 87
  postural alignment in, 94–97, 97c
Spatial relations test, 229, *230*
Spatial skills, facilitation of, 251
Speech. *See* Language and articulation
Spirituality, 470–471
Splint, for keyboarding, 584
Stability
  central, facilitation of, 292–312
  development of, 261
  evaluation of, 103–104, 537, 590–591
  mobility and, 86, 91–93, *94–96*, 95c, 261
  positional, 92–93, *94–96*, 95c
  proximal, facilitation of, 596
Standardized assessment tools, for quality of movement, 104–105
Standing position, 268
  support for, 309–312, *310*, *312*
Stiffness, 86–87, 91, *92*
Straps, for stander, 311–312, *312*
Stress, 432–433
  causes of, 433
  coping with, 341–342, 432. *See also* Coping
  definition of, 432
  developmental disabilities and, 441–443
  positive aspects of, 432
  response to, 432–433
  whole-body reactions and, 271
Stressors, 433
Suck-blow activities, 195–196, *197*
Suck-swallow-breathe synchrony, 136, 150c
  evaluation of, 593
  facilitation of, 195–196
Summary feedback, 414

Supine flexion, 188, 189, *191*
Supine position, postural control in, 262, 262–264, *263*, 282–283
    facilitation of, 292
Supine stander, 311–312, *312*
Surface support, muscle tone and, 272
Swallowing. *See* Suck-swallow-breathe synchrony
Switch activation
    evaluation of, 288, 579
    facilitation of, 317–319
    function/dysfunction indicators for, 277–278, 278c
Systems theory
    definition of, 43
    family and cultural contexts in, 47–50
    health and education contexts in, 43–45
    macrosystem in, 47
    microsystem in, 47

Tactile defensiveness, 127, 131–132, 591, 593
Tactile discrimination, 126, 136
    evaluation of, 154c, 593
    function/dysfunction indicators for, 150c
Tactile system, 126–127
    evaluation of, 591
    function/dysfunction indicators for, 148c
Tasks
    analysis of, 405
    closed, 407, *408*
    components of, 405
    definition of, 405
    environment for, 406
    evaluation of, 420
    functional, 405
    meaning of, 405
    open, 407, *409*
    performance of. *See also* Motor skill acquisition frame of reference; Skill acquisition
        facilitation of, 422–427
    regulatory conditions for, 406–408
    variability in, 406–408, *407*, 425
    whole, 425
Teaching/learning process
    as legitimate tool, 37
    principles of, 234t
    for visual information analysis, 235
Team approach, in occupational therapy, 61–62
Technology, assistive. *See* Assistive technology
Technology Related Assistance for Individuals with Disabilities Act of 1988 (Tech Act), 31
Temperament, innate, 324–325
Temperament adaptation
    facilitation of, 358–359
    function/dysfunction indicators for, 344, 345c
    postulates regarding change for, 355–356
Temperature, muscle tone and, 272
Temporal adaptation, 21–22
Temporal performance context, 18, 21–22
Test of Playfulness, 353
Test of Visual Motor Skills, 230
Test of Visual Perceptual Skills, 227, 228
Theoretical base

for frame of reference, 68–73
    example of, 70–73
    organization of, 73
Theory(ies)
    acquisitional, 69
    assumptions underlying, 71
    concepts in, 71
    constant, 69
    definition of, 68
    definitions in, 72
    developmental, 69, 70
    dynamic, 69
    hypotheses of, 72–73
    integration of with practice, 69
    maturational, 69
    operational, 69
    postulates of, 72
    purpose of, 68
Theory-based interventions, 68–73
Therapeutic environment, 523–524
Therapeutic listening, 184
Therapeutic relationship, 523
Thigh supports, 302, *302*
Toddler Infant Motor Evaluation (TIME), 104
Toileting, 486t, 486–487
    evaluation of, 287–288, 579
    facilitation of, 317, *318*, *587*, 587–588
    function/dysfunction indicators for, 277, 277c
Tone. *See* Muscle tone; Postural tone
Tonic labyrinthine reflex, *285*
Tonic muscles, functions of, 272
Tonic neck reflex, 259, 262
    asymmetrical, 271
    symmetrical, 271
Tools
    definition of, 27
    legitimate, 27–38. *See also* Legitimate tools
Toys. *See also* Play
    as legitimate tools, *31*, 39
    mouth, 196, *197*
Traction, in preparation and facilitation, 110
Travel, 493t
Tricycles, 314, *316*
Tripod sitting, 267
Trunk control, 261–268
    evaluation of, 282, 282–284, *283*, 576
    function/dysfunction indicators for, 274–275, 276c
    in prone position, 264–265, *265*
    in sidelying position, 265–266, *266*
    in sitting position, 266–268, *267*
    in standing position, 268
    in supine position, 262–264, *263*
Trunk supports, 302–304, *304*
Tufts Assessment of Motor Performance, 104

Unconditional positive regard, 378, 386, 523
Underarousal, 147, 148c–149c
    hyperactivity and, 181
Underreactivity, sensory system, 135, 135t
Uniform Terminology (AOTA), 10

Utricle, 127

Values, coping and, 439, 445–446, 447c, 452–453, 458
Variety of movement, 87–88, 97–98, 100c
    evaluation of, 104, 538, 591
    postulates regarding change for, 106–107
Verbal contact. *See also* Language and articulation
    function/dysfunction indicators for, 75–76, 76t
Vestibular ocular reflex movements, definition of, 256
Vestibular system, 127–128. *See also* Balance and equilibrium
    sensitivity to movement and, 134–135
    visual system and, 128
Vicarious reinforcement, 382–383
Vigilance, in visual attention, 211
    facilitation of, 239–242
    function/dysfunction indicators for, 220–221, 221c
Vision
    central, definition of, 256
    motor aspects of, 256
    peripheral, definition of, 256
    sensory aspects of, 256
    terminology for, 256
Vision examination, 224
Visual arousal, 134, 148c
Visual attention, 210–211
    arousal/alerting in, 210
        facilitation of, 236–237, *237*
    evaluation of, 224–227
    facilitation of, 235–242
    function/dysfunction indicators for, 219–220
    selective, 210–211
        facilitation of, 237–239, *239–243*
    vigilance in, 211
        facilitation of, 239–242
        function/dysfunction indicators for, 220–221,
            221c
Visual defensiveness, 134
Visual discrimination, 135, 150c, 214–217, *215–217*,
        246–247
    categorization in, 214–216, *216*, *217*, 249, 249–250
    detecting relationships in, 217, *218*, 250, 250–252, *251*
    evaluation of, 227–232, *230–232*
    facilitation of, 246–252
    function/dysfunction indicators for, 222–223, *223*
    matching in, 214, *215*, *216*, 229, 247–249
    postulates regarding change for, 234
    recognition in, 214, *215*, 247, *248*
Visual information analysis, 205–253
    application to practice of, 235–252
    cognitive analysis skills and, 209–217
    definition of, 205
    evaluation in, 223–232
        checklist for, *225*
    function/dysfunction continua in, 219–233
    information processing model in, 207, 207–209, *210*
    in learning, 217–219
    postulates regarding change in, 233–235
    processing skills and, 209
    terminology for, 256

theoretical base of, 206–219
    visual attention in, 210–211. *See also* Visual attention
    visual discrimination in, 214–217, *215–217*. *See also*
        Visual discrimination
    visual input and, 207, 208, *210*
    visual memory in, 211–212. *See also* Visual memory
    visual output and, 207, 209, *210*
Visual input, from environmental stimuli, 207, 208, *210*
Visual memory, 211–212
    coding in, 212, 245–246
    evaluation of, 227
    facilitation of, 243–246
    function/dysfunction indicators for, 221, 222c
    postulates regarding change for, 233–234
    registration in, 244–245
    retrieval in, 211, 212, 246
Visual motor tasks, problems with, 222–223
Visual perception frame of reference. *See* Visual informa-
        tion analysis
Visual perceptual deficits, perceptual and motor effects of,
        206
Visual receptors, 207, 208–209
Visual system
    function/dysfunction indicators for, 148c
    in sensory integration, 128
Voiding. *See* Toileting
Volunteer activities, as occupation, 487–490

Walkers, 578, *578*, 582
Waterbed, 187, *187*
Wedge, 109, *110*
    prone, 293–294, *294*, *295*
Weightbearing, 111–113, *113*, *114*
    facilitation of, 542–543
Weightshifting, 111–113, *113*, *114*, 261
    development of, 264
    facilitation of, 542–543
    in prone position, 264
    in sitting position, 267–268
Wheelchairs, 314–315, 580–581, 582–583
    laptray for, 304–306, 307, 583, 584, *585*, 586
Whole-body reactions
    effort/stress and, 271
    head position and, 271
Wilbarger Protocol, 181–182
Work
    function/dysfunction indicators for, 499–500, 501c
    as occupation, 487–488, 487–490
    as performance area, 12
    play and, 338–341
Work behaviors, 340–341
Work skills, group activities for, 365–366. *See also* Activity
        groups
Workmanship, 339
Worksheets, modification of, for selective attention
        deficit, 238, 239, *241*
Writing, hand control for, 202, 203

Zone of proximal development, 404, 413